Gynecology in Primary Care

Gynecology in Primary Care

ROGER P. SMITH, M.D.

Professor
Chief, Section of General Gynecology and Obstetrics
Department of Obstetrics and Gynecology
Medical College of Georgia
Augusta, Georgia

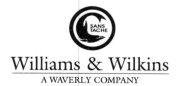

Williams & Wilkins

A WAVERLY COMPANY

BALTIMORE • PHILADELPHIA • LONDON • PARIS • BANGKOK
BUENOS AIRES • HONG KONG • MUNICH • SYDNEY • TOKYO • WROCLAW

Editor: Charles W. Mitchell
Managing Editor: Grace E. Miller
Production Coordinator: Kim Nawrozki
Designer: Silverchair
Illustration Planner: Lorraine Wrzosek
Typesetter: Peirce Graphic Services, Inc.
Manufacturer: R.R. Donnelley

Copyright © 1997 Williams & Wilkins

351 West Camden Street
Baltimore, Maryland 21201-2436 USA

Rose Tree Corporate Center
1400 North Providence Road
Building II, Suite 5025
Media, Pennsylvania 19063-2043 USA

Accurate indications, adverse reactions and dosage schedules for drugs are provided in this book, but it is possible that they may change. The reader is urged to review the package information data of the manufacturers of the medications mentioned.

Printed in the United States of America

Library of Congress Cataloging-in-Publication Data
Smith, Roger P. (Roger Perry), 1949–
   Gynecology in primary care / Roger P. Smith
      p.   cm. — (Primary care ; 1)
   ISBN 0–683–07779–1
   1. Gynecology.   2. Generative organs, Female—Diseases.
3. Primary care (Medicine)   I. Title.   II. Series: Primary Care
(Baltimore, MD.) ; 1.
   [DNLM: 1. Genital Diseases, Female.   2. Pregnancy.   3. Primary
Health Care.   WP 140 S658g 1996]
   RG101.S645   1996
   618.1—dc20
   DNLM/DLC
   for Library of Congress   96-13603
                                                                CIP

The publishers have made every effort to trace the copyright holders for borrowed material. If they have inadvertently overlooked any, they will be pleased to make the necessary arrangements at the first opportunity.

96 97 98 99 00
1 2 3 4 5 6 7 8 9 10

Visit Williams & Wilkins on the Internet
http://www.wwilkins.com

To purchase additional copies of this book, call our customer service department at (800)638-0672 or fax orders to (800)447-8438. Outside the United States, please call (410)528-4000. Williams & Wilkins customer service representatives are available from 8:45 am to 6:00 pm, EST, Monday through Friday. For other book services, including chapter reprints and large quantity sales, ask for the Special Sales Department.

Dedication

To my father who taught the "Art of medicine,"
To my mother who taught humanism beyond medicine,
To my wife who endures my evangelism of these principles, and to my sons whom, I
hope, will also learn these lessons to apply to their lives.

Preface

Why a book on gynecology for health-care providers who don't want to be gynecologists? First, more than half of the patients using our health care system are female. Women obviously have health care requirements that differ from men. With unique physiologic problems and special medical concerns, women are different and the potential for gynecologic considerations in any routine medical encounter is great. Understanding gynecologic problems is mandatory if women are part of our care.

But why *this* book? There are many sources for information about the practice of obstetrics and gynecology. The standard textbooks offer exhaustive discussions and extensive science as they chronicle in detail the history and diagnosis of a given condition, its therapies and controversies. These texts are excellent for readers who have time and seek depth, but offer less help with the practical "What do I do now?" kinds of questions. Student texts are more streamlined. They are designed to get the student through a 6-week rotation and the final test, but are too basic and lack the clinical expertise (and experience) to be helpful in direct patient care. There are pocket manuals and review-type question books written for trainees in obstetrics and gynecology, but they have a crisis mentality geared to surviving an inpatient experience or the out-of-body experience of "The Boards." There are procedure oriented books that provide information about specific aspects of gynecologic care, but these tend to follow narrow procedure oriented specialty areas and fail to cover the broad sweep of women's health issues that are encountered in the primary care setting.

This book sets out to provide a balance between the science that gives us understanding of disease and its rational treatment, and the practical, "seat-of-the-pants," approach of day-in-day-out clinical medicine. Here, it is hoped, you will find not only the whys, but the tips and secrets learned through years of clinical experience, coupled with current science and useful answers to common questions. Above all, perhaps this book will help you find a renewed comfort and joy in the care of all of your patients.

When I was a student at Northwestern University Medical School, my first clinical rotation was at Wesley Hospital (since made a wing of Northwestern Memorial Hospital) on the General Surgery service. In one corner of the operating room complex was a small room used as a "surgeon's lounge." What made it memorable was not its dilapidated couches with tufts of stuffing protruding from every surface, but the very small, and very old brass plaque next to the door. It read: "To a wise, kind surgeon." That overlooked plaque said more about what we do and who we are as providers of medical care, than any lecture by the Dean. In subsequent years, my father (also an obstetrician and gynecologist) demonstrated this maxim with what he calls "the art of medicine." Through example and discussion he emphasized that we must care about our patients, not just for them. It is this principle of practical, human-to-human care that I have tried to instill in these pages. We are accorded the rare privilege of helping care for women throughout their lives; care as they and their families grow. We come to know them as people, and are in a position to provide true primary care. No matter our job description or title, if we lose site of this privilege, we lose a precious gift of opportunity.

Acknowledgments

Though this is a "single author" text, it is by no means the work of one person. Charley Mitchell and Grace Miller, of Williams & Wilkins, have been at once giving and forgiving as they have guided me through the complex process that brings a work to publication. I must also thank my wife and children who have given up a lot of evenings and weekends while I went to "work on the computer." Last, I must thank the electronics industry that has made it possible to develop this manuscript in hotel rooms, airplanes, and waiting areas all over the country.

Contents

I

The Basics

1

Pelvic Anatomy and Embryology

We tend to think of anatomy as the province of the pelvic surgeon, but anyone caring for women in an ambulatory setting can apply the benefits a better understanding of anatomy and embryology provides. A medical career often begins with the study of gross anatomy. New terms, smells, sensations, and sometimes concerns about our career choices, assail us. For many, the embryology and anatomy of the female pelvis is especially difficult to comprehend. To fully understand the complex interrelationships present in this area, it is necessary to visualize the structures abstractly, and in three dimensions. A daunting task at best, and often impossible until some degree of clinical experience has been gained. Without experience as a framework, vital information stays with some of us only until the final examination. As we deal with patients in the real world of ambulatory care, some of that lost knowledge can be quite handy.

BACKGROUND AND SCIENCE

For the purposes of this book, it is assumed that the reader has had basic exposure to embryology and anatomy, and that a review of key points with their clinical correlation is all that is appropriate. For a more in-depth discussion of these topics, please see one of the general sources listed at the end of the chapter.

Embryology

The developing embryo begins as sexually indifferent, neither male nor female, although genetic sex has been assigned at the time of fertilization. The urogenital track begins to differentiate into male and female structures at about 6 to 7 weeks after ovulation. In the absence of a Y chromosome and the sexual differentiation factors it produces (müllerian inhibiting factor [MIF], among others), the gonads and genital tract will differentiate into female structures. The rare exception to this is testicular feminization syndrome, in which normal testes are formed but a failure of the appropriate hormone receptors on target cells results in the development of the default (female) urogenital structures. Although the development of female sexual structures happens as the default condition, it requires two X chromosomes for complete development of the ovary. In individuals who are 45,X karyotype, the ovaries develop but accelerated atresia of oocytes results in their complete loss by birth, resulting in only a fibrous streak gonad.

Most of the genital tract develops from embryonic intermediate mesoderm (Figure 1.1). This mesoderm folds inward to form the urogenital ridges which are covered by celomic epithelium. The primitive gonad begins its development at about the fifth week but does not differentiate into male or female until approximately the eighth week. During the sixth week of development the primordial germ cells migrate to the genital ridge and the primary sex

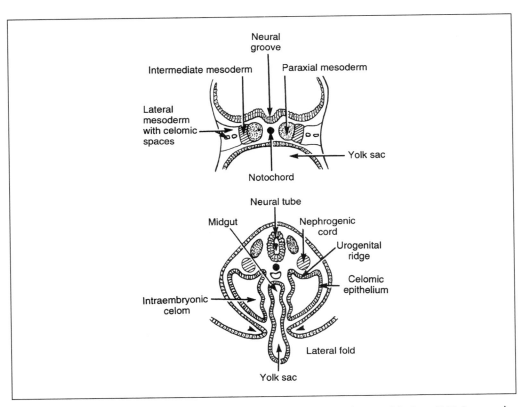

Figure 1.1. Early development of urogenital system. (From Beckmann RB, Ling FW, Barzansky BM, et al. Obstetrics and gynecology. 2nd ed. Baltimore: Williams & Wilkins, 1995:32.)

cords subsequently to become the oogonia. The oogonia rapidly proliferate through mitotic cell division until they reach a maximum of roughly 2.5 million by 20 weeks of development. During the same period, some of the oogonia undergo the first meiotic division, becoming oocytes. By 20 weeks development, there are roughly 5 million oocytes in primitive follicles located in the cortical cords of the ovary. After the 20th week, the oogonia undergo atresia, disappearing by the time of birth. Similarly, there is a steady loss of oocytes, so that at birth roughly 1 to 2 million remain, with half of these showing signs of degeneration. No further germ cells will be formed. The final maturation of ovarian follicles does not occur until puberty or after. (See Chapter 7, Pediatric and Adolescent Care.)

During the undifferentiated stage of embryonic development, two sets of genital ducts

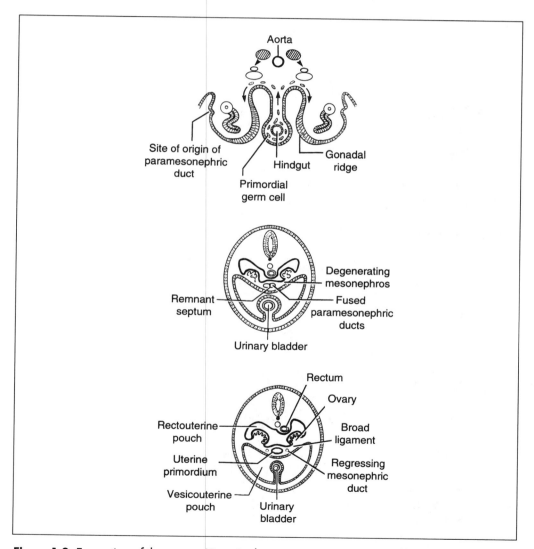

Figure 1.2. Formation of the uterus. (From Beckmann RB, Ling FW, Barzansky BM, et al. Obstetrics and gynecology. 2nd ed. Baltimore: Williams & Wilkins, 1995:33.)

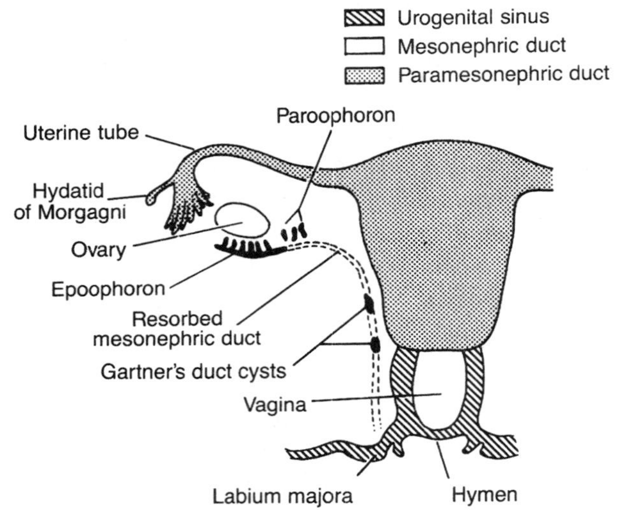

Figure 1.3. Functional and vestigial structures of the upper genital tract. (From Jones HW, Wentz AC, Burnett LS. Novak's textbook of gynecology. 11th ed. Baltimore: Williams & Wilkins, 1988:94.)

develop: the mesonephric ducts (wolffian) and the paramesonephric ducts (müllerian). In the absence of male factors, the mesonephric ducts almost completely disappear and the paramesonephric ducts fuse to become the uterus and fallopian tubes (Figure 1.2). When these processes are incomplete, mesonephric duct remnants may remain (paratubal and paraovarian cysts, Gartner's duct cysts, lateral vaginal wall cysts), or there may be incomplete fusion resulting in uterine and cervical anomalies (duplications, bicornuate uterus, septate uterus, and so forth). Fusion of the paramesonephric ducts also brings together two folds of peritoneum which become the broad ligaments of the uterus. The functional and vestigial structures of the upper genital tract and their origins are shown in Figure 1.3.

The vagina develops from the endoderm of the urogenital sinus and the sinovaginal bulbs. These structures grow caudally toward the distal ends of the fused paramesonephric ducts (the uterovaginal primordium). The paired sinovaginal bulbs then cannulate to form the vaginal canal. Failure of this process may lead to complete vaginal agenesis, transverse or longitudinal septa, or an imperforate hymen. The urogenital sinus also gives rise to the epithelium of the bladder, urethra, vestibular glands, and hymeneal plate, which normally canalizes late in gestation.

The external genitalia also pass through an undifferentiated stage (Figure 1.4). The genital tubercle is formed by the fourth week of development but does not become fully differentiated into either a phallus or clitoris until the twelfth week. In the absence of male factors, the urogenital folds remain unfused, becoming the labia minora. The labia majora are formed from the unfused labioscrotal swellings. When these processes fail or the fetus is exposed to androgens (exogenous or from the fetal adrenal gland, as in adrenogenital syndrome), intersex or pseudohermaphrodism may result.

The main features of sexual development and differentiation are shown in Figure 1.5.

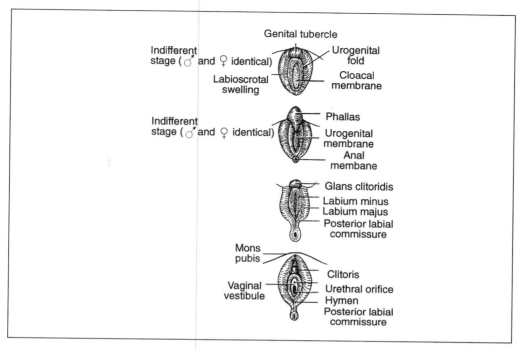

Figure 1.4. Development of the external genitalia. (From Beckmann RB, Ling FW, Barzansky BM, et al. Obstetrics and gynecology. 2nd ed. Baltimore: Williams & Wilkins, 1995:33.)

Pelvic anatomy

A basic concept of the structure of the pelvis and its contents greatly assists in the detection and interpretation of findings made at the time of pelvic examination or through imaging techniques such as ultrasonography, computed tomography, magnetic resonance imaging, and others. Again, a basic familiarity with the pelvic anatomy is assumed and this discussion focuses on relationships and clinically significant considerations that may present on a recurring basis.

Bones

The bony pelvis is made up of the paired innominate bones and the sacrum, joined at the symphysis anteriorly and at the bilateral sacroiliac joints posteriorly (Figure 1.6). Around the time of puberty, the innominate bones fuse from their three constituent parts (ilium, ischium, pubis), which renders the pelvis relatively rigid. Although flexion and limited movement in response to significant force is possible via the three joints, it is generally done with significant discomfort. Despite popular folklore, the symphysis is a strong, relatively inflexible joint that does not separate during pregnancy. Indeed, when there is rupture of this joint, significant pelvic instability results making even ambulation difficult.

Clinically the pelvis is divided into the true pelvis (pelvis minor) and the false pelvis (pelvis major), separated by the linea terminalis. The false pelvis lies above the pelvic brim, bounded by the lumber vertebra posteriorly, the iliac fossa laterally, and the abdominal

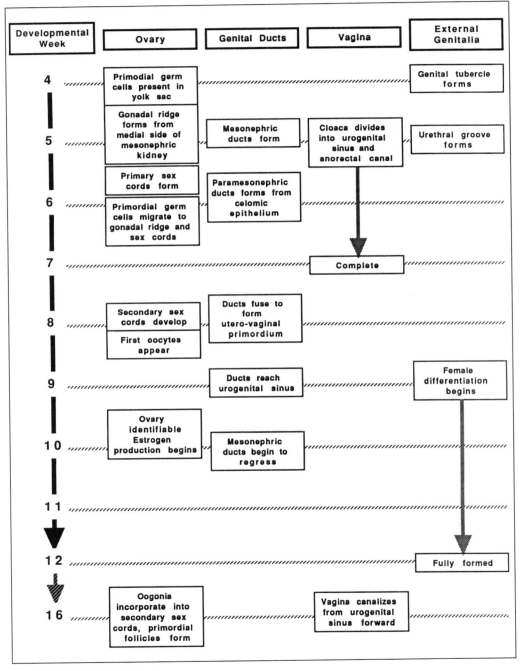

Figure 1.5. Development sequence of genital structures.

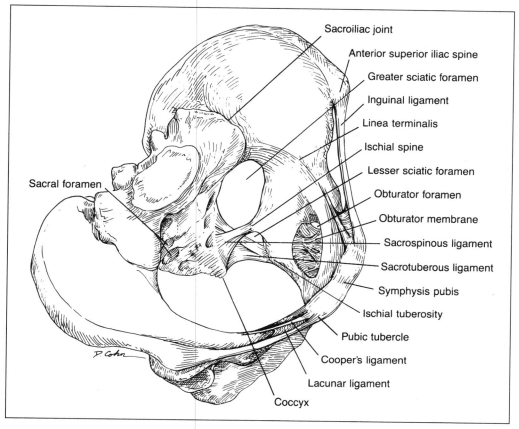

Sacroiliac joint

Anterior superior iliac spine

Greater sciatic foramen

Inguinal ligament

Linea terminalis

Ischial spine

Lesser sciatic foramen

Obturator foramen

Obturator membrane

Sacrospinous ligament

Sacrotuberous ligament

Symphysis pubis

Ischial tuberosity

Pubic tubercle

Cooper's ligament

Lacunar ligament

Coccyx

Sacral foramen

P. Cohn

Figure 1.6. Bony pelvis. View of the pelvis from above, showing bones, joints, ligaments, and foramina. (From Beckmann RB, Ling FW, Barzansky BM, et al. Obstetrics and gynecology. 2nd ed. Baltimore: Williams & Wilkins, 1995:34.)

wall anteriorly. This is the pelvis that supports the pregnant uterus and the "pelvis" of pelvic-abdominal pain. The true pelvis is the bony passage that the fetus must traverse during labor. Although it is uncommon for the true pelvis to be sufficiently distorted that vaginal delivery is unlikely (such as found in patients with damage due to rickets), a passing understanding of the dimensions of the true pelvis is valuable (Figure 1.7). The most important of these dimensions is the midplane, bounded by the lower border of the pubis and the lower sacrum, at the level of the ischial spines, representing the narrowest point of passage for a delivery. Most of the bony landmarks and foramina can be palpated during vaginal or rectovaginal examination and will be clearly visible on radiographic studies.

Muscles

Large and small muscles line, traverse, or define the pelvis and its functions (Figure 1.8). Many of these are involved with erect posture and locomotion and affect gynecologic care only in passing. For the most part, familiarity with their form and functions is no different for the care of women than it is for the care of men. Of greatest significance to gyne-

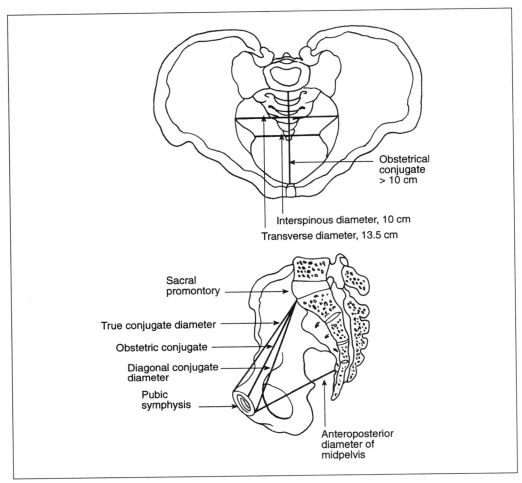

Obstetrical
conjugate
> 10 cm

Interspinous diameter, 10 cm
Transverse diameter, 13.5 cm

Sacral
promontory

True conjugate diameter

Obstetric conjugate

Diagonal conjugate
diameter

Pubic
symphysis

Anteroposterior
diameter of
midpelvis

Figure 1.7. Dimensions of a gynecoid pelvis. (From Beckmann RB, Ling FW, Barzansky BM, et al. Obstetrics and gynecology. 2nd ed. Baltimore: Williams & Wilkins, 1995:35.)

cologic care are the muscles of the pelvic floor and the support structures of the reproductive system.

The pelvic floor, perineum, and urogenital diaphragm are a complex collection of muscles that support the abdominal contents at their most dependent point (Figures 1.9 and 1.10). This muscular sling is perforated by the anus, the vaginal opening, and the urethra. The openings made to accommodate these structures provide potential routes for herniation and support failure. It is the muscles of the perineum and pelvic floor that are most involved in the Kegel exercises often prescribed as a part of the management of stress urinary incontinence.

Support for the upper genital tract is provided by a diffuse web of endopelvic fascia and a system of ligaments that support the uterus (Figures 1.11 and 1.12). The main supports for the uterus come from the cardinal ligaments, located as a condensation of connective tissue in the base of the broad ligament at the level of the inner cervical os, and the uterosacral ligaments that traverse the peritoneum posteriorly to the sacrum. Little functional support is provided by the infundibulopelvic, utero-ovarian, round, or broad liga-

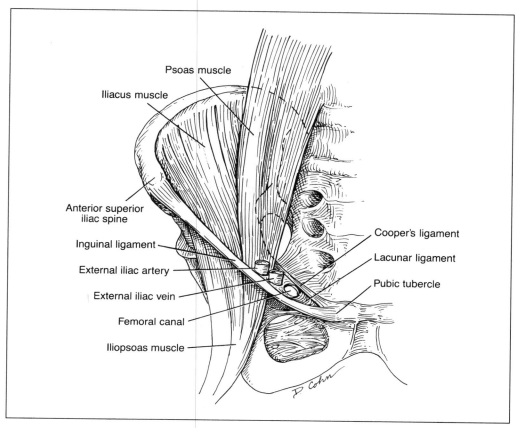

Figure 1.8. Musculature of the true and false pelvis. (From Jones HW, Wentz AC, Burnett LS. Novak's textbook of gynecology. 11th ed. Baltimore: Williams & Wilkins, 1988:44.)

ments. Teleologically, this allows for continuing support in the face of the massive uterine enlargement necessitated by pregnancy.

Support for the vaginal barrel is provided by the endopelvic fascia. This is a false fascia that is neither tough nor readily identifiable and, therefore, there is an increased risk of rupture or failure with childbirth, obesity, advancing age, chronic cough, or heavy lifting; it is difficult to provide lasting surgical repairs for these failures. Failure of the anterior vaginal wall supports results in a cystocele, urethrocele, or both. Posterior vaginal wall failure results in a rectocele. The posterior cul-de-sac, bounded by the posterior vaginal wall and fornix anteriorly, the rectum posteriorly, and the uterosacral ligaments laterally, provides an area of anatomic weakness that may result in an enterocele.

Nerves

The nerve supply of the pelvis is rich, consisting of sensory, motor, and visceral nerves (Figures 1.13 and 1.14). Although most of the enervation of pelvic and perineal structures arises from the lower lumbar and upper sacral levels, multiple interconnections exist, allowing nerves from levels L_1 to S_5 to be involved. This broad-based supply, and even more diffuse autonomic pathways, make assigning specific routes to any location or sensation diffi-

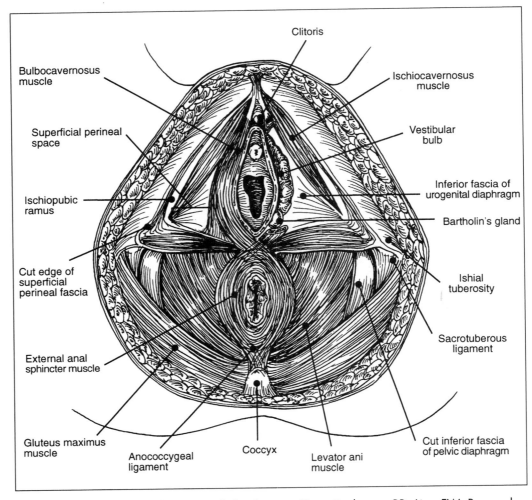

Figure 1.9. Perineum and urogenital diaphragm. (From Beckmann RB, Ling FW, Barzansky BM, et al. Obstetrics and gynecology. 2nd ed. Baltimore: Williams & Wilkins, 1995:38.)

cult. The location of nerve branches and bundles is exploited to provide local or regional anesthesia for clinical procedures. These tracts also provide the justification for presacral neurectomy or ablation of the uterosacral ligaments, used by some to treat pelvic pain.

Enervation is supplied to the vulva from three separate sources: the lumbar plexus (iliohypogastric, ilioinguinal, and genitofemoral nerves) that serve the anterior vulva and mons; the pudendal nerve serving the clitoris, vestibule, and most of the labia; and lastly, the perineal branch of the posterior femoral cutaneous nerve (a branch of the sacral plexus) supplying the lateral perineum, the posterior vulva, and the perianal area. If local anesthesia of the entire vulva is desired, this triple enervation must be taken into account.

The upper two thirds of the vagina are relatively poorly supplied with sensory nerve fibers, via the pudendal nerve. This accounts for the possibility of foreign body retention (e.g., tampons) without symptoms.

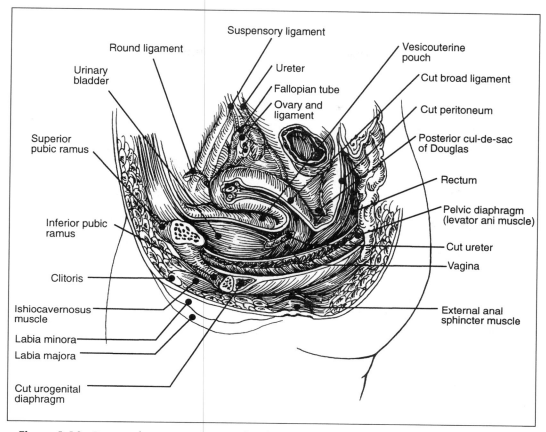

Round ligament

Suspensory ligament

Urinary bladder

Ureter

Fallopian tube

Ovary and ligament

Vesicouterine pouch

Cut broad ligament

Superior pubic ramus

Cut peritoneum

Posterior cul-de-sac of Douglas

Rectum

Inferior pubic ramus

Pelvic diaphragm (levator ani muscle)

Cut ureter

Clitoris

Vagina

Ishiocavernosus muscle

External anal sphincter muscle

Labia minora

Labia majora

Cut urogenital diaphragm

Figure 1.10. Paramedian sagittal view of pelvic viscera and perineum.(From Beckmann RB, Ling FW, Barzansky BM, et al. Obstetrics and gynecology. 2nd ed. Baltimore: Williams & Wilkins, 1995:40.)

Vessels

As with the neural supply of the pelvis, the pelvic organs are richly supplied with blood (Figures 1.15 and 1.16). Although the presence of large vessels and multiple anastomoses ensures a good blood supply to the uterus for pregnancy (Figure 1.17), it also means that vascular injury in the pelvis may be catastrophic. The extensive plexus of veins that drain the pelvis may be the focus of phlebitis and thrombosis, which are most likely to arise after pelvic surgery or childbirth, but may also complicate extensive pelvic cellulitis.

There are multiple anastomoses between pelvic veins and the portal circulation (via the hemorrhoidal plexus), the presacral, and the lumbar veins. These latter connections allow thrombus or tumor embolization directly to the brain without the normal pulmonary filtration taking place.

External genitalia

The form and function of the external genitalia reflect both the underlying bone and muscle, and also the unique aspects of the soft tissues from which they are constituted (Figure 1.18). The skin of the perineum is similar to that elsewhere in the body, but is subjected

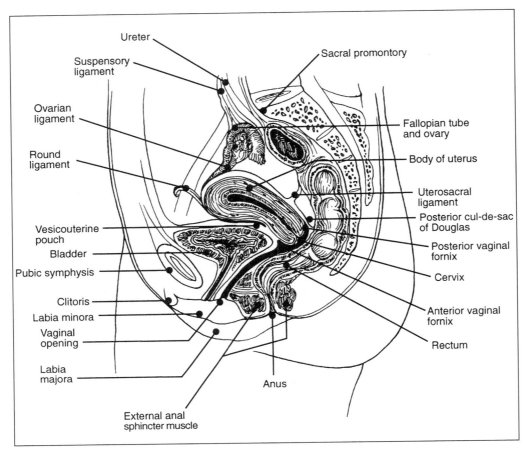

Figure 1.11. Midsagittal view of pelvic viscera and perineum. (The cardinal ligament lies in the base of the broad ligament, both of which lie at right angles to the plane of this illustration.) (From Beckmann RB, Ling FW, Barzansky BM, et al. Obstetrics and gynecology. 2nd ed. Baltimore: Williams & Wilkins, 1995:39.)

to moisture and trauma because of its location. The skin of the labia and vaginal introitus are less keratinized than that further from the vaginal opening or elsewhere on the body, making it both more sensitive and more vulnerable. Sebaceous glands and hair follicles are a part of the skin of the perineum; like keratinization, they become more common further away from the vaginal opening. (The inner aspects of the labia majora have many sebaceous and sweat glands but no hair follicles. Hair follicles are found on the outer, lateral aspects of the labia majora.) The skin of the vulva is sensitive to cortisone and testosterone, but not to topical estrogen.

The vaginal vestibule is the lowest remnant of the urogenital sinus, bounded by clitoris, posterior fourchette, and the labia minora. The vestibule encompasses the vaginal and urethral openings as well as the ducts from the Bartholin's and Skene's glands, and numerous small mucinous glands. It is these small mucinous glands that are involved in vulvar vestibulitis. Both the Bartholin's and Skene's glands may become infected, leading to discharge or cyst and abscess formation. Because there is significant individual variation in the size and shape of the vaginal vestibule, great care must be taken in the assessment of alleged sexual abuse in children and adolescent patients. (See also Chapter 23, Sexual Assault and Abuse.)

Internal genitalia

The vaginal barrel connects the external and internal genitalia. This distensible, fibromuscular tube runs along the anterior wall of the rectum in a nearly horizontal axis when a woman is standing upright. The vaginal canal curves anteriorly in its upper third, following the contour of the pelvis itself. This normal axis must be considered when accomplishing a pelvic examination. Ignorance of this axis may contribute to dyspareunia for some couples.

Despite the appearance provided by most illustrations, the vaginal and uterine cavities are potential spaces unless distended by some influence (such as a speculum, pregnancy, polyp, or the like). Transverse folds (rugae) are most prominent in the lower one third of the vagina, and are lost after menopause if hormones levels are not maintained. Vaginal epithelium is similar to epithelium elsewhere on the body, with the notable absence of glands. For this reason, the common term "vaginal mucosa" is incorrect. Despite the absence of glands, the vagina is able to secrete lubrication during sexual arousal because of engorgement of the vascular plexus surrounding the vaginal barrel, resulting in a transudation of fluid.

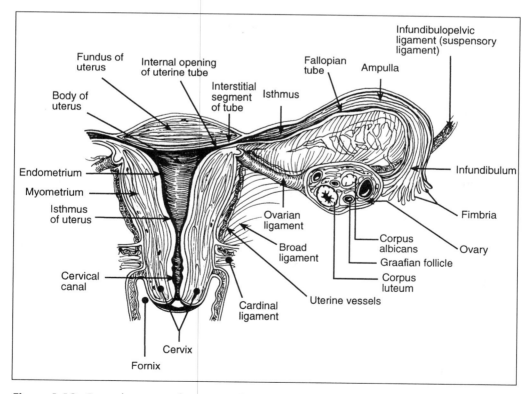

Figure 1.12. Frontal section of uterus and adnexa. (From Beckmann RB, Ling FW, Barzansky BM, et al. Obstetrics and gynecology. 2nd ed. Baltimore: Williams & Wilkins, 1995:41.)

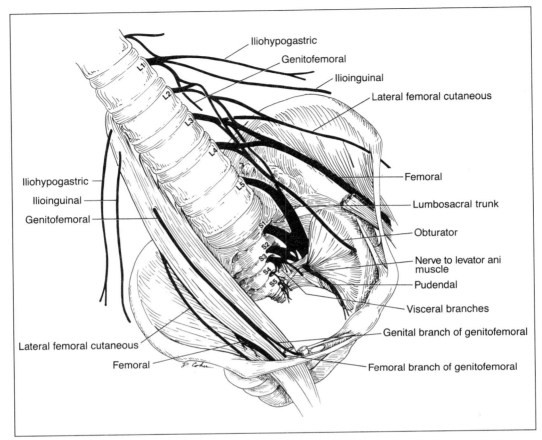

Figure 1.13. Lumbar and sacral plexuses. (Left: the psoas muscle has been removed.) (From Jones HW, Wentz AC, Burnett LS. Novak's textbook of gynecology. 11th ed. Baltimore: Williams & Wilkins, 1988:52.)

The uterus and cervix enter the apex of the anterior wall of the vagina at roughly a 90° angle. The relatively larger posterior fornix directly abuts the pelvic peritoneum in the posterior cul-de-sac. This close approximation provides a point of access for culdocentesis and many operative procedures, such as vaginal tubal ligation.

The uterus is generally one half to two thirds the size of a fist (40 to 80 g), with parous women occupying the upper end of the normal range. Although the uterus is wider than it is thick, it should be shaped symmetrically. Distortions of size, shape, or position suggest intrinsic or extrinsic pathology that warrants further investigation.

The uterine muscle is composed of interlaced bundles of smooth muscle. This muscular wall is capable of generating most of the expulsive forces of labor and may create pressures in excess of 400 mm Hg during dysmenorrheic menstruation. It is only the thin, inner endometrial lining that is significantly responsive to hormonal changes. With the increased resolution afforded by transvaginal ultrasonography, this layer can often be visualized and measured, although the clinical application of such measures remains experimental.

The term "adnexa" loosely refers to the ovary and fallopian tube and their supporting structures. For the most part, these structures will not be clinically identifiable except in the most cooperative, thin patient. The thin mesenteries and axial suspensory ligaments supporting the adnexal structures place them at risk for torsion, which is is most likely when a cystic or solid mass is present. Ultrasonography can often visualize adnexal structures, including small ovarian cysts; however, these visualizations are generally of no clinical significance. Correlation with the phase of the menstrual cycle at the time of the study often helps confirm the physiologic nature of these findings. (See Chapter 2, Physiology of Menstruation.) Paratubal cysts, embryonic remnants of the wolffian system, may also be found and are of little consequence unless they are symptomatic, large, or cannot be differentiated from ovarian pathologies.

The relationship of the ureters and other pelvic structures is clinically significant. The close proximity of the ureter to the cervix and the uterine blood supply must be borne in mind any time sutures are placed for cervical hemostasis (cervical biopsy, conization). In addition, displacement of the ureters caused by uterine descensus or prolapse may place them outside the introitus, exposing them to trauma or obstruction.

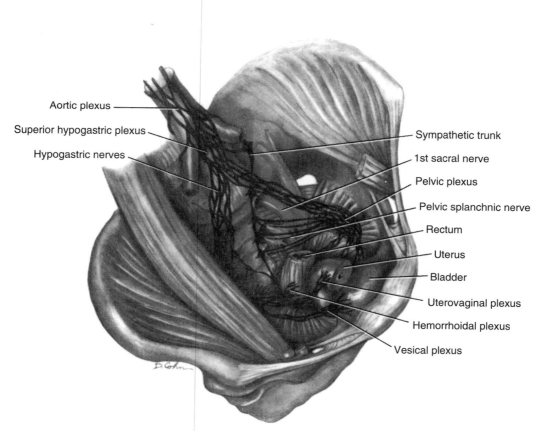

Figure 1.14. Visceral nervous system in the pelvis. (From Jones HW, Wentz AC, Burnett LS. Novak's textbook of gynecology. 11th ed. Baltimore: Williams & Wilkins, 1988:54.)

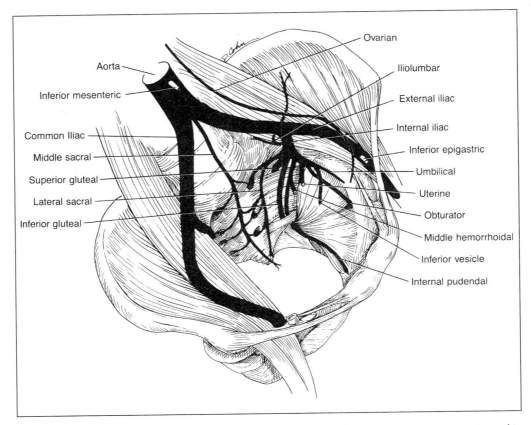

Figure 1.15. Arteries of the female pelvis. (From Jones HW, Wentz AC, Burnett LS. Novak's textbook of gynecology. 11th ed. Baltimore: Williams & Wilkins, 1988:47.)

A summary of normal measurements for selected gynecologic structures that may be helpful when evaluating clinical or imaging findings, is shown in Table 1.1.

CLINICAL APPLICATION

Anatomic variations

For most patients, small skin tags (carunculae myrtiformes) are the only remnant of the hymeneal membrane. Failure of the distal endodermal tissues separating the vagina lumen and the urogenital sinus to partially or completely canalize late in fetal life results in hymeneal abnormalities ranging from an imperforate hymen to cribriform or stenotic openings. With the exception of the imperforate hymen, these will be of limited clinical significance. It is only when stenosis, scarring, or discomfort limit tampon use, menstrual fluid egress, or intercourse that any therapeutic intervention should be considered.

Nabothian cysts are asymptomatic mucous-filled cystic masses found on the ecto-cervix. They are not embryologic remnants, like Gartner's duct cysts of the vagina, but rather are endocervical glands whose openings have been covered over by squamous meta-plasia, resulting in blockage and cyst formation. They are benign and require no therapy. Rapid growth, evidence of bleeding, or an irregular or ulcerated surface should suggest more sinister diagnoses and should prompt a referral.

Perineal hair patterns show a moderate degree of normal variation, including those induced by shaving or depilation. Up to one fourth of normal women exhibit a diamond-shaped (male pattern) escutcheon.

The clitoris is the homologue of the male phallus and, like the penis, it is erectile, but highly variable in size in both the erect and flaccid state, although on average it is rough-ly 1.5 to 2.5 cm in overall length. Similarly, the degree to which the clitoris is covered by the clitoral hood (an extension of the labia minora) is variable, although for most women the glans of the clitoris is covered except when erect. When significant enlargement is pre-sent, the possibility of virilization should be considered. (See Chapter 19, No Periods [Amenorrhea].)

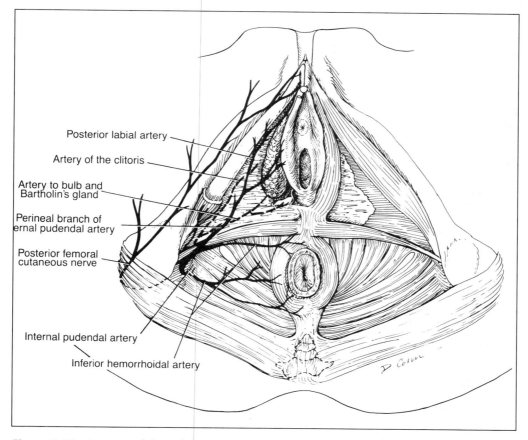

Figure 1.16. Arteries of the vulva and perineum. (The posterior femoral cutaneous nerve is also shown.) (From Jones HW, Wentz AC, Burnett LS. Novak's textbook of gynecology. 11th ed. Baltimore: Williams & Wilkins, 1988:50.)

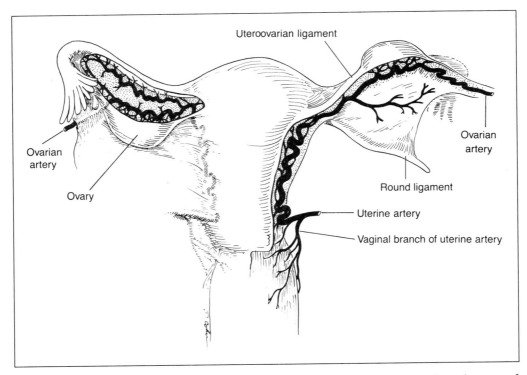

Figure 1.17. Arteries supplying the vagina, uterus, tubes, and ovaries. (Selected areas of peritoneum have been removed.) (From Jones HW, Wentz AC, Burnett LS. Novak's textbook of gynecology. 11th ed. Baltimore: Williams & Wilkins, 1988:50.)

Clinical considerations

Clinically identifiable changes in the shape of the bony pelvis or factors that alter the functional dimensions of the various pelvic planes, such as an anteriorly displaced fractured coccyx, affect both obstetric management and planning for some types of pelvic surgery. The angle of the subpubic arch, the distance to the sacral promontory, and other factors may help determine the route chosen for hysterectomy or the best method of suspending a prolapsed vaginal vault. Although the surgeon makes these decisions based on multiple factors unique to the individual, the primary care team should be aware of these aspects of the patient's anatomy to assist in counseling and to answer patient or family questions. If routine obstetric care is a part of the services provided in the primary care setting, it is essential to be familiar with pelvic dimensions, such as the midplane, and to be able to clinically assess them.

Presacral neurectomy is designed to interrupt the afferent nerves of the superior hypogastric plexus. When this is accomplished it may also disrupt the afferent and efferent autonomic fibers of the splanchnic nerves, causing bladder or bowel dysfunction. Similarly, ablation of the uterosacral ligaments is occasionally attempted to interrupt fibers from the hemorrhoidal plexus and the posterior portions of the pelvic plexus. Although neurologic dysfunction is less common with this procedure, the multiple paths taken by the pelvic nerves limit its success.

In the clinical setting the most significant neural tracts are those of the pudendal nerve and the cutaneous enervation of the perineum. For the most part, the nerves supplying the vulva and perineum follow the vascular bundles shown in Figure 1.16. Because of this, when local anesthetics are used for procedures, such as vulvar biopsies, infiltration of the tissues lateral and inferior to the site of biopsy provides the greatest analgesia. It should also be apparent that when large neural bundles are to be infiltrated with local anesthetics for wider blocks, such as a pudendal anesthetic, care must be taken to aspirate to check for the possibility of vascular puncture prior to injecting the anesthetic agent.

Trauma to the vulva may result in large hematoma formation, due to the rich vascular supply and loose connective tissue stoma present. The vascular supply and abundant cellularity present, contribute to the rapid healing and relative resistance to infection exemplified in episiotomy healing. Because the tissues of the external genital structures sit atop a potential fascial space, the possibility of rapid and distant spread must always be considered if an infection does become established. Necrotizing fasciitis arising in the vulva, perineum, or groins carries mortality rates of 30% to 50% even with aggressive surgical intervention.

Swellings in the labia are often attributed to the Bartholin's glands, but care must be taken to consider other sources. As noted in Figure 1.18, the Bartholin's glands are located low in the base of the labia minora, at roughly the four and eight o'clock positions. Swellings that occur in the labia majora or more anteriorly in the labia minora should be

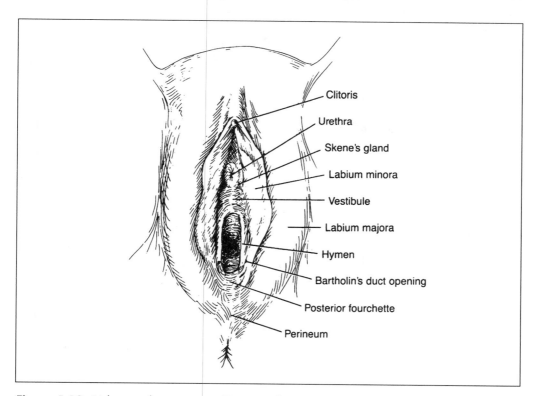

Clitoris

Urethra

Skene's gland

Labium minora

Vestibule

Labium majora

Hymen

Bartholin's duct opening

Posterior fourchette

Perineum

Figure 1.18. Vulva and perineum. (From Beckmann RB, Ling FW, Barzansky BM, et al. Obstetrics and gynecology. 2nd ed. Baltimore: Williams & Wilkins, 1995:37.)

Table 1.1. Normal Sizes of Pelvic Organs (Reproductive Years)

Structure	Length (cm)	Width	Thickness
Uterus (total)	7–8	4–5 cm	2–4 cm
Fallopian tubes	10–14	1–6 mm (internal diameter)	<1 cm
Endometrium	4–6	1.5–3 cm	1–6 mm
Cervix	2–3	2 cm	2 cm
Cervical canal	2–3	7–8 mm	—
Ovary	3–5	2–3 cm	1–3 cm
Postmenopausal	2–3	1–2 cm	1–2 cm
Vagina	8–14*	3–5 cm (distensible to 10+)	—
Labia majora	7–8	2–3† cm	—
Clitoris	1.5–2.5	<1 cm	—
Urethra	3.5–5	4–6 mm (meatus)	—

*Anterior wall 2–3 cm shorter owing to cervix.
†Variable, based on body fat.

suspected to be of other origin and evaluated appropriately. (See Chapter 28, Vulvitis and Vaginal Infections.)

The junction between the squamous epithelium of the external cervix and the columnar epithelium of the endocervical canal is the most frequent site of metaplasia, dysplasia, and malignant change. The exact location of this junction is variable, and care must be taken to obtain cervical cytology specimens from this junction. In parous women, the relatively more open cervix may allow more of the columnar epithelium to be visible, giving the cervix a red, raw appearance (eversion). This may also be seen in young, nulliparous women using hormonal contraception. Despite the inflammatory look that this gives the cervix, it is normal and requires no therapy.

The cervix is well supplied with autonomic nerve endings, but comparatively less well supplied with sensory fibers. As a result, the cervix may be cauterized with heat or cold with only relatively mild discomfort, but dilatation of the cervix may result in vasovagal symptoms, including bradycardia and syncope. This must be kept in mind when the cervix must be instrumented for endometrial biopsy or intrauterine contraceptive device placement.

Because the principal support for the uterus comes from the cardinal ligaments and the uterosacral ligaments, the fundus of the uterus is free to pivot about the plane of the inner cervical os. It is for this reason that retroversion of the uterus is of no clinical significance unless it occurs owing to the effects of scarring or a mass. Retroflexion, when the axis of the uterus is rotated posterior to that of the cervix, occurs in roughly 25% of patients and is not significant.

The lymphatic drainage of the vagina, uterus, and adnexa roughly parallels the vascular supply. This means that tumors from the upper reproductive tract may quickly reach the aortic nodes near the renal vessels (ovarian vascular paths), or the nearby internal iliac nodes. Lymphatic channels to the external iliac and inguinal nodes drain the external genitalia, vagina, and even the cervix. It is this lymphatic abundance that makes the treatment of genital tract malignancies so difficult.

The close proximity of the distal right fallopian tube, right ovary, and appendix makes differentiating these structures difficult even with ultrasonography. Ovarian masses tend to be symmetric or spherical, whereas tubal enlargement (hydrosalpinx) is more likely to be fusiform. Appendiceal abscesses tend to be diffuse and more laterally adherent than are those of adnexal origin.

SUGGESTED READINGS

General references

England MA. Color Atlas of Life Before Birth. Chicago: Year Book Medical Publishers, 1983.

Moore KL. The Developing Human: Clinically Oriented Embryology, 4th ed. Philadelphia: WB Saunders, 1988;246.

Moore KL, Persaud TVN. Before We are Born, 4th ed. Philadelphia: WB Saunders, 1993.

Moore KL, Persaud TVN, Shiota K. Color Atlas of Clinical Embryology. Philadelphia: WB Saunders, 1994.

Muckle CW. Developmental abnormalities of the female reproductive organs. In: Sciarra JJ, ed. Gynecology and Obstetrics, Vol 1, Chapter 4. Philadelphia: JB Lippincott, 1995; 1.

2

Physiology of Menstruation

Little defines being a woman more than the regular process of ovulation, menstruation, and the possibility of childbearing. The average women will ovulate and menstruate 12 to 14 times a year. This occurs on a regular basis for 35 to 40 years, except when interrupted by pregnancy, lactation, and some forms of contraception. The hormonal changes that take place to bring about this monthly cycle have profound, and sometimes unwanted, effects on more than just the ovary, the uterus, and reproductive ability. It is this ever-changing hormonal environment that women find themselves in for half of their expected life span. Although often taken for granted, this rhythmic phenomenon is the result of very complex positive and negative feedback processes that involve a number of hormones and structures. When the system works well, these changes form a background to the activities of life; when dysfunctional, these changes can provide a recurring curse instead. Disturbances in any part of the system may lead to a disruption of the menstrual cycle, resulting in the loss of periods, irregular periods, or random bleeding. Understanding some of the complexity involved in this process is vital to understanding any dysfunction and implementating effective therapy.

BACKGROUND AND SCIENCE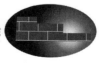

On the surface, the complex interactions outlined below seem far removed from the day-to-day problems of patient care. Once some of the subtle interactions involved in the regulation of menstruation are understood, processes such as exercise or stress-induced amenorrhea, long-acting hormonal contraception, irregular menstrual cycles, or menopause become easier to understand, diagnose, and properly treat. To understand the complex interactions involved in rhythmic menstruation, it is useful to separate the structures, signals (hormones), and feedback processes involved. This pseudoengineering approach allows a degree of simplification and organization that can facilitate clinical application to problems of menstruation.

THE PLAYERS

Structures

Traditionally, the control of cyclic menstruation is attributed to the "hypothalamic-pituitary-ovarian axis" (Figure 2.1). These three structures provide the hormonal signals involved in the positive and negative feedback controls that result in cyclic function. Strong evidence has accumulated to show that it is the developing follicle that controls its own fate.

Hypothalamus

The production and release of follicle stimulating hormone (FSH) and luteinizing hormone (LH) from the pituitary into the blood stream is regulated by the action of the hypothalamus by way of gonadotropin-releasing hormones (primarily GnRH) and poorly understood neurologic signals. The hypothalamus, which is part of the oldest structures of the brain (the diencephalon), is located at the base of the brain, forming part of the floor and lateral walls of the third ventricle. The hypothalamus integrates information from several sources. In addition to responding to circulating estrogen and progesterone levels, the hypothalamus gets extensive information from nerve connections within the brain. These connections have the ability to modify hypothalamic function. Stress, emotional factors,

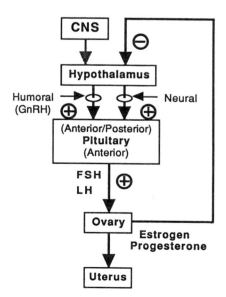

Figure 2.1. Traditional block diagram of feedback and control of menstruation. Traditionally, control of menstruation is based on a simple feedback loop involving the hypothalamic-pituitary-ovarian axis. This view is giving way to evidence that the follicle itself controls the cyclic process.

and even light and dark cycles may play at least a small role in the regulation of hypothalamic function. This hormonal and neural information is integrated by the hypothalamus to determine its output of GnRH. Similar mechanisms exist for the regulation of thyroid-stimulating hormone (TSH), adrenocorticotropin hormone (ACTH), and the control over the production of growth hormone, prolactin (by inhibiting secretion), and others.

Gonadotropin releasing hormones are secreted from the arcuate nucleus within the hypothalamus in a very specific pulsatile fashion. The frequency and amplitude of these fluctuations is critical to the correct function of the system. This release is under the influence of an array of neurotransmitters including dopamine, norepinephrine, endorphin, serotonin, and melatonin. A simplified block diagram of this control system is shown in Figure 2.2.

Pituitary

The pituitary gland functions by receiving chemical and neurologic signals from the circulatory system and brain. The anterior pituitary is chemically controlled, whereas the posterior pituitary is primarily controlled by nerve signals. The pituitary receives and sends its chemical messages by way of the lacy portal network of blood vessels that surround it and connect it to the basal areas of the brain. The pituitary controls ovarian production of estrogen, progesterone, and the ovulation process through the secretion of FSH and LH. These, in turn, are controlled by the pulsatile release of GnRH delivered from the hypothalamus via the portal vessels.

Both FSH and LH are secreted by the same type of cell, the gonadotrope. These are primarily located in the lateral portions of the pituitary. Secretion of FSH and LH is complexly controlled by internal second messengers such as calmodulin, protein kinase, calcium, inositol 1,4,5-triphosphate (IP_3), and others. GnRH receptors on these cells are sensitive to GnRH regulation, inhibin, activin, and sex steroids. Exposure of these cells to GnRH plus estrogen produces an enhanced response to further GnRH stimulation, providing a positive feedback and setting the stage for the midcycle surge in FSH and LH that is vital to the ovulation process. Prolonged, tonic stimulation of GnRH receptors results in a desensitization and uncoupling process that results in decreased secretion. This is

Figure 2.2. Neuroendocrine control of gonadotropin secretion. Pulsatile release of GnRH is modulated by a balance between the positive influences of norepinephrine and the inhibitory effects of dopamine.

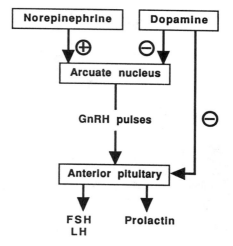

exploited clinically when GnRH analogs (leuprolide acetate [Lupron], nufarelin acetate [Synarel], goserelin acetate [Zoladex]) are used to induce reversible menopause for the treatment of endometriosis, fibroids, premenstral syndrome (PMS), or pelvic pain.

Ovary

Although the ovaries are relatively inactive before and after a woman's reproductive years, their dual function of hormone production and egg release are critical for reproduction and menstruation. Hormonal secretions takes place in both the follicular elements and the ovarian stroma. Estrogen and progesterone are made primarily in the cortical and follicular elements of the ovary and are created through the cooperative efforts of both theca and granulosa cells (Figure 2.3).

The process of follicular maturation is central to both fertility and hormone production (Figure 2.4). Immature follicles, made up of an egg and its surrounding coat of granulosa cells, undergo a series of changes controlled by estrogen, FSH, and LH. Under the influence of FSH and gradually rising estrogen six to eight immature follicles begin to develop during the first few days of the follicular phase of the cycle. As the follicle develops, theca cells differentiate from the surrounding ovarian stroma, forming an outer ring of cells surrounding the granulosa layer and the oocyte. These continue to produce the substrates for estrogen production by the granulosa cells. At the same time, the granulosa cells become increasingly sensitive to both estrogen and FSH, further enhancing follicular growth and estrogen production. In response to FSH, granulosa cells also express LH receptors, beginning the transition to luteinization and promoting further development. At some point, this reinforcement results in one follicle becoming dominant. The other follicles undergo atresia as FSH declines under the influence of rising estrogen and inhibin produced by the dominant follicle. It is this dominant follicle that will rupture, releas-

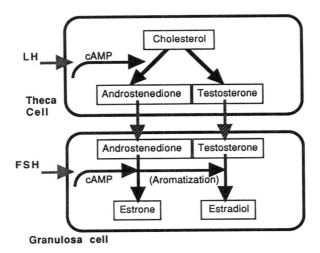

Figure 2.3. Two-stage process of estrogen production in the ovary. Estrogen production in the follicle is now recognized as a two-cell process that begins with the synthesis of androstenedione and testosterone from cholesterol under the control of LH. This diffuses to the granulosa cells where aromatization to estrogens occurs under the stimulus of FSH.

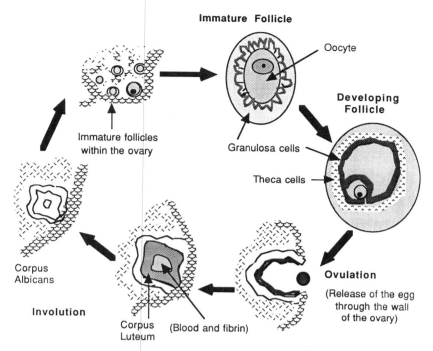

Figure 2.4. Cyclic changes in ovarian follicle development. Follicular maturation begins with the recruitment of several primordial follicles that enter into the preantral stage in which theca and granulosa layers develop. By day 5, a dominant follicle emerges and the other follicles undergo atresia. The dominant follicle then develops a fluid-filled antrum containing a rich protein liquid filled with estrogen secreted by the granulosa cell layer. This follicle will swell to 2 cm or greater at the time of ovulation. After ovulation, the follicle becomes luteinized, producing high levels of progesterone. If pregnancy does not occur, involution of the corpus luteum occurs, resulting in the formation of the scarred corpora albicans.

ing the oocyte, and undergo transformation into the progesterone-producing corpus luteum.

After ovulation, the follicle undergoes transformation into the corpus luteum, which produces both estrogen and progesterone. Once the corpus luteum's function has ended, it undergoes involution and scarring, becoming the corpus albicans.

Menopause occurs when no more follicles are available or are able to develop. The loss of inhibin and estrogen production results in tonically elevated gonadotropins and the beginning of systemic symptoms of estrogen withdrawal. (See Chapter 12, Menopause.)

Uterus

The lining of the uterus undergoes cyclic changes each month in preparation for the possibility of pregnancy (Figure 2.5). During the first half of the cycle, the endometrium regenerates through the stimulation of rising estrogen. This reaches a peak 1 to 2 days before ovulation occurs. After ovulation, progesterone from the corpus luteum causes the glands of the endometrium to become secretory, vessels become tortuous, and vascular lakes appear in the edematous stroma. These changes prepare the endometrium to sup-

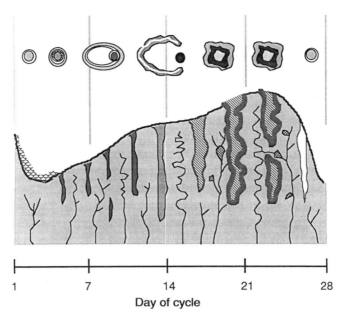

Day of cycle

Figure 2.5. Endometrial changes associated with cyclic follicle development. During the follicular phase of the menstrual cycle, regeneration and proliferation occur, glands that are straight and relatively inactive develop, and vessels regrow. Once ovulation occurs, glands become filled with secretions, vessels become tortuous and show small lakes and hemorrhages, and the supporting stroma becomes edematous.

port the implantation of a fertilized egg. When the corpus luteum undergoes involution, hormone levels fall and the lining sloughs off to start another cycle.

At the beginning of menstruation, the endometrium has become unstable and undergone cellular death due to the effects of declining hormone levels. Over the course of the first 2 to 3 days, most of the lining sloughs off revealing a denuded basal layer. This basal, or lower, layer is the area that is responsible for the monthly regeneration process. This layer is not lost in the monthly sloughing process. The sloughing process slows and stops in 4 to 7 days because of the rising levels of estrogen being made as a new group of follicles begin development.

Traditionally, the uterus has been seen as a passive participant in the menstrual cycle, lending only its response in preparation for pregnancy and the slough of the endometrium as markers for the rhythmic processes going on in the rest of the system. This view is changing as new evidence from nonprimate animal studies suggests that prostaglandins made by the endometrium may be responsible for luteolysis, which terminates the cycle when pregnancy does not occur.

Hormones

Gonadotropin-Releasing Hormone (GnRH)
Gonadotropin-releasing hormone (GnRH) is a short molecule of 10 amino acids that has a remarkable homology of structure among most mammals. Similarities across species sug-

gest that it has existed for more than 500 million years. It is sent from the hypothalamus to the pituitary through neural secretion and delivered by the network of portal vessels. GnRH, which is released in a pulsatile fashion, has an extremely short half-life (2 to 4 minutes). Pulsatile GnRH stimulates the anterior pituitary to secrete both FSH and LH, but the response is modulated by circulating levels of estrogen and progesterone. Control of this pulsatile secretion is through both positive and negative feedback from the ovaries, the pituitary, and the hypothalamus itself.

Pulsatile secretion of GnRH begins just before puberty with nighttime pulsations that grow in both frequency and amplitude. As puberty progresses, this becomes more regular and extends to the daytime until the adult, 24-hour pattern of pulsatile secretion of GnRh is established. (See Chapter 7, Pediatric and Adolescent Care.) This pulsation must be in a narrow range of both frequency and amplitude to elicit an appropriate response from the pituitary. Faster or slower pulses are not only less effective, but they also result in a decreased number of GnRH receptors on the gonadotrophs, further lessening the effectiveness of the GnRH present.

Because of the very low levels of GnRH released and the extreme dilution that occurs as the molecules leave the pituitary portal system, LH pulsations are often used as a surrogate marker for GnRH secretion. Pulse frequency and the amplitude of LH secretion during the menstrual cycle are shown in Table 2.1.

Gonatropin-releasing hormone has three main actions in the process of gonadotropin regulation: GnRH stimulates the synthesis and storage of gonadotropins by the gonadotropes; it promotes the activation, or movement of the formed gonadotropins from a reserve pool within the cell to a pool ready for secretion; and it promotes the direct release of gonadotropins from this prerelease pool. The degree to which these three activities take place is modulated by the effects of estrogen and progesterone.

Follicle-Stimulating Hormone (FSH) and Luteinizing Hormone (LH)

Follicle-stimulating hormone and LH are both formed by two chains of glycoprotein: alpha and beta. The alpha chains of FSH and LH are identical; they are made up of 89 amino acids. The alpha chains are identical to alpha chains found in thyroid-stimulating hormone (TSH) and human chorionic gonadotropin (HCG). They are homologous to alpha chains found in similar hormones in many animals. It is the beta chain that determines the differences and functions of these hormones. The beta chains of FSH and LH are much longer sequences of amino acids (118 amino acids for LH and 127 for FSH) and

Table 2.1. Characteristics of LH Pulses During the Normal Menstrual Cycle (Means)

Phase	Amplitude (IU/L)	Frequency (Minutes)
Early follicular	6.5	94
Mid follicular	5.1	
Late follicular	7.2	71
Early luteal	14.9	103
Mid luteal	12.2	
Late luteal	7.6	216

Data from: Speroff L, Glass RH, Kase NG. Clinical Gynecologic Endocrinology and Infertility, 5th ed. Baltimore: Williams & Wilkins, 1994; 192.

carry one or two sites of carbohydrate attachment. Even within the beta chains there are large numbers of similarities, leading to the speculation that they may have evolved from a single genetic source (i.e., they may have evolved from a single parent hormone as humans themselves have evolved).

LH is primarily responsible for promoting the initial conversion of cholesterol to pregnenolone, which takes place in the theca cells or the corpus luteum (see Figure 2.3). FSH regulates the conversion of androgens to estrogens through aromatization, which happens mainly in granulosa cells. Because of the sequential nature of sex steroid formation, the action of FSH requires the antecedent effects of LH, although LH can act independently as the prime regulator of steroidogenesis. Early in the follicular phase of the cycle, receptors for LH are only located on the theca cells, whereas FSH receptors are limited to the granulosa cells. Later in the cycle, FSH causes the luteinized granulosa cells to gain LH receptors, which allows continued control of progesterone secretion.

Production, storage, and secretion of gonadotropins varies throughout the menstrual cycle. Early in the cycle, when circulating estrogen is low, both the secretion and storage pools of gonadotropin are depleted. As estrogen increases, production replenishes these storage pools but there is little change in the amounts of gonadotropins available for secretion (Figure 2.6). The replenished storage pools ensure that when larger amounts of gonadotropins are needed for the midcycle surge, they will have already been formed. Rising GnRH levels near midcycle move gonadotropins from the storage pool to the secretion pool in preparation for release.

Studies in primates suggest that the main site for controlling the midcycle surge in gonadotropins is not the hypothalamus, but the pituitary. Hypothalamic GnRH appears

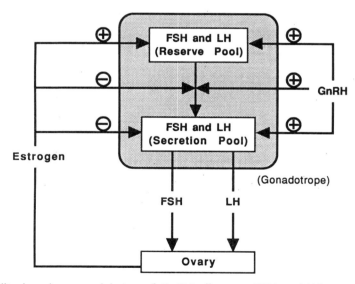

Figure 2.6. Follicular phase modulation of GnRH effects on FSH and LH secretion. Early in the follicular phase, low levels of estrogen potentiate the production and storage processes stimulated by GnRH pulses arriving from the hypothalamus. Low levels of estrogen also modulate the release of formed gonadotropins, resulting in stockpiles that will be released as part of the midcycle surge.

to play a more permissive, rather than controlling role, than was once thought. Although GnRH pulsations of the correct amplitude and frequency are required, modulation by sex steroids appears to provide the necessary feedback to create the gonadotropin surge at the correct time and in the appropriate amount. Because the production of sex steroids is under the control of the dominant follicle, it is the follicle itself that is responsible for the direction of its own destiny.

Estrogens

"Estrogen" is not really a single hormone, but rather three hormones with similar functions and that are generally lumped together. These three hormones are β-estradiol, estrone, and estriol, in order of potency. Both β-estradiol and estrone are made in large amounts by the ovary (in the follicles), whereas estriol is a breakdown product formed by the liver in the process of metabolism of the other two molecules. For this discussion, it is acceptable to lump these three hormones together under the term "estrogen."

The principal function of estrogen is to cause cellular proliferation and growth in the tissues of the genital tract and in other tissues related to reproduction. The uterus responds to estrogen by enlarging twofold during puberty, and changing slightly throughout the menstrual cycle owing to changes in cellular fluid and endometrial proliferation. The fallopian tubes respond to estrogen by thickening and increasing the number of ciliated lining cells. These cells are responsible for the eventual transportation of the egg toward the uterus. The mucus made by the cervical glands becomes thin and watery as the estrogen increases. This is why some women notice an increase in vaginal discharge at the time of ovulation.

Estrogen affects the vagina by causing an increase in vaginal size during puberty and by altering the character of the wall of the vagina. Under the influence of estrogen, the wall of the vagina thickens and undergoes changes that increase its resistance to trauma and infection. This estrogen-dependent thickening also results in the formation of the characteristic vaginal rugae. The monthly surge of estrogen keeps the vagina supple and facilitates the formation of lubricating fluid during intercourse. Estrogens are responsible for causing the labia to thicken and grow to adult form during puberty.

The increasing estrogen of puberty induces fat deposition in the breast and the development of an extensive ductile system. The ability of the nipple to become erect and the increase in the pigmentation of the areola are also under the control of estrogen. Estrogen stimulates the lobules and glandular tissue of the breast to develop to a limited extent. Estrogen is responsible only for developing the female contour of the breast and putting in place the basic structures necessary for milk production. This development will be completed by the effects of progesterone. Indeed, large quantities of estrogen, such as found during early to midpregnancy, may inhibit the production of milk. When estrogen levels decline in menopause the contour of the breast flattens and support lessens, leading to sagging.

In addition to generalized growth, estrogen also causes an increase in the amount of calcium stored in growing bone by inhibiting its reabsorption. With decreased amounts of estrogen after menopause, calcium may be lost. Studies show that estrogen confers some degree of protection from cardiovascular disease and heart attack. There are cultural and racial differences, but in general the heart attack rate for women lags 10 to 15 years behind that of men. This difference is only present when estrogen levels are in the normal premenopausal range, and comes from more than just an altered ratio of phospholipids in the blood stream; it includes direct effects of estrogen on vascular epithelium that result in altered prostacyclin production, reduced platelet adhesion, and other protective mechanisms. Studies show that this protection may be maintained after menopause by the administration of replacement estrogens. (See Chapter 12, Menopause.)

Under the influence of estrogen there is an increased deposition of excess calories into fat rather than protein (muscle). This gives women a slightly thicker, fatty layer and the feminine "curves" that come about when fat is laid down in the hips and buttocks. Estrogens cause the skin to develop a softer and generally smoother texture, in spite of the fact that the skin becomes slightly thicker. The skin also becomes more vascular, causing a slight blush and increased warmth. Because of this, women may bleed slightly more from superficial cuts that do men. Estrogen does not have any great effect on hair in any other part of the body other than the pubic region. Here estrogen causes the distribution of pubic hair to take on the feminine inverted triangular shape with a flat upper border. Men have a more diamond shaped distribution with a point that may extend to the navel, although this pattern may be seen in up to 25% of normal women.

Progesterone

Unlike estrogen, there is really only one progesterone. Progesterone is secreted primarily by the corpus luteum; it is made in much larger amounts than is estrogen, but is weaker in its effectiveness. Like estrogen, progesterone is rapidly metabolized in the liver into inactive compounds (primarily pregnanediol).

Progesterone has its greatest effects on the endometrium. Here its function is to promote secretory changes that prepare the endometrium for implantation of the fertilized egg. Progesterone can cause these changes only when the endometrium has had enough stimulation ("priming") by estrogen. Progesterone also calms the uterine muscles, decreasing the normal mild uterine contractions that are present. Teleologically, this may help to lessen the chance of expulsion of a fertilized egg. Secretory changes also take place in the fallopian tube that cause an increase in nutrients available for the egg during transport toward the uterus. During this journey, the fertilized egg undergoes initial cell division and growth. The added secretions from the fallopian tube may be important for this process to continue normally. Progesterone causes the mucus made by the cervix to become thick and sticky, effectively sealing the cervix and uterus against infection.

Progesterone provides the final stimulus for the development of the lobules and glandular tissue of the breast. It causes the breast glands to enlarge and become secretory, but does not induce milk production. Milk production is set in motion by prolactin (PRL). Progesterone causes the breast to swell, owing to the stimulation of the glands and the deposition of water in the tissues below the skin. This is why many women experience breast fullness, tenderness, and soreness when progesterone levels are high near the end of their menstrual cycle, just before their period. This fluid storage may be felt in other parts of the body as well, causing shoes to pinch and rings no longer to fit. This storage of fluid comes about because of an increase in reabsorption of sodium, chloride, and water in the kidney. Restricting sodium (salt) before periods can be helpful for some women in combating this problem.

Progesterone is a catabolic hormone, promoting the breakdown of protein into glucose for metabolism by the body. Progesterone also directly affects the hypothalamus and the thermoregulatory system. Although these effects are slight, a change in metabolic activity may be detected by small variations of the body's resting temperature. This is the basis of the "basal body temperature graphs" that are used to detect the presence and time of ovulation (Figure 2.7). After ovulation when there is a rise in progesterone levels there is a slight rise in the body's resting temperature. Knowing when ovulation occurred can be useful for either promoting or preventing pregnancy. The temperature rises only when progesterone rises, which is 24 to 48 hours after the actual ovulation takes place. Therefore, temperature graphs give information only after the fact.

Other Hormones

ACTIVIN, INHIBIN, AND FOLLISTATIN. Activin, inhibin, and follistatin are small peptide hormones that are members of the transforming growth factor-β family. These hormones are primarily secreted by granulosa cells in response to FSH stimulation, although they may be made by many tissues throughout the body. All three act as autocrine and paracrine regulators of cellular functions, although inhibin also acts remotely in the regulation of gonadotropin secretion. Activin is found in three forms, whereas inhibin has two forms. Activin increases GnRH receptors, augments FSH release, and inhibits the production of prolactin and growth hormone. Activin promote the effects of FSH on granulosa cells, resulting in proliferation, enhanced aromatization of androgens to form estrogens, the production of inhibin, and the induction of further FSH and LH receptor formation (Figure 2.8). Activin secreted by immature granulosa cells tends to suppress androgen production by local theca cells, moving the follicle toward the estrogen predominant environment necessary for continued development. Early and mid follicular phase activin action helps to prevent premature luteinization of the follicle and delay progesterone production.

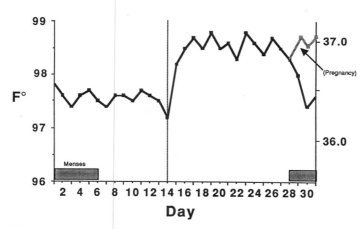

Figure 2.7. Basal body temperature (BBT) changes during the normal menstrual cycle. Measurement of resting BBT may be used to infer that ovulation has taken place. This is based on the slight thermogenic properties of progesterone and its elevation following ovulation. The basal temperature will rise 24 to 48 hours after ovulation and will drop back with the start of menses if a pregnancy does not occur.

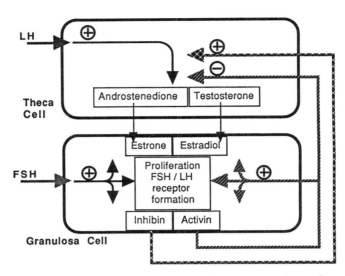

Figure 2.8. Early follicular phase effects of activin and inhibin. In the early and mid portions of the follicular phase, activin and inhibin perform important feedback functions to augment that of the emerging dominate follicle while promoting the atresia of competing follicles. In the immature follicle, activin production predominates to augment the growth of the follicle. When inhibin secretion increases in the more mature follicle, it serves to enhance steroidogenesis in the mature follicle while overandrogenizing competing follicles, ensuring their failure.

Inhibin is secreted by the granulosa cells of the maturing follicle and acts to inhibit FSH secretion, but it has little effect on the production of LH. High concentrations of inhibin can suppress FSH synthesis, promote intracellular degradation of pre-formed gonadotropins, and reduce the numbers and sensitivity of GnRH receptors. Production of inhibin by the dominant follicle promotes the action of LH and the formation of androgens in immature follicles, further acting to suppress the response of these follicles, helping to ensure their atresia, and guaranteeing dominance. Inhibin levels rise slowly during the follicular phase, reaching a peak at the same time as the gonadotropin surge. Late follicular phase production of inhibin causes the theca cells to increase androgen production and, thus, promotes late follicular and luteal phase estrogen production. Once the luteal phase begins, inhibin production comes under the control of LH, rising again to a maximal level at midluteal phase that is roughly twofold higher than that found at ovulation.

Follistatin is a single chain peptide that reduces FSH activity through binding activin. It is primarily found in preovulatory follicles and in the pituitary, where it acts in a similar way to inhibin.

INSULIN-LIKE GROWTH FACTOR (IGF). Insulin-like growth factors (IGF) (also called somatomedins) are peptides with structures similar to insulin that medicate the action of growth hormones. These factors act at the level of the granulosa and theca cells to promote DNA synthesis, steroidogenesis, aromatase activity, inhibin production, and the production of LH receptors on the cell surface. These factors also stimulate granulosa cell proliferation. Insulin-like growth factors act in synergy with FSH, and to a lesser extent LH, to promote sex steroid production. Because these factors are made by the theca cells under the influence of LH itself, they can act as a short-loop (paracrine) feedback system to enhance their own production and assist in the control of steroid synthesis. As granulosa cells grow, growth hormone, FSH, and estradiol enhance granulosa cell production of IGF, resulting in further stimulation of steroid production. It appears that the overall role of IGF is one of facilitation, with other hormones playing the governing role.

ENDOGENOUS OPIOIDS. The endogenous opioids of the brain are a group of molecules that have important roles as neurotransmitters. There are three classes of endogenous opiates: enkephalins, endorphin, and dynorphin. Each of these groups is derived from specific precursor molecules that are cleaved to produce the active agents. In general, the endogenous opiates inhibit FSH and LH secretion by suppressing GnRH release from the hypothalamus.

It appears that much of the negative feedback effect of estrogen and progesterone on the secretion of FSH and LH may be mediated by endorphins. Endorphin secretion is increased through a synergistic effect of estrogen and progesterone. This stimulation is lost in postmenopausal women, unless estrogen is replaced, and is enhanced by the relatively high hormones found during the late luteal phase and pregnancy. It is probable that when clomiphene is used clinically to induce ovulation, it is its action as an estrogen agonist that decreases endogenous opiate levels, allowing LH secretion and ovulation. The role of endorphin and the catecholestrogens in the release of GnRH is shown in Figure 2.9.

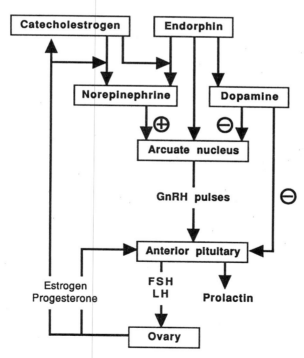

Figure 2.9. Central control of GnRH pulsatile release. The modulation of GnRH secretion is now recognized as the result of a complex interaction of stimulation and inhibition that is, itself, modulated by estrogen, progesterone, endorphins, and catecholestrogens.

THE PROCESS

Feedback and Control

The menstrual cycle involves the interaction of the hypothalamus, the pituitary, the theca and granulosa cells of ovarian follicle, and the uterus. Once thought to be a simple feedback loop involving cyclic centers in the hypothalamus subject to downregulation by increased estrogen and progesterone, the picture of control that has emerged from recent studies indicates a much richer system. The cycle may be divided into three phases that differ widely in their function, control systems, and outcomes: the follicular phase in which a follicle is recruited and matures; ovulation that results in the liberation of the egg; and the transition process to the final stage, the luteal phase during which progesterone dominates the functions of the ovary.

Normal Sequence of Events

Follicular Phase Events

Communication between the higher centers and the ovary is by way of FSH and LH, with feedback control being provided by ovarian production of estrogen, progesterone, activin, and inhibin. Soon after menstruation, freed from the suppression of high circulating estrogen and inhibin, FSH levels rise. This rise in FSH appears critical to inducing the first changes from primordial follicle to primary follicle. Low levels of LH stimulate the maturing theca cells, causing them to grow and convert cholesterol into pregnenolone, androstenedione, and testosterone. The conversion of these precursors into estrogens is completed by the inner layer of cells surrounding the egg, the granulosa cells (see Figure 2.3). The granulosa cells respond to FSH by proliferating and increasing the rate of aromatization, forming β-estradiol and estrone. The production of estrogen then helps to increase the sensitivity of the surrounding granulosa cells to FSH, thus augmenting and continuing the process while the egg develops. This reinforcement of FSH receptor binding, which stimulates estrogen and activin production, which increases FSH and LH receptors and allows FSH and LH binding, which promotes estrogen production, and so forth, is part of what ensures that one follicle will become the dominant follicle. In many ways, it is the follicle that attains the strongest degree of aromatization activity and LH receptor induction in response to FSH that becomes the dominant follicle. It is also the attainment of adequate numbers of LH receptors that ensures successful functioning of the future corpus luteum. Follicles that begin development when LH levels are high and FSH is low, or those that are unable to make the transition from androgen precursor production to estrogen synthesis, are doomed to become atretic.

At the hypothalamus, low levels of estrogen are insufficient to suppress GnRH release. Low levels of both estrogen and progesterone stimulate further FSH and LH production and storage in preparation for the midcycle surge (Figure 2.10). During this time, the egg quadruples in size as it stores the cellular material needed for early development should fertilization take place. There is also an accumulation of follicular fluid, rich in estrogen, that enlarges the size of the follicle.

As levels of estrogen and inhibin rise, the hypothalamus begins to decreases its secretion of GnRH and the amount of FSH released by the pituitary begins to fall. There is a slight rise in LH, which occurs because of altered pituitary response to GnRH brought on

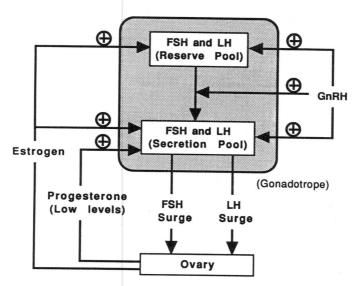

Figure 2.10. Midcycle modulation of GnRH effects on FSH and LH secretion. GnRH encourages the production, movement, and secretion of FSH and LH. This is potentiated in the late follicular phase by positive feedback from estrogen and progesterone.

by prolonged exposure to estrogen, resulting in stimulatory rather than inhibitory feedback. The presence of FSH in the early parts of the cycle causes the granulosa cells to become increasingly sensitive to the effects of LH through the induction of LH receptor formation. Later, when the level of LH causes increasing androgen precursor production by the theca cells, LH stimulation causes the granulosa cells to secrete their estrogen into the blood stream. By the late follicular phase, LH causes the granulosa cells to produce progesterone under the modulation of activin, itself stimulated by LH. Until ovulation occurs, full-scale secretion of progesterone into the blood stream is inhibited. The interplay of feedback and production is summarized in Figure 2.11.

The increasing rate of rise and the amount of estrogen in the blood stream appears to promote a rapid rise in LH due to a special stimulated hypothalamic secretion of GnRH and altered responses of the pituitary to GnRH stimuli. This hypothalamic stimulation appears to occur because of nerve signals coming from an area above and in front of the hypothalamus. This area is thought to be sensitive to the rate of change and the amount of estrogen present. It sends a neurologic signal to the hypothalamus to overcome the normal suppressive effects of estrogen, yielding a brief increase of GnRH. Because of this increase and the altered response from the pituitary due to the effects of estrogen, the pituitary responds with a surge that is predominantly made up of LH. This surge in LH, which is the trigger that causes the follicle to rupture and the egg to be expelled, generally lasts for 48 to 50 hours. Ovulation generally occurs between 10 and 12 hours after the crest of this surge in LH or between 24 to 36 hours after the peak in estradiol. The LH surge is blunted, or possibly terminated, by rising progesterone production by the granulosa cells as they undergo luteinization. The ability of the follicle itself to control the LH surge ensures that it will occur at the optimum time for ovulation.

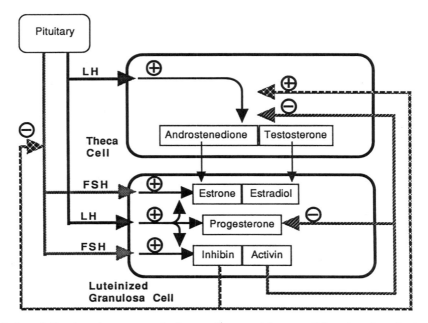

Figure 2.11. Late follicular phase control of granulosa and theca cell function. Late in the follicular phase, the granulosa cell LH receptors have been induced; however, FSH-based production of activin holds progesterone secretion to a minimum. Increasing production of inhibin plays an important role in suppressing FSH, which prevents the development of other follicles and enhances the maturation of the dominant follicle, which can respond to rising levels of LH. Although FSH levels decline in the late follicular phase, an increased sensitivity to FSH and LH and increased production of androgens by the theca supplying a large quantity of substrate for estrogen production ensures continued estrogen production in the granulosa cells.

Ovulation

Just prior to ovulation the oocyte resumes meiosis, approaching completion of its reduction division. (Meiosis will not be completed until after the sperm has entered the egg and the second polar body is expelled.) During the preovulation phase, the granulosa cells of the follicle enlarge and acquire lipid inclusions and the theca layer develops a rich vascular supply while the cells undergo vacuolization. There is also a transfer of inhibin production to LH control, ensuring continued function as FSH levels drop.

Ovulation occurs because of a rapid increase in the follicular fluid and the direct action of proteolytic enzymes and prostaglandins. Follicular fluid accumulates gradually as the follicle grows, but rapidly increases in response to the LH surge and to a change in follicular wall elasticity. At ovulation, the amount of follicular fluid is between 1 and 3 mL. In addition to the expansion in the size of the follicle, the theca cells surrounding the follicle begin to erode through the overlying epithelial covering of the ovary with the help of proteases, collagenase, plasmin, and prostaglandins E_2, $F_{2\alpha}$, and other eicosanoids. These weaken the capsule and stimulate smooth muscle contractions in the cortex of the ovary, facilitating rupture of the follicle and the expulsion of the egg. The slight progesterone-mediated rise in FSH seen just after the LH surge is thought to help induce proteases that help free the oocyte from its surrounding follicular attachments. The LH surge, by itself, is inadequate to induce ovulation in a follicle that has not undergone sufficient maturation.

Luteal Phase Events

The remnant of the follicle, with its LH-sensitized (luteinized) granulosa cells, is the corpus luteum; it is responsible for continued hormone production. Following the release of the egg, the center of the follicle becomes filled by blood clot and fibrin into which small blood vessels start to grow. Along these vessels there is a proliferation of the luteinized granulosa cells to fill the cavity. The luteinized cells take on a yellow color due to the accumulation of a yellow pigment in lipoid granules. These granules contain progesterone and its precursors, cholesterol and carotene. The corpus luteum reaches maximal production of estrogen and progesterone at about 10 days after ovulation. If conception has not occurred, the corpus luteum begins to regress, ending its function by about 14 to 15 days after ovulation. The exact reason for this involution is unknown, but only rescue by human chorionic gonadotropin (HCG) can prevent its occurrence.

Although the LH sensitized granulosa cells produce increasing amounts of both estrogen and progesterone, there is a slight fall in the levels of estrogen around the time of ovulation as production from the mature follicle ends and the luteinized granulosa cells begin to increase their production. This slight dip in estrogen may be enough to cause some women to experience slight bleeding or spotting at the time of ovulation. Peak progesterone levels occur at about 8 days after ovulation.

It is the continued production of estrogen, progesterone, and inhibin that suppresses the hypothalamus, decreasing its GnRH production (Figure 2.12). This, in turn, decreases

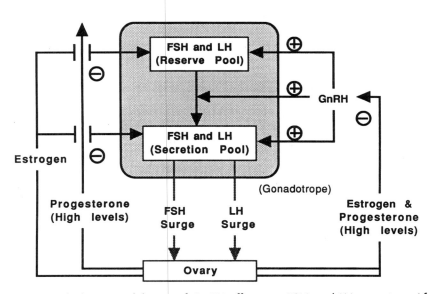

Figure 2.12. Luteal phase modulation of GnRH effects on FSH and LH secretion. After ovulation, rising levels of both estrogen and progesterone suppress the production of GnRH and decrease the gonadotrope's responsiveness to GnRH stimulation, reducing the production and release of FSH and LH.

the release of FSH and LH from the pituitary, further preventing other follicles from maturing and releasing their eggs. This self-limiting process generally ensures that there is only one egg that can be fertilized each month. Failure of this system to inhibit addition-al follicles, or the nearly simultaneous rupture of more than one follicle, can set the stage for fraternal twinning.

As the follicles that failed to reach dominance become atretic, the activated theca cells once again become part of the ovarian stroma, but their increased gonadotropin sensitivity continues to induce androgen production. This, combined with androgen production by the rest of the ovarian stroma, results in a midcycle rise in androgens, which results in a very slight rise in libido that accompanies ovulation. The complex behaviors that dictate sexual expression tend to mask this effect, although it may be demonstrated in controlled studies.

While the corpus luteum is functioning, the high levels of estrogen, progesterone, and inhibin produced continue to suppress the hypothalamus and, hence, the release of FSH and LH by the pituitary. When the corpus luteum regresses at 9 to 11 days after ovulation and these levels fall, this inhibition is removed, FSH and LH levels rise, and the cycle starts again. Each hormone follows its own cycle of rising and falling because of the intricate control of stimulation and inhibition built into the elements of the system (Figure 2.13).

Some of the important events in the sequencing of the menstrual cycle are summa-rized in Figure 2.14.

Results

Hormone changes leading to ovulation are obviously necessary for reproduction, but little comes of a fertilization if the uterus has not been made ready for the implantation and growth of the egg. While all of the changes have been taking place in the ovary, estrogen and progesterone have caused very profound changes in the uterus (see Figure 2.5). Indeed, it is these changes that yield the most observable evidence of the menstrual cycle, menstruation itself.

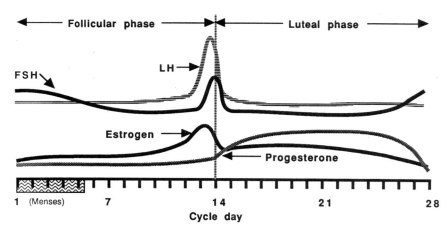

Figure 2.13. Hormonal and gonadotrophin changes during the normal menstrual cycle. Relative levels of FSH, LH, estrogen, and progesterone are shown as they vary throughout the menstrual cycle (not to scale).

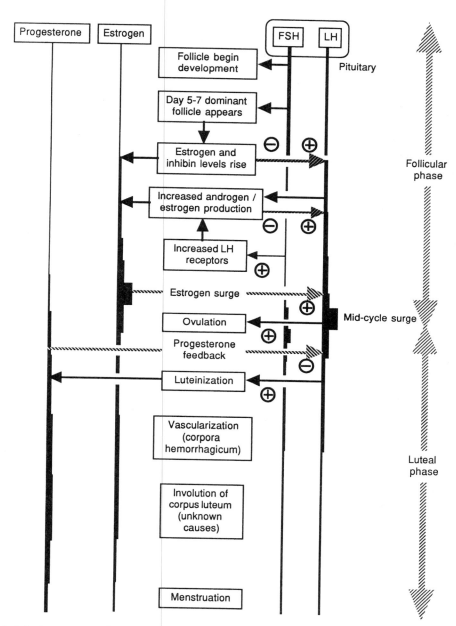

Figure 2.14. Sequence of events in a normal menstrual cycle. The sequence of events involved in the normal menstrual cycle involves a complex interaction between ovarian steroids and gonadotropins.

By about 1 week into the cycle, the surface layer of cells has been replenished by an outgrowth of cells from glands left behind in the compact basal layer after the prior menstrual slough. For the next 5 to 7 days, the endometrium thickens and many straight, test tubelike, glands develop. This growth takes place under the influence of estrogen, with the proliferation reaching its peak at about the same time the peak in estrogen occurs. In addition to glands and supporting stroma, there is rapid growth of blood vessels to nourish the new tissue. The arteries supplying the superficial layers of the endometrium grow faster than the stromal tissue, causing the arteries to spiral and become convoluted. These spiral arteries play an important part in providing blood to a placenta or in causing the surface of the endometrium to slough during menstruation. There is a practical limit to the amount of growth that the lining can undergo under the influence of estrogen alone, and this limit is reached at about the same time ovulation takes place. If no ovulation occurs for a prolonged time, continuing gradual growth may result in hypertrophy and irregular shedding of the endometrium in the form of dysfunctional bleeding.

After ovulation and the formation of the corpus luteum, the secretion of progesterone causes a characteristic differentiation to begin. These endometrial changes can be seen as early as 48 hours after ovulation occurs. Under the influence of progesterone the endometrial glands begin to form and secrete glycogen. The first sign of this activity is an accumulation of the glycogen-rich secretions at the base of the cells lining the walls of the endometrial glands. As more of the secretions form, the secretions move upward in the cell and are discharged into the cavity of the gland. This secretory activity causes the glands to swell and become twisted and convoluted. Extra capillaries appear and dilated veins filled with blood ("venous lakes") become common. The supportive tissues become pale when seen under the microscope as the cells begin to swell with fluid and nutrients in preparation for a possible pregnancy. All the changes that take place under the influence of both estrogen and progesterone are sufficiently predictable that the specific stage in the menstrual cycle can be determined by examining an endometrial biopsy. This is clinically important in determining hormone function and whether or not ovulation has taken place.

Cervical mucous production changes in response to the varying hormonal conditions throughout the menstrual cycle. Under the influence of estrogen, cervical mucus become copious, thin, and watery, facilitating sperm capture and transport. When progesterone dominates after ovulation, cervical mucous production declines and it becomes thick, tenacious, and opaque.

If no pregnancy is established, hormone levels fall as the corpus luteum begins to fail and the supportive tissues of the endometrium swell with fluid, white blood cells begin to invade the tissue, and the spiral arteries become spasmodic, causing anoxia and cell death. Menstruation begins as red blood cells leak from the capillaries and portions of the upper layers of endometrium begin to slough off.

HINTS AND COMMON QUESTIONS

Although we speak of a "normal" cycle of 28 days from the first day of flow to the next first day of flow, there is no real normal. There is, however, an average made from observations of large populations of women. Although the "average" menstrual cycle is between 26 and 29 days long, there is wide variation from person to person. Cycles between 21 and 35 days long are considered to be in the average range and are normal, with less than 1% of women falling outside of this range. Even this average range varies with age (Figure 2.15). The best gauge is whatever is normal for the individual. If a patient's cycles have

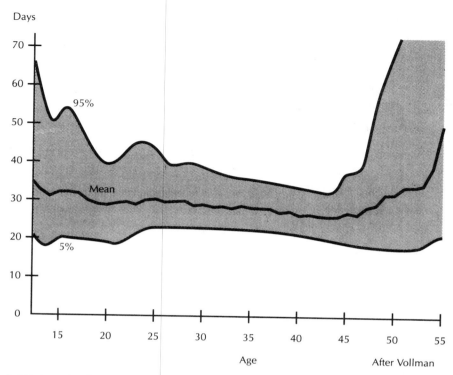

Figure 2.15. Length of menstrual cycle by age. (From: Vollman RF. The menstrual cycle. In: Friedman E, ed. Major Problems in Obstetrics and Gynecology. Philadelphia: WB Saunders, 1977.) (From Wollman RF, The menstrual cycle, in Friedman E, editor, Major problems in obstetrics and gynecology. Philadelphia: W.B. Saunders Co., 1977.)

always been 32 days, then 32 days is normal for her. Only when there are sudden, large changes from normal should there be concern.

Even if the average menstrual period lasts 4 to 7 days, 80% of menstrual blood loss occurs in the first 48 hours. The average blood loss is between 30 and 50 mL.

The control mechanisms involved the regulation of menses are very delicate, so any significant deviation from normal effectively destroys the regularity of the system. Therefore, if menstrual periods are reasonably regular, there is little chance of a hormonal imbalance.

If estrogen is administered after a dominant follicle develops and before ovulation can occur, FSH levels will drop below that necessary to sustain follicular maturation and the dominant follicle itself will undergo atresia. This necessitates beginning the process of recruitment all over with a new group of primordial follicles, potentially delaying the onset of the next menses.

For two thirds of women, the LH surge occurs between midnight and 7:30 AM, with the average being 3 AM. There are seasonal variations in the time of ovulation, with ovulation occurring primarily in the morning during the spring and in the evening during the fall and winter. Studies indicate that in the northern hemisphere, roughly 50% of women ovulate between midnight and 11 AM during the spring and 90% of women ovulate between 4 and 7 AM from July to February. This information is derived from data in assisted reproduction programs. It has not been established if this information could be of help to couples planning their own conceptions.

By recording the body's temperature for 5 minutes the first thing in the morning (before arising), it is possible to make some guess about the time of ovulation. Although there is often a slight dip in temperature at the time of ovulation itself, the more reliable change in temperature is the rise in temperature seen 1 to 2 days later. The information in this graph can be very useful in evaluating infertility or in trying to determine "safe" times for intercourse using the "rhythm" method of birth control.

Although there is some theoretic basis for predicting that ovulation should alternate between ovaries from month to month, there is no clinical evidence to support this. It appears that determining the ovary that is the source of ovulation on a given month is random and based on the complex processes that select the dominant follicle.

Because ovulation involves breeching the capsule of the ovary, it is sometimes accompanied by vague lower abdominal pain. This pain is poorly localized owing to the character of visceral pain sensation. This midcycle pain ("mittelschmerz") is generally mild, but for some patients may be sufficient to cause difficulty. Analgesics or nonsteroidal anti-inflammatory agents may be used if the patient is not actively pursuing conception.

In animals, exposure to light and dark affects estrous and breeding cycles. Prolonged periods of darkness result in increased production of melatonin, which suppresses GnRH production. This effect is thought to be mediated through the pineal gland. Although variations in melatonin levels may be documented in humans in response to seasons and jet travel, any effect on menstruation remains conjectural. Melatonin may contribute to jet lag, however.

Although the "average" interval from ovulation to menstruation is 14 days, intervals from 11 to 17 days may be considered normal. Only about 5% of women have true short luteal phase cycles.

As the follicle undergoes conversion into a corpus luteum, blood and fibrin clot fills the vacated antrum and significant bleeding can occur. Patients who are anticoagulated are at particular risk, making ovulation suppression an important consideration.

If there has been adequate amounts of estrogen, low levels of progesterone can provide a positive feedback response at the level of the pituitary, which may result in an LH surge. This may explain the surprising onset of ovulation found in some anovulatory patients treated with a progesterone challenge.

Because of the central role of prostaglandins in the production of proteases and direct stimulation of the ovulation process, infertility patients should be advised to avoid the use of nonsteroidal anti-inflammatory agents near the time of possible ovulation.

Hormones, in general, and estrogens specifically, do not "make you gain weight." Estrogen does have an effect on where the calories will be stored when intake exceeds use.

In patients well beyond the onset of menopause, measurement of FSH or LH levels to determine the effectiveness of estrogen therapy may be misleading or inaccurate. Estrogen, by itself, is insufficient to suppress FSH and LH release without inhibin. The absence of inhibin production by the ovary results in incomplete blockage of gonadotropin release. Inhibin is most effective in blocking LH release. As a result, as inhibin levels begin to fall prior to menopause, there may be an early, preferential increase in FSH, as seen in some women even before the loss of menstruation.

SUGGESTED READINGS

General References

Jones HW III. Cyclic histology and cytology of the genital tract. In: Jones HW III, Wentz AC, Burnett LS, eds. Novak's Textbook of Gynecology, 11th ed. Baltimore: Williams & Wilkins, 1988;68.

Speroff L, Glass RH, Kase NG. Clinical Gynecologic Endocrinology and Infertility, 5th ed. Baltimore: Williams & Wilkins, 1994;183.

Vollman RF. The menstrual cycle. In: Friedman E, ed. Major Problems in Obstetrics and Gynecology. Philadelphia: WB Saunders, 1977.

Specific References

Adams DB, Gold AR. Rise in female-initiated sexual activity at ovulation and its suppression by oral contraceptives. N Engl J Med 1978;229:1145.

Barreca A, Artini PG, Del Monte P, et al. In vivo and in vitro effect of growth hormone on estradiol secretion by human granulosa cell. J Clin Endocrinol Metab 1993;77:61.

Bicsak TA, Tucker EM, Cappel S, et al. Hormonal regulation of granulosa cell inhibin biosynthesis. Endocrinology 1986;119:2711.

Chikasawa K, Araki S, Tameda T. Morphological and endocrinological studies on follicular development during the human menstrual cycle. J Clin Endocrinol Metab 1986;62:305.

Collet ME, Wertenberger GE, Fiske VM. The effect of age upon the pattern of the menstrual cycle. Fertil Steril 1954;5:437.

Couzinet B, Brailly S, Bouchard P, Schaison G. Progesterone stimulates luteinizing hormone secretion by acting directly on the pituitary. J Clin Endocrinol Metab 1992;74:374.

Filicori M, Santoro N, Merrian GR, Crowley WF Jr. Characterization of the physilogical pattern of episodic gonadotropin secretion throughout the human menstrual cycle. J Clin Endocrinol Metab 1986;62:1136.

Fritz AM, McLachlan RI, Cohen NL, Dahl KD, Bremner WJ, Soules MR. Onset and characteristics of the mid-cycle surge in bioactive and immunoactive luteinizing hormone secretion in normal women: influence of physiological variations in periovulatory ovarian steroid hormone secretion. J Clin Endocrinol Metab 1992;75:489.

Gougeon A, Lefevre B. Histological evidence of alternating ovulation in women. J Reprod Fertil 1984;70:7.

Grimes RW, Samaras SE, Barber JA, Shimasaki S, Ling N, Hammond JM. Gonadotropin and cyclic-AMP modulation of insulin-like growth factor-binding protein production in ovarian granulosa cells. Am J Physiol 1992;262:E497.

Hendricks C, Piccinino LJ, Udry JR, Chimbira THK. Peak coital rate coincides with onset of luteinizing hormone surge. Fertil Steril 1987;48:234.

Hillier SG, Wickings EJ, Illingworth PI, et al. Control of immunoactive inhibin production by human granulosa cells. Clin Endocrinol 1991;35:71.

Laatikainen T, Raisanen I, Tulenheimo A, Salminen K. Plasma β-endorphines and the menstrual cycle. Fertil Steril 1985;44:206.

Le Nestour E, Marraoui J, Lahlou N, Roger M, de Siegler D, Bouchard PH. Role of estradiol in the rise in follicle-stimulating hormone levels during the luteal-follicular transition. J Clin Endocrinol Metab 1993;77:439.

Lenton EA, de Kretser DM, Woodward AJ, Rogertson DM. Inhibin concentrations throughout the menstrual cycles of normal, infertile, and older women compared with those during spontaneous conception cycles. J Clin Endocrinol Metab 1991;73:1180.

Lenton EA, Landgren B, Sexton L, Harper R. Normal variation in the length of the follicular phase of the menstrual cycle: Effect of chronological age. Br J Obstet Gynaecol 1984;91:681.

Lenton EA, Landgren B, Sexton L. Normal variation in the length of the luteal phase of the menstrual cycle: Identification of the short luteal phase. Br J Obstet Gynaecol 1984;91:685.

MacNaughton J, Banah M, McCloud P, Hee J, Burger H. Age related changes in follicle stimulating hormone, luteinizing hormone, oestradiol and immunoreactive inhibin in women of reproductive age. Clin Endocrinol 1992;36:339.

Mais V, Kazer RR, Ctel NS, Rivier J, Vale W, Yen SSC. The dependency of folliculogenesis and corpus luteum function on pulsatile gonadotropin secretion in cycling women using a gonadotropin-releasing hormone antagonist as a probe. J Clin Endocrinol Metab 1986;62:1250.

McLachlin RI, Cohen ML, Vale WE, et al. The importance of luteinizing hormone in the control of inhibin and progesterone secretion by the human corpus luteum. J Clin Endocrinol Metab 1989;68:1078.

McNatty KP, Makris A, DeGrazia C, Osathanondh R, Ryan KJ. The production of progesterone, androgens, and estrogens by granulosa cell, thecal tissue, and stromal tissue from human ovaries in vitro. J Clin Endocrinol Metab 1979;49:687.

McNatty KP, Smith DM, Makris A, Osathanondh R, Ryan KJ. The microenvironment of the human antral follicle; inter-relationships among the steroid levels in antral fluid, the population of granulosa cells, and the status of the oocyte in vivo and in vitro. J Clin Endocrinol Metab 1979;49:851.

Miro F, Hillier SG. Relative effects of activin and inhibin on steroid hormone synthesis in primate granulosa cells. J Clin Endocrinol Metab 1992;75:1556.

Mortola JF, Laughlin GA, Yen SSC. A circadian rhythm of serum follicle-stimulating hormone in women. J Clin Endocrinol Metab 1992;75:861.

Munster K, Schjmidt L, Helm P. Length and variation in the menstrual cycle—a cross-sectional study from a Danish county. Br J Obstet Gynaecol 1992;99:422.

Nippold TB, Reame NE, Kelch RP, Marshall JC. The roles of estradiol and progesterone in decreasing luteinizing hormone pulse frequency in the luteal phase of the menstrual cycle. J Clin Endocrinol Metab 1989;69:67.

Richards JS, Jahansen T, Hedin L, et al. Ovarian follicular development: From physiology to molecular biology. Recent Prog Horm Res 1987;43:231.

Sherman BM, Koreman SG. Hormonal characteristics of the human menstrual cycle throughout reproductive life. J Clin Invest 1975;55:699.

Testart J, Frydman R, Roger M. Seasonal influence of diurnal rhythms in the onset of the plasma luteinizing hormone surge in women. J Clin Endocrinol Metab 1982;55:374.

Treloar AE, Boynton RE, Borghild GB, Brown BW. Variation of the human menstrual cycle through reproductive life. Int J Fertil 1967;12:77.

Urban RJ, Veldhuis JD, Dufau ML. Estrogen regulates the gonadotropin-releasing hormone-stimulated secretion of biologically active luteinizing hormone. J Clin Endocrinol Metab 1991;72:660.

Vermesh M, Kletzky OA. Longitudinal evaluation of the luteal phase and its transition into the follicular phase. J Clin Endocrinol Metab 1987;65:653.

Yamoto M, Shima K, Nakano R. Gonadortopin receptors in human ovarian follicles and corpora lutea throughout the menstrual cycle. Horm Res 1992;37(suppl 1):5.

Yong EL, Baird DT, Yates R, Reichert LE Jr, Hillier SG. Hormonal regulation of the growth and steroidogenic function of human granulosa cells. J Clin Endocrinol Metab 1992;74:842.

Yoshimura Y, Wallach EE. Studies on the mechanism(s) of mammalian ovulation. Fertil Steril 1987;47:22.

3

Secrets of the Gynecologic History and Physical Examination

There are a limited number of elements that set apart the gynecologic history and physical from an examination performed for any patient of either gender. These differences not only define the field of gynecologic care, but the manner of their execution can mean the difference between successful care and a nonproductive ordeal. If we are going to provide health care to women, we must be prepared to perform the requisite history and physical assessments in an efficient, but compassionate manner. To do otherwise is to breach the sacred contract we make with our female patients.

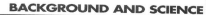 **BACKGROUND AND SCIENCE**

Obstetric and Gynecologic History

The evaluation of a gynecologic concern, be it the assessment of a problem or routine screening for health maintenance and risk reduction, begins with a thorough history. This history must, of course, include the normal inquiries that frame good care for any patient. In addition, special attention must be given to those aspects of a woman's physiology that make her care unique: breast health, menstruation, and reproductive function. The basic structure of a gynecologic history is shown in Table 3.1, although the sequence in which the material is covered and recorded is a matter of individual preference, modified by the nature of the patient's complaint. Details of the gynecologic history applicable to evaluating specific presenting complaints are contained in subsequent chapters.

Table 3.1. Generalized Elements of the Gynecologic History

Chief complaint
Menstrual history
    Last menstrual period (LMP)
    Previous menstrual period (PMP)
    Normal
    Menarche
    Usual menstrual pattern (frequency, duration, character)
    Abnormal periods
    [Menopause—Onset, symptoms, postmenopausal bleeding]
Obstetric history (may be abbreviated in "GaPbcde" form)
    [Dates/Duration/Outcome/Complications]
Gynecologic history
    Abuse/Incest/Rape
    Breast disease
    Contraception (present, past, problems)
    Gynecologic diseases
    Sexuality (activity, satisfaction, problems, partner(s), high-risk behaviors)
    Sexually transmitted disease
    Surgeries
    Treatments
    Urinary tract problems (including incontinence)
Family history (especially breast and gynecologic disease)
General history and review of systems (with emphasis on breast and pelvic organs, including
    use of breast and genital self-examinations)

For those aspects of the general history not related to the patient's presenting concerns, the history may be obtained by a questionnaire, computer software, or screening by an experienced health professional. This will be based on the preferences in the individual practice and the geographic custom. If the history is obtained in this manner, it must be reviewed by the provider and the patient to ensure accuracy and completeness.

Breast Health

Questions unique to the evaluation of the female breasts must include the obvious exploration of signs or symptoms, family history, and breast health practices, such as mammography and breast self-examination. Women with a first-degree relative with breast cancer are at increased risk of developing breast cancer. If that cancer was diagnosed before menopause, the woman's lifetime risk may exceed 50%. Recording the family history may be facilitated by using a family tree diagram such as that shown in Figure 3.1, made up of commonly agreed-on symbols (Figure 3.2).

As a part of the review of breast symptoms, check for the presence of cyclic mastalgia, localized pain, masses or thickenings, skin changes, or nipple discharge. A review of the patient's use of breast self-examination (BSE) may establish a dialogue and allow for health promotion. Mammography, baseline or periodic screening, should be reviewed and encouraged as appropriate.

Menstruation

Based on the character of the patient's concerns, portions of the menstrual history may be covered in exploring and recording the chief compliant. In addition, the menstrual history

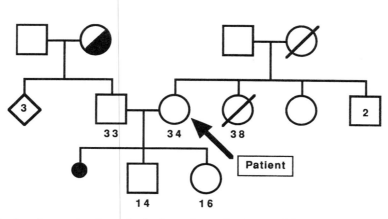

Figure 3.1. The family tree (pedigree) of a hypothetical 34-year-old G3 P2012 woman with a sister who died of breast cancer at age 38, whose father is alive, and mother has died. She has two other living brothers and a living sister. The patient's husband has three siblings (gender not specified) and it is indicated that his mother is a carrier of a genetically determined disease.

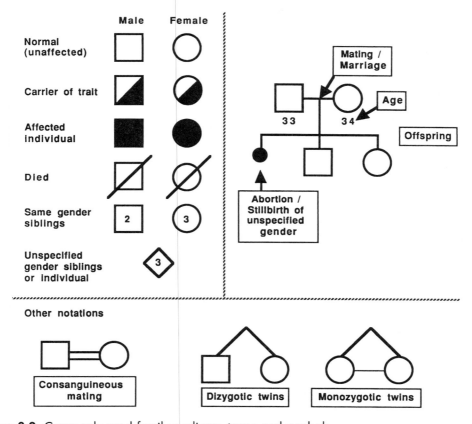

Figure 3.2. Commonly used family pedigree terms and symbols.

section of the patient's evaluation must chronicle menarche, typical menstrual cycling (including interval, duration, and character), the date of the most recent and previous menses, and the events of menopause, if appropriate. Premenstrual or menstrual complaints, and any medication used for them, should be entered with the rest of the menstrual history if germane to the presenting complaint. The presence of any postcoital bleeding should be noted.

Closely related to the menstrual history is the more general gynecologic history. This includes previous pelvic surgeries and gynecologic diseases, such as endometriosis, dysfunctional bleeding, infertility, and sexually transmitted disease along with their treatments. Any breast complaints and the patient's contraceptive experience should be chronicled. The latter should include both the patient's current method and previous experiences, problems, and degree of satisfaction. The placement of this particular information within the menstrual history, medication list (for hormonal contraception), or a separate gynecologic history is a matter of personal preference.

The date of the patient's last cytologic screening and results should be ascertained. The regularity with which the patient has had Pap smears and whether any have been abnormal should be determined. Hygienic practices, such as douching, the use of feminine hygiene sprays, and the use of talc on the vulva or perineum should be recorded. (Douching is associated with vaginal and upper genital tract infections, sprays may cause chemical vulvitis, and the use of talc may be linked to a higher incidence of ovarian cancer.)

Patients who have undergone a hysterectomy should have the year, indication, type of procedure (with special emphasis on whether the ovaries remain), and the use of hormonal replacement recorded in their history. Elements of this may be included in a surgical review or in a medication list. If the hysterectomy was performed for cervical or uterine malignancy, this should be noted because it affects the frequency and type of follow-up the patient should receive.

Reproductive Function
The review of the patient's sexual function is a necessary and vital part of any gynecologic history (see Chapter 8, Sexuality and Contraception; and Chapters 23–25, Sexual Assault and Abuse, Sexual Dysfunction, and Sexual Pain). For some clinicians, this aspect of the patient's history is an area of discomfort, resulting in value. If this discussion is included as a part of the general review of systems and carried out in a matter-of-fact manner, this discomfort may be minimized, though the value of the discussion cannot. Consideration of sexuality and sexual function may be included in the

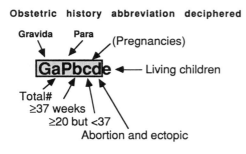

Obstetric history abbreviation deciphered

Figure 3.3. Obstetric history abbreviation deciphered. "G" represents the "Gravida" of older abbreviations, while "P" is the "Para."

Table 3.2. Common Obstetric Descriptive Terms

Gravida	One who is or has been pregnant
Nulligravida	One who has never been pregnant
Primigravida	One who is in or has had her first pregnancy
Multigravida	One who has been pregnant more than once
Nullipara	One who has never had a pregnancy progress beyond 20 weeks duration
Primipara	One who has delivered one pregnancy of greater than 20 weeks gestation, regardless of number of fetuses
Multipara	One who has delivered two or more pregnancies of greater than 20 weeks duration
Parturient	One who is currently in labor
Puerpera	One who has recently given birth

more general discussion of current and past contraception, providing a natural transition to the subject.

One confusing element of the obstetric history is the commonly used abbreviation representing the patient's experience with, and outcome of, previous pregnancies. This shorthand information contains the number of times the patient has been pregnant and the number of term and preterm births, miscarriages, and currently living children (Figure 3.3). In all but the last of these numbers, the referent is the number of pregnancies, not the number of infants involved. For this reason, a patient who has been pregnant only once with a twin pregnancy delivered at term, and whose children are still living, would be described as being "G1P1002." In all cases, the number following the "G" must equal the sum of the first three numbers following the "P" for women who are not pregnant, and exceed it by exactly one for those who are currently pregnant.

For the patient who has been pregnant, her experiences in previous pregnancies, such as complications of the gestation, route of birth, or postpartum complications will all have a bearing on the management of future pregnancies. For pregnancies that have been lost, any medical or surgical therapies that were required, causes for the loss that may have been established, and the patient's feelings about the events are appropriate lines of inquiry.

A number of descriptive terms are applied to women based on their obstetric history. Although definitions of these terms are well established (Table 3.2), when in doubt, a narrative description is less likely to be incorrectly interpreted.

Physical Assessment

As with the gynecologic history, the physical evaluation of women is premised on the same principles that govern any physical assessment: respect, care, thoroughness, and professionalism. The very nature of the areas pivotal to gynecologic care gives these examinations a social and personal significance that sets them apart. In many ways, a gynecologic examination should be viewed as an invasive procedure. It is a very special privilege that we are accorded, and it should be treated as such.

As with the history, three elements set apart the physical examination of women: the breast, abdomen, and pelvic areas. These are summarized in Table 3.3.

Table 3.3. Generalized Elements of the Gynecologic Examination*

Basic data
    Height, weight, blood pressure
Breast examination
    Masses, tenderness, skin changes
Abdominal examination
    Masses, tenderness, skin changes, back, and lymphatics
Pelvic examination
    Vulva and vaginal opening
    [Clitoris: separate notation if appropriate]
    Bartholin's, urethral, and Skene's glands (BUS)
    Vagina
    Cervix: lesions, eversion, discharge, Pap smear
    Uterus: size, shape, configuration
    Adnexa: masses, tenderness
    Rectovaginal: masses, tenderness, guaiac

*In addition to other physical evaluations as appropriate.

Examination of the Breast

Office examination of the breast remains one of the most cost-effective methods of detecting breast cancer. To fulfill this role, however, it must be done as a routine part of every periodic examination, and must be supported by the judicious use of mammography, ultrasonography, and biopsy. The value of clinical examination is well established for women over the age of 40, but debate continues about its effectiveness for younger women. Because it carries little direct cost and is minimally invasive, it should probably remain a part of all routine examinations. In addition to its screening benefit, the breast examination provides an opportunity to instruct and reinforce the techniques of breast self-examination.

Inspection of the breasts begins the examination. This should be done with the patient sitting comfortably with her arms at her sides (Figure 3.4). The presence of discoloration, skin changes, puckering, or retraction is sought. Inspection is then repeated with the patient pressing her hand into her hips and then with her arms raised over her head. Some asymmetry is common, but marked differences or recent changes deserve further attention.

Palpation of the breast is carried out while the patient is sitting with her arms raised and then repeated while she is supine. Palpation is conducted using the flat portion of the fingers, exploiting the sensitivity of the distal finger pads. A combination of small spirals and wavelike finger palpations give the best examination of the breast tissue. These maneuvers must be done slowly, carefully, gently, and thoroughly, covering all quadrants of the breast and the axilla. Some examiners use a radial spiral working outward from the areola to ensure that all areas are palpated, whereas others examine each quadrant in sequence (Figure 3.5). This is a matter of personal preference.

Some authors have advocated the used of adjuncts such as powder, liquid soap, or a rubber membrane to improve sensitivity during breast palpation. Although the advocates of these techniques claim they are superior, no unbiased studies are available, leaving the decision to use one of the methods a matter of personal choice.

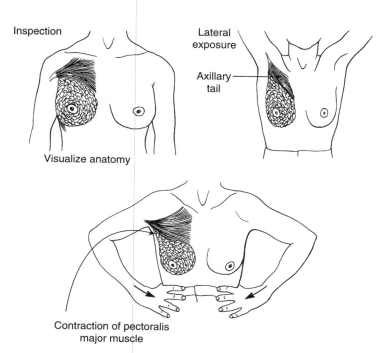

Inspection

Visualize anatomy

Lateral exposure

Axillary tail

Contraction of pectoralis major muscle

Figure 3.4. Inspection of the breast is carried out with the patient sitting with arms at her sides (A), raised over head (B), and with the pectoralis major muscles contracted (C). (From Beckmann RB, Ling FW, Barzansky BM, et al. Obstetrics and gynecology. 2nd ed. Baltimore: Williams & Wilkins, 1995:9.)

Breast palpation techniques

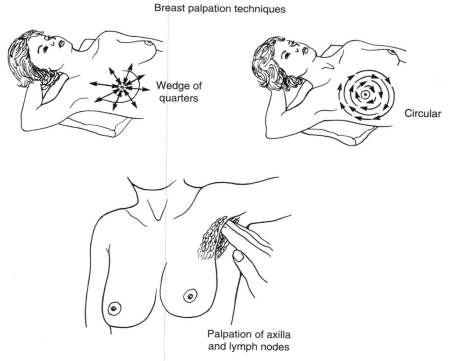

Wedge of quarters

Circular

Palpation of axilla and lymph nodes

Figure 3.5. Palpation of the breast can be done in many ways as long as all of the breast tissue is systematically examined. (From Beckmann RB, Ling FW, Barzansky BM, et al. Obstetrics and gynecology. 2nd ed. Baltimore: Williams & Wilkins, 1995:9.)

If any anomalies are found, their location, size, shape, consistency, and mobility should be noted. This is often best recorded in the form of a quick sketch or drawing entered in the patient's chart. If this is done, care must be taken to indicate only discrete masses with discrete symbols (Figure 3.6). If there is only an area of diffuse thickening, the use of symbols suggestive of a discrete mass is misleading and may lead to unnecessary liability exposure.

Once general palpation is completed, the areola and nipple must be examined for sub-areolar masses, discharges, or exudates. Gentle pressure downward, then inward and upward on the base of the nipple will express discharge without undue discomfort (Figure 3.7). If the patient has noted discharge in the past, you may choose to have the patient herself express the discharge. Clear or milky discharges may be ignored, whereas bloody discharge must be further evaluated.

Examination of the Abdomen

The abdominal examination of women is carried out, for the most part, in the same way as that for men. The main difference is the extra attention paid to the lower abdomen and suprapubic areas. Gentle palpation of these areas may reveal uterine or adnexal enlargement, tenderness, or abdominal wall abnormalities. As with any abdominal examination, the presence of scars, protuberances, skin lesions or discoloration, abnormal hair patterns, or striations should be noted. Gentle palpation may reveal organomegaly, tenderness, guarding, rigidity, or the presence of fluid. Palpation of the inguinal lymph nodes should not be overlooked. Percussion and auscultation complete the examination.

For patients who are ticklish, the abdominal examination is not humorous; it may be very uncomfortable. This may be overcome by having the patient place her hand on top of that of the examiner as the examiner moves from one location to the next. This not only gives the patient an indication of where palpation is to be performed, but "confuses" the brain into thinking that the hand is the patient's own. Because it is virtually impossible for

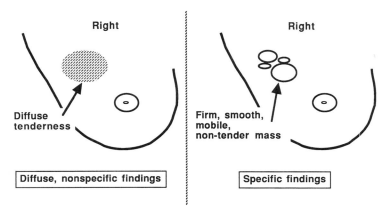

Figure 3.6. Appropriate methods of recording breast findings. Any nonspecific changes should be indicated in a manner appropriate to their tentative character. Conversely, specific findings must be carefully documented to allow comparison with later examinations. Implying greater or less precision by the manner that the findings are recorded contravenes the purpose of the record entry and may unnecessarily invite questions of management and liability.

Figure 3.7. Expression of nipple discharge. Nipple discharge can be expressed by gentle pressure in an inward and upward direction. (From Beckmann RB, Ling FW, Barzansky BM, et al. Obstetrics and gynecology. 2nd ed. Baltimore: Williams & Wilkins, 1995:9.)

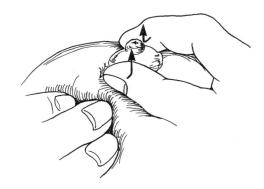

someone to tickle themselves, the patient will remain relaxed and comfortable, allowing a productive examination with a minimum of distress.

The Pelvic Examination

EQUIPMENT. The equipment necessary to perform a pelvic examination is sufficiently simple that care in its selection or its ready availability is often overlooked. The examination room should be warm and provide sufficient privacy to promote confidence. A curtained area for changing and clothing storage should be provided. Stocking this area with tissues, sanitary pads or tampons, a wastebasket, and mirror will be greatly appreciated by all patients. The foot of the examining table should never face the door, even when a screen or curtain is provided. If the room has windows, they must be covered by drapery or blinds during the examination, and preferably at any time the patient is not in her normal clothing.

A good light source that can be easily adjusted is indispensable. It should provide a bright, white light and it should not cause an inadvertent burn to either the patient or the staff. This should be positioned just below the line of sight for the examiner; care should be taken to avoid adjustments of the light with contaminated gloves.

The speculum to be used should be selected based on the anticipated anatomy and the planned procedures (Figure 3.8). Most commonly used is the Graves speculum. This speculum works well for most patients; it is available in three sizes to allow some flexibility in meeting the needs of the specific patient. The Pederson speculum is slightly narrower and better suited for virginal patients, those with atrophic stenosis, or those with vulvar or vaginal conditions that might predispose to increased discomfort. Some practitioners prefer the Pederson speculum for most examinations, although it may prove inadequate for the multiparous patient with significant vaginal relaxation or for the obese patient. Plastic versions of the Graves speculum are available. These offer the ability to visualize the vaginal wall through the blades, albeit in a distorted manner, and less heat conduction, making them feel less cold. These disposable specula do carry the risk of sharp edges left over from the molding process, and a smaller range of adjustments that are possible. Ultimately, the decision of the type of speculum to use will be based on experience, custom, and the individual needs of the patient at hand. A selection of sizes and types should be readily available.

PREPARATION. To optimize the sensitivity of the pelvic examination and to provide maximal comfort for the patient, ask the patient to empty her bladder immediately before the examination begins. If a urine specimen is desired, it may be obtained at this time.

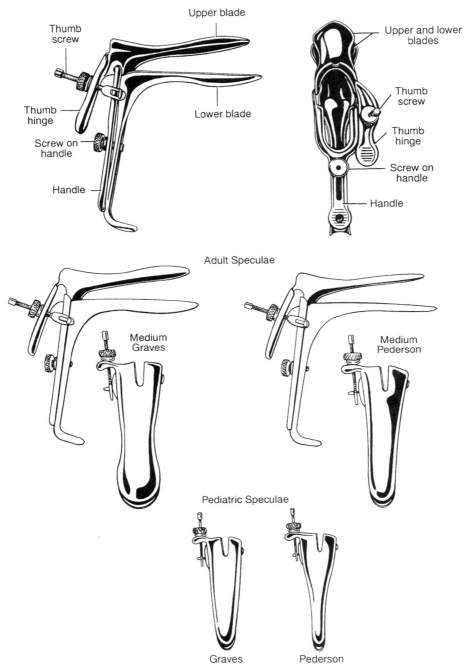

Figure 3.8. Vaginal specula. The most common type of vaginal speculum is the Graves (left). The Pederson speculum is narrower and better suited to patients who are virginal, have atrophic narrowing, or have significant perineal disease that would create pain or spasm. (From Beckmann RB, Ling FW, Barzansky BM, et al. Obstetrics and gynecology. 2nd ed. Baltimore: Williams & Wilkins, 1995:12.)

Just prior to the examination, patients should be asked to disrobe and don the gown provided. Under most circumstances, they should disrobe completely, although for focused examinations the patient may be able to remain in street clothes (e.g., routine prenatal visits) or only partially disrobe (e.g., an episodic examination for vaginitis). The gown offered for the patient's use should provide warmth, comfort, and a sense of modesty. Cloth is preferred to paper, if possible. Unresolved is the age-old question "does the opening go in the front or the back?" Although some suggest that more discreet coverage is possible during abdominal and pelvic examinations if the opening is in the back, the final choice is probably moot and subject to personal preference.

Because of the character of the pelvic examination and to help provide assistance with specimen preparation, most examiners (of either gender) have an assistant present during all pelvic examinations. Many have this assistant present during the breast and abdominal examinations as well. Prudence and propriety endorse the wisdom of this policy.

For most pelvic examinations, the patient should be draped with a sheet to provide as much modesty as possible. This should cover the lower abdomen and legs, but be arranged so that eye contact can be maintained. A few patients will request that the sheet be dispensed with and this request, although infrequent, should be honored. In situations where a hand mirror is used to provide instruction to the patient, the drape may have to be readjusted or dispensed with as well.

Elevating the head of the examining table facilitates eye contact and abdominal wall relaxation. The value of eye contact cannot be overlooked for it provides direct feedback to the examiner while reducing the dehumanizing aspects of the examination. Despite repeated instructions, many patients are reluctant to express discomfort during an examination. Facial expressions often provide clues that would otherwise be missed.

Because much of the pelvic examination takes place out of the direct view (but not experience) of the patient, a good rule of thumb is to "talk before you touch."" By providing a warning of what to expect, relaxation and cooperation will be greatest. This may be as simple as saying "you'll feel me touch you now," or "this will be cold and gooey." A running conversation provides both information about what is being performed and a distraction. Reassurance is also provided by giving control to the patient in the form of statements such as "stop me if I cause too much discomfort," or "tell me which hand causes the least discomfort and I will try to do more of the examination using that hand." Few positions in life are as helpless as being naked in the lithotomy position, so any control that can be returned to the patient will go a long way toward establishing rapport and garnering cooperation.

Appropriate warning about portions of the examination that may create distress should be provided, but this must be done in such a way as not to cause undue anticipatory concern. Depending on the practitioner's individual style, this may even be done with humor: "As I go near the ovaries they may be somewhat tender. Not too bad—a bit like being backed into by a city bus."

The common admonition to relax is both futile and the fodder of stand-up comedy routines. Relaxation of relevant muscle groups is vital to the success and comfort of the examination, but this is best accomplished by specific suggestion. Asking the patient to take regular shallow breaths or to let her abdominal wall cave in like "someone has placed a book on your stomach," will provide the specifics the patient needs to cooperate. Perineal relaxation may be obtained by placing the examining finger against the perineum, pressing gently, and asking the patient to "feel these muscles and try to gradually relax them so I don't pinch."

THE EXAMINATION. Inspection of the perineum is the often-omitted first step in a pelvic examination. Once visible structures are inspected, the labia should be gently separated to allow the introitus to be visualized. This is best accomplished by touching the patient's inner thigh with the back of the examining hand, then rolling the hand into position to make contact with the vulva. This allows the first contact to be in a less threatening area and gives the patient a physical indication of what is coming, which augments the verbal information simultaneously provided. Inspection should include the mons, labia, urethral meatus, perineum, and perianal areas. The condition of the Skene's and Bartholin's glands should be noted. Asking the patient to bear down, cough, or strain while the labia are gently separated will often demonstrate the presence and magnitude of a cystocele, rectocele, or uterine prolapse.

Following inspection, single-handed (sometime called a "monomanual") examination should proceed. Gentle palpation of the labia, perineal body, anterior and posterior vaginal walls, and the distal urethra should be included. The presence of any discharges from accessory glands or the distal urethra should be noted and cultured, if necessary. Some examiners palpate the upper vagina and locate the cervix to facilitate the subsequent speculum examination. If this is done, only water should be used as a lubricant.

Speculum examination should not proceed without preparation. Whichever type and size of speculum is selected, it should be inspected for integrity and functionality, and warmed prior to use. Warming can be accomplished with a warmer, a heating pad, or the use of warm water. The latter has the additional advantage of providing a modicum of lubrication. (Water-soluble lubricants are necessary for the bimanual examination, but must not be used during the speculum examination because they may interfere with cultures and cytologic evaluations.) If water is used to warm the speculum, excess should be gently shaken off and the temperature checked against the hand or wrist, or the patient's thigh prior to insertion. Because what feels nice to the hands may not feel the same when applied to the perineum, the patient should be told something to the effect that "this should be warm and you may feel some pressure as I look inside. If this is too warm, let me know and I will let it cool a little."

Insertion of the speculum is best accomplished by using the fingers of one hand to separate the labia and retract the pubic hair while the other hand positions the speculum. The speculum should be inserted with the blades in a horizontal position and the posterior blade resting on the posterior fourchette. In most parous women, the speculum can be balanced on the extended thumb and allowed to slide into the vagina at a 45° downward angle under the influence of its own weight. Gentle pressure can be applied along this axis, if needed. If more assistance with insertion is needed, pressure should be applied only in a posterior direction. This is the only direction in which soft tissues can yield to pressure. Any pressure applied anteriorly will result in trapping the urethra between the speculum and the symphysis, resulting in significant discomfort.

The cervix can be most easily visualized by inserting the speculum into the posterior fornix and then gently separating the blades. This allows the cervix to drop into the opening of the speculum. A patient with a significant retroversion or other displacement (such as seen with pelvic scarring or extensive leiomyomas) may have a cervix that is difficult to locate. A slight withdrawal of the speculum, with the blades partially separated, may give an indication of the location of the cervix. Asking the patient to gently bear down while the speculum is stabilized in the open position often causes the cervix to enter the field of view.

Once the cervix is located, the blades of the speculum should be held open by adjusting one or both screws or ratchets. Care must be taken to secure these adjustments because uncontrolled closure of either the distal or proximal portions of the speculum may result in entrapment of tissues and significant pain.

Once cytologic or microbiologic specimens have been obtained, the speculum can be removed. This must be done slowly, with the distal portion of the blades in the partially open position. This avoids pinching the tissues and facilitates a very important, but often omitted, portion of the examination: the inspection of the vaginal walls. As with insertion, any pressure applied during removal must be in a posterior direction.

Bimanual examination of the uterus and adnexa is next performed by inserting either the index finger or the index and third fingers into the vagina. Here, a water-soluble lubricant is a must. The choice of which hand to palpate abdominally and which to place in the vagina is a matter of regional training and personal preference. Some examiners even switch the roles of the hands midway through the procedure to facilitate palpation of the adnexa. Whatever the preference, a more stable examination is obtained if the elbow of the arm used for the vaginal portion is rested on the knee of the examiner's ipsilateral leg, raised to an appropriate level by a step or lift. This position also provides some relaxation of the examiner's own low back, thereby reducing strain.

The fingers inserted in the vagina should be placed in the posterior fornix. This allows elevation of the uterus and adnexal structures toward the abdominal wall and the external palpating hand (Figure 3.9). As with the other steps in the process, a running discussion of what is being done and the sensations that are likely to occur is vital. This is mandatory

Figure 3.9. Bimanual palpation of the pelvic viscera. (From Jones HW, Wentz AC, Burnett LS. Novak's textbook of gynecology. 11th ed. Baltimore: Williams & Wilkins, 1988:11.)

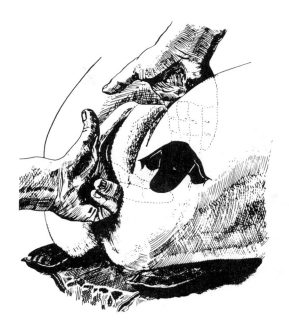

during palpation of the adnexal structures. Ovaries are like testes; even gentle palpation produces moderate discomfort, bordering on nausea. Care is the watchword.

The pelvic examination concludes with the rectal examination. As with the vaginal evaluation, inspection must precede the introduction of the examining finger (one only; typically the third finger). The glove used for the vaginal examination should not be used for the rectal portion. The soiled glove must be removed and replaced by a clean glove. Placement of the rectal finger can be facilitated by asking the patient to gently bear down during the process of insertion. Simultaneous palpation from the rectal and vaginal sides of the rectovaginal septum is valuable and may be done with the same glove so long as the fingers are not removed and reinserted, which would necessitate a new glove. Occult blood testing of any stool present on the glove at the close of the rectal examination should be based on the presence of symptoms, findings, or screening guidelines. (See Chapter 10, Cancer Screening.)

At the conclusion of the examination, the patient should be offered a hand to regain the sitting position. A soft wash cloth is always preferable to tissues, or worse a paper towel, for removing excess lubricant. Wherever possible, discussion of any findings, as with the initial history, should be done when the patient has once again dressed in street clothes.

HINTS AND COMMON QUESTIONS

Care must be taken when obtaining a menstrual history that menstrual interval is measured from first day of flow to the next first day of flow. Many patients will interpret the question of interval as the bleeding-free period. It is fundamental that both the provider and the patient use the same measure to avoid confusion.

It is difficult to assess the amount of menstrual flow a woman experiences. It is appropriate to ask about the use of tampons or pads, the number used per period, the frequency with which they must be changed, or the presence of clots. These give a broad indication of the amount of flow; however, objective studies have shown a poor correlation with the actual measured blood loss. If anemia is present without any other source of blood loss apparent, heavy flow (menorrhagia) may be inferred.

It is always wise to be alert to the possibility of a "hidden agenda" when a patient presents with seemingly trivial or chronic nonspecific complaints. These patients may be seeking help for problems they do not know how to express or discuss. These concerns run the gamut from orgasmic dysfunction and sexual orientation to abuse, rape, and worries over sexually transmitted disease.

To facilitate inspection of patients with large or pendulous breasts, have the patient lean forward slightly. This will move the breast away from the chest wall, making inspection easier and increasing the probability of detecting skin retraction or dimpling.

Women with large breasts often have a thicken, nontender ridge of tissue palpable, which runs transversely below the lower edge of the breast. This is the inframammary ridge, which is normal.

Nipple discharge that is expressed from only one duct suggests a localized condition that will require further investigation. When the discharge is present at the opening of more than one duct, the underlying process is diffuse, and reassurance is appropriate in most cases.

When in doubt about the normality of a breast finding, compare the analogous area (mirror image) to the opposite breast. When a similar finding is made, it is safe to assume that the finding is physiologic or developmental, and therefore is normal.

Oven mitts with a central thumb (ambidextrous) make good covering for office stirrups; they are soft, warmer than uncovered stirrups, and may be washed. If a stirrup cover is not used, you may wish to have the patient keep her shoes on for comfort.

Before using a heating pad to warm specula, check local fire and electrical codes. In many areas, the use of heating pads (especially inside of storage drawers) is against fire regulations. Special grounding may be required for any device, including an ordinary heating pad, that is used in patient care areas. Checking these regulations in advance will prevent problems and minimize risk. When in doubt, use warm water instead.

Because it is desirable to change gloves between the vaginal and rectal portions of the pelvic examination, begin with two gloves on the hand that will do the internal portions of the examination to facilitate the process. Once the vaginal examination is concluded, the vaginal glove can be removed, quickly exposing the clean glove for the rectal examination, optimizing speed and minimizing the risk of contamination for all involved.

When attempting to perform a speculum examination on an obese patient or a patient with significant vaginal laxity, you may find the lateral vaginal walls often intrude through the side openings of the speculum, making visualization of the cervix or vaginal apex impossible. Placing a latex condom, or the finger of a glove (with the tip removed), over the speculum, provides the lateral retraction required to accomplish the examination.

For the unusual patient who cannot abduct her hips, the pelvic examination can be accomplished in either the Sims' (lateral) position or in the knee-chest position.

Insertion of a speculum in the vertical plane, with rotation to the horizontal once one third to one half the speculum is inside the vaginal canal, is advocated by some. This is to be avoided. The vaginal opening is a potential space, thus providing no advantage to the vertical (parallel to the labia) orientation. Rotation, or any other unnecessary movements of the speculum, only increases the likelihood of discomfort and should be avoided.

Some examiners insert the vaginal speculum over a finger placed at the posterior vaginal fourchette. This allows the finger to displace the posterior vaginal opening and provides feedback about the degree of perineal muscle relaxation. It has the disadvantage of increasing the volume of materials that must be contained in the vaginal opening, potentially complicating insertion and compromising comfort.

Plastic specula produce a large variety of cracking, popping, and snapping noises when they are opened or locked into position. This can be very disconcerting to the patient if she has not been warned that this will happen.

SUGGESTED READINGS

General References

Beckmann CRB, Ling FW, Barzansky BM, et al, eds. Obstetrics and Gynecology, 2nd ed. Baltimore: Williams & Wilkins, 1995;1.

Sapira JD. The Art and Science of Bedside Diagnosis. Baltimore: Williams & Wilkins, 1990;399.

Specific References

Granberg S, Wikland M. A comparison between ultrasound and gynecologic examination for detection of enlarged ovaries in a group of women at risk for ovarian carcinoma. J Ultrasound Med 1988;7:59.

Magee J. The pelvic examination: A view from the other end of the table. Ann Intern Med 1975;83:563.

Wilbanks GD. Changing gloves between vaginal and rectal examination: Reinstitution of old practices for new diseases. JAMA 1986;256:1893.

II

Ambulatory Obstetrics

4

Early Pregnancy

In the United states, there are over 4 million births annually and more than 90% of American women bear children during their lifetime. The care these women receive during this special phase of their lives is critical both to their health and to the success of the pregnancy. Although not all primary care providers wish to provide obstetric service, many do provide routine prenatal care in conjunction with others who will supervise the final delivery.

The goal of prenatal care is to ensure the health of both the mother and the baby, although it must be recognized that achieving this goal cannot be guaranteed. It is reasonable to set forth realistic objectives for prenatal care (Table 4.1) and to develop a systematic approach to achieving them. When successfully implemented, prenatal care is an excellent example of preventive medicine; when it is not, it is an opportunity squandered, often with tragic results.

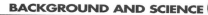 **BACKGROUND AND SCIENCE**

Preconception

For many couples, prenatal care begins with prepregnancy testing. This may take the form of a general health check or screening for specific conditions that could modify either the desirability of pregnancy or its course. General evaluations are directed toward establishing optimal maternal health, providing nutritional counseling, and instituting appropriate

Table 4.1. Objectives of Prenatal Care

Evaluation of the health of mother and baby
Assessment of gestational age and development
Identification and minimization of risk where possible
Prevention of complications
Patient education and communication

prophylaxis. Screening is based on the general principles of cost-effective detection and the ability to intervene to improve the outcome of an involved process or disease. In the case of prenatal testing, this generally takes the form of genetic screening or the detection of maternal diseases, such as diabetes, that will alter or be altered by a future pregnancy.

Ideal preconception care is predicated on obtaining a realistic appraisal of those risks that cannot be altered and modifying those factors that can be changed to decrease risk or optimize outcome. The most common form of risk appraisal is genetic counseling. Based on age, ethnic origin, race, or family history couples can be identified who have an increased risk of having children with chromosomal or enzymatic abnormalities (Table 4.2). Screening couples in groups at risk allows an appraisal of the degree of risk and may suggest the need for later testing, such as amniocentesis or chorionic villus sampling. Indications for prenatal counseling or genetic screening are shown in Table 4.3.

Before pregnancy is the optimal time for rubella immunization and baseline laboratory testing. Anemia, hypothyroidism, urinary tract infections, and other conditions may be identified and treated prior to conception. Nutritional and weight reduction counseling may be accomplished before pregnancy, with admonitions about the risks of using medications, drugs, alcohol, and tobacco products during early pregnancy. If the patient has significant medical problems, the impact of pregnancy on these problems and the implications for the pregnancy may be determined in an unhurried manner, allowing pragmatic assessment and nonjudgmental counseling to facilitate informed decisions. When appropriate, referrals may be made to specialists for risk assessment or management to ensure early evaluation and continuity of care.

The most common reason for genetic testing is advanced maternal age. There is a well-established relationship between maternal age at delivery and the risk of chromosomal abnormalities (Fig. 4.1). The geometric nature of this relationship may be most easily seen when a logarithmic scale is used (Fig. 4.2). When plotted in this manner, an accel-

Table 4.2. Genetic Screening Based on Ethnicity

Disorder	High-Risk group	Parental test	Fetal test
Tay-Sachs disease	Ashkenazi Jews	Serum hexosaminidase-A	CVS or amniocentesis for enzyme analysis
Sickle-cell disease	Blacks	Hemoglobin electrophoresis	CVS or amniocentesis for genotype
β-Thalassemia	Mediterranean peoples	MCV <80, then hemoglobin electrophoresis	CVS or amniocentesis for genotype
α-Thalassemia	Southeast Asians and Chinese	MCV <80, then hemoglobin electrophoresis	CVS or amniocentesis for genotype

MCV = Mean corpuscular volume; CVS = chorionic villus sampling.

Table 4.3. Indications for Prenatal Counseling and Diagnosis

- Maternal age ≥35 y
- Parental chromosomal rearrangements
- Previous child with chromosomal abnormality
- Abnormally high or low maternal serum α-fetoprotein (MSAFP)
- Family history of single-gene defect
- Significant risk of neural tube defect
- Significant risk of multifactorial disorder
- Fetal anomalies found by ultrasonography

erated rate of abnormalities may be clearly seen beginning at around age 32. By age 35, the risk of a major chromosomal defect exceeds the risk of most tests used to detect fetal genetic anomalies, prompting a recommendation for screening of all women who are at or beyond age 35 at the time of expected delivery.

Physiology of pregnancy

General Changes

An increase in maternal weight during pregnancy is desirable and is a consequence of the normal physiology of pregnancy. The average weight gained during pregnancy is between 11 and 13 kg (25 to 30 lb). This gain is unequally distributed across the duration of pregnancy,

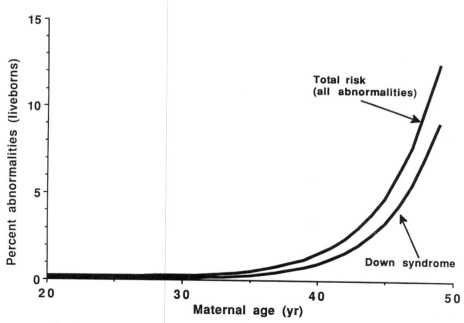

Figure 4.1. Risk of chromosomal abnormalities in live-born infants by maternal age. The risk of chromosomal abnormalities in live-born infants is a geometric function of maternal age. Data from: Hook EB, Cross PK, Schreinemachers DM. Chromosomal abnormality rates at amniocentesis and in live-born infants. JAMA 1983;249:2034; and Hook EB. Rates of chromosomal abnormalities at different maternal ages. Obstet Gynecol 1981;58:282.

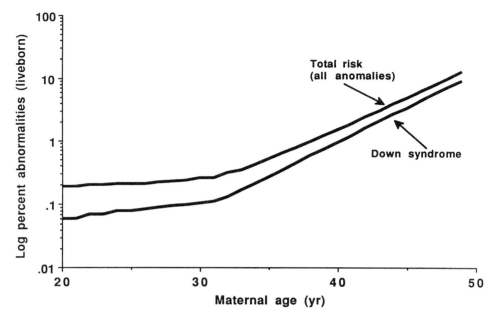

Figure 4.2. Risk of chromosomal abnormalities in live-born infants by maternal age (logarithmic). The relationship between risk of chromosomal abnormality and increasing age becomes more apparent when graphed in a logarithmic manner. Note how risk becomes an exponential function after the age of 32. Data from: Hook EB, Cross PK, Schreinemachers DM. Chromosomal abnormality rates at amniocentesis and in live-born infants. JAMA 1983;249:2034; and Hook EB. Rates of chromosomal abnormalities at different maternal ages. Obstet Gynecol 1981;58:282.

with about 1 kg gained during the first trimester, and 5 kg gained during each of the last trimesters. This weight gain comes mainly from the uterus and its contents, increased volume of the breasts, and fluid storage in the form of expanded blood volume and extracellular fluid (Table 4.4). Within limits, the recommended weight gain during pregnancy is predicated on the patient's prepregnant weight, with underweight patients expected to gain more than patients who are overweight (Fig. 4.3). There appears to be a linear relationship between excessive weight gain (greater than 5.1 body mass index units) and the risk of fetal macrosomia and cesarean delivery, underscoring the importance of careful monitoring and counseling. There is also good evidence that young mothers who gain more than 1.5 lb a week between the 20th and 30th week of gestation weigh an average of 10% to 15% more 6 months after birth than they did during pregnancy.

METABOLIC CHANGES. In addition to changes in weight, pregnant women experience changes in the metabolism of water, protein, and carbohydrates. As pregnancy progresses, water retention ensues, mediated in part by a fall in plasma osmolality. This fluid storage is predominantly responsible for the weight gains noted above; at term, the water content of the fetus, placenta, and uterus is about 3.5 L, with an additional 3 L of fluid accumulated in increased maternal blood volume and uterine and breast size. Pathologic retention of sodium and water is found in patients with pregnancy-induced hypertension.

Table 4.4. Components of Weight Gain During Pregnancy (Normal Singleton, at Term)

	Weight (g)	
Maternal	7650	
Fat		3345
Water (circulatory and extracellular)		1680
Blood		1250
Uterus		970
Breasts		405
Fetoplacental	4650	
Fetus		3400
Amniotic fluid		800
Placenta		650
Total	12500	

During pregnancy there is a gain of about 1 kg of protein that is equally divided between gains by the mother and the protein laid down in the fetus and placenta. Maternal protein gains take the form of increased uterine muscle, breast glandular tissue, and blood. Because the efficiency of protein utilization is estimated to be about 25%, pregnant patients must be advised to maintain or increase dietary protein during pregnancy to cover these demands.

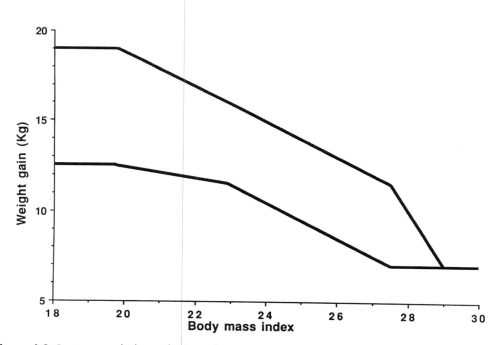

Figure 4.3. Recommended weight gain during pregnancy based on body mass index (BMI). Shown are the upper and lower limits of recommended weight gain for a singleton pregnancy based on prepregnant body mass index.

Pregnancy is potentially a diabetogenic state. Patients who are diabetic may become worse, those who are borderline may become frankly diabetic, and normal patients may be stressed sufficiently to become borderline or worse. Normal pregnancy is characterized by a slight fasting hypoglycemia, a postprandial hyperglycemia, and hyperinsulinemia, the latter of which helps explain the former. Although there is debate to the hormonal mechanisms involved, beta cell hypertrophy, hyperplasia, and hypersecretion are well documented in pregnant women.

The growing conceptus' requirements for iron and the changes in maternal iron utilization are considerable. The average young woman is estimated to have iron stores on the order of 300 mg compared with the estimated total iron requirement of 1 g for the duration of pregnancy. Of this total, about 300 mg are transferred to the fetus, 200 mg are lost by various routes, and 500 mg are retained by the mother in the form of increased maternal red cell mass. The average blood loss associated with the vaginal delivery of a single fetus is estimated to be between 500 and 600 mL and 1 L for cesarean deliveries. This includes losses via lochia during the postpartum period.

Most of the iron demand comes in the last half of pregnancy when daily requirements may be as high as 6 to 7 mg. These demands must be supplied by external sources or maternal hemoglobin will fall. In general, the amount of iron absorbed from the diet and mobilized from maternal stores is inadequate to supply all the needs of pregnancy, resulting in maternal depletion and progressive deficit with each subsequent pregnancy, unless nutrition is supplemented and sustained.

During pregnancy there is a 50% increase in plasma fibrinogen (factor I). This contributes to the large increase in the erythrocyte sedimentation rate, which renders this test of limited value during pregnancy. Increases in other clotting factors (VII, VIII, IX, and X) contribute to the relative hypercoagulable state that is found during pregnancy.

ENDOCRINE CHANGES. During pregnancy the pituitary gland increases by about 135%. Although uncommon, this increase may be sufficient to compress the optic chiasma, resulting in visual field defects. Despite this enlargement, the pituitary is not necessary for the maintenance of pregnancy, save for its role in regulating thyroid and glucocorticoids, whose absence would be potentially lethal.

Maternal serum prolactin levels rise tenfold during the course of pregnancy (Fig. 4.4). This increase disappears rapidly after delivery, even for women who choose to breast-feed. The principal action of prolactin appears to be to prepare the breast for nursing. Prolactin stimulates proliferation of glandular cells and the presecretory alveolar cells of the breast. Prolactin also induces DNA, RNA, and enzyme production to promote galactopoiesis. During lactation, pulsatile release of prolactin occurs in response to suckling. Although the exact function is unknown, amniotic fluid levels of prolactin may reach as high as 10,000 ng/mL at their peak, between 20 and 26 weeks of gestation.

Pregnancy causes a marked increase in maternal thyroxine-binding globulin, which plateaus at a twice-normal level around 20 weeks of gestation. Reduced maternal iodine (due to increased renal clearance), and a proposed direct effect of chorionic gonadotropin on thyroid production, further influence thyroid physiology during pregnancy. As a result of these changes, a moderate enlargement of the thyroid gland and a slight decline in free thyroid hormones (T_3 and T_4) are common during pregnancy.

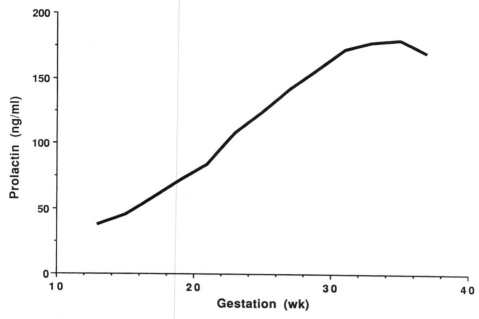

Figure 4.4. Changes in maternal serum prolactin during pregnancy. During pregnancy there is a steady rise in prolactin levels until near term. These levels peak at roughly ten times the levels found in nonpregnant women. (Based on: Kletzky OA, Rossman F, Bertolli SI, Platt LD, Mischell DR. Dynamics of human chorionic gonadotropin, prolactin, and growth hormone in serum and amniotic fluid throughout normal human pregnancy. Am J Obstet Gynecol 1985;151:878.)

A rise in maternal serum cortisol and a fall in adrenocorticotropic hormone (ACTH) is found during pregnancy. Although much of the increased cortisol is bound to transcortin, an increased half-life of cortisol maintains functional balance.

Early in pregnancy, the corpus luteum produces both progesterone and estrogen, but this synthesis is taken over by the placenta beginning at 6 to 8 weeks gestation. Because of the active production of progesterone by the placenta, progesterone levels in pregnancy are six to eight times higher than in the normal luteal phase. Placental estrogen comes from androgen precursors supplied by the maternal and fetal adrenal glands.

CARDIOVASCULAR AND PULMONARY CHANGES. A number of changes are found in the cardio-vascular and respiratory system during pregnancy. Pulse rate and cardiac output change over the course of pregnancy (Fig. 4.5). Pulse rate rises by 10 to 15 beats per minute, reaching a maximal change at term. Cardiac output rises initially, reaching a peak between 28 and 32 weeks of gestation, then declining to term. During pregnancy there is a decrease in maternal peripheral vascular resistance, resulting in a decrease in blood pressure despite increased cardiac stroke volume. Cardiac function changes revert to prepregnant values very rapidly after delivery.

Circulation dynamics in pregnancy are strongly affected by posture and position. Enlargement of the uterus causes impingement on the inferior vena cava, which can result in significant decreases in venous return, potentially creating positional hypotension. In late pregnancy, the weight of the uterus is sufficient that partial compression of the aorta may also occur, compromising arterial supply to distal structures, including the uterus itself. This is most likely to take place late in pregnancy when the patient is in the supine position. Left lateral deviation of the uterus, or use of the lateral recumbent position, is advised to avoid this problem.

Elevation of the diaphragms caused by the expanding uterus results in upward and leftward rotation of the heart, giving it an enlarged appearance on standard chest roentograms. In addition, there is roughly a 10% increase (75 mL) in true cardiac volume, which correlates with the increased stroke volume also found during pregnancy. Combined, these make the detection of true cardiac enlargement more difficult as pregnancy progresses. There is not normally any significant change in the electrocardiogram, save for a minor shift of the electrical axis to the left.

Pregnancy induces changes in the cardiac sounds heard during auscultation. Ninety percent of pregnant women develop a systolic flow murmur that intensifies during inspiration. Up to one fifth of pregnant women also develop a soft, blowing diastolic murmur as well. Pregnancy is associated with an exaggerated splitting of the first heart sound, with an increase in the volume of both components.

During pregnancy the diaphragm rises an average of 4 cm. The subcostal angle widens as the transverse diameter of the chest cage increases by about 2 cm. This increase in diam-

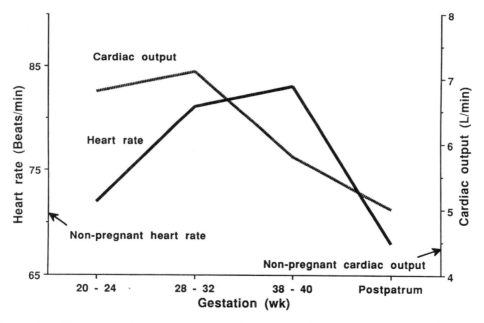

Figure 4.5. Changes in heart rate and cardiac output during pregnancy. Cardiac output reaches its peak at between 28 and 32 weeks of gestation. Exclusive of the physical exertion of labor, this is the time of greatest risk for patients with cardiac disease. Values shown are for lateral recumbent position. Values measured while sitting or supine are lower, with supine values often reduced by .20%.

Table 4.5. Pregnancy-induced Changes in Pulmonary Function Tests

Function (mL)	Nonpregnant	Pregnant
Tidal volume	485	680
Minute ventilation	7270	10,340
Vital capacity	3260	3310
Residual volume	965	770

eter results in a 6-cm increase in circumference, which may contribute to the often-encountered need for pregnant women to change bra size, even when cup size remains comfortable. Despite the anatomic changes in the chest, there is a reduction in residual lung volume. Increased diaphragmatic excursion results in an increase in tidal volume during pregnancy (Table 4.5). A slight sensation of dyspnea is common even in the early phases of pregnancy.

RENAL AND URINARY TRACT CHANGES. During the course of pregnancy the kidneys increase in length by roughly 1.5 cm. Both glomerular filtration rate (GFR) and renal plasma flow (RPF) increase early in pregnancy. By the second trimester, GFR can increase by as much as 50%. As a result of these changes, creatinine clearance is typically on the order of 140 mL/min. Awareness of this elevation is important to correctly interpret clinical tests.

The presence of glucose in the urine during pregnancy is not necessarily abnormal. The increase in GFR and impaired tubal reabsorption of filtered glucose is sufficient to allow some glucose to be present in the urine. Except following vigorous activity, protein is not generally present in any significant amounts. The presence of albuminuria, therefore, suggests a pathologic process, such as renal disease or infection.

As the uterus rises from the pelvis, the ureters are compressed at the level of the pelvic brim. Because of dextrorotation of the uterus as it grows and a slight cushioning effect by the sigmoid, there is a greater degree of compression on the right ureter than on the left. Because of this compression, some degree of hydroureter and hydronephrosis greater on the right than on the left is common.

From the fourth month of pregnancy on, the enlargement of the uterus, pelvic hyperemia, and hyperplasia of pelvic connective tissue all contribute to cause an elevation of the bladder trigone and a thickening of its posterior portion. Increased bladder pressure is compensated for by increases in urethral pressure and length, allowing the patient to maintain continence. Bladder capacity is reduced and residual volume declines.

GASTROINTESTINAL AND HEPATIC SYSTEM IMPACT. Displacement of the stomach and intestines by the enlarging uterus contributes to the development of common symptoms, such as fullness, flatulence, dyspepsia, and heartburn, and confounds the diagnosis of gastrointestinal pathologies. For example, the appendix is displaced upward and laterally during the course of pregnancy, resulting in a significant shift in the location of symptoms when inflammation is present.

Whether due to mechanical or hormonal factors, gastric emptying and gastrointestinal transit time are delayed during pregnancy. This notably increases the risk of aspiration of food or stomach acid should a general anesthetic be administered. These changes in gastric and intestinal function, and a reduced lower esophageal sphincter tone, are responsible for the esophageal reflux and heartburn that plagues women in the later stages of pregnancy.

There appear to be no morphologic changes in the liver attributable to normal pregnancy. Many laboratory evaluations of hepatic function, however, are significantly altered by pregnancy. These alterations are somewhat consistent with hepatic disease, making interpretation difficult. Total alkaline phosphatase activity doubles during pregnancy, partially owing to placental production. Plasma albumen decreases during pregnancy, dropping to an average of about 3 g/dL (4.3 g/dL normal, nonpregnant). There is a slight decline in plasma cholinesterase activity, roughly paralleling the changes found in serum albumen. There is a threefold increase in serum levels of leucine aminopeptidase by term.

During pregnancy, the gallbladder is slow to empty, maintaining an increased residual volume of bile. This stasis, combined with alterations in the concentration of bile salts and a doubling of bile secretion, markedly increases the risk of cholesterol stone formation during and after pregnancy. Between 3% and 4% of patients will develop gallbladder problems during the course of pregnancy. Because of this, cholecystectomy is second only to appendectomy as the most common nonobstetric surgery performed during gestation. Fortunately, less than 3% of those afflicted have to undergo surgical therapy during gestation. When performed, such surgery carries a 5% fetal mortality, rising to 60% if pancreatitis is present. Of women who enter pregnancy with known asymptomatic gallstones, more than 40% will develop symptoms during pregnancy, and over 30% will develop symptoms subsequent to pregnancy. Cholestasis, which is worse late in pregnancy, is often responsible for the common complaint of skin itching.

MUSCULOSKELETAL CHANGES. The mechanical demands of a growing uterus results in a progressive lordosis, which shifts the maternal center of gravity, compensating for the bulk of the growing uterus. There is an increased mobility of the sacroiliac, sacrococcygeal, and pubic joints, which is thought to be due to hormonal influences that cause a general laxity of connective tissue. This laxity and altered body dynamics predispose the woman to sprains, strains, and falls.

Dependent edema is common in the later phases of pregnancy. Facial edema, or edema found in the first or second trimester, may portend toxemia and should be aggressively evaluated, including the possibility of consultation.

Uterus and Contents

No other organ undergoes as dramatic a change in form or function as does the uterus during pregnancy. During pregnancy it changes from an almost solid 70-gm muscular organ, with a cavity of 10 mL or less, into a thin-walled organ capable of containing the fetus, placenta, and amniotic fluid that can range in volume to 20 L or more during multiple gestations. This 500 to 1000 times increase is associated with an increase in organ weight, bringing its mass to approximately 1100 gm. Most of the enlargement of the uterus is due to a mixture of stretch and hypertrophy of the uterine muscle, with some increase in connective tissue as well.

The uterus grows too large to be contained in the true pelvis by 12 weeks of gestation. As it continues to grow, it displaces the intestines laterally and superiorly, coming in contact with the anterior abdominal wall. Tension on the broad and round ligaments contributes to the lower abdominal and groin achelike pain often experienced by primigravid patients. Rotation of the uterus to the right as it grows makes right groin discomfort more prevalent.

By approximately 20 weeks of gestation, the fundus of the uterus reaches the level of the umbilicus, with maximal uterine height reached between 36 and 38 weeks (Fig. 4.6). The uterus continues to grow after this point, but descent into the pelvis offsets or exceeds this growth, causing an apparent reduction in size. Because this descent is accompanied by a downward and backward displacement of the center of gravity, with a concomitant reduction in pressure on the diaphragm, this process is often referred to as "lightening."

From the time of conception on, the uterus undergoes periodic contractions. Early in pregnancy these may be perceived as lower abdominal achelike or crampy discomfort if felt at all. Later in pregnancy these contraction may be perceived as a tightening of the uterus, often accompanied by the uterus pushing forward against the abdominal wall, making it appear to "stand up." Late in pregnancy, these contractions become more frequent, although they are still irregular (the Braxton-Hicks contractions of false labor). These irregular contractions eventually evolve into the rhythmic, productive contractions of true labor. The distinctions between Braxton-Hicks contractions and true labor are subtle and semantic. Often, the only difference between true and false labor is the outcome.

The pivotal role of the placenta in supporting the metabolic and waste removal needs of the growing fetus requires a significant diversion of maternal blood flow. Blood flow to and through the uterus increases progressively throughout pregnancy, reaching a peak of

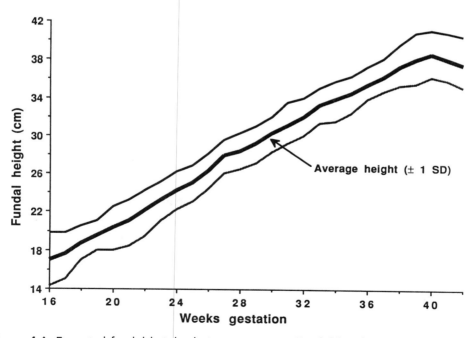

Figure 4.6. Expected fundal height during pregnancy. Fundal height, measured from symphysis to fundus with empty bladder, parallels gestation's age. Any significant change from this expected rate of growth suggests the possibility of a problem with the pregnancy, warranting investigation and possible consultation.

500 to 650 mL/min during late pregnancy. While blood freely bathes the placental tissues in the intervillous space, there is normally no direct mingling of blood between mother and baby. Perfusion of the intervillous space is dependent on many factors but broadly follows maternal blood pressure. Catacholamines, angiotensin II, the quality of venous return to the heart, and other factors all contribute to this dynamic process. This high-volume, low-resistance flow is offset by the increases in cardiac output and intravascular volume, allowing the maintenance of perfusion to other maternal organs.

Amniotic fluid provides a cushion against trauma for the developing fetus and acts as a heat sink to help maintain a stable temperature. The production of amniotic fluid begins early in gestation, reaching a volume of roughly 50 mL by the end of the first trimester. By 20 weeks gestation, this volume has increased to approximately 400 mL, reaching its peak of 1000 mL at 36 to 38 weeks of gestation. The increasing amount of amniotic fluid contributes significantly to the growth of the uterus and to maternal weight gain, accounting for roughly a kilogram of weight at the peak of fluid volume. When amniotic fluid levels are inadequate, physical deformities and developmental problems, such as club foot or pulmonary hypoplasia, may result.

The cervix undergoes softening and a change in blood flow that results in mild cyanosis, which may be an early physical sign of pregnancy (Chadwick's sign). The glands of the cervix undergo hypertrophy until late in pregnancy, when the glands occupy almost one half of the tissue of the cervix. Soon after conception, a thick plug of mucus blocks the cervical canal. This is expelled late in pregnancy or at the onset of labor; it is sometimes detected by the patient (the plug itself) or it is lost in the presence of a variable amount of vaginal bleeding (bloody show).

During pregnancy, the volume of vaginal secretions may increase slightly in response to the hormones present, although the consistency of these secretions is often thicker. The resulting increase in vaginal secretions may be distressing to the patient and must be distinguished from pathologic increases due to intercurrent infections. The pH of the vagina remains acidic (3.5 to 6).

ANTEPARTUM CARE

Initial Assessment

Often the first part of prenatal care is the diagnosis of pregnancy itself. Although there are many home urine pregnancy tests available, many couples prefer to have the diagnosis made or confirmed by the provider or hospital. Home pregnancy test kits are reliable, but they are slightly less sensitive than the office or hospital laboratory tests. As a result, patients may be assured that if their home test was positive, they are most likely pregnant. As with any test, a negative test, even when performed in the hospital laboratory, does not rule out the possibility of pregnancy. Many serum-based hospital tests can detect the presence of human chorionic gonadotrophin before the patient has missed her first period, although this type of testing is generally reserved for research or assisted fertility programs. For practical purposes, most patients should be advised to wait for a few days to a week after their anticipated menstrual period before testing is done. This will reduce the number of tests performed for women whose periods have only been delayed and will increase the likelihood of detecting an early pregnancy with a single test.

The initial assessment of the pregnant patient is the most comprehensive one. At the first encounter, all of the elements of a routine history and physical examination must be employed, augmented by those that are specific to the conduct of a safe and healthy pregnancy. Previous pregnancy experience and outcomes should be recorded. If not performed during prepregnant evaluations, social, demographic, occupational, and family risk factors should be determined. Baseline and screening laboratory tests should be ordered (Table 4.6), and the need for continuing follow-up reinforced.

The initial physical assessment of the pregnant patient should be thorough. It is directed toward detecting processes that may adversely affect the patient or pregnancy during gestation or those that themselves will be altered by the presence of the pregnancy. In addition to the normal procedures of a physical examination, clinical pelvimetry should be performed to determine the adequacy of the pelvis. Pelvic examination should also help establish or confirm the gestational age of the fetus. Discrepancies between uterine size and the last menstrual period should prompt an ultrasonographic evaluation of the health and age of the gestation.

The initial encounter also offers a chance to address educational and emotional needs of the patient. Nutritional counseling, discussions of sexually transmitted disease, high-risk behaviors, and parenting and employment skills, may all be included. These may be of par-

Table 4.6. Recommended Timing of Routine and Special Testing in Pregnancy

Time (wks)	Laboratory Blood	Cultures	Immunology	Imaging	Other*
Initial visit	Hemoglobin/ hematocrit Type & Rh	Chlamydia Gonorrhea Urine screen	Antibody screen Rubella titer Syphilis screen Hepatitis B screen HIV screen		Pap smear (if not done in past year) Hemoglobin electrophoresis Tuberculin skin testing
8–18	Maternal serum AFP or triple screen (MSAFP, βHCG, estriol)			Ultrasonography (for dates)	Amniocentesis/ chorionic villus sampling (based on maternal age) Amniotic fluid AFP (based on maternal AFP)
24–28	Diabetes screen Hemoglobin/ hematocrit		Repeat Rh screen (if Rh negative)		Prophylactic D immune globulin (unsensitized Rh negative patients)
32–36		Gonorrhea	Syphilis screen	Ultrasonography (dates and growth)	Hemoglobin/ hematocrit (if at risk for anemia)

*As needed or based on specific indications.
HIV = human immunodeficiency virus; MSAFP/AFP = maternal serum α-feto-protein; βHCG = beta subunit human chorionic gonadotropin.

ticular value for the first-time parent, the teenager, or the older patient, all of whom may have special needs or concerns.

Laboratory and Imaging

Most of the laboratory evaluation of the pregnant patient occurs at the time of the first prenatal visit (see Table 4.6). For most patients, follow-up laboratory assessments are carried out at about 24 to 28 weeks, and should include a measurement of hemoglobin or hematocrit, a screening test for diabetes, and, for Rh-negative mothers, a repeat test of antibody status, should be performed. At this stage of pregnance, unsensitized Rh-negative patients should receive prophylactic Rh immunoglobulin. Follow-up cultures, serologic tests, or other evaluations should be based on the individual needs of the patient.

The term sonography literally means "sound writing". Ultrasonography uses very short bursts of low energy, high frequency sound waves in the 2 to 9 MHz range to provide images of the interface between two tissues that transmit sound differently. At such an interface, some of the sound energy is reflected back toward the sound source. The returning sound waves are detected, with the distance from the sensor deduced using the elapsed time from transmission to reception. This information is displayed graphically as a cross-sectional view of the structure encountered by the beam.

Ultrasonography uses low energy sound waves and, therefore, is considered safe for use in pregnancy. Because of its reliance on subtle tissue differences to produce detectable echoes, ultrasonography is limited in its ability to distinguish some tissue planes. It is subject to interference from factors that absorb or reflect sound, such as bowel gas. Despite these limitations, ultrasonography is very good at most fetal assessments. Measures of fetal anatomy are frequently obtained to infer age and weight and to evaluate fetal structures such as heart, brain, spinal column, or kidneys. Fetal gender may often be guessed at an early age.

Improved resolution for visualizing intrauterine and adnexal structures may be obtained by the use of higher frequency sound and the placement of the ultrasound transducer inside the vagina, closer to the objects of interest. The higher frequencies of sound used for transvaginal imaging improve resolution, but limit the depth of penetration and consequently the applicability of transvaginal ultrasound to those structures located near the apex of the vagina. As a result, the greatest application of transvaginal ultrasonography is in gynecology, with obstetrical applications limited to the very earliest stages of pregnancy.

Another form of ultrasonography is Doppler ultrasound. Doppler evaluations use changes in the frequency of the reflected sound, not just the presence of the echo. These systems use this information to infer motion of the reflecting surface. This is useful in detecting fetal cardiac motion or assessing umbilical blood flow. A change in blood flow patterns in the umbilical vessels can be an indication of fetal stress, although these studies remain in the evaluation stage and are not yet ready for wide clinical application.

Nutrition and Weight Gain

An important aspect of prenatal care is the encouragement of adequate, balanced nutrition. This must focus on the quantity and quality of food ingested, as well as special needs caused by the pregnancy or other medical conditions, such as diabetes. For the most part, good general nutrition is good prenatal nutrition as well, with the recommended daily intake of most vitamins and mineral either unchanged or minimally changed by pregnancy. Only iron, folate, and vitamin D require significant adjustments. Other changes in the recommended diet necessitated by pregnancy are minimal as shown in Table 4.7.

Because the recommended daily intake of iron is not generally met by diet alone, daily supplementation with 30 mg ferrous iron is suggested. This may be accomplished using 150 mg ferrous sulfate, 300 mg ferrous gluconate, or 100 mg of ferrous fumarate. Taking this supplement between meals increases iron absorption.

Patients should be encouraged to eat four or more servings each of fruits and vegetables, grains, and milk or milk products. In addition, they should have three or more servings of proteins such as meat, fish, poultry, eggs, nuts, or beans. Pregnant patients should avoid uncooked meat because of the (slight) risk of toxoplasmosis. Pregnant women require roughly 15% more kilocalories per day (300 to 500 kcal) compared with their baseline needs.

As noted previously, a target weight gain of 25 to 30 lbs for the duration of pregnancy is best for most patients, with this target adjusted based on prepregnant weight, activity, medical condition, and other needs of the individual patient. If a patient has not gained about 10 lbs by midpregnancy, her overall nutritional status should be carefully evaluated and her fetus monitored closely for growth restriction. Rapid weight gain, especially late in pregnancy, should suggest the possibility of fluid storage and impending toxemia. These patients should be closely monitored for peripheral edema, proteinuria, and hypertension.

Exercise and Physical Activity

Most patients may, and should, maintain normal physical activities during pregnancy. Recreational and avocational activities that are not excessive or do not place the patient at

Table 4.7. Changes In Recommended Dietary Allowances Caused by Pregnancy and Lactation*

	Nonpregnant women[†]	Pregnant women	Lactating women
Energy (kcal)		+ 300–500	+ 500
Protein (g)	45–50	60	65
Vitamin E (mg TE)	8	10	12
Vitamin C (mg)	60	70	95
Vitamin D (μg)	5	10	10
Vitamin B_6 (mg)	1.5–1.6	2.2	2.1
Niacin (Mg NE)	15	17	20
Folate (μg)	180	400	280
Calcium (mg)	800–1200	1200	1200
Iron (mg)	15	30	15
Iodine (μg)	150	175	200
Zinc (mg)	12	15	19

*Based on: National Academy of Sciences: Recommended Dietary Allowances, 10th ed. Washington, DC: National Academy Press, 1989.
†Age 19–24.

physical risk, may be maintained by most pregnant women. Healthy patients may work until delivery. Strenuous activities, prolonged standing, or heavy lifting should be avoided, which occasionally may necessitate changing work assignments for part or all of pregnancy. Any activity should be discontinued if discomfort, significant shortness of breath, or pain in the chest or abdomen appears.

Smoking, Alcohol, and Drugs

Approximately one third of all women continue some level of alcohol consumption during their pregnancy. It is estimated that 7% to 10% of women seeking prenatal care are alcohol abusers. Somewhere between 19% and 30% of pregnant women continue to smoke during pregnancy despite the well-documented association between smoking and pregnancy complications, such as low birth weight, that has been heavily publicized in the lay press. Similarly, drug use and abuse, most notably cocaine, continues to be a major source of morbidity for both mother and fetus. Careful screening for the use of licit and illicit substance is important during the first prenatal visit and at subsequent visits. Support services should be made available and their use encouraged for any patient who is a substance user or abuser. A more complete discussion of the effects of alcohol and tobacco in pregnancy, along with suggestions for diagnostic and therapeutic intervention is contained in Chapter 11, Periodic Testing and Health Maintenance.

Continuing Care

Traditionally, prenatal visits for a normally progressing pregnancy have been scheduled every 4 weeks for the first 28 weeks, every 2 to 3 weeks until 36 weeks, and weekly thereafter. It has been suggested that this schedule may be relaxed for normal parous women; however, studies supporting this are lacking. In the absence of definitive studies, no specific guidelines seem forthcoming, although flexibility seems warranted to avoid scheduling during family vacations, holidays, and so forth. Patients who manifest abnormalities in any parameter of prenatal evaluations, at the very least, require more frequent evaluations or consultation to ensure the continuing health and safety of the mother and baby.

At each routine visit the patient should be questioned about any medical or psychosocial changes that may have taken place in the intervening period. Weight, blood pressure, fundal height, the presence and quality of fetal heart tones, and the presence of peripheral edema should be assessed at each visit and recorded on a prenatal flow chart, many of which are available from commercial sources and The American College of Obstetricians and Gynecologists. A flow-chart type of record makes it easier to detect trends and changes in blood pressure, weight, or fundal height that may suggest the development of problems.

During the later stages of pregnancy, the fetal presentation and position should be determined. Near the expected date of delivery, a copy of the prenatal record should be made available to the facility where delivery is planned; this record should be continuously updated until delivery is accomplished.

Traditionally, a screening evaluation of voided urine for protein and glucose has been included as a part of each routine visit. This practice has been questioned for its cost effectiveness. Certainly any patient at risk for diabetes, renal disease, hypertension, toxemia, or other condition detectable by this screening should be accorded it. This screening should be at the discretion of the care giver for other low-risk patients.

Pelvic examinations are generally performed only at the first prenatal visit and are not routinely repeated. Patients at risk for premature delivery or those with a history of in utero exposure to diethylstilbestrol (DES), may require frequent cervical evaluations. Any patient who reports significant uterine contractile activity should also have the status of her cervix evaluated prior to determining an appropriate disposition.

At every routine prenatal visit the patient or her family should be given an opportunity to discuss any questions they may have, to be counseled about health matters, to be alerted to warning signs that should be immediately reported, and to prepare the patient for the onset of labor and the process of delivery. The involvement of families in the prenatal evaluation process should be encouraged, but it should be tempered by the constraints of time and space imposed by the care setting.

Preparation for Childbirth

Childbirth education, in any number of forms, can have a beneficial impact on the conduct of labor and delivery. Ideally, preparation for childbirth should be an extension of education that continues throughout the course of the pregnancy. In late pregnancy, the focus of education should shift toward the recognition of labor, hospital, labor and delivery procedures, and techniques to aid the birth process. This should include warning signs and symptoms that require immediate attention (Table 4.8). Because many aspects of the labor and delivery suggestions are specific to the site of the eventual delivery, many primary care providers who do not perform deliveries choose to defer this part of the educational process to those who do so. Whether it is in the primary care setting or not, childbirth education should be encouraged.

Special Procedures or Considerations

Much of antenatal diagnosis is based on the ability to obtain fetal tissue or blood via amniocentesis or chorionic villus sampling. These procedures are often even beyond the scope of care given by general obstetricians, but the primary care provider should be familiar with what they entail and their strengths and shortcomings so that counseling and referral may be appropriately made.

As noted, amniocentesis or chorionic villus sampling are often carried out in patients over the age of 35 because of the increased incidence of genetic abnormalities in this age group. Because these tests carry a 0.5% to 0.8% risk of fetal loss, they are usually reserved

Table 4.8. Warning Signs and Symptoms Requiring Immediate Attention

Abdominal pain
Fever or chills
Fluid loss from the vagina
Marked changes in fetal activity
Painful urination (dysuria)
Persistent vomiting
Severe or continuous headache
Swelling of the face or fingers
Vaginal bleeding
Visual changes (dimness or blurring)

for patients whose risk of abnormality is greater than the risk of the procedure. Bleeding, infection, or fetal loss is infrequent, but possible, complications with either technique.

Amniocentesis

Amniocentesis is the percutaneous withdrawal of fluid from the amniotic sac. Fluid and cells obtained can be used for a variety of tests aimed at the assessment of fetal status or genetic make-up. Biochemical studies can indicate the presence of physiologic markers (e.g., Tay-Sachs disease) or the presence of substances indicating fetal abnormalities (e.g., alpha fetoprotein in neural tube defects or bilirubin in Rh incompatibility). Tissue culture of cells obtained by amniocentesis allows the genetic complement of the fetus to be studied.

In later pregnancy, amniocentesis is used to obtain fluid to assess fetal lung maturity. A number of tests allow the presence and efficacy of pulmonary surfactants to be evaluated. This indication of fetal lung readiness is extremely valuable in the management of premature labor or in the timing of delivery for patients with medical complications.

Chorionic Villus Sampling

Chorionic villus sampling is a technique used to obtain fetal tissue early in gestation (generally 9 to 12 weeks). This is accomplished using a small cannula passed through the cervix to aspirate villus cells under ultrasound guidance. Cells can also be acquired via transabdominal or transvaginal aspiration. The cells obtained are then cultured for genetic studies.

HINTS AND COMMON QUESTIONS

Pregnancy is a time of great expectation and worry. Many times, the areas that concern expectant patients can be anticipated and addressed in a positive, pre-emptive manner. Most patient concerns stem from the physiologic changes of pregnancy and can be resolved with information and reassurance. Arranged alphabetically below is a partial list of such issues.

Abdominal Pain

Low abdominal pain, especially in the groin early in the course of pregnancy, is frequently related to stretch of the round ligaments (round ligament pain). Tenderness over the inguinal ligament is confirmatory. This source of discomfort generally resolves later in pregnancy. When this type of pain is encountered late in pregnancy, other possible sources (e.g., urinary tract infections, muscle strains or pulls, hernias, and possible premature uterine activity) must all be considered. Pain elsewhere in the abdomen should be evaluated as appropriate for patients who are not pregnant.

Alcohol

The use of alcohol during pregnancy should be discouraged. Although fetal alcohol syndrome is generally not seen with ingestion rates of less than 1 oz of alcohol per day, there does not seem to be a safe threshold below which alcohol consumption is completely safe. Occasional use, such as a glass of wine on an anniversary, is acceptable; however, as with most things, the less the better.

Automobile Passenger Restraints

The use of lap and shoulder restraints should be strongly encouraged for all patients, even those who are pregnant. The greatest injuries arise when a pregnant women is not restrained during an automobile accident, not from damage caused by the restraints. Indeed, the most common cause of fetal death in automobile accidents is the death of the mother. Lap belts should be worn low; over the hips and shoulder restraints should rest comfortably between the breasts. The use of approved infant seats to transport the newborn home and for all subsequent travel must also be supported in the strongest terms.

Backache

As the uterus grows, the center of gravity of the patient moves progressively upward and outward. To counteract the tendency to fall forward that this would normally cause, women adopt a characteristic pelvis-forward, "duck waddle." This posture places increased strain on the muscles, ligaments, and joints of the low back and hips, resulting in chronic backache. Some relief is gained when the fetus descends into the pelvis in the last days of the gestation, but the sudden return to upright and the constant bending of caring for the newborn make this improvement short-lived.

The backache of pregnancy may be reduced through the use of low back support, good posture, sensible shoes, and muscle-strengthening exercises, such as the pelvic tilt. (If the latter is used, it must not be performed in the supine position late in pregnancy or by women whose activities must be restricted.) A maternity girdle or slacks that are a bit tight may help. Where possible, elevating legs while sitting or slightly raising one leg while standing will result in flattening of the low back, easing strain. Massage, heat, and analgesics can be used to relieve the symptoms when they occur.

Bathing

Patients frequently ask about the use of tub baths during pregnancy. They may be used safely throughout pregnancy without restriction. Care in entering and exiting the tub should be encouraged to avoid falls, which occur more frequently owing to the woman's altered center of gravity and partially obstructed view of the floor in late pregnancy. There is no evidence that bath water enters the vagina under normal bathing practices.

Bleeding Gums

Hyperemia and softening of the gums is common during pregnancy. As a result, bleeding from mild trauma, such as toothbrushing, is common and not a cause for concern. When in doubt, consultation with the patient's dentist is appropriate.

Breast Changes

Often one of the first signs of pregnancy is a tingling sensation in the breasts, tenderness, and increased breast size. By the second month of pregnancy, hypertrophy of the alveoli results in a nodular texture to the breast tissue. Increased vascular patterns become visible on the skin and striae may appear as the pregnancy enters the third trimester. In addition to darkening, the areola and nipples become larger and more erectile. By the middle of gestation, straw colored, thick fluid (colostrum) may be expressed from the nipple. Hypertroph of sebaceous gland in the periphery of the areola results in increased prominence of Montgomery's glands.

Breast enlargement during gestation is frequently sufficient to require a change in bra size. When this happens, patients should be counseled to keep their old bras, as the breasts generally return to close to their prepregnancy size after delivery.

Breast Feeding

There are many reasons to encourage breast feeding and, with help, almost all patients can enjoy some measure of success. Despite this, some women cannot or will not be successful; their decision to abandon nursing or to use bottles from the onset, should be supported and they should not be made to feel they are "second class mothers."

Women who wish to try nursing may be encouraged to toughen the nipples prior to delivery, although studies suggest that this is not necessary for successful nursing. Toughening is most easily accomplished by exposing the breasts to the air and gentle stimulation from clothing or a dry wash cloth. If the latter is used, gentle circular massage of the nipple and areola nightly is all that is required. Vigorous rubbing or the use of more abrasive materials is neither necessary nor productive. Soap and drying agents may cause cracking of the nipples; they should be washed using only water.

The expression of colostrum from the breast prior to delivery is not necessary to induce milk production or to prepare the breast for successful nursing. Some authors argue that the loss of the antibody-rich colostrum may even be detrimental to the long-term health benefits derived from nursing. In the absence of a consensus, expressing milk or colostrum prior to delivery should be an individual choice.

Colds and "Flu"

Viral illnesses tend to have stronger symptoms and last longer during pregnancy. Fluids, rest, fruit juices, and mild symptomatic treatments (e.g., acetaminophen, salt-water gargles, and throat sprays) are safe and should be encouraged. When used in moderation, most over-the-counter cough and cold preparations are safe, but the patient should check with the health care team before using them.

Some studies suggest that increasing the daily intake of vitamin C may reduce the severity and duration of upper respiratory infections. This may be advised, within reason.

Constipation

Constipation is common throughout pregnancy. Decreased intestinal motility begins the process and the iatrogenic effects of iron therapy often make it worse. Encouraging dietary measures, such as fiber and fluids, forms the first line of therapy, with stool softeners and enemas reserved for difficult cases. Laxatives should be avoided owing to the moderate likelihood of habituation.

Dental Care

Routine dental care should be encouraged for all pregnant patients. Dental x-ray studies may be performed with appropriate abdominal shielding. If medications, such as antibiotics, are to be prescribed, the dentist or hygienist should be made aware of the pregnancy so that the medications are chosen accordingly. There is no evidence that pregnancy increases the likelihood of tooth decay.

Diastasis Recti

Separation of the rectus muscles in the midline is a not infrequent occurrence during pregnancy. When this separation is small, it may only be detected by noting a slight bulge when the patient tenses the abdominal wall while in the supine position (as when attempting to lift her head). In extreme cases, separation of the muscles results in the fundus of the uterus being covered only by skin, attenuated fascias, and peritoneum, in much the same manner as a hernia sac. A maternity girdle or other support may reduce the symptoms of this diastasis, which generally resolves spontaneously after the infant is delivered.

Drugs and Medications

The patient should be advised to avoid all unnecessary medication, prescription or over-the-counter, during pregnancy. When in doubt, the patient should check with the health care team for specific advice. The common use of nonprescription medications makes reinforcing this admonition advisable. A list of common drugs that have serious consequences when used in pregnancy is shown in Table 4.9.

Table 4.9. Common Drugs Contraindicated During Pregnancy*

Agent	Risk
Androgenic hormones	Clitoral enlargement if used before 13 weeks.
Anticoagulants (warfarin, coumarin)	Major and minor malformations in 25% of fetuses exposed in first trimester.
Antithyroid drugs (propylthiouracil, methimazole, iodide)	Fetal hypothyroidism. Methimazole may produce fetal scalp defects.
Anticonvulsants (diphenylhydantoin, trimethadione, paramethadione, carbamazepine)	Abnormal facies, cleft lip or palate, microcephaly, growth deficiency, congenital heart disease, and mental retardation in 10% to 30% of exposed fetuses. With trimethadione or paramethadione, spontaneous abortion rate ~ 60% to 80%. Carbamazepine carries a 1% risk of spina bifida.
Diethylstilbestrol	Vaginal adenosis found in 50% of females exposed in utero prior to the ninth week of gestation. Genitourinary tract abnormalities in 25% of males exposed in utero.
Lithium	Malformation in 5% to 10% of exposed offspring; usually heart and great vessels.
Vitamin A & congeners	
High-dose Vitamin A	Risk at >25,000 IU/d, malformation at >40,000 IU/d.
Etretinate	Detectable for up to 2 years after use, with malformation reported up to 18 months after use. Congenital abnormalities similar to Isotretinoin.
Isotretinoin	Major malformations in 35% of exposed fetuses.

*This is a representative listing only; the safety of any drug should be ascertained before it is used in pregnancy.

Fatigue

Fatigue is common, especially during the early and late phases of gestation. The cause of this fatigue in the first few weeks is uncertain, but its impact can be profound. Toward the end of pregnancy, the mechanical effort of carrying the added weight of the pregnancy may add to other hormonal factors to cause this chronic tiredness. Except in unusual cases, this is normal and carries no prognostic significance. No special tests or therapies beyond rest and reassurance are indicated.

Fainting (syncope)

Venous pooling when standing or compression of the vena cava by the enlarging uterus, may both lead to fainting. Support stockings and exercising the calf muscles to promote venous return, and avoiding the supine position (late in pregnancy) help reduce this risk.

Haircare and Hair Loss

Many patients will ask about the safety of hair coloring or permanent wave treatments during pregnancy. There is evidence that the chemicals used are absorbed through the skin and pose a theoretic risk, although it is minimal. As a result, occasional use of these products is probably safe, but excessive use should be discouraged. Normal shampoos and rinses can be used without restriction.

Often in the early stages of pregnancy or in the immediate postpartum period, patients experience hair loss. For some, this may be of sufficient volume to cause concern or cosmetic problems. Accelerated hair loss of this type may come about anytime there is an abrupt change in hormonal patterns and is the result of a higher number of hair follicles entering into the resting, or telogen, phase of hair growth. Hair follicles follow a cycle: growth (anagen), a resting phase (telogen) of 3 to 9 months, and resumption of normal growth. Alterations in hormones may induce an increased number of follicles to enter telogen. If this is the situation, the lost hair will be regained in time. To tell the difference between this type of loss and loss due to pathologic processes, examine the base of a few lost hair shafts. If the shaft is smooth, it came from natural (telogen) loss; if the base has the follicular bulb still attached (a white swelling at the end), the loss may be due to dermatologic or other disease conditions and consultation is suggested.

Heartburn

Increased acid production, a relaxation of the cardiac (esophageal) sphincter under hormonal influence, and a decreased rate of gastric emptying, result in the common complaint of heartburn and excessive gas. Patients should be encouraged to avoid large meals before bedtime, use a bed wedge or extra pillows and antacids as needed. Antacids that coat (liquids) and those that tend to float on the surface of the stomach contents, such as Gaviscon, provide better heartburn relief than other agents.

Hemorrhoids

Hemorrhoids are an occupational hazard of pregnancy. Increased pelvic congestion and a laxity of connective tissues result in vericosities of vessels. In the perineum, this takes the form of hemorrhoids. The tendency toward constipation, which is also a part of pregnancy, further aggravates this dilatation of the hemorrhoidal vessels. Topical therapy with over-the-counter or prescription medications, sitz baths, and maintenace of bowel regularity will all be of some help. Hemorrhoids symptoms usually improve after delivery, although some degree of persistence is common.

Immunizations

Many immunizations can be carried out during pregnancy (Table 4.10). Most live, attenuated virus vaccines are contraindicated. Patients who are immunized against rubella (a live virus vaccine) should be advised not to conceive within 3 months, although no adverse outcomes have been reported thus far in pregnancies that have been exposed to the vaccine. Measles, mumps, and rubella vaccines can be safely given to other members of the family without risk to the pregnant mother. There appears to be no risk associated with the use of inactivated virus vaccines, bacterial vaccines, toxoids, or tetanus immunoglobulin; they may be used as indicated.

Leg Cramps

Leg cramps are common in the second and third trimester of pregnancy, with a predilection for evenings and nights. Debate over a role for altered calcium levels or calcium metabolism has not resolved either the cause or best prophylaxis. Massage, heat, and analgesics when needed are the best management available.

Table 4.10. Recommendations Regarding Immunization and Prophylaxis During Pregnancy

Contraindicated
    Measles
    Mumps
    Rubella
Not recommended
    Poliomyelitis
    Typhoid
    Yellow fever
Unchanged by pregnancy
    Pneumococcus
    Tetanus-diphtheria
Based on travel or high risk
    Cholera
    Hepatitis B
    Influenza
    Plague
Prophylaxis
    Hepatitis A
    Hepatitis B
    Measles
    Rabies
    Tetanus
    Varicella (within 96 h)

Morning Sickness

Nausea or vomiting in early pregnancy is common, but highly variable. Not every patient will have it, not every pregnancy will produce it for a given patient, and it varies from mild queasiness to all-day misery. Symptoms generally begin between the fourth and eight week, lasting until 16 weeks or longer. The initial treatment is nonpharmacologic, consisting of small, frequent feedings with bland foods (crackers, toast, and so forth). Spicy or greasy foods should be avoided; some advocate a protein snack at bedtime. Medical therapy with vitamin B_6, antiemetics, or intravenous hydration should be reserved for patients who do not respond to simple support. If the symptoms are excessive, the possibility of an abnormality of pregnancy (trophoblastic disease, multiple gestation) or psychological overlay should be considered.

Painting and Redecoration

Patients frequently ask if they may paint or be around paint fumes during pregnancy. Patients should be counseled that the only precautions necessary are those that would be appropriate for anyone, pregnant or not: avoid prolonged exposure and maintain adequate ventilation. Similarly, there are no special restrictions for wallpapering, furniture staining, or most other activities. Patients should be warned about the risks accompanying most redecoration projects, such as falls and injury from certain tools.

Round Ligament Pain

Sharp groin pains, more frequent on the right than the left, and more abundant in primiparous patients, are common from the late first trimester onward. They are the results of stretch and spasms in the round ligament as it increases in length to reach the enlarging uterus. These pains will be noted most often after activity or late in the day. They respond well to rest, heat, and the occasional use of analgesics. If the pains are persistent, a maternity girdle or clothing that provides some additional support for the lower abdomen will reduce the frequency and severity of symptoms.

Sexuality

Common during pregnancy are concerns about sexuality and sexual activity. For almost all patients, there should be no restriction on normal sexual activities. The mechanics of the enlarging uterus and changes in body image, for both partners, result in changes in desire and comfort, resulting in altered coital frequency and the use of different forms of sexual expression. Cuddling, holding, and caressing become more common forms of sexual expression as the pregnancy nears term. As long as the couple is comfortable with the activity or sexual position, there is little risk of harm.

Many women notice some uterine contractions after intercourse. The source of these contractions is debated, but their presence is not. Except for the rare patient with a history of recurrent premature labors, these contractions are of no significance and can be ignored.

Skin Changes

Because of a strong degree of homology between human chorionic gonadotropin and melanocyte stimulating hormone (MSH) combined with a slight rise in MSH level itself, many pregnancy women will experience a darkening of their nipples, the formation of a brownish-black midline abdominal streak (linea nigra), and irregular dark patches on the face and neck (chloasma, melasma gravidarum, mask of pregnancy). These changes will regress significantly or disappear after delivery.

The growing fetus generates a great deal of metabolic heat that must be dissipated by the maternal circulation. As a result, during pregnancy there is an increase in cutaneous blood flow to the forearms, thighs, chest, and face. This increased blood flow and the rosy color it imparts to fair-skinned women is partly responsible for the "glow of pregnancy."

Small vascular angiomas (spider nevi) develop in two thirds of white women and one tenth of black women. These small, red, raised lesions have radiating radicles that blanch if compressed with a microscope slide. Roughly two thirds of white women and one third of black women also develop palmar erythema. Both of these conditions are not clinically significant and are thought to arise from the high levels of estrogen present during pregnancy.

Stretch Marks

About half of pregnant women develop reddish, slightly depressed streaks in the skin of the abdomen, breasts, or thighs. These become silvery, glistening striae that persist indefinitely after the end of the pregnancy. Many patients use skin creams, softeners, or vitamin preparations to try to prevent the formation of these striae. While there is little harm in the use of most of these preparations, there are few data to suggest significant benefit. Recommendation and use should be at the discretion of the provider and patient.

Swelling

Increased sodium and water retention is a normal part of pregnancy. When complicated by the pressure on the vena cava from the enlarging uterus, this retention results in an increased incidence of dependent edema, which worsens as the pregnancy progresses. Pitting edema of the ankles and feet is seen in a large proportion of pregnant patients as they near term. Reassurance and elevation of dependent extremities, when feasible, are the only therapies that are appropriate. Diuretics should not be used.

Travel

At some point in pregnancy, almost all patients ask about travel restrictions. For patients without special risks, no restrictions need be made. Patients will find that they fatigue more quickly and have a markedly diminished bladder capacity, making more frequent stops both desirable and necessary. Air travel by commercial carrier is safe at any stage of pregnancy, however, most carriers discourage long flights in the late stages of pregnancy to avoid the slight chance of an unanticipated midair birth. Because of the increased risk of venous stasis, prolonged sitting during travel by any mode should be avoided. Patients traveling far from home late in pregnancy should consider carrying a copy of their prenatal record to facilitate care should it be required.

Sometimes the reason for the question is a desire not to travel. The physical exertion of travel, the emotional stresses of late pregnancy and a family gathering, and some individual trepidation about travel often result in the patient hoping that the provider will supply a convenient excuse to avoid the obligation. ("Gee, Aunt Ethel, we would love to come for the holidays, but my doctor won't let me. . . . ") Sensitivity to this possibility is appropriate, with the best response based on the individual needs of the patient and the personal preferences of the health care provider.

Urinary Changes

Increasing pressure by the growing uterus early in pregnancy causes decreased bladder capacity, resulting in frequency and urgency. As the uterus rises out of the pelvis this improves, only to worsen again at the end of pregnancy when the presenting part again impinges on the back of the bladder. The urine may be more concentrated during pregnancy, resulting in a darker color and more intense odor, which are normal, and the patient may be reassured. Pain with urination suggests the possibility of infection and should be investigated by urinalysis or culture.

Vaginal Discharge

The high hormones of pregnancy cause a noticeable change in vaginal discharge. Cervical mucus, which makes up a large part of the liquid phase of the secretions, becomes thick and viscous early in pregnancy. Toward the end of pregnancy, there is an increase in vaginal wetness that may be particularly distressing in hot, humid weather. If the discharge reported by the patient is clear and nonirritating, it is probably physiologic and reassurance is in order. Anytime there is doubt, the vaginal secretions should be examined to assess the possibility of an intercurrent vaginal infection. (See Chapter 28, Vulvitis and Vaginal Infections.)

Varicose Veins

Venous stasis, increasing pressure on the inferior vena cava and pelvic veins, and a loss of connective tissue elasticity significantly increase the risk of developing varicose veins during pregnancy. Wearing support stockings, limiting unnecessary standing, periodic exercising of calf muscles, and elevating the legs, when practical, may all help to reduce this risk.

Vision Changes

Owing to changes in corneal thickness and intraocular pressure, pregnant patients who use corrective eye wear may notice a change in their visual acuity or prescription during pregnancy. This will often regress after delivery. Therefore, minor changes in visual acuity should be tolerated to avoid the necessity of re-refraction after delivery.

Work During Pregnancy

As with travel, there are few medical reasons to restrict work-related activities during normal pregnancies. The mechanical changes that occur owing to postural alterations and increased laxity of the joints suggest limiting certain activities, such as heavy lifting or those that require good balance, near the end of pregnancy. Exposure to harmful or dangerous activities or substances ideally should be evaluated and limited before the pregnancy begins.

The extent to which employers may provide this type of safety has been limited somewhat by recent court decisions, but the patient can request reassignment on an individual basis. Intervention by the health care team can help facilitate this form of risk reduction. Most authors suggest that keeping the patient active in her work provides benefits, both economic and physical, that transcend any theoretic risks. Patients with a history of vaginal bleeding, an incompetent cervix, uterine malformation associated with fetal loss, pregnancy-induced hypertension, abnormalities of fetal growth, preterm deliveries, maternal illness, or multifetal gestations may require limitation or curtailment of work obligations.

At one time, a 6-week postpartum recovery period was standard and accepted by most employers. Changing practices, insurance, and economic pressures have all resulted in shorter and shorter postpartal leaves. From the medical standpoint, a gradual return to work beginning in 2 to 3 weeks is not dangerous, but should be governed by the overall health of the mother, the type of delivery, and her postdelivery course. This should be individualized, taking into account the occupation of the patient and her specific needs. A good general guide is the amount of lochia present. If the lochia increases, the patient is probably overdoing activities (work or otherwise) and should cut back; if the lochia is average and decreasing, activity may continue and be increased gradually.

X-rays

Diagnostic radiologic studies may be performed during pregnancy based on need. Elective imaging should be delayed until the completion of pregnancy; semielective studies should be delayed until the second half of gestation; and urgent or emergent imaging should be performed as needed, without regard to gestational age. For most radiologic studies, there is very little risk to the developing fetus. In the earliest stages of pregnancy, moderate to large dose x-ray exposure carries an all or nothing impact, resulting in pregnancy loss or no effect at all.

SUGGESTED READINGS

General References

American Academy of Pediatrics, American College of Obstetricians and Gynecologists. Guidelines for Prenatal Care, 3rd ed. Elk Grove Village, Illinois:AAP. Washington, DC:ACOG, 1992.

American College of Obstetricians and Gynecologists. Immunization during pregnancy. ACOG Technical Bulletin 160. Washington, DC:ACOG, 1991.

American College of Obstetricians and Gynecologists. Nutrition during pregnancy. ACOG Technical Bulletin 179. Washington, DC:ACOG, 1993.

American College of Obstetricians and Gynecologists. Exercise during pregnancy and the postpartum period. ACOG Technical Bulletin 189. Washington, DC:ACOG, 1994.

American College of Obstetricians and Gynecologists. Preconceptional care. ACOG Technical Bulletin 205. Washington, DC:ACOG, 1994.

Caring for Our Future: The Content of Prenatal Care. Public Health Service Expert Panel Report. Washington, DC:PHS-DHHS, 1989.

Everson GT, McKinley C, Kern F JR. Mechanisms of gallstone formation in women. J Clin Invest 1991;87:237.

Hook EB, Cross PK, Schreinemachers DM. Chromosomal abnormality rates at amniocentesis and in live-born infants. JAMA 1983;249:2034.

Hook EB. Rates of chromosomal abnormalities at different maternal ages. Obstet Gynecol 1981;58:282.

Johnson TRB, Walker MA, Niebyl JR. Preconception and prenatal care. In Gabbe SG, Niebyl JR, Simpson JL (eds.) Obstetrics: Normal & Problem Pregnancies. New York:Churchill Livingstone, 1991, p 209.

New York State Department of Health, AIDS Institute. Clinical guidelines for the use of zidovudine therapy in pregnancy to reduce perinatal transmission of HIV. October 1994.

Prenatal care. In: Cunningham FG, MacDonald PC, Gant NF, Leneno KJ, Gilstrap LC III (eds.) Williams Obstetrics, 19th ed. Norwalk, Connecticut: Appleton & Lange, 1993, p 247.

Specific References

Genetic Counseling, Risk Assessment

American College of Obstetricians and Gynecologists. Alpha-fetoprotein. ACOG Technical Bulletin 154. Washington, DC:ACOG, 1991.

Burton BK, Prins GS, Verp MS. A prospective trial of prenatal screening for Down Syndrome by means of maternal serum alpha-fetoprotein, human chorionic gonadotropin, and unconjugated estriol. Am J Obstet Gynecol 1993;169:526.

Canadian Collaborative CVS-Amniocentesis Clinical Trial Group. Multicenter randomised clinical trial of chorion villus sampling and amniocentesis. Lancet 1989;1:1.

Cheng EY, Luthy DA, Zebelman AM, Williams MA, Lieppman RE, Hickok DE. A prospective evaluation of a second-trimester screening test for fetal Down syndrome using maternal serum alpha-fetoprotein, hCG, and unconjugated estriol. Obstet Gynecol 1993;81:72.

Crandall BF, Hanson FW, Keener S, Matsumoto M, Miller W. Maternal serum screening for alpha-fetoprotein, unconjugated estriol, and human chorionic gonadotropin between 11 and 15 weeks of pregnancy to detect fetal chromosomal abnormalities. Am J Obstet Gynecol 1993;168:1864.

Firth HV, Boyd PA, Chamberlain P, MacKinzie IZ, Lindenbaum RH, Huson SM. Severe limb abnormalities after chorion villus sampling at 56–66 days' gestation. Lancet 1991;337:762.

Foster UG, Baird PA. Limb reduction defects and chorionic villus sampling. Lancet 1993;328:114.

Jackson LG, Zachary JM. Prenatal diagnosis. N Engl J Med 1993;328:114.

Ledbetter DH, Martin AO, Verlinsky Y, et al. Cytogenetic results of chorionic villus sampling: high success rate and diagnostic accuracy in the United States collaborative study. Am J Obstet Gynecol 1990;162:495.

Serdula M, Williamson DF, Kendrick JS, Anda RF, Byers T. Trends in alcohol consumption by pregnant women: 1985 through 1989. JAMA 1991;265:876.

Teitelman AM, Welch LS, Hellenbrand KG, Bracken MB. Effect of maternal work activity on preterm birth and low birth-weight. Am J Epidemiol 1990;131:104.

Physiologic Changes

Aboul-Khair SA, Crooks J, Turnbull AC, Hytten FE. The physiological changes in thyroid function during pregnancy. Clin Sci 1964;27:195.

Assali NS, Douglass RA, Baird WW, Nicholson DB, Suyemoto R. Measurement of uterine blood flow and uterine metabolism. IV. Results in normal pregnancy. Am J Obstet Gynecol 1960;79:86.

Bender HS, Chickering WR. Minireview: Pregnancy and diabetes: The maternal response. Life Sci 1985;37:1.

Bolton FG, Street MJ, Pace AJ. Changes in erythrocyte volume and shape in pregnancy. Br J Obstet Gynaecol 1982;89:1018.

Braverman DZ, Johnson ML, Kern F JR. Effects of pregnancy and contraceptive steroids on gallbladder function. N Engl J Med 1980;302:362.

Brown MA, Gallery EDM, Ross MR, Esber RP. Sodium excretion in normal and hypertensive pregnancy: a prospective study. Am J Obstet Gynecol 1988;159:297.

Burt RL, Davidson IWF. Insulin half-life and utilization in normal pregnancy. Obstet Gynecol 1974;43:161.

Carter J. Serum bile acids in normal pregnancy. Br J Obstet Gynecol 1991;98:540.

Cohen S. The sluggish gallbladder of pregnancy. N Engl J Med 1980;302:397.

Cutforth R, MacDonald CB. Heart sounds and murmurs in pregnancy. Am Heart J 1966;71:741.

Darmady JM, Postle AD. Lipid metabolism in pregnancy. Br J Obstet Gynaecol 1982;89:211.

Davison JM, Hytten FE. Glomerular filtration during and after pregnancy. Br J Obstet Gynaecol 1974;81:588.

Dennis KJ, Bytheway WR. Changes in the body weight after delivery. Br J Obstet Gynaecol 1965;72:94.

Easterling TR, Schmucker BC, Benedetti TJ. The hemodynamic effects of orthostatic stress during pregnancy. Obstet Gynecol 1988;72:550.

Ezimokhai M, Davison JM, Philips PR, Dunlop W. Non-postural serial changes in renal function during the third trimester of normal human pregnancy. Br J Obstet Gynaecol 1981;88:465.

Glinoer D, DeNayer P, Bourdoux P, et al. Regulation of maternal thyroid during pregnancy. J Clin Endocrinol Metab 1990;71:276.

Gonzalez JG, Elizondon G, Saldivar D, Nanez H, Todd LE, Villarreal JZ. Pituitary gland growth during normal pregnancy: an in vivo study using magnetic resonance imaging. Am J Med 1988;85:217.

Howard BK, Goodson JH, Mengert WF. Supine hypotensive syndrome in late pregnancy. Obstet Gynecol 1953; 1:371.

Iosif S, Ingemarsson I, Ulmsten U. Urodynamic studies in normal pregnancy and the puerperium. Am J Obstet Gynecol 1980;137:696.

Kennedy RL, Darne J. The role of hCG in regulation of the thyroid gland in normal and abnormal pregnancy. Obstet Gynecol 1991;78:298.

Kletzky OA, Rossman F, Bertolli SI, Platt LD, Mischell DR. Dynamics of human chorionic gonadotropin, prolactin and growth hormone in serum and amniotic fluid throughout normal human pregnancy. Am J Obstet Gynecol 1985;151:878.

Levy RP, Newman DM, Rejali LS, Barford DAG. The myth of goiter in pregnancy. Am J Obstet Gynecol 1980;137:701.

Lind T. Metabolic changes in pregnancy relavent to diabetes mellitus. Postgrad Med J 1979;55:353.

Macfie AG, Magides AP, Richmond MN, Reilly CS. Gastric empyting in pregnancy. Br J Anaesth 1991;67:54.

Metcalfe J, Romney SL, Ramsey LH, Reid DE, Burwell CS. Estimation of uterine blood flow during late pregnancy. J Clin Invest 1957;34:1632.

Milne JS, Howie AD, Pack AI. Dyspnea during normal pregnancy. Br J Obstet Gynaecol 1978;85:260.

Peake SL, Roxburgh HB, Langlois SLP. Ultrasonic assessment of hydronephrosis of pregnancy. Radiology 1983;146:167.

Pipe NGJ, Smith T, Halliday D, Edmonds CJ, Williams C, Coltart TM. Changes in fat, fat free mass and body water in human normal pregnancy. Br J Obstet Gynaecol 1979;86:929.

Pitkin RM, Reynolds WA, Williams GA, Hargis GK. Calcium metabolism in pregnancy: a longitudinal study. Am J Obstet Gynecol 1985;151:99.

Pritchard JA. Changes in the blood volume during pregnancy and delivery. Anesthesiology 1965;26:393.

Scheithauer BW, Sano T, Kovacs KT, Young WF JR, Ryan N, Randah RV. The pituitary gland in pregnancy: a clinicopathologic and immunohistochemical study of 69 cases. Mayo Clin Proc 1990;65:461.

Scholl T, Hediger M, Schall J, et al. Gestational weight gain, pregnancy outcome, and postpartum weight retention. Obstet Gynecol 1995;86:423.

Song CS, Kappas A. The influence of estrogens, progestins and pregnancy on the liver. Vitam Horm 1968;26:147.

Sunness JS. The pregnant woman's eye. Surv Ophthalmol 1988;32:219.

Ueland K, Metcalfe J. Circulatory changes in pregnancy. Clin Obstet Gynecol 1975;18:41.

Health Maintenance, Prevention and Screening

American College of Obstetricians and Gynecologists. Cocaine in pregnancy. ACOG Committee Opinion 114. Washington, DC:ACOG, 1992.

American College of Obstetricians and Gynecologists. Prevention of D isoimmunization. ACOG Technical Bulletin 147. Washington, DC:ACOG, 1990.

American College of Obstetricians and Gynecologists. Automobile passenger restraints for children and pregnant women. ACOG Technical Bulletin 151. Washington, DC:ACOG, 1991.

American College of Obstetricians and Gynecologists. Group B Streptococcal infections in pregnancy. ACOG Technical Bulletin 170. Washington, DC:ACOG, 1992.

American College of Obstetricians and Gynecologists. Rubella and pregnancy. ACOG Technical Bulletin 171. Washington, DC:ACOG, 1992.

American College of Obstetricians and Gynecologists. Hepatitis in pregnancy. ACOG Technical Bulletin 174. Washington, DC:ACOG, 1992.

American College of Obstetricians and Gynecologists. Substance abuse in pregnancy. ACOG Technical Bulletin 195. Washington, DC:ACOG, 1994.

Ayoola EA, Johnson AOD. Hepatitis B vaccine in pregnancy: immunogenicity, safety and transfer of antibodies to infants. Int J Gynaecol Obstet 1987;25:297.

British Medical Research Council Vitamin Study Research Group. Prevention of neural tube defects: results of the medical research council vitamin-study. Lancet 1991;338:131.

Calvert JP, Crean EE, Newcombe RG, Pearson JF. Antenatal screening of measurement of symphysis-fundis height. Br Med J 1982;285:846.

Centers for Disease Control and Prevention. Use of folic acid for prevention of spina bifida and other neural tube defects 1983–1991. MMWR 1991;40:513.

Centers for Disease Control and Prevention. Recommendations for the use of folic acid to reduce the number of cases of spina bifida and other neural tube defects. MMWR 1992;41:1.

Colmorgan GHC, Johnson C, Zazzarino MA, Durinzi K. Routine urine drug screening at the first prenatal visit. Am J Obstet Gynecol 1987;166:588.

Connor EM, Sperling RS, Gelber R, et al. Reduction of maternal-infant transmission of human immunodeficiency virus type 1 with zidovudine treatment. N Engl J Med 1994;331:1173.

Czeizel AE, Dudas I. Prevention of the first occurrence of neural-tube defects by periconceptional vitamin supplementation. N Engl J Med 1992;327:1832.

Dawes MC, Green J, Ashurst H. Routine weighing in pregnancy. Br Med J 1992;304:487.

Ernhart CB, Sokil RJ, Martier S, et al. Alcohol teratogenicity in the human: a detailed assessment of specificity, critical period, and threshold. Am J Obstet Gynecol 1987;156:33.

Ewigman BG, Crane JP, Frigoletto FD, LeFevre ML, Bain RP, McNellis D. Effect of prenatal ultrasound screening on prenatal outcome: RADIUS study group. N Engl J Med 1993;329:821.

Foulon W, Naessens A, Lauwers S, De Meuter F, Amy JJ. Impact of primary prevention on the incidence of toxoplasmosis during pregnancy. Obstet Gynecol 1988;72:363.

Gibbs RS, McDuffie RS JR, McNabb F, Fryer G, Miyoshi T, Merestein G. Neonatal group B streptococcal sepsis during 2 years of a universal screening program. Obstet Gynecol 1994;84:496.

Gillogley KM, Evans AT, Hansen RL, Samuels SJ, Batra KK. The perinatal impact of cocaine, amphetamine, and opiate use detected by universal intrapartum screening. Am J Obstet Gynecol 1990;163:1535.

Institute of Medicine, Subcommittee of Nutritional Status and Weight Gain during Pregnancy. Nutrition during pregnancy. Washington, DC:National Academy Press, 1990.

Kitchens JM. Does this patient have an alcohol problem? JAMA 1994;272:1782.

Little BB, Snell LM, Klein VR, Gilstrap LC. Cocaine abuse during pregnancy: maternal and fetal implications. Obstet Gynecol 1989;73:157.

Mamelle N, Laumon B, Lazar P. Prematurity and occupational activity during pregnancy. Am J Epidemiol 1984;119:309.

Mills JL, Knopp RH, Simpson JL, et al. Lack of relation of increased malformation rates in infants of diabetic mothers to glycemic control during organogenesis. N Eng J Med 1988;318:671.

Mills JL, Rhoads GG, Simpson JL, et al. The absence of a relation between the periconceptional use of vitamins and neural-tube defects. N Engl J Med 1989;321:430.

Milunsky A, Jick H, Jick S, et al. Multivitamin/folic acid supplementation in early pregnancy reduces the prevalence of neural tube defects. JAMA 1989;262:2847.

Minkoff HL, Henderson C, Mendez H. Pregnancy outcomes among mothers infected with human immunodeficiency virus and uninfected control subjects. Am J Obstet Gynecol 1990;163:1598.

MRC Vitamin Study Research Group. Prevention of neural tube defects: results of the Medical Research Council Vitamin Study. Lancet 1991;338:131.

Mueller-Heubach E, Buzik DS. Evaluation of risk scoring in a preterm birth prevention study of indigent patients. Obstet Gynecol 1989;160:829.

Mulinare J, Cordero JF, Erickson JD, Berry RJ. Periconceptional use of mulitvitamins and the occurrence of neural tube defects. JAMA 1988;260:3141.

National Academy of Sciences. Recommended Dietary Allowances, 10th ed. Washington, DC:National Academy Press, 1989.

Pastorek JG. Hepatitis in pregnancy. In Pastorek JG (ed). Obstetrics and Gynecologic Infectious Disease. New York:Raven Press, 1994, p 315.

Pastorek JG, Miller JM, Summers PR. The effect of hepatitis B antigenemia on pregnancy outcome. Am J Obstet Gynecol 1988;158:486.

Piper JM, Ray WA, Rosa FW. Pregnancy outcome following exposure to angiotensin-converting enzyme ihnibitors. Obstet Gynecol 1992;80:429.

Rosen MG, Merkatz IR, Hill JG. Caring for our future: A report by the expert panel on the content of prenatal care. Obstet Gynecol 1991;77:782.

Saari-Kemppainen A, Karjalainen O, Ylöstalo P, Heinonen OP. Ultrasound screening and perinatal mortality: controlled trial of systematic one-stage screening in pregnancy. Lancet 1990;336:387.

Streissguth AP, Grant TM, Barr HM, et al. Cocaine and the use of alcohol and other drugs during pregnancy. Am J Obstet Gynecol 1991;164:1239.

Yancey MK, Duff P, Clark P, Kurtzer T, Horn Frentzen B, Kubilis P. Peripartum infection associated with vaginal group B streptococcal colonization. Obstet Gynecol 1994;84:816.

Miscellaneous

American Institute of Ultrasound in Medicine. Bioeffects and safety of diagnostic ultrasound. Rockville, Maryland:AIUM, 1993.

Annas GJ. Fetal protection and employment discrimination—The Johnson controls case. N Engl J Med 1991;325:740.

Aronson ME, Nelson PK. Fatal air embolism in pregnancy resulting from an unusual sex act. Obstet Gynecol 1967;30:127.

Benowitz NL. Nicotine replacement therapy during pregnancy. JAMA 1991;266:3174.

Brown MS, Hurloch JT. Preparation of the breast for breast feeding. Nurs Res 1975;24:449.

Buekens P, Alexander S, Boutsen M, et al. Randomised controlled trial of routine cervical examinations in pregnancy. Lancet 1994;344:841.

Kovelesky RA, Minor JR. Antiretroviral therapy during pregnancy. Am J Hosp Pharm 1994;51:2187.

O'Sullivan MJ, Boyer PJJ, Scott GB, et al. The pharmacokinetics and safety of zidovudine in the third trimester of pregnancy for women infected with human innumodeficiency virus and their infants: Phase I Acquired Immunodeficiency Syndrome Clinical Trials Group Study (Protocol 082). Am J Obstet Gynecol 1993;168:1510.

Perkins RP. Sexuality during pregnancy: myths, mysteries, and realities. Female Patient 1992;17:37–46.

Scialli AR. Fetal protection policies in the United States. Semin Perinatol 1993;17:50.

5

Complications of Early Pregnancy

Most primary care providers will encounter women early in the course of pregnancy and some choose to provide the initial care these women need. In this capacity, it is necessary that the clinician be aware of complications that may jeopardize either the pregnancy or the health of the mother herself. These complications include abortion, extrauterine pregnancy, and the less common molar pregnancy.

BACKGROUND AND SCIENCE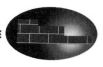

Abortion is the termination of a pregnancy prior to the age of viability. Abortion is typically defined as occuring at less than 20 weeks from the first day of the last normal menstrual period or involving a fetus weighing less than 500 g, although some countries use weights of up to 1000 g. Whether spontaneous or induced, abortion has profound medical and emotional implications. It is necessary to recognize these factors to intervene promptly or avoid unneeded treatment, as appropriate.

Ectopic pregnancy is the leading cause of pregnancy-related death during the first trimester and the second leading cause of maternal death overall. The risk of death from extrauterine pregnancy is ten times greater than for a vaginal delivery and 50 times greater than for an elective abortion. In 1989, ectopic pregnancy was responsible for 34 maternal deaths resulting in a fatality rate of 3.8 deaths per 10,000 ectopic pregnancies. The number of ectopic pregnancies has progressivly increased from a rate of 4.5 per 1000 pregnancies in

1970 to 16.1 in 1989, accounting for roughly 88,000 hospital admissions in that year. For nonwhite women, the rate may be up to 30 per 1000 pregnancies.

New diagnostic tools, such as sensitive biochemical measures and transvaginal ultrasonography, are available to aid in the diagnosis of ectopic pregnancy. These allow for earlier and more accurate diagnoses. The ability to diagnose ectopic pregnancies well in advance of rupture makes the possibility of nonsurgical therapies feasible. The risk posed by ectopic implantation, as well as the new therapies available when early diagnosis is established, make it imperative that those involved in the care of women early in the course of pregnancy be familiar with the diagnosis and therapy of ectopic pregnancy.

Pregnancy Loss

A number of terms are used to describe pregnancy loss in its various stages, resulting in possible confusion for provider and patient alike. Common terms are summarized in Figure 5.1. With the exception of threatened abortions, the jeopardy to the pregnancy is high.

A threatened abortion, as the name implies, is a pregnancy that is at risk for some reason. Most often this applies to any pregnancy in which vaginal bleeding or uterine cramping takes place, but no cervical changes have occurred. This happens in up to 25% of pregnant women, with approximately one half of these patients going on to lose the pregnancy in a spontaneous abortion. Those who go on to carry the pregnancy to viability are at greater risk for preterm delivery, a low birth weight infant, and a higher incidence of perinatal mortality. There does not, however, appear to be a higher incidence of congenital malformations in these newborns.

An inevitable abortion is one in which rupture of the membranes or cervical dilatation takes place during the first half of pregnancy. Uterine contractions typically follow, ending in spontaneous loss of the pregnancy for most patients. For those who do not spon-

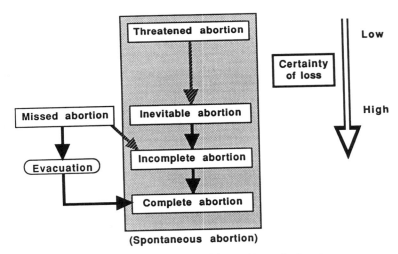

Figure 5.1. Types of abortion and certainty of loss. Missed abortions may spontaneously abort, progressing through incomplete to complete stages, or may be evacuated. Septic abortions are a variant of incomplete abortion in which infection of the uterus and its contents has occurred.

taneously lose the pregnancy, infection or bleeding often ensues, requiring evacuation of the uterus. Conservative management of these patients is seldom successful and should be reserved for only the most special cases.

Spontaneous passage of some, but not all, of the products of conception (incomplete abortion) is associated with uniform pregnancy loss. Incomplete abortions are more common after the tenth week of gestation when fetal and placental tissues tend to be passed separately. Although most of these patient go on to pass the remaining tissue (complete abortion) spontaneously, bleeding, cramping, and the risk of infections associated with expectant management generally mitigate in favor of surgical evacuation.

When an incomplete abortion becomes infected (septic abortion) emergency evacuation of the uterine contents is mandatory because of the significant threat it represents. Septic abortion rarely occurs with a legal abortion; however, it is often associated with "criminal (illegal) abortions," done under unsterile conditions by persons who may have little or no knowledge of medicine or anatomy. The patient can present with severe hemorrhage, bacteremia, septic shock, and renal failure. Broad spectrum parenteral antibiotics, fluid therapy, and prompt evacuation of the uterus are indicated. The possibility of trauma, including perforation of the uterus or vagina, must also be considered.

The wide application of ultrasonography early in pregnancy has led to an increase in the number of doomed pregnancies that are detected before symptoms herald their status as a threatened or incomplete abortion. Traditionally, a missed abortion is the retention of a failed intrauterine pregnancy for an extended period; however, with ultrasound studies, a missed abortion is often detected significantly before it could have been done on clinical grounds alone. These patients typically present with decreased or minimal uterine growth early in pregnancy. Some lose early symptoms of pregnancy, such as breast fullness or morning sickness. Although rare, disseminated intravascular coagulopathy (DIC) can occur when a second trimester intrauterine fetal demise has been retained beyond 6 weeks after the death of the fetus. Evacuation of the uterus can be accomplished either through dilatation and evacuation (D&E) or with the use prostaglandin suppositories and should be based on the stage of the pregnancy and other considerations.

The terms "recurrent" or "habitual" abortion (aborter) are used when a woman has had two consecutive, or three total, first trimester spontaneous pregnancy losses. For these patients, the possibility of a recurring cause is sufficient to warrant an evaluation so that appropriate counseling or intervention may be provided. When the losses have been early in gestation, there is a greater likelihood of a chromosomal abnormality being the cause, whereas in later abortions, a maternal cause, such as a uterine anomaly, is more likely. Although most chromosomal abnormalities result from disorders of meiosis in gamete formation or in mitosis after fertilization, 5% of couples who experience recurrent abortion will have a detectable parental chromosomal abnormality. Therefore, karyotyping of both parents is recommended when recurrent early abortions have occurred. The possibility of maternal medical conditions or anatomic defects should be evaluated for those patients with recurrent late abortions. These include surgically correctable uterine abnormalities, an incompetent cervix, or intrauterine synechiae. Uterine anomalies are found in 10% to 15% of women with recurrent abortion. The possibility of immunologic factors as a cause of recurrent losses should also be evaluated. Referral for specialized evaluation and counseling is appropriate.

Spontaneous Abortion

The true incidence of spontaneous abortion is not known but has been estimated to be as high at 50% to 60% of all conceptions. This is based on the assumption that many fertilizations terminate before pregnancy is recognized. Of women who know they are pregnant, between 10% and 15% (possibly higher in first pregnancies) will be lost to spontaneous abortion, with approximately 80% of these occurring during the first 12 weeks of gestation. The risk of pregnancy loss subsequent to a spontaneous abortion rises slightly (Fig. 5.2), although much of this rise may result from selection of those with factors that mitigate against successful pregnancy.

A number of factors may be responsible for the loss of a pregnancy (Table 5.1). Roughly 50% to 70% of early abortions are caused by chromosomal abnormalities, most common of which is trisomy, which occurs in approximately 40% to 50% of cases. When the losses are due to aneuploidy or polyploidy, they tend to happen earlier in gestation (75% before 8 weeks) and are more likely to recur in subsequent pregnancies. Additional risk factors for spontaneous abortion include increasing parity, advanced maternal and paternal age, and a short interval between pregnancies. Abnormal development of the early pregnancy, including the zygote, embryo, fetus, or placenta, is common in spontaneous abortion. Expulsion of the pregnancy is almost always preceded by the death of the embryo or fetus.

Second trimester abortions are less likely to be due to chromosomal factors (20%-30%) and much more likely to be due to a maternal systemic disease, abnormal placentation, or uterine anomalies. Maternal conditions associated with spontaneous abortion

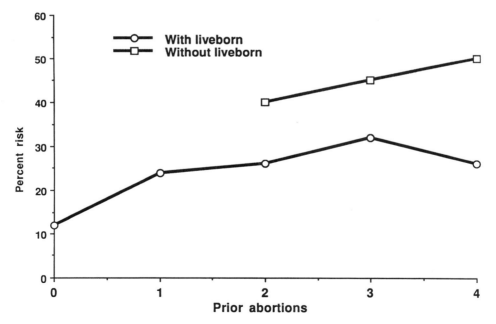

Figure 5.2. Recurrence risk of spontaneous abortion based on previous liveborn and spontaneous abortion history. Data from: Warburton D, Fraser FC. Spontaneous abortion risks in man: Data from reproductive histories collected in a medical genetics unit. Am J Human Genet 1964;16:1; and Poland BJ, Miller JR, Jones DC, Trimble BK. Reproductive counseling in patients who have had a spontaneous abortion. Am J Obstet Gynecol 1977;127:685.

Table 5.1. Causes of spontaneous abortion

Endocrine abnormalities (25%–50%)
    Hyperandrogenism
    In utero DES exposure
    Luteal phase defect
    Thyroid disease
Genetic factors (10%–70%)
    (Balanced translocation/carrier state, nondisjunction) Trisomy (40%–50%) (Trisomy 16
        most common, any possible except trisomy 1) Monosomy X (15%–25%)
    Triploidy (15%)
    Tetraploidy (5%)
Reproductive tract abnormalities (6%–12%)
    Abnormality of placentation
    Bicornuate or unicornuate uterus
    Incompetent cervix
    Intrauterine adhesions (Asherman's syndrome)
    In utero DES exposure
    Leiomyomata uteri (submucous)
    Septate uterus
Infection
    Mycoplasma hominis
    Syphilis
    Toxoplasmosis
    Ureaplasma urealyticus
    ?Chlamydia
    ?Herpes
Systemic disease
    Chronic cardiovascular disease
    Chronic renal disease
    Diabetes mellitus
    Systemic lupus/lupus anticoagulant
Environmental factors
    Alcohol
    Anesthetic gases
    Drug use
    Radiation
    Smoking
    Toxins
Other factors
    Advanced maternal age
    Delayed fertilization (old egg)
    Trauma

DES = diethylstilbestrol.

include systemic infections such as *Mycoplasma hominis,* ureaplasma ureolyticum, and toxoplasmosis. Although uncommon, uncorrected medical conditions such as hyperthyroidism and diabetes may cause spontaneous abortion. Insufficient secretion of progesterone by the corpus luteum or the placenta has also been implicated in spontaneous abortion, although controversy about the prevalence of this exists. Spontaneous abortion may also be caused by environmental toxins, radiation, or immunologic factors. These causes of spontaneous abortion are potentially treatable and, therefore, preventing recurrent spontaneous abortion is potentially possible as well.

Spontaneous abortion can be caused by congenital or acquired abnormalities of the uterus, such as a unicornuate or septate uterus, leiomyomata, or Asherman's syndrome. Roughly 20% to 30% of women with unicornuate or septate uteruses have recurrent pregnancy loss. In utero exposure to diethylstilbestrol (DES) has been associated with abnormally shaped uteri as well as cervical incompetence, both of which may increase a woman's risk of miscarriage. Intrauterine synechiae (Asherman's syndrome) has been linked to spontaneous abortion due to insufficient endometrial tissue to support implantation. This condition, which is rare, typically occurs after an overly vigorous uterine curettage or with an infection following abortion, curettage, or birth, resulting in subsequent destruction and scarring of the endometrial cavity (see also Chapter 19, No Periods [Amenorrhea]). Submucous leiomyomata have been associated with spontaneous abortion, but it is uncommon for subserous or intramucosal leiomyomata to be a causative factor in abortion. Myomectomy is justifiable only if it can be determined that pregnancy wastage has been caused by this anatomic distortion.

Toxins encountered at work or in the environment have been implicated in increased rates of spontaneous abortion. Industrial toxins such as arsenic, lead, formaldehyde, benzene, and ethylene oxide all increase the risk of abortion. Some studies have indicated an increased risk for women exposed to anesthetic gases, although other studies have not demonstrated this risk. Recent studies indicate that video display terminals (computer screens), shortwaves, and ultrasound are not implicated in any increased risk.

Both smoking and alcohol consumption are linked to miscarriages. Women who smoke more than one pack per day of cigarettes have an approximately twofold increase in their rate of spontaneous pregnancy loss; women who drink more than 2 days per week during early pregnancy experience twice the abortion rate of those who do not. There is some evidence that caffeine consumption, in excess of four cups per day, increases the risk of early pregnancy loss.

Induced Abortion

Although not a complication of early pregnancy, a few words about induced abortion and its medical consequences are in order.

Termination of an intact pregnancy prior to viability can be done to safeguard the health of the mother or on a purely elective basis. Prior to choosing an elective abortion, patients must be aware that choices are available, including continuation of pregnancy with subsequent adoption, continuation of pregnancy and rearing the child, and termination of the pregnancy during either the first or second trimester. Complications are attendant with all of these choices. The lowest rate of medical complications occurs with first trimester elective abortion, which carries fewer risks than are associated with carrying a pregnancy to term. First trimester pregnancies are typically terminated by means of suction curettage. Second trimester abortions convey greater risk; they are most commonly performed through suction, destructive forceps, or by the use of prostaglandins to induce uterine contractions. Other techniques used to terminate pregnancy include hysterectomy, intrauterine infusion of hypersonic solutions (such as saline or urea), and the not currently approved antiprogesterone RU-486.

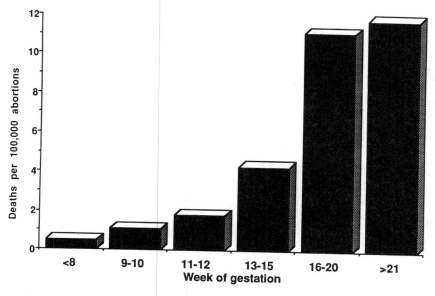

Figure 5.3. Mortality rate for legal abortions by weeks of gestation, United States, 1972–1980. From: Atrash HK, MacKay T, Binkin NJ, Hogue CJR. Legal abortion mortality in the United States: 1972–1982. Am J Obstet Gynecol 1987;156:605.

The risk of death due to abortion during the first 8 weeks of pregnancy is less than 1 per 100,000 procedures, with the risk increasing with gestational age (Fig. 5.3). There is no apparent risk to future pregnancies if the termination is uncomplicated. There appears to be a slight increase risk of premature delivery if more than three first trimester pregnancies are electively terminated.

It is often assumed that elective abortion is most commonly chosen by teenage unwed women, but statistics indicate that the highest percent is among women between the ages of 20 and 24 years (Fig. 5.4). A high rate of pregnancy terminations also occurs among married women under the age of 20 (Fig. 5.5). No matter what motivates the individual patient to choose this route, nonjudgmental counseling should be provided while the decision is being made as well as medical follow-up as for a complete spontaneous miscarriage.

Ectopic Pregnancy

Ectopic pregnancy is the global term used for any pregnancy that implants outside of the usual location in the uterine cavity. The incidence of ectopic pregnancy is steadily rising in the United States (Fig. 5.6), with the highest rate in older, nonwhite patients (Fig. 5.7). Women age 35 to 44 have a three times greater rate of extrauterine gestations than women between the ages of 15 and 24, although the largest number of ectopic pregnancies occur for women between the ages of 20 and 29 (>40%). Nonwhite patients have both a greater incidence of ectopic pregnancies (1.5 times) and a greater case fatality rate (3.5 times). Despite the threat that rising rates of ectopic pregnancy pose, hospital stays have decreased. This may be due to better diagnostic tests, early use of ultrasonography, laparoscopic management of the unruptured ectopic pregnancy, and the use of outpatient methotrexate.

Previous pelvic infection is the most common risk factor for ectopic pregnancy, resulting

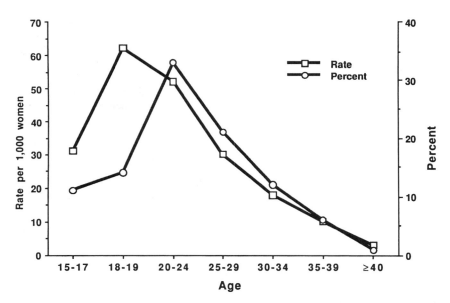

Figure 5.4. Rate and percent distribution by age of legal abortions in the United States, 1987. Data from: Henshaw SK, Koonin LM, Smith JC. Characteristics of U.S. women having abortions. Fam Plann Perspect 1991;23:75.

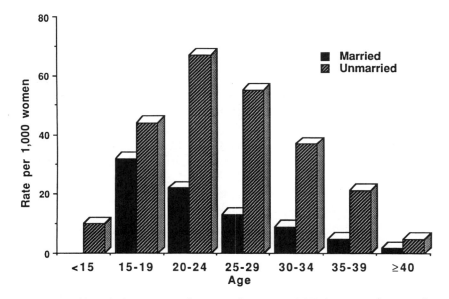

Figure 5.5. Rate of legal abortions in the United States, 1987, by marital status. Data from: Henshaw SK, Koonin LM, Smith JC. Characteristics of U.S. women having abortions. Fam Plann Perspect 1991;23:75.

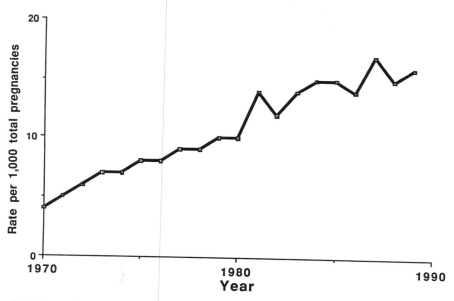

Figure 5.6. Rates of ectopic pregnancy in the United States, 1970–1989. From: Goldner TE, Lawson HW, Xia Z, Atrash HK. Surveillance for ectopic pregnancy—United States, 1970–1989. MMWR CDC Surveill Summ 1993;42(SS-6):73.

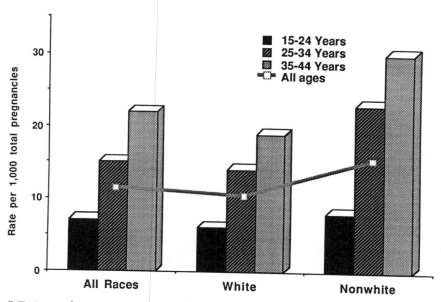

Figure 5.7. Rate of ectopic pregnancy by race and age. From: Goldner TE, Lawson HW, Xia Z, Atrash HK. Surveillance for ectopic pregnancy—United States, 1970–1989. MMWR CDC Surveill Summ 1993;42(SS-6):73.

in a sixfold increase in risk. Other common risk factors include maternal age, multiparity, previous intrauterine contraceptive device (IUCD) usage, and previous fallopian tube surgery. A patient with a prior ectopic pregnancy, has a tenfold increase in her risk of a future ectopic implantation and should be assessed accordingly. Some authors suggest that up to 75% of pregnancies that occur after tubal ligation will be ectopic. The presence of risk factors should alert the clinician to the prospect of an ectopic pregnancy, but the absence of clinically identifiable risk does not rule out its possibility. Risk factors for ectopic pregnancy are summarized in Table 5.2.

Because the tissues on which extrauterine pregnancies implant are not well suited to supporting the gestation, one of several outcomes will occur: the tissues will be unable to support the implantation and the pregnancy will die; the pregnancy will implant and grow briefly, outgrow space or blood supply and be aborted from the site (tubal or fimbrial abortion); the pregnancy will grow until the confining structure ruptures; or the pregnancy will grow to term (the rare situation in abdominal implantation). The symptoms encountered and the risks to the pregnancy and mother vary with each of the possible courses.

Invasion of local blood vessels is common to all sites and results in bleeding that varies from small to massive. Bleeding, combined with stretch of tissues when the implantation is in a confined space, generally produce pain. Because the hormonal changes of pregnancy will be similar to what are normal in the early stages of an extrauterine pregnancy, uterine softening, mild enlargement, and endometrial thickening all occur regardless of the site of implantation. The extent of these changes is dictated by the relative health and longevity of the gestation.

Most ectopic gestations are tubal, with the ampulla (78%) and isthmus (12%) most common (Fig. 5.8). Tubal pregnancies are associated with rupture in 40% to 90% of cases, often leading to intense sudden pain or catastrophic bleeding. Because there are implantation sites other than the fallopian tube (such as ovary, cervix, or abdomen), a persistently elevated beta human chorionic gonadotropin level (β-HCG) requires further evaluation, including the possibility for exploratory laparotomy. Ectopic pregnancies have

Table 5.2. Risk Factors for Ectopic Pregnancy

Age >35 years (three-fold increased risk)
Assisted reproduction procedures (GIFT, IVF, ovum transfer)
Cigarette smoking at time of conception
Congenital abnormalities of the uterus and tubes
Endometriosis
History of intrauterine contraceptive device use
In utero exposure to DES
Multiparity
Multiple induced abortions
Nonwhite race
Ovulation induction, especially with human menopausal gonadotropins
Pelvic inflammatory disease (six-fold increased risk)
Previous ectopic pregnancy (ten-fold increased risk)
Prior pelvic surgery (especially with infection)
Tubal ligation
Tubal reversal surgery

DES = diethylstilbertrol. GIFT = gamete intrafallopian transfer; IVF = in vitro fertilization.

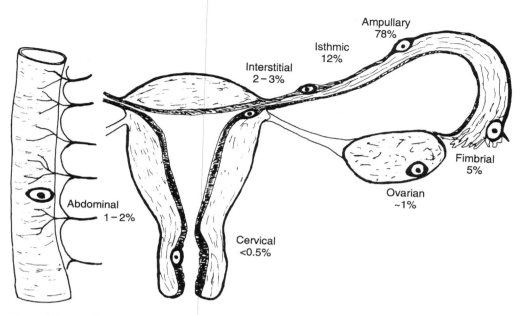

Figure 5.8. Incidence of types of ectopic pregnancy by location. (From Beckmann RB, Ling FW, Barzansky BM, et al. Obstetrics and gynecology. 2nd ed. Baltimore: Williams & Wilkins, 1995:322.)

been reported even after hysterectomy, usually from an impregnation just prior to surgery or tubal fistula to the apex of the vagina.

The risk of heterotrophic gestations (simultaneous intrauterine and extrauterine gestations) varies from 1 per 30,000 pregnancies to as high as 2% to 3% of pregnancies conceived through assisted reproduction techniques. Higher rates than expected also occur for women with recurrent abortion. Extra care should be taken to consider ectopic implantation in those at increased risk.

Molar Pregnancy

A molar pregnancy (hydatidiform mole) is a part of a group of gestational trophoblastic diseases that include choriocarcinoma. These uncommon variants of pregnancy arise entirely from abnormal placental proliferation. They are classified as being either complete, in which no fetus is present, or incomplete, where both fetus and molar tissue are present. A comparison of these two entities is shown in Table 5.3.

Gestational trophoblastic neoplasia (GTN) is notable for the possibility of malignant transformation, although less than 10% of patients develop malignant changes. These abnormalities of pregnancy always present as a pregnancy, but are associated with more profound hormonal changes, leading to exaggerated symptoms of pregnancy in many cases. These hormonal changes also present the opportunity to use β-HCG as a tumor marker to follow the results of therapy. These tumors generally have a characteristic genetic make-up and are very sensitive to chemotherapy.

The cause of GTN is unknown, although racial and regional differences in prevalence suggest both a genetic and environmental predilection. Asian women living in Asia have a

Table 5.3. Comparison of Complete and Incomplete Molar Pregnancies

	Complete	Incomplete
Synonymous	True, classic	Partial
Percent prevalence	90%	10%
Embryo	None	Abnormal
Karyotype	Mostly 46, XX	Triploid (69, XXY or XXX)
Genetic origin	Paternal (blighted ovum + haploid sperm; reduplicated)	Mixed (maternal + duplication of 1 sperm or 2 haploid sperm)
β–HCG level	Very high	Moderate to high
Histology		
Villi	All edematous	Some normal
Capillaries	Few	Some
Fetal red cells	None	Present
Cell of origin	Syncytiotrophoblast	Cytotrophoblast
Malignant potential	15%–20%	<5%–10%
Medical complications	Frequent	Rare

rate of GTN that approaches 1 of 120 to 200 pregnancies, whereas white women living in Europe or the United States have a rate that is ten times lower (1 of 2000). Overall estimates of incidence in the United States cite a rate of 1 of 600 therapeutic abortions and 1 of 1000 to 1500 pregnancies. Gestational trophoblastic disease is more common both early and late in a woman's reproductive years; it is more common for patients with folic acid deficiencies; and has a recurrence rate of approximately 2%. Choriocarcinoma occurs in roughly 1 per 20,000 pregnancies in the United States.

ESTABLISHING THE DIAGNOSIS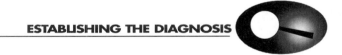

Spontaneous Abortion

For most patients, the first indication of a threatened abortion is vaginal bleeding, which may be bright to dark red in color. Lower abdominal cramping may follow in a few hours to a few days; it is generally rhythmic and may be accompanied by pelvic or low back pressure symptoms. The symptom of pain is a more ominous sign for the pregnancy than bleeding alone.

The differential diagnosis of vaginal bleeding in the first trimester of pregnancy must include ectopic pregnancy, cervical polyps, cervicitis, and molar pregnancy. Cervical sources of bleeding are more likely to be painless. To establish a diagnosis, the patient should undergo a speculum and bimanual examination whenever bleeding occurs. In the absence of other findings, any bleeding in the first half of an intrauterine pregnancy is presumptively called a threatened abortion. Some patients experience bleeding at the time of their expected menses, sometimes referred to as the placental sign or implantation bleeding. This is probably due to ruptured blood vessels in the endometrium or small separations between the placenta and decidual layers as implantation is occurring. This type of bleeding carries little significance for future pregnancy complications.

Ultrasound examinations, which detect an intact early gestation, can be reassuring for patients with bleeding early in pregnancy, but the presence of an early gestation does not ensure successful completion. In addition, the inability to identify a gestational sac does not rule out a viable pregnancy. Ultrasonography, in conjunction with quantitative β-HCG, may be used to suggest the viability of pregnancies where bleeding is encountered. For this a combination of serial β-HCG determinations, and either transvaginal or transabdominal ultrasonography is best. Transabdominal ultrasonography is generally able to identify an intact gestation if the quantitative β-HCG exceeds 5000 to 6500 (mIU/mL, International Reference Preparation), whereas transvaginal ultrasonography should identify an early pregnancy at levels of 1500 (mIU/mL). The absence of an identifiable sac under these conditions is diagnostic in 85% to 90% of cases. Unfortunately, fewer than 25% of ectopic pregnancies will have β-HCG values above 6000 mIU at the time of initial evaluation, making ectopic pregnancy a diagnosis that must always be considered. Transvaginal ultrasonography can often identify a gestational sac by menstrual day 35. By menstrual day 45 fetal heart activity can generally be demonstrated in a normal pregnancy.

Measurement of serum hormone levels may help in evaluating patients with complications of early pregnancy. If serial determinations of quantitative β-HCG do not show at least a 66% increase every 48 hours, the outlook for the pregnancy is poor. Serum progesterone has been proposed as a marker for abnormal pregnancies. Values below 5 to 10 ng/mL, when a gestational sac is seen on ultrasonography or β-HCG values >1000 mIU/mL, are associated with abnormal pregnancies and few, if any, of these, will survive. These values do not differentiate between doomed intrauterine implantation and ectopic pregnancies, however.

If speculum and bimanual examination identify significant cervical dilatation or if tissue is seen at the cervix, a diagnosis of inevitable or incomplete abortion is established, and treatment must be instituted accordingly.

Ectopic Pregnancy

The availability of improved assays and imaging tools has resulted the in earlier diagnosis of ectopic pregnancy, in most cases. As a consequence, the incidence of tubal rupture is now less than 20% in many centers. The most important factor in making a timely diagnosis is considering ectopic as a possibility, if not probability, for all patients with abdominal pain who might be pregnant. Delayed or inaccurate diagnosis is a factor in roughly half of maternal deaths due to ectopic pregnancy. In one study one third of women with extrauterine pregnancies had been seen once and 11% seen twice before the diagnosis was established.

Patients with an ectopic pregnancy have a wide array of history, signs, and symptoms. Classically, these patients present with a history of amenorrhea, abdominal pain, and vaginal bleeding. The pain experienced by these patients is generally described as being dull, crampy, or colicky. The pain may be unilateral but may not be located on the same side as the implantation. Intra-abdominal bleeding, present in 20% of patients, may give rise to

Table 5.4. Common Symptoms of Ectopic Pregnancy

Symptom	Prevalence (%)
Abdominal pain	95–100
Generalized	50
Unilateral pelvic	35
Shoulder (referred)	20
Back	5–10
History of amenorrhea	75–95
2 weeks or less	45
2–6 weeks	35
up to 12 weeks	15
Abnormal vaginal bleeding	60–85
Hemodynamic symptoms	
Dizziness	20–58
Syncope	10–18
Pregnancy symptoms ("feel pregnant")	10–20
Gastrointestinal symptoms	80
Nausea	15
Tenesmus	5–15

pain referred to the back or shoulders. The symptoms of an ectopic pregnancy are often variable in presence and intensity, making diagnosis difficult in the early stages of the process (Table 5.4). Other diagnoses that should be considered are summarized in Table 5.5. Diagnoses that may be confused with ectopic pregnancy are summarized in Table 5.6.

The physical condition of a patient with an ectopic pregnancy may range from normal to life-threatening hypovolemic shock. Fortunately, the latter occurs in only about 5% of patients. As with the symptoms of ectopic pregnancy, the physical findings present are varied and nonspecific (Table 5.7). Although findings such as an adnexal mass support the diagnosis of ectopic implantation, its absence does not rule out the possibility.

The production of β-HCG is directly correlated with the proliferation of trophoblastic tissue, making serial determinationis of β-HCG levels useful in assessing the health of a pregnancy. A single β-HCG value is of little use unless it is negative. The general rule of thumb is that a doubling in value should occur in just over 48 hours, but the time may range from 1.4 to 3.5 days in normal pregnancies (Fig. 5.9). Tubal pregnancies generally plateau or

Table 5.5. Differential Diagnosis in Ectopic Pregnancy

Appendicitis
Degenerating fibroid
Dysfunctional uterine bleeding
Endometriosis
Gastroenteritis
Ovulation
Ruptured corpus luteum cyst
Salpingitis
Septic abortion
Threatened or incomplete abortion
Torsion of an adnexal mass

Table 5.6. Misdiagnoses in Fatal Ectopic Pregnancies in the United States, 1979–1980

Misdiagnosis	Occurrences (%)*
Gastrointestinal disorder	25
Normal pregnancy	18
Pelvic inflammatory disease	14
Psychiatric disorder	9
Spontaneous abortions	9
Complications of induced abortion	7
Urinary tract infection	7
Adnexal cyst	4
Dysfunctional uterine bleeding	4
Fetal death	2
Placenta previa or abruption	2

*Total greater than 100 due to rounding
Data from: Dorfman SF, Grimes DA, Cates W JR, Binkin NJ, Kafrissen ME, O'Reilly KR. Ectopic pregnancy mortality, United States, 1979 to 1980: Clinical aspects. Obstet Gynecol 1984;64:386.

have a decline in β-HCG levels, although this is not uniform. As noted, this is also seen with a nonviable intrauterine pregnancy. Being able to document a decline in β-HCG levels is critical to following patients who are treated conservatively (observation only), with methotrexate or linear salpingostomy. By 72 hours of surgical removal, levels should be 20% of preoperative levels.

The early diagnosis of ectopic pregnancy has been greatly aided by high-resolution transvaginal ultrasonography. Transabdominal ultrasound consistently shows a gestational sac at 5 weeks, a fetal pole at 6 weeks, and cardiac activity at 7 weeks in the presence of a

Table 5.7. Common Physical Findings in Ectopic Pregnancy

Finding	Prevalence (%)
Abdominal tenderness	80–90
Adnexal tenderness	75–90
Bilateral	50–75
Unilateral	40–75
Cervical motion tenderness	50–75
Peritoneal signs (e.g., rebound tenderness)	
Ruptured pregnancies	50
Unruptured pregnancies	5
Pelvic examination	
"Normal"	10
Adnexal mass	30–50
Contralateral	20
Uterus	
Normal size	70–75
Enlarged	15–30
Hemodynamics	
Orthostatic changes	10–15
Hypovolemia	5
Temperature >37°C	5–10
Vomiting	15

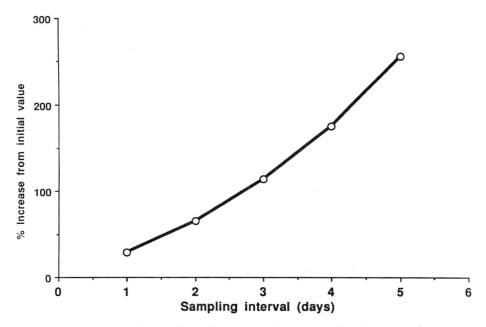

Figure 5.9. Lower limits of normal rise for percent rise in β-HCG during early intrauterine pregnancy. From: Kadar N, Caldwell BV, Romero R. A method of screening for ectopic pregnancy and its indications. Obstet Gynecol 1981;58:162.

normal gestation. Reliable transabdominal ultrasonographic images of an intrauterine gestation should be possible when the β-HCG level reaches 5000 to 6000 mIU/mL. Transvaginal ultrasonography generally identifies a gestational sac at 4 to 5 weeks, a yolk sac at 5 weeks, and fetal cardiac activity around 6 weeks. Transvaginal imaging of an intrauterine pregnancy should be routinely possible after the β-HCG level reaches 1500 mIU/mL. Because the diagnosis of ectopic pregnancy is made prior to 7 weeks in over one half of the cases, few patients benefit from conventional transabdominal examination, making transvaginal ultrasonography the procedure of choice. Color or pulsed Doppler ultrasound techniques hold promise for enhanced diagnosis, but limited availability and experience with these techniques confine their use to specialized centers and research settings.

Typical findings in ectopic pregnancy include a noncystic adnexal mass, cardiac activity in the adnexa (found in 20% to 25% of scans), and an empty uterine cavity (Fig. 5.10). If a complex echogenic adnexal mass is identified by ultrasonography, the positive predictive value for ectopic pregnancy is 94%. Free intraperitoneal fluid may be helpful in the diagnosis of ectopic pregnancy, but it is nonspecific.

Culdocentesis was once a standard tool in the evaluation of possible ectopic pregnancies, but the rapid evolution of sensitive serum pregnancy testing and high-resolution ultrasonography has lessened its importance Even in the best hands, the procedure still is associated with a certain amount of pain and results that are nonspecific. For these reasons, culdocentesis has fallen out of favor even among specialists and should not be attempted in the primary care setting.

Dilatation and curettage can be helpful in the diagnosis of abnormal pregnancy. When

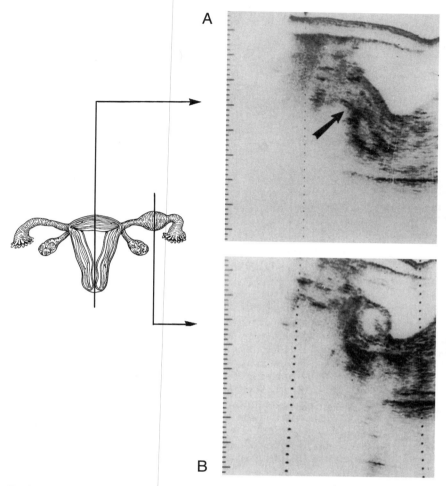

Figure 5.10. Sonographic findings in tubal ectopic pregnancy. **A,** Midline view through empty uterus. **B,** Paramidline view showing cystic mass in area of fallopian tube. (From Beckmann RB, Ling FW, Barzansky BM, et al. Obstetrics and gynecology. 2nd ed. Baltimore: Williams & Wilkins, 1995:325.)

products of conception (chorionic villi) are found, ectopic pregnancy is essentially ruled out. In the case of a missed abortion or blighted ovum, β-HCG levels are usually stable or decreasing and chorionic villi will be found.

An algorithm for the evaluation and management of patients suspected of having an ectopic pregnancy is shown in Figure 5.11.

Molar Pregnancy

Patients with molar pregnancies typically have exaggerated symptoms of pregnancy, a uterus that is different in size than expected for gestational age (usually larger), and most often (95%) painless vaginal bleeding suggestive of threatened abortion. Patients may also experience marked hypertension, pre-eclampsia, proteinuria, nausea and vomiting, visual

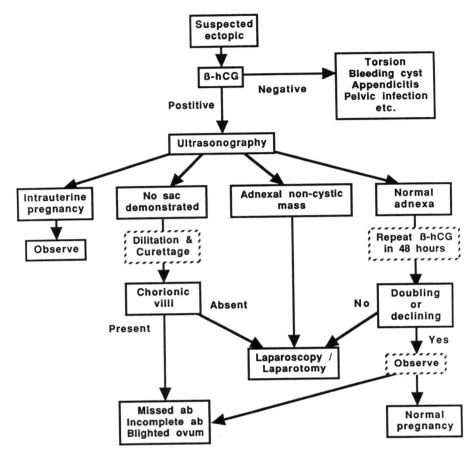

Figure 5.11. Management algorithm for suspected ectopic pregnancy.

changes, tachycardia, and shortness of breath. Pregnancy-induced hypertension in the first trimester of pregnancy is virtually diagnostic of molar pregnancy. Edematous trophoblastic fragments may be passed vaginally through a partially dilated cervical os, alerting the clinician to the diagnosis.

Physical examination will reveal a uterine size-date discrepancy and an absence of heart sounds (in a complete mole). Bilateral adnexal masses (theca lutein cysts) occur in 15% to 20% of patients and result from hormonal hyperstimulation of the ovaries. Ultrasonographic examination is usually diagnostic, revealing a pathognomic "snowstorm" appearance (Fig. 5.12).

Once a molar pregnancy is diagnosed, a quantitative β-HCG value must be obtained to help establish the patient's risk category and to allow monitoring of disease response to therapy. A baseline chest roentogram to check for metastatic disease and a complete blood count should also be obtained. The patient's blood type and Rh should be established to allow for Rh immune globulin therapy (if needed) and to prepare for the possibility of blood replacement due to bleeding or surgical losses during evacuation of the uterine contents. Clotting function studies are advisable.

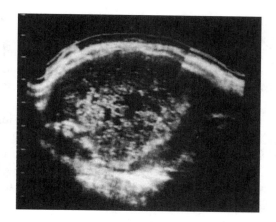

Figure 5.12. Ultrasonographic appearance of hydatidiform mole. (From Beckmann RB, Ling FW, Barzansky BM, et al. Obstetrics and gynecology. 2nd ed. Baltimore: Williams & Wilkins, 1995: 469.)

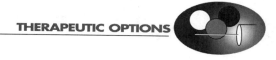

THERAPEUTIC OPTIONS

Spontaneous Abortion

Intervention for patients with threatened abortion should be minimal, even when bleeding is accompanied by low abdominal pain and cramping. If there is no evidence of cervical change, the patient can be reassured and encouraged to continue normal activities. Although frequently recommended, a short period of bed rest has no documented benefit. Intercourse is usually proscribed for 2 to 3 weeks, or longer, although probably this also provides more psychological support than medical effect. Regardless of β-HCG level or ultrasonography findings, if significant pain or bleeding persist, especially bleeding leading to hemodynamic alterations, evacuation of the uterus should be carried out. Chromosomal evaluation of spontaneously passed tissue is not recommended except in the case of recurrent abortion.

Once it is apparent that loss of pregnancy has occurred or is occurring, treatment is based on both the immediate and long-term needs of the patient. Immediate considerations include control of bleeding, prevention of infection, pain relief (if needed), and emotional support. Bleeding is controlled by ensuring that all the products of the conception have been expelled from the uterus. This is presumed in the case of complete abortion, but must be accomplished through curettage in cases of incomplete, inevitable, missed, or septic abortions. Hemostasis is augmented through uterine contraction, encouraged through the use of intravenous (IV) oxytocin (10–20 U/L IV fluids) or intramuscular (IM) methylergonovine maleate (Methergine) (0.2 mg IM). Removal of the products of conception, combined with vaginal rest (no tampons, douches, or intercourse), provides adequate infection protection in most cases. A mild analgesic may be required and should be offered. Rh negative mothers should receive Rh immune globulin as prophylaxis against sensitization. Because ovulation may occur as early as 2 weeks after an abortion, a discussion of contraception is warranted.

If low-grade fever, bleeding, and pain are present after an abortion, infection should be suspected and treated with oral antibiotic and ergot. The possibility of retained tissue must be strongly considered. If retained tissue is present or cannot be ruled out, curettage must be promptly performed. Significant infection, such as found in septic abortions, must be treated aggressively with combination intravenous antibiotics (such as ampicillin, clindamycin, and gentamycin). Once antibiotics have been started, uterine evacuation must be performed.

It is importance for both the short- and long-term well-being of the patient that emotional support be a part of the care provided. No matter how well prepared for the possibility of pregnancy loss a couple is, the loss of a pregnancy represents a significant calamity. When appropriate, the couple should be reassured that the loss was not induced by anything that they did or did not do; there was nothing that they could have done to prevent the loss and nothing they could have done to have caused it. There is a natural tendency to try to find a reason for the loss of a pregnancy. This is often expressed in thoughts or expression such as "if we hadn't made love 2 weeks ago," or "if I hadn't let her pick up the grocery bag." These are clearly unrelated to the cause of most abortions, but can easily lead to further stress at a time when both partners need support the most. Couples are often reluctant to raise these issues; therefore, they should be raised directly by the clinician.

Patients who have chosen an elective termination of pregnancy require the same type of follow-up as those who suffer a spontaneous loss. In addition to protection from Rh immunization and observation for bleeding and infections, the possibility of perforation, coexistent ectopic pregnancy, or incomplete extraction of the products of conception must be kept in mind.

Four to 6 weeks after miscarriage the patient should return to be evaluated for uterine involution and the return of menses, and to discuss reproductive plans. Reiteration of the causes (or lack of causes) of the pregnancy loss and its impact on future childbearing should be a part of this visit. Contraceptive options should again be offered as appropriate.

Couples who experience recurrent abortion must be counseled and treated based on the results of their medical and genetic evaluation. Those with parental chromosomal anomalies may be offered donor oocytes or artificial insemination with donor sperm. Uterine anomalies or submucous fibroids may be treated, although care must be taken to recognize the possibility of continued failure for other reasons.

Ectopic Pregnancy

Surgical therapy has been the mainstay of treatment for ectopic gestations. In the past decade, new surgical techniques and the emergence of medical therapies have changed the way these patients are managed. Management now depends on the location and size of the pregnancy, the presence of disease in the pelvis, and the technical abilities of the surgeon. Although most of the management of patients with ectopic pregnancies falls outside the realm of primary care, the primary care provider must be familiar with current therapy to provide counseling and to assist with global care.

Salpingectomy has been traditionally performed for ectopic gestations and is still appropriate in many situations. The patient with a prior tubal ligation who desires no future fertility or the patient who is hemodynamically unstable should still undergo salpingectomy. The patient with a ruptured tubal pregnancy resulting in an irreparable fallopian tube should receive a unilateral salpingectomy. Removal of the ipsilateral ovary should be based on ovarian viability and not performed routinely. Salpingectomy done via laparotomy is associated with a contralateral tubal patency rate of 80% to 90%, intrauterine pregnancy rates of 40% to 50%, repeat ectopic pregnancy rates of 10% to 25%, and infertility rates of 25% to 30%.

Conservative procedures are becoming more feasible with earlier recognition of ectopic pregnancies. Partial salpingectomy or linear salpingotomy has become more commonly performed. Several recent reports have introduced the use of laparoscopic injection of prostaglandin $PGF_{2\alpha}$ or hyperosmolar glucose into the gestation to cause death of the pregnancy and involution. The use of a laparoscopic surgical approach is feasible in 70% to 95% of cases. Patients who undergo these more conservative operations should be followed by serial β-HCG titers, because up to 5% may need a second operation for persistent trophoblastic tissue. Conservative procedures give similar pregnancy rates to salpingectomy.

Medical management of patients with ectopic pregnancies is an option for selected patients. Chemotherapeutic agents such as methotrexate and actinomycin D may be used to medically treat the pregnancy, resulting in involution and reabsorption. Methotrexate has been most commonly used and may be given orally, intramuscularly, or injected into the pregnancy via a transvaginal route with ultrasonic guidance or via laparoscopy. Intramuscular therapy has been provided by the administration of the first dose of methotrexate on an inpatient basis, followed by outpatient therapy for up to four additional doses given in combination with citrovorum rescue. More recent reports suggest that total outpatient therapy is possible for centers experienced with this technique. Patient selection criteria for this therapy include a tubal gestation no greater than 3 cm, β-HCG levels below 15,000 mUI/mL, and hemodynamic stability. Patients with a history of active hepatic or renal disease, fetal cardiac activity demonstrated in the ectopic gestation, active ulcer disease, or significant alterations in white blood count (<3000, platelet count (<100,000) are not candidates for this therapy. Laparoscopy or laparotomy are still possible for those patients who do not respond or who experience complications before medical therapy can be effective, which occurs in between 5% and 10% of cases. Rhesus status of the patient should be determined; if negative, appropriate therapy should be provided.

Molar Pregnancy

Molar pregnancies are treated with surgical evacuation of the uterine contents, which is most often accomplished via suction curettage. Because of the large size of some molar pregnancies and a tendency toward uterine atony, concomitant oxytocin administration is advisable and blood for transfusion must be available, should it be needed. Induction of labor or hysterectomy may be required in extreme cases, but suction evacuation is preferred. In general, the larger or more advanced the molar pregnancy, the greater the risk of pulmonary complications, bleeding, trophoblastic emboli, or fluid overload. The treatment of these patients requires special expertise.

Once the uterus has been emptied, the patient must be closely followed for at least 1 year for the possibility of recurrent benign or malignant disease. The follow-up of these patients is summarized in Table 5.8. Any change in the patient's examination, a rise in β-HCG titers, or a failure of the β-HCG value to fall below 10 mIU/mL by 12 weeks after

Table 5.8. Posttreatment Follow-up for Molar Pregnancy

- General physical and pelvic examination at 2 weeks (baseline chest roentogram if not done at time of diagnosis)
- Quantitative β–HCG every 2 weeks until <10mIU/mL, monthly thereafter for 1 year
- Reliable contraception (oral contraceptives preferred) for 1 year
- Early ultrasonography and quantitative β–HCG for any future pregnancy

evacuation must be evaluated for the possibility of recurrent benign or malignant disease. Roughly 80% of patients diagnosed with molar pregnancies have a benign course after initial therapy. Between 15% and 25% of patients develop invasive disease and 3% to 5% eventually have metastatic lesions.

Primary or recurrent malignant trophoblastic disease is generally treated with chemotherapy (methotrexate, actinomycin, or chlorambucil, singly or in combination). The prognosis for these patients is generally good (90% cure rate). Successful pregnancies after treatment for choriocarcinoma are common and studies suggest that these patients do not have any higher rate of abortions, stillbirths, congenital anomalies, prematurity, or other complications.

HINTS AND COMMON QUESTIONS

Cervical polyps, cervical eversion or cervicitis, or other cervical lesions may cause bleeding in early pregnancy. The lack of lower abdominal cramping and the results of vaginal speculum examination help identify these imitators of threatened abortion.

Rarely, a cast of the uterine cavity may be passed during normal menstruation. This is generally accompanied by moderate to strong cramping. It may be differentiated from a spontaneous abortion histologically or by the negative pregnancy test. If the pregnancy test is positive, suspect an ectopic pregnancy.

When abortion is threatened, it is often difficult to tell by history if tissue has been passed. If the patient reports tissue that is dark red and "liverlike," it is probably just a blood clot. If the tissue is described as shaggy or like a bloody wash cloth, it is more likely to be products of conception. The best situation is to have the patient bring in any questionable material for examination.

Progesterone therapy for threatened abortions is of no benefit and may potentially result in virilization of a fetus or in a missed abortion. It should not be used.

Ultrasonography may be useful in distinguishing between complete and incomplete abortions. Be aware that an intrauterine clot may appear like retained tissue.

When trying to distinguish between a decidual reaction and an intrauterine gestation on ultrasonography, it is useful to remember that decidual reactions are generally symmetric whereas gestations tend to have asymmetric thickening due to the placenta and fetal tissues.

Fever above 38°C or a white blood count of >20,000/dL is rare in patients with ectopic pregnancies. The presence of either should suggest the possibility of a pelvic infection, including septic abortion.

Pain is a common complaint for patients with both spontaneous abortions and extrauterine gestations. Patients with miscarriages tend to note a more rhythmic pattern of less severe pain, whereas patients with an ectopic pregnancy are more likely to have severe, unremitting complaints.

Serum progesterone determinations are of little or no value in evaluating pregnancies conceived through the use of clomiphene- or menotropin-stimulated ovulation owing to the formation of multiple corpora lutea.

Following two ectopic pregnancies, only one third of patients achieve successful pregnancy with out-assisted reproductive technologies. The risk of ectopic pregnancy in these patients is also dramatically increased.

If a patient is receiving methotrexate therapy she should not take multivitamins with folic acid (e.g., prenatal vitamins) as they will defeat the effects of the methotrexate.

The theca lutein cysts often found in molar pregnancies may take several months to regress following evacuation of the uterine contents.

SUGGESTED READINGS

General References

Abortion. In: Cunningham FG, MacDonald PC, Gant NF, Leveno KJ, Gilstrap LC III (eds). Williams Obstetrics, 19th ed. Norwalk, CT: Appleton & Lange, 1993, p 661.
Buckley JD. The epidemiology of molar pregnancy and choriocarcinoma. Clin Obstet Gynecol 1984;27:153.
Cartwright PS. Ectopic Pregnancy. In Jones HW III, Wentz AC, Burnett LS (eds). Novak's Textbook of Gynecology, 11th ed. Baltimore: Williams & Wilkins, 1988, p 479.
Ectopic pregnancy. In Cunningham FG, MacDonald PC, Gant NF, Leveno KJ, Gilstrap LC III (eds). Williams Obstetrics, 19th ed. Norwalk, CT: Appleton & Lange, 1993, p 691.
Hammond CB, ed. Trophoblastic disease. Obstet Gynecol Clin North Am 1988;15:435.
Hammond CB, Soper JT. Gestational trophoblastic diseases. In Sciarra JJ (ed). Gynecology and Obstetrics, Vol 4. Philadelphia: JB Lippincott, 1993, p 1.
Russell JB. The etiology of ectopic pregnancy. Clin Obstet Gynecol 1987;30:181.

Specific References

Miscarriage/Abortion

Armstrong BG, McDonald AD, Sloan M. Cigarette, alcohol, and coffee consumption and spontaneous abortion. Am J Public Health 1992;82:85.
Atrash HK, MacKay T, Binkin NJ, Hogue CJR. Legal abortion mortality in the United States: 1972–1982. Am J Obstet Gynecol 1987;156:605.
Baird DT, Normal JE, Thong KJ, Glasier AF. Misoprostol, mifepristone, and abortion. Lancet 1992;339:313.
Barlow S, Sullivan FM. Reproductive hazards of industrial chemicals: an evaluation of animal and human data. New York: Academic Press, 1982.
Batzofin JH, Fielding WI, Friedman EA. Effect of vaginal bleeding in early pregnancy on outcome. Obstet Gynecol 1984;63:515.
Boklage CE. Survival probability of human conceptions from fertilization to term. Int J Fertil 1990;35:75.
Byrne JLB, Ward K. Genetic factors in recurrent abortion. Clin Obstet Gynecol 1994;37:693.
Fossum GT, Davajan V, Kletzky OA. Early detection of pregnancy with transvaginal ultrasound. Fertil Steril 1988;49:788.
Funderburk SJ, Guthrie D, Meldrum D. Outcome of pregnancies complicated by early vaginal bleeding. Br J Obstet Gynecol 1980;87:100.
Goldstein SR. Sonography in early pregnancy failure. Clin Obstet Gynecol 1994;37:681.
Hahlin M, Wallin A, Sjoblom P, Lindblom B. Single progesterone assay for early recognition of abnormal pregnancy. Hum Reprod 1990;5:662.

Hakim-Elahie E, Tovell HM, Burnhill MS. Complications of first-trimester abortions: a report of 170,000 cases. Obstet Gynecol 1990;76:129.

Harlap S, Shiono PH. Alcohol, smoking, and incidence of spontateous abortions in the first and second trimester. Lancet 1980;2:173.

Hatasaka HH. Recurrent miscarriage: epidemiologic factors, definitions, and incidence. Clin Obstet Gynecol 1994;37:625.

Henshaw SK, Koonin LM, Smith JC. Characteristics of U.S. women having abortions. Fam Plann Perspect 1991;23:75.

Hogue CJR. Impact of abortion on subsequent fecundity. Clin Obstet Gynecol 1986;13:95.

Mackenzie WE, Holmes DS, Newton JR. Spontaneous abortion rate in ultrasonographically viable pregnancies. Obstet Gynecol 1988;71:81.

Ohno M, Maeda T, Matsunobu A. A cytogenetic study of spontaneous abortions with direct analysis of chorionic villi. Obstet Gynecol 1991;77:394.

Poland BJ, Miller JR, Jones DC, Trimble BK. Reproductive counseling in patients who have had a spontaneous abortion. Am J Obstet Gynecol 1977;127:685.

Schnorr TM, Grajewski BA, Hornung RW, et al. Video display terminals and the risk of spontaneous abortion. N Engl J Med 1991;324:727.

Scott JR. Recurrent miscarriage: overview and recommendations. Clin Obstet Gynecol 1994;37:768.

Stubblefield PG, Grimes DA. Septic abortion. N Engl J Med 1994;331:310.

Taskinen H, Kyyrönen P, Hemminki K. Effects of ultrasound, shortwaves, and physical exertion on pregnancy outcome in physiotherapists. J Epidemiol Community Health 1990;44:196.

Thom DH, Nelson LM, Vaughan TL. Spontaneous abortion and subsequent adverse birth outcomes. Am J Obstet Gynecol 1992;166:111.

Warburton D, Fraser FC. Spontaneous abortion risks in man: data from reproductive histories collected in a medical genetics unit. Am J Human Genet 1964;16:1.

Ectopic Pregnancy

Ankum WM, Van der Veen F, Hamerlynck JVTH, Lammes FB. Suspected ectopic pregnancy: what to do when human chorionic gonadotropin levels are below the discrimination zone. J Reprod Med 1995;40:525.

Asseryanis E, Frigo P, Schurz B, Huber J. A new diagnostic method to detect ectopic pregnancy at a very early stage. Am J Obstet Gynecol 1995;173:236.

Blumenfeld Z, Rottem S, Elgali S, Timor-Tritsch IE. Transvaginal sonographic assessment of early embryological development. In Timor-Tritsch IE, Rotten S (eds). Transvaginal Sonography. New York: Elsevier, 1988, p 87.

Brumsted J, Kessler C, Gibson C, Nakajima S, Riddick DH, Gibson M. A comparison of laparoscopy and laparotomy for the treatment of ectopic pregnancy. Obstet Gynecol 1988;71:889.

Budowick M, Johnson TR JR, Genadry R, Parmely TH, Woodruff JD. The histopathology of the developing tubal ectopic pregnancy. Fertil Steril 1980;34:169.

Centers for Disease Control and Prevention. Ectopic pregnancy–United States, 1988–1989. MMWR 1992;41:591.

Chambers SE, Muir BB, Haddad NG. Ultrasound evaluation of ectopic pregnancy including correlation with human chorionic gonadotrophin levels. Br J Radiol 1990;63:748.

DeCherney A, Kase N. The conservative surgical management of unruptured ectopic pregnancy. Obstet Gynecol 1979;54:451.

DeCherney AH, Diamond MP. Laparoscopic salpingostomy for ectopic pregnancy. Obstet Gynecol 1987;70:948.

DeCherney AH, Maheaux R, Naftolin F. Salpingostomy for ectopic pregnancy in the sole patent oviduct: reproductive outcome. Fertil Steril 1982;37:619.

Diamond MP, DeCherney AH. Surgical techniques in the management of ectopic pregnancy. Clin Obstet Gynecol 1987;39:200.

Dimitry ES, Subak-Sharpe R, Mills M, Margara R, Winston R. Nine cases of heterotropic pregnancies in 4 years of in vitro fertilization. Fertil Steril 1990;53:107.

Dorfman SF, Grimes DA, Cates W JR, Binkin NJ, Kafrissen ME, O'Reilly KR. Ectopic pregnancy mortality, United States, 1979 to 1980: Clinical aspects. Obstet Gynecol 1984;64:386.

Dubuisson JB, Aubriot FX, Cardone V. Laparoscopic salpingectomy for tubal pregnancy. Fertil Steril 1987;47:225.

Emerson DS, Cartier MS, Altierie LA, et al. Diagnostic efficacy of endovaginal color Doppler flow imaging in an ectopic pregnancy screening program. Radiology 1992;183:413.

Fedele L, Acaia B, Parazzini F, Ricciardiello O, Candiani GB. Ectopic pregnancy and recurrent spontaneous abortion: two associated reproductive failures. Obstet Gynecol 1989;73:206.

Goldner TE, Lawson HW, Xia Z, Atrash HK. Surveillance for ectopic pregnancy–United States, 1970–1989. MMWR CDC Surveill Summ 1993;42(SS-6):73.

Kadar N, Caldwell BV, Romero R. A method of screening for ectopic pregnancy and its indications. Obstet Gynecol 1981;58:162.

Kamrava MM, Taymor ML, Berger MJ, Thompson IE, Seibel MM. Disappearance of human chorionic gonadotropin following removal of ectopic pregnancy. Obstet Gynecol 1983;62:486.

Langer R, Bukovsky I, Herman A, Lifshits Y, Caspi E. "Milking"-A conservative surgical technique for a tubal gestation. Int J Fertil 1983;28(1):49.

Leeton J, Davison G. Nonsurgical management of unruptured tubal pregnancy with intra-amniotic methotrexate: preliminary report of two cases. Fertil Steril 1988;59:167.

Mashiach S, Carp HJA, Serr DM. Nonoperative management of ectopic pregnancy: a preliminary report. J Reprod Med 1982;27:127.

Nehra PC, Loginsky SJ. Pregnancy after vaginal hysterectomy. Obstet Gynecol 1984;64:735.

Pansky M, Bukovsky I, Golan A, Langer R, Schneider D, Arieli S, Caspi E. Local methotrexate injection: a non-surgical treatment of ectopic pregnancy. Am J Obstet Gynecol 1989;161:393.

Paulsson G, Kvint S, Labecker B-M, Lofstrand T, Lindblom B. Laparoscopic prostaglandin injection in ectopic pregnancy: success rates according to endocrine activity. Fertil Steril 1995;63:473.

Pittaway DE, Reish RL, Wentz AC. Doubling times of human chorionic gonadotropin increase in early viable intrauterine pregnancies. Am J Obstet Gynecol 1985;152:299.

Pouly JL, Mahnes H, Mage G, Canis M, Bruhat MA. Conservative laparoscopic treatment of 321 ectopic pregnancies. Fertil Steril 1988;50:580.

Reece EA, Petrie RH, Sirmans MF, Finster M, Todd WD. Combined intrauterine and extrauterine gestations: review. Am J Obstet Gynecol 1983;146:323.

Reich H, Freifeld ML, McGlynn F, et al. Laparoscopic treatment of tubal pregnancy. Obstet Gynecol 1987;69:275.

Russell JB. The etiology of ectopic pregnancy. Clin Obstet Gynecol 1987;30:181.

Stovall TG, Kellerman AL, Ling FW, Buster JE. Emergency department diagnosis of ectopic pregnancy. Ann Emerg Med 1990;19:1098.

Stovall TG, Ling FW, Buster JE. Outpatient chemotherapy of unruptured ectopic pregnancy. Fertil Steril 1989;51:435.

Stovall TG, Ling FW, Cope BJ, Buster JE. Preventing ruptured ectopic pregnancy with a single serum progesterone. Am J Obstet Gynecol 1989;160:1425.

Timonen S, Neiminen U. Tubal pregnancy, choice of operative method of treatment. Acta Obstet Gynecol Scand 1967;46:327.

Timor-Tritsch IE, Yeh MN, Peisner DB, Lesser KB, Slavik TA. The use of transvaginal ultrasonography in the diagnosis of ectopic pregnancy. Am J Obstet Gynecol 1989;161:157.

Trio D, Strobelt N, Picciolo C, Lapinski RH, Ghidini A. Prognostic factors for successful expectant management of ectopic pregnancy. Fertil Steril 1995;63:469.

Yeko TR, Mayer JC, Parsons AK, Maroulis GB. A prospective series of unruptured ectopic pregnancies treated by tubal injection with hyperosmolar glucose. Obstet Gynecol 1995;85:265.

Molar Pregnancy

Craighill MC, Cramer DW. Epidemiology of complete molar pregnancy. J Reprod Med 1984;29:784.

Curry SL, Hammond CB, Tyrey L, Creasman WT, Parker RT. Hydatidiform mole (diagnosis, management and long-term follow-up of 347 patients). Obstet Gynecol 1975;45:1.

Lurain JR, Casanova LA, Miller DS, Rademaker AW. Prognostic factors in gestational trophoblastic tumors: a proposed new scoring system based on multivariate analysis. Am J Obstet Gynecol 1991;164:611.

Messerli ML, Lilienfeld AM, Parmeley T, Woodruff JD, Rosenshein NB. Risk factors for gestational trophoblastic neoplasia. Am J Obstet Gynecol 1985;153:294.

Romero R, Horgan JG, Kohorn EI, Kadar N, Taylor KJW, Hobbins JC. New criteria for the diagnosis of gestational trophoblastic disease. Obstet Gynecol 1985;66:553.

Wong LC, Choo YC, Ma HK. Methotrexate with citrovorum factor rescue in gestational trophoblastic disease. Am J Obstet Gynecol 1985;152:59.

6

When Low Risk becomes High Risk (Medical and Surgical Complications of Pregnancy)

In many ways, all pregnancies are high risk. With current diagnostic and therapeutic modalities has come a complacency about pregnancy. Near the turn of this century, pregnancy was successful if mother survived the childbirth process. By the middle of the century it was presumed that mother would survive and success was measured by a living baby. As the century comes to a close, we not only presume a happy, healthy mother and baby, but expect it to be a community experience akin to the barn-raisings that occurred a century before.

There are a number of medical and surgical conditions that place a "routine" pregnancy at higher risk for complications. Most may be detected in the primary care setting. Many will not require a transfer of care, only a greater degree of vigilance or collaboration. It is not the purpose of this chapter to set out all the possible factors that can make a pregnancy high risk, but rather to alert the primary care team to a number of commonly encountered situations that require special care. Specifically not addressed are issues of intrapartum management, premature labor, premature rupture of the membranes, post-term pregnancy, significant vaginal bleeding, or other situations that clearly call for collaborative management or transfer of care.

BACKGROUND AND SCIENCE

Anemias

As noted in Chapter 4, Early Pregnancy, there is a large increase in plasma volume (1000 mL) during the course of pregnancy. While there is a concomitant increase in red cell mass (300 mL), the increase in plasma is proportionately greater, resulting in a "physiologic", or dilutional change in hemoglobin and hematocrit. During normal pregnancy, these values decrease by roughly 2 g/dL and 6% to 8%, respectively. Because total blood volume is increased, these changes in laboratory parameters do not reflect a true anemia.

True anemia can result when the iron demands of pregnancy outstrip maternal iron stores available or when there is a deficiency of folate in the diet. Although iron absorption increases from about 10% before pregnancy up to around 30% near the end of gestation, normal dietary supplies are generally inadequate without the support of good maternal stores, making iron supplementation desirable for most patients. Folic acid requirements roughly triple during pregnancy and when not met result in a megaloblastic anemia. Medications, such as phenytoin, nitrofurantoin, pyrimethamine, or trimethoprim, or excessive alcohol use may also result in folate deficiency. Between 10% and 25% of pregnant women have low serum folate levels.

Hereditary hemolytic anemias can also cause anemia during pregnancy. Most common of these are sickle-cell disease and trait, α- and β-thalassemias, and sickle-thalassemia. These vary in prevalence from sickle trait, found in 1 of 12 black Americans, to the very rare major and minor thalassemias. When one of these anemias is present or suspected, consultation with a specialist in high risk pregnancy is warranted.

Cancer

Cancer complicates roughly 1 of 1000 pregnancies. The most common cancers encountered are cervical cancer, breast cancer, melanoma, ovarian cancer, leukemia or lymphoma, and colorectal cancer. The management of these patients is a delicate balance of the maternal risks of the malignancy and its treatment versus the risks posed to the fetus.

Abnormal cervical cytology, dysplasia, and cervical cancer occur in declining frequency, with about 3% of pregnant women having abnormal cytology, a small number of whom have dysplasia, and an even smaller number of whom have cervical carcinoma. It appears that when matched stage for stage, pregnant patients have no different cervical cancer outcome. It is unclear whether vaginal delivery through a cervix affected by cancer changes the prognosis. Because of this uncertainty and the need for definitive surgical treatment, abdominal delivery is often advocated in cases of frank carcinoma.

Breast cancer is an infrequent finding with an uncertain relationship with pregnancy. Current data suggest that there is no difference in the stage-for-stage prognosis for these patients, but a delay in diagnosis due to pregnancy-induced breast changes is often encountered. There is no evidence that breast cancer, by itself, adversely affects pregnancy.

Ovarian malignancies are rare during pregnancy, but must be considered in the evaluation of adnexal masses found in early pregnancy. The possibility of a malignancy is greater in a solid mass, making more aggressive evaluation of these masses advisable.

Although rare, melanoma is adversely affected by pregnancy. The presence of estrogen receptors on some melanoma cells and the increase in melanocyte-stimulating hormone brought on by pregnancy, may all contribute to this finding. Whereas any malignant metastasis to the fetus is rare, melanomas represent up to a third of all cases found.

Hodgkin's disease is the most common form of lymphoma encountered during pregnancy. This malignancy is unaffected by pregnancy and, in turn, has no direct effect on the outcome of the pregnancy. Hodgkin's lymphomas are responsive to radiotherapy and chemotherapy, depending on the stage, allowing some flexibility in treatment. Therapy can often be adjusted to allow treatment to continue with a minimal risk to the fetus. Non-Hodgkin's lymphoma cases have risen in the past few years in parallel with the rate of AIDS.

Cardiac Disease

Cardiac disease complicates approximately 1% of all pregnancies and is one of the major causes of nonobstetric maternal mortality. Where once patients with congenital heart disease did not survive to reproductive age, it is now common for these patients to face a pregnancy, be it planned or unplanned. As a result, only about half the pregnant patients with cardiac disease have rheumatic or acquired valvular disease. As noted in Chapter 4, Early Pregnancy, pregnancy causes a 40% increase in cardiac output by midpregnancy. For patients with cardiac disease, this increase in demand may be potentially fatal, making pre-conceptional assessment and counseling vital for these patients. Even when patients tolerate the processes of pregnancy and labor, pregnancy-induced risk does not end with delivery. Cardiac output manifests an additional rise in the immediate postpartum period, as up to 500 mL of additional blood enters the maternal circulation owing to uterine contractions and rapid loss of uterine volume. Even after the high-risk events of the immediate postpartum period have passed, cardiac complications such as peripartum cardiomyopathy can occur up to 6 months after delivery.

The New York Heart Association classification of heart disease is a useful guide to the risk of pregnancy, because it is based on functional impact, rather than on the type of heart disease (Table 6.1). Patients with class I or II disease, such as those with septal defects, patent ductus arteriosus, or mild mitral or aortic valvular disease, generally do well during pregnancy, although their fetuses are at greater risk of prematurity and low birth weight. Patient with class III or IV disease owing to primary pulmonary hypertension, uncorrected tetralogy of Fallot, Eisenmenger syndrome, or other conditions, rarely do well, with pregnancy inducing a significant risk of death, often in excess of 50%. Patients with this degree of cardiac decompensation should be advised to avoid pregnancy or to consider termination, based on careful consultation with specialists in both cardiology and high-risk obstetrics.

Table 6.1. New York Heart Association Classification of Heart Disease

Class I	No cardiac decompensation
Class II	No symptoms of decompensation at rest
	Minor limitations of physical activity
Class III	No symptoms of decompensation at rest
	Marked limitations of physical activity
Class IV	Symptoms of decompensation at rest
	Discomfort with any physical activity

Valvular heart disease is the most commonly encountered cardiac complication of pregnancy. Rheumatic heart disease accounts for most of the valvular damage encountered. The severity of the associated valvular lesion determines the degree of risk associated with pregnancy. These patients are at increased risk of thromboembolic disease, subacute bacterial endocarditis, cardiac failure, and pulmonary edema. These women have a high rate of fetal loss early in pregnancy. Roughly 90% of these patients have mitral stenosis, which may result in worsening obstruction as cardiac output increases during the pregnancy. When severe or when associated with atrial fibrillation, the risk of cardiac failure during pregnancy increases.

It is estimated that mitral valve prolapse may be found in 5% to 7% of pregnant women. This condition is generally asymptomatic, except for a late systolic murmur or late systolic click, although arrhythmias or bacterial endocarditis may occur. Most patients with mitral valve prolapse do well and need little additional monitoring. The rare patient with left atrial and ventricular enlargement may develop dysfunction during the course of pregnancy. The severity of the disease and impact on the atrium and ventricle can be assessed by echocardiography.

Peripartum cardiomyopathy is a rare, but uniformly severe, pregnancy-associated cardiac condition. Occurring predominately in the last month of pregnancy or the first 6 months following delivery, it is similar to other cardiomyopathies in symptoms and findings. Most often a specific cause, such as myocarditis, is not identified and the etiology remains unknown. Peripartum cardiomyopathy presents an especially grave risk, necessitating early awareness and aggressive consultative management. Patients at highest risk are those in their 30s, who are multiparous, black, and who have had twins or pre-eclampsia.

Unusual cardiac conditions, such as idiopathic hypertrophic subaortic stenosis (IHSS) and the structural anomalies associated with Marfan's syndrome, are associated with maternal moralities of 25% to 50%, or greater. The presence of such conditions demands realistic preconception counseling and early transfer for specialized care should a pregnancy occur.

Diabetes and Glucose Metabolism

Approximately 1 of 50 pregnancies is complicated by either new or antecedent diabetes, in roughly equal proportions. Diabetes and pregnancy have profound effects on each other, making a familiarity with the interactions between mother, fetus, and the diabetic process necessary to provide optimal care.

The severity of diabetes can be classified by either the American Diabetic Association (ADA) classification (Table 6.2) or by the White classification schemes (Table 6.3), although

Table 6.2. American Diabetic Association Classification of Diabetes Mellitus

Type I	Childhood: often brittle, control difficult
Type II	Adult-onset
Gestational	Glucose intolerance identified during pregnancy

the latter has been rendered less useful by improvements in fetal assessment, neonatal care, and the metabolic management of the pregnant patient. The use of these classifications makes comparisons of published data meaningful and may help to predict the relative risk to the pregnant mother and fetus. Patients with ADA type I diabetes tend to be brittle, with an increased risk of diabetic ketoacidosis (DKA). These patients have a greater number of both maternal and fetal complications (Table 6.4). Patients with ADA type II disease are often overweight and may be controlled with strict diet or with minimal insulin therapy. Gestational diabetes is reversible, although these patients have a greater incidence of glucose intolerance in subsequent pregnancies or with aging. Patients with both type II and gestational diabetes have lower rates of maternal and fetal complications; however, both groups are at increased risk compared with the general population.

Effects of Pregnancy on Glucose Metabolism

Pregnancy results in significant disruptions in glucose metabolism. In early pregnancy nausea, vomiting, and changes in food preferences alter dietary patterns. Human placental lactogen (HPL), made in abundance by the growing placenta, promotes lipolysis and decreases glucose uptake and gluconeogenesis. This anti-insulin effect is sufficient to tip borderline patients into a diabetic state or prompt readjustments in the insulin dosage used by insulin-dependent diabetics. Estrogen, progesterone, and placental insulinase further complicate the management of diabetes, making diabetic ketoacidosis more common.

Effects of Diabetes on the Mother

High renal plasma flow and diffusion rates that exceed tubular reabsorption result in a physiologic glucosuria of approximately 300 mg/d. This physiologic glucosuria, combined with the poor correlation between urinary glucose and blood glucose levels, makes the use of urinary sugar screening useless to detect or monitor diabetes. This increase in urinary sugar also provides nutrients that promote urinary tract infection, resulting in a twofold increase in the rate of these infections for diabetic women during pregnancy. Diabetic

Table 6.3. White Classification of Diabetes Mellitus

Class	Onset	Duration	Vascular disease
A	Gestational	—	—
B	After age 20	<10 years	No disease
C	Age 10–19	10–19 years	No disease
D	Under age 10	≥20 years	Some, retina, legs
E	Pelvic arteriosclerosis by x-ray study		
F	Vascular nephritis		
R	Proliferative retinopathy		
T	Transplant		

Table 6.4. Maternal and Fetal Complications Associated with Maternal Diabetes

Maternal effects/risks
    Diabetic ketoacidosis
    Glucosuria
    Hyperglycemia
    Polyhydramios
    Pre-eclampsia
    Pregnancy-induced hypertension
    Preterm labor
    Retinopathy
    Urinary tract infections
    Uterine atony

Fetal or neonatal effects/risks
    Congenital anomalies
    Fetal demise
    Hydramnios
    Hyperbilirubinemia
    Hypocalcemia
    Hypoglycemia
    Macrosomia
    Polycythemia
    Prematurity
    Respiratory distress syndrome
    Spontaneous abortion

women have roughly twice the risk of developing pregnancy-induced hypertension or pre-eclampsia compared with nondiabetic patients. Diabetic retinopathy worsens in about 15% of pregnant diabetics, which can lead to proliferative retinopathy and vision loss if untreated. Roughly half of the patients with gestational diabetes will develop diabetes mellitus within 20 years.

Effects of Diabetes on the Fetus

The offspring of diabetic women are at a threefold greater risk of congenital anomalies (3% to 6%) than are those of nondiabetic mothers (1% to 2%). Most common among these anomalies are cardiac and limb deformities. Fetal macrosomia, with its attendant delivery risks, is more common in diabetic pregnancies because glucose readily crosses the placenta, whereas insulin does not. As a result, these fetuses develop hyperglycemia with increased weight gain. These neonates are at greater risk of hypoglycemia in the first few hours of life owing to compensatory (increased) insulin production by the fetal pancreas. After birth, this insulin production overshoots the amount required because of the sudden decrease in glucose supply available after separation from the sugar-rich maternal circulation. These infants have increased rates of neonatal hyperbilirubinemia, hypocalcemia, and polycythemia. Infants born of diabetic mothers have a greater incidence of respiratory distress syndrome, even when the effects of gestational age are taken into account.

Diabetic pregnancies are at significantly greater risk of spontaneous abortion, intrauterine fetal demise, and stillbirth, with fetal and neonatal mortality rates that are between 2% and 5%. These complications are less likely when glucose control is good but even with the best of control these patients' risks are still elevated compared with nondiabetic mothers. Pregnant diabetic patients are at greater risk of polyhydramnios (>2000 mL of amniotic fluid). This increase in amniotic fluid and the increased fetal weight common for these pregnancies result in overdistension of the uterus and a greater prevalence of placental abruption, preterm labor, and postpartum uterine atony.

Gastrointestinal Disease

Hormonal and physical changes induced by pregnancy have profound effects on the gastrointestinal tract and its function, often resulting in the development or worsening of gastrointestinal complaints (Table 6.5).

Nausea, vomiting, and heartburn affect more than 50% of patients during the early phases of pregnancy. Most of the symptoms are self-limited and respond to simple interventions. Intractable nausea and vomiting (hyperemesis gravidarum) occurs in about 1 of every 250 pregnancies. The possibility of other gastrointestinal pathology or abnormalities of pregnancy must be considered for these patients. Except in extreme cases, morning sickness, repeated emesis, or gastroesophageal reflux pose no threat except to the well-being of the mother.

New peptic ulcer disease and pancreatitis are rare complications of pregnancy. Existing peptic ulcers often improve during pregnancy. When pancreatitis is encountered during pregnancy, it usually happens in the third trimester and is associated with cholelithiasis, alcohol abuse, pregnancy-induced hypertension, or pre-existing liver disease. Pancreatitis is associated with significant maternal morbidity (congestive heart failure, pulmonary effusion, hypotension, hyperglycemia, and acidosis), mortality (10%), and perinatal mortality (10% to 40%).

Appendicitis complicates roughly 0.1% of pregnancies, constituting the most com-

Table 6.5. Gastrointestinal Changes During Pregnancy and Their Clinical Manifestations

Site	Physiologic changes	Clinical manifestation
Esophagus	Reduced lower sphincter pressure	Gastroesophageal reflux
		Heartburn
	Decreased motility	Erosive esophagitis
Stomach	Decreased emptying	Increased risk of aspiration during anesthesia
	Increased residual volume	
		Decreased incidence of duodenal ulcer
Small bowel	Decreased motility	Stasis
	Increased transit time	Bacterial overgrowth
	Increased activity and efficiency of brush borders	Pseudo-obstruction
		Sequestration of bile salts
		Increased nutrient absorption (some types)
Large bowel	Reduced contractility	Constipation
	Increased water and sodium absorption	Pseudo-obstruction

mon surgical emergency during pregnancy. Because of difficulty making the diagnosis and the attendant risks of surgery during pregnancy, morbidity due to appendicitis is greater during pregnancy. For these reasons, maternal mortality in the first and second trimesters is 2% and rises to as high as 10% in the third trimester. This is compared to a mortality rate of 0.25% for nonpregnant patients. Premature labor, induced by the appendicitis or its treatment, threatens the well-being of the fetus.

Inflammatory bowel disease (ulcerative colitis and Crohn's disease) has little impact on pregnancy; however, 15% to 30% of patients with these disorders experience exacerbation of their symptoms during pregnancy.

Hepatobilliary Disease and Cholelithiasis

Hepatitis is the major cause of jaundice during pregnancy. Hepatitis A accounts for 10% of cases in pregnancy, with hepatitis C, D, and E accounting for an additional 10%. The majority of cases of hepatitis encountered during pregnancy are hepatitis B, with rates that range from 1–2/1000 for acute disease to 5–15/1000 for chronic hepatitis. Groups at greatest risk for hepatitis B are intravenous drug users, hemophiliacs, homosexuals, and health care workers (Table 6.6). The course of hepatitis B is not significantly different during pregnancy and, as in the nonpregnant patient, symptoms can vary widely. Vertical transmission of the infection to the developing fetus can pose a significant risk. Untreated, the majority of infants become chronic carriers, capable of infecting others. These infants are also at increased risk of cirrhosis and hepatic cancer.

Gallbladder disease is a common affliction of women and, therefore, there is a significant risk of gallbladder disease complicating pregnancy. Gallbladder disease affects 20,000,000 people a year in the United States, which is approximately 10% of the population. Each year 1 million new cases are diagnosed, resulting in an estimated one-half million surgical cases and more than $5 billion in health care expenditures.

Although gallbladder disease occurs most frequently in individuals over the age of 40, age is only one of the major risk factors in the development of cholelithiasis (Table 6.7). The effects of pregnancy, estrogen (both natural and pharmacologic), and other unique female factors result in a disease rate that is three times higher in women than in men. Parity plays a role in the development of gallstones with 75% of affected patients having one or more

Table 6.6. Risk Factors for Hepatitis B

Blood component therapy
High-risk ethnic group (Eskimos, Asians)
History of a tattoo
Homosexual or bisexual males
Household contact with carrier
Illicit drug (past or present)
Multiple sexual partners
Occupational exposure (health care, public safety,
  developmentally disabled institution, detention facilities)
Sexual partner of infected male
Sexually transmitted disease

Table 6.7. Risk Factors for Cholelithiasis

Age >40
Cirrhosis
Crohn's disease
Diabetes
Diet and medications
Family history
Obesity
Oral contraceptives
Oral estrogen replacement
Pregnancy
Sex (female:male = 3:1)

pregnancies. During pregnancy, bile secretion roughly doubles while the rate of gallbladder emptying decreases. Of preganant patients, 3% to 4% will have symptomatic gallstones; cholecystectomy ranks second to appendectomy as the most common nonobstetric surgery performed during pregnancy. Cholecystectomy during pregnancy is associated with a fetal loss rate of 5%, which rises to about 60% if pancreatitis is present at the time of surgery.

Intrahepatic cholestasis is not uncommon during pregnancy, usually presenting during the third trimester as mild pruritus that begins at night and progresses to severe, unrelenting itching. Cholestasis of pregnancy tends to recur in subsequent pregnancies. It is associated with an increased frequency of prematurity, fetal distress, and fetal mortality.

Human Immunodeficiency Virus (HIV)

More than 10% of Americans infected with the human immunodeficiency virus (HIV) are women, although this percentage is rapidly rising. Of those women infected, over half are of childbearing age. Most women acquire the HIV infection through intravenous drug use or through sexual relations with an infected partner. More than 80% of pediatric HIV infections are acquired by vertical transmission from mother to fetus during pregnancy.

Independent of other risk factors, such as drug abuse, HIV infection does not seem to have any direct effect on the course of pregnancy. However, pregnancy does have an impact on the course of the HIV infection, slightly accelerating the process and worsening the prognosis. Between one quarter and one third of all fetuses born to HIV-infected mothers become HIV infected via transplacental passage of the virus. This is independent of the route of delivery.

Hypertension

Pregnancy can induce or further complicate pre-existent hypertension. Pregnancy-induced changes in blood pressure may be one of the early signs of pre-eclampsia and as such requires continued monitoring of blood pressure and prompt intervention when changes occur. The classification of hypertension during pregnancy is shown in Table 6.8. The term "toxemia" has been dropped in favor of more descriptive terms.

The etiology of pregnancy-induced hypertension (PIH) is unknown, although patterns of risk have been well described. Primigravid women, women with multiple gesta-

Table 6.8. Classification of Hypertension Complicating Pregnancy

Pregnancy-induced hypertension (PIH)
    Pre-eclampsia
      Mild
      Severe
    Eclampsia
Chronic hypertension preceding pregnancy
Chronic hypertension with superimposed PIH
    Superimposed pre-eclampsia
    Superimposed eclampsia

tions, hydatidiform molar pregnancies, lupus erythematosus, renal disease, or insulin-dependent diabetes are at greatest risk. When PIH is present, peripheral vasospasm, combined with the increased cardiac output of normal pregnancy, results in increased blood pressure, unpredictable changes in renal and hepatic perfusion, and reduced placental perfusion. This reduction in placental perfusion and the adverse maternal effects also caused by hypertension place the fetus at risk for intrauterine growth restriction, placental complications (e.g., abruption), and premature delivery.

Infections

A number of infections take on special significance to mother or fetus when they occur during pregnancy. The impact of these infections varies from congenital malformations, increased fetal loss, and premature labor to maternal morbidity. Most of the involved infections are common outside of pregnancy, although pregnancy notably alters their consequences.

Bacterial Vaginosis

As noted in Chapter 28, Vulvitis and Vaginal Infections, bacterial vaginosis may occur in up to one in five women, half of whom are asymptomatic. The presence of bacterial vaginosis is associated with an increased risk of complications during pregnancy, labor, and the postpartum period (Table 6.9). The diagnosis and management of bacterial vaginosis is unchanged by pregnancy. It is reviewed in Chapter 28, Vulvitis and Vaginal Infections.

Cytomegalovirus

Cytomegalovirus (CMV) infection affects 1% of births in the United States, making it the most common congenital infection. CMV can be transmitted by saliva, semen, cervical secretions, breast milk, blood, or urine. Infection with CMV is often asymptomatic, although a short nondescript febrile illness may occur. CMV is a DNA virus, which as is the case with its relative, herpes, may lie dormant for long periods. Maternal infection with CMV is associated with a 0.5% to 1.5% risk of fetal transmission. When this occurs, it is associated with roughly a 10% risk of congenital anomalies, including microcephaly, intrauterine growth restriction, or hepatosplenomegaly. About 10% of asymptomatic CMV-infected infants go on to develop sensorineural hearing loss, chorioretinitis, neurologic effects, and dental defects.

Table 6.9. Pregnancy Complications Associated with Bacterial Vaginosis

	Relative risk
Postabortal pelvic infection	3.0
Preterm delivery	1.4–3.8
Low birthweight	1.5
Premature rupture of membranes	2.4
Chorioamnionitis	1.5–2.6
Postpartum endometritis	2.2–5.8

Genital Herpes

Infection by the herpes simplex virus (HSV) poses a significant threat to the newborn. Primary maternal infections pose the greatest threat because of the greater number of virus particles present. Delivery through the lower genital tract when it is primarily infected by HSV is associated with a neonatal infection rate of more than 50%. Of those infected, neonatal mortality rates approach 50%, with serious neurologic sequella in 75% of survivors.

Gonorrhea

Infection by *Neisseria gonorrhoeae* is sufficiently common that routine screening will be positive in 1% to 8% of cases, depending on the population being served. Infection of the upper genital tract and fallopian tubes is unusual after the first few weeks of gestation, when the growing pregnancy blocks access to ascending infection. Infection present at the time of delivery is associated with gonococcal ophthalmia in the neonate, which can lead to blindness if untreated.

Group B Streptococcus

Asymptomatic colonization of the cervix by group B streptococcus occurs in about one third of all pregnancies. Half of infants born to colonized mothers will become infected. For most of these infants, the colonization is inconsequential; however, 2 to 3 infants per 1000 live births may develop septicemia, septic shock, pneumonia, or meningitis. The risk of these manifestations is greatest for premature infants, although any newborn can be affected. Signs of infection may appear up to 4 weeks after delivery. When clinical infection is present, perinatal mortality may reach 50%. Septic meningitis, caused by group B streptococcus, carries a 25% mortality.

Maternal infection, in the form of postpartum endometritis, may result from group B streptococcus. When this occurs, it is marked by sudden onset of significant fever and tachycardia, generally within 24 hours of delivery. Generalized sepsis may follow unless aggressive therapy is instituted.

Rubella

Rubella (German, or 3-day measles) can have devastating effects if infection occurs during early pregnancy. Approximately 15% of reproductive age women lack immunity to rubella, making them susceptible to infection. When immunity is present, it is lifelong. The incubation period for rubella is 14 to 21 days, with a period of communicability that ranges from 7 days before the development of a rash to 4 days after the rash appears.

Table 6.10. Clinical Manifestations of Congenital Rubella Syndrome

Congenital heart disease
Deafness
Developmental delays
Hemolytic anemia
Hepatosplenomegaly
Intrauterine growth restriction
Mental retardation
Microcephaly
Ocular abnormalities
Pneumonia
Thrombocytopenia

Rubella infections early in pregnancy are associated with an increased risk of spontaneous pregnancy loss and congenital rubella syndrome. Common defects associated with congenital rubella infection include congenital heart disease (patent ductus arteriosus), mental retardation, deafness, and cataracts (Table 6.10). Between 50% and 70% of affected infants will appear normal at birth, only subsequently showing signs of congenital infection. The risk of congenital rubella syndrome is inversely related to the gestational age of the pregnancy at the time of maternal infection (Fig 6.1).

Syphilis

Syphilis remains a significant risk to the developing fetus. The prevalence of syphilis is steady or increasing in most areas of the United States. Abortion, stillbirth, and neonatal death are

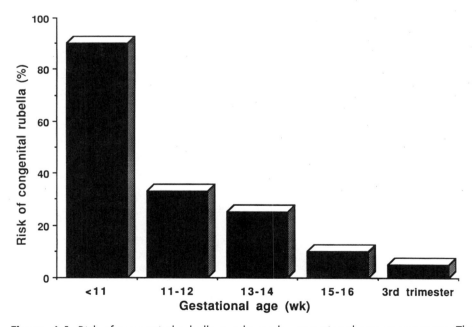

Figure. 6.1. Risk of congenital rubella syndrome by gestational age at exposure. The risk of acquiring congenital rubella syndrome is inversely related to the gestational age at which the mother is infected.

more common in any untreated patient, whereas neonatal infection is greatest in patients in the primary or secondary stages of the infection. *Treponema pallidum* crosses the placenta after 16 weeks gestation, resulting in congenital infection. Infants born with congenital syphilis show classic stigmata of infection, although most will be asymptomatic for at least the first 10 to 14 days after delivery. Early signs of infections include a maculopapular rash, sniffles, mucous patches in the mouth and oropharynx, hepatosplenomegaly, jaundice, lymphadenopathy, and chorioretinitis. Later manifestations include Hutchinson's incisors, mulberry molars, saddle nose deformity, and saber shins.

Toxoplasmosis

The ingestion of insufficiently cooked meat or contact with the infected feces of cats can result in infection by the intracellular parasite, *Toxoplasma gondii*. Domestic cats, who do not hunt and kill their own food, are not generally infected and pose little risk. Cats that are allowed to roam may become infected and their droppings may remain infectious for more than a year. Asymptomatic human infections are common, with approximately one third of reproductive age women having antibody indications of prior infection. Infection by toxoplasmosis in the first trimester of pregnancy can result in mental retardation with chorioretinitis, blindness, epilepsy, intracranial calcifications, and hydrocephalus. Roughly 60% of infants of infected mothers show serologic evidence of infection themselves. Of these, three quarters show no gross evidence of infection at the time of birth.

Multiple Gestation

Multifetal gestations occur in 1% to 2% of all pregnancies. Two thirds of twin gestations arise from fertilization of two separate ova, resulting in dizygotic (fraternal) twins. The incidence of polyzygotic, multifetal gestations varies with ethnic and racial background, heredity, maternal age, and parity. This type of twinning is more common in mothers who are themselves a dizygotic twin. The rate of dizygotic twinning is not increased if the father is a twin. In the United States, the rate of multiple gestations is highest in women who have required assisted reproduction techniques to achieve their pregnancy. The remaining third of twin gestations result from the division of a single ova fertilized by a single sperm. The point after fertilization at which division occurs determines the form that the membranes, placenta, and amniotic cavities take (Table 6.11). This type of twinning occurs at a relatively constant rate of 1 set per 250 births, independent of race, heredity, age, or parity.

Multiple gestation places both the mother and the fetuses in jeopardy for a number of complications that occur at rates that are two to six times greater than for a singleton

Table 6.11. Mechanisms of Twin Gestation Formation

Mechanism	Resulting twin pregnancy
Two ova, two sperm	Dizygotic (fraternal)
Single ova, single sperm	Monozygotic ("identical")
Division within 72 h	Diamniotic, dichorionic
Division between 4 and 8 d*	Diamniotic, monochorionic
Division 8 to 13 d	Monoamniotic, monochorionic
Division after 10 to 13 d	Conjoined twins

*Days after fertilization.

Table 6.12. Pregnancy Complications Associated with Multifetal Gestation

Abnormal fetal presentation
Cerebral palsy
Cord entwinement/entanglement
Cord prolapse
Fetal-fetal hemorrhage (resulting in hypovolemia, hypervolemia, anemia,
    hyperviscosity, cerebral injury)
Hydramnios/polyhydramnios
Increased rate of cesarean delivery
Ineffective labor
Intrauterine fetal growth restriction
Low birth weight
Malformations
Maternal anemia
Microcephaly
Obstructive uropathy
Perinatal mortality
Placenta previa
Placental abruption
Postpartum hemorrhage
Pre-eclampsia/eclampsia
Pregnancy-induced hypertension
Preterm labor and delivery
Spontaneous abortion
Uterine atony
Vasa previa

pregnancy (Table 6.12). These risks vary based on the type of twinning involved, as evidenced by the observation that monozygotic twins experience complications at a rate that is two to three times higher than that of dizygotic pregnancies. Monoamniotic twins, which account for 1% of twin pregnancies, have a 50% mortality rate.

Multiple gestations are associated with intrauterine growth restriction and the possibility of discordant growth. When there is a discrepancy of more than 25% in the weight of the fetuses, there is a threefold increase in the rate of perinatal mortality. Multifetal pregnancies are also associated with a twofold increase in the rate of congenital malformation.

Neurologic Disease and Headaches

Seizure disorders are the most common neurologic problems to coexist with pregnancy. Some studies have indicated that seizure control deteriorates during pregnancy; however, more recent experience suggests that when careful monitoring and adjustment of medication is carried out, this need not be the case. Hepatic changes induced by pregnancy result in accelerated metabolism of many of the drugs used to treat seizures, necessitating increased doses to maintain therapeutic blood levels. These adjustments may be on the order of a twofold increase.

Both untreated and treated epilepsy appear to be associated with an increased risk of fetal malformations. The use of phenytoin in pregnancy is associated with microcephaly, mild to moderate mental retardation, developmental delay, facial dysmorphisms and clefts, limb abnormalities, and genital malformations. This collection of changes is often referred to as the "fetal hydantoin syndrome," and may be found in over 10% of infants born to mothers who use phenytoin. Other drugs commonly used to control seizures have an associated risk of cranial, facial, and neural tube defects. The risk of these malformations is higher than the background rate, but the risk of treatment is generally seen to be outweighed by the risks of the untreated seizure disorder.

Between 15% and 20% of pregnant women experience migraine headaches. The effect of pregnancy on the frequency and severity of migraine headaches is somewhat unpredictable, as some women experience improvement and others find their symptoms worsen. Patients who experience their worst headaches around the time of menstruation are often the most likely to improve; smokers are those most likely to experience a worsening.

Respiratory Disease and Asthma

Asthma is found in roughly 1% of pregnant patients, approximately 15% of whom will have one or more severe asthma attacks during pregnancy. Pregnancy has little effect for about half of pregnant asthmatics, with roughly equal proportions of the remaining patients experiencing worsening or improvement in their symptoms. Pregnancy-induced changes, such as bronchial wall edema, thickened airway secretions, and smooth muscle contraction, constrict airway diameter, resulting in increased airway resistance, decreased expiratory air flow, increased respiratory effort, and altered blood gasses. The effects of asthma on pregnancy are highly variable, but may include chronic hypoxia, intrauterine growth restriction, and, rarely, fetal death. When asthma attacks are kept to a minimum and there is maximal air exchange, the impact on the fetus may be negligible, which are the goals to which asthma treatment during pregnancy is directed.

Affecting over 40% of Americans every year, the symptoms of the common cold are familiar to us all. Although the prevalence of the common cold is unchanged during pregnancy, the sneezing, runny nose, and malaise generally last longer than the usual 6 to 10 days, and may range up to 26 days. Coryza (rhinorrhea and sneezing) affects 50% to 66% of patients, with almost 50% of patients experiencing pharyngitis. Hoarseness and cough develop in 25% to 50% of patients. Between 25% and 45% of patients experience headache, muscular aches, lethargy, and malaise, although only 15% to 30% of patients actually develop fever or chills. It is important to differentiate the common cold from more sinister problems such as influenza, *Mycoplasma pneumoniae,* streptococcal pharyngitis, and the very dangerous, although relatively rare, varicella pneumonia. Pneumonia during pregnancy is uncommon, but carries a 3% to 4% maternal mortality.

Substance Abuse

The use of legal and illicit drugs and substances that pose a threat to the pregnant mother and fetus has risen. It is now likely that almost all patients will encounter one or more medications, over-the-counter remedies, alcohol-containing products or drinks, or tobacco-products at some time during the course of a pregnancy.

Any patient who is, or may become pregnant, must be aware of the possible adverse effects that substances and medications can have on a pregnancy. These patients should be advised to alert all health care providers of their pregnancy status when medications are prescribed. They should also read all labels on over-the-counter medications, checking with the health care team if there is any question about safety or the availabilty of alternate treatments.

Cocaine use has become more widespread as cost has gone down and accessibility has risen. Cocaine is highly addictive and associated with a number of adverse health effects, both directly and through the associated behavioral and lifestyle changes associated with its use. Spontaneous abortion, intrauterine fetal death, premature rupture of the membranes (20%), preterm labor and delivery (25%), intrauterine growth restriction (30%), predelivery meconium passage (30%), and placental abruption (6% to 10%) are all potential complications that result from cocaine use in pregnancy. Congenital malformations, such as segmental intestinal atresia, limb-reduction defects, disruptive brain anomalies, congenital heart defects, prune-belly syndrome, and urinary tract abnormalities, have been associated with cocaine use during pregnancy. Surviving infants of cocaine-using mothers are at higher risk for sudden infant death syndrome (SIDS), poor learning and school performance, and behavioral problems.

The use of marijuana, opiates, or hallucinogens during pregnancy is associated with significant fetal risk. It is estimated that between 5% and 15% of pregnant women may use marijuana or hashish during pregnancy. In animals, the active compounds in marijuana are teratogenic, although the human effects are less clear cut. Heroin abuse during pregnancy is associated with rates of stillbirth, fetal growth restriction, and premature labor and delivery that are three times higher than those in the general population. Newborn narcotic withdrawal, which appears 1 to 2 days after birth and is potentially fatal, is seen in two thirds of infants born to narcotic users.

Two thirds of women of childbearing age report being current drinkers, with approximately one third of all women continuing some level of alcohol consumption during pregnancy. It is estimated that between 7% and 10% of women seeking prenatal care are alcohol abusers. Alcohol is both a morphologic and behavioral teratogen, with an estimated 5000 births per year affected by fetal alcohol syndrome. Morphologic and behavioral sequelae can result from in utero exposure to chronic alcohol intake (see Chapter 11, Periodic Testing and Health Maintenance, Table 11.5). Alcohol use is the most commonly identifiable cause of mental retardation for children born in the United States. Fetal alcohol syndrome is usually seen in children of women who consume 3 oz or more of alcohol per day during pregnancy, but there does not appear to be a threshold below which alcohol is completely safe. The greatest jeopardy arises through exposure during the first trimester.

Roughly one quarter of all American women of reproductive age smoke. This proportion rises to 35% for women between age 18 and 25. Up to a third of pregnant women continue to smoke during pregnancy, resulting in higher rates of pregnancy complications. Pregnant smokers are more likely to have premature rupture of the membranes, premature birth, intrauterine growth restriction, and a low birth weight infant. These effects come about owing to the effects of carbon monoxide and the vasoconstriction caused by nicotine.

Surgical Conditions and Trauma

Surgical emergencies are neither more nor less common in pregnancy. Only the problem of dealing with two patients simultaneously affects the diagnosis and management of these cases. When a surgical emergency arises, care is directed toward rapid diagnosis and intervention as needed. Radiologic studies may be carried out as needed, for the risk of misdiagnosis far outweighs the minimal risk of radiation exposure. The only considerations that pregnancy requires are periodic assessment of the fetal status and an awareness of maternal physiologic changes. This latter is helpful to avoid such things as supine hypotension, caused by vena cava compression by the pregnant uterus, aspiration of gastric contents during the induction of anesthesia, or ventilatory compromise due to the reduced functional reserve induced by pregnancy.

The two most common forms of trauma encountered during pregnancy are domestic abuse and motor vehicle accidents. The incidence of domestic abuse does not diminish during pregnancy; it is estimated to occur to 10% or more of pregnant women. Most of the injuries found jeopardize the health and safety of the mother; direct fetal or uterine injury is uncommon, but has been reported. Domestic abuse remains a major source of life-threatening injury or homicide and, as such, threatens the safety of the pregnancy.

The greatest danger of injury during a motor vehicle accident occurs to unrestrained passengers. Even with the use of seat and shoulder restraints, separation of the placenta from the uterine wall may result from the shearing forces involved in abrupt deceleration. Fetal-maternal bleeding occurs in 5% to 25% of trauma cases, but the volume of bleeding is generally small. This transfer of fetal cells may be sufficient to induce Rh sensitization, making it important to provide Rh immune globulin for Rh-negative mothers. Uterine rupture is associated with severe direct trauma to the abdomen. Fetal death is rare, except as a result of maternal death or compromise.

Thrombophlebitis and Embolism

The risk of superficial and deep vein phlebitis and of pulmonary embolism is increased during pregnancy and the postpartum period owing to increases in key coagulation factors, venous stasis, and peripheral vascular pooling brought on by pregnancy. Superficial thrombophlebitis is the most common of these phenomena, occurring roughly in 1 of 500 to 750 pregnancies. Most of these cases happen in the first 72 hours following delivery. Superficial thrombophlebitis offers little risk beyond maternal discomfort.

Deep venous thrombophlebitis is less common, but potentially more serious. Deep vein thrombophlebitis is estimated to happen in between 0.15% to 3% of pregnancies and, as with superficial thrombophlebitis, is found most often in the postpartum period. Recent studies using sophisticated new technology suggest that these estimates of frequency may be very low compared with the true incidence of asymptomatic disease. Although frequently unapparent, deep vein thrombophlebitis is often the forerunner of pulmonary embolism. Pulmonary embolism represents a potentially catastrophic mishap, with two thirds of fatalities within 30 minutes of the acute event. With rapid diagnosis and prompt anticoagulation, mortality can be reduced to less than 1%.

Septic pelvic thrombophlebitis may be found in postpartum patients with bacterial infections of the uterus. These infections spread to the ovarian veins, setting in motion the process that results in septic thrombophlebitis. Septic thrombophlebitis is more common in the right ovarian vein than the left, but either or both may be involved. Like deep vein thrombophlebitis, septic thrombophlebitis represents a risk for pulmonary embolism and must be diagnosed and treated aggressively.

Urinary Tract Infection and Renal Disease

Urinary stasis, decreased ureteral tone and motility, a relatively more alkaline urine, mild glucosuria, and the mechanical effects of the growing uterus all conspire to place pregnant women at increased risk for urinary tract infection. Urinary tract infections and pyelonephritis frequently provoke significant morbidity during pregnancy and are very common medical complications found in pregnancy. Asymptomatic bacteriuria occurs in 4% to 8% of pregnant women, whereas acute cystitis complicates 1% to 3% of pregnancies. It is estimated that 40% of women with untreated asymptomatic bacteriuria will develop pyelonephritis. Pyelonephritis affects 2% of all pregnant women, resulting in acute illness with fever, costovertebral tenderness, malaise, and dehydration. About 1 of 5 patients will have uterine irritability or preterm labor and 1 of 10 patients will have positive blood cultures.

Acute cystitis and symptomatic bacteriuria are more common, although less threatening complications of pregnancy. Of women with asymptomatic bacteriuria, 40% will go on to develop symptoms. Even with treatment, 25% to 30% of these patients will progress to symptomatic infections. Recurrent infections, or those that fail to respond to appropriate therapy, should prompt a suspicion of other urinary tract disease. Evaluation of this possibility can generally be deferred until 6 weeks after delivery.

Urinary calculi are found in roughly 1 of 1500 pregnant women. Recurrent symptoms of pyelonephritis, urinary tract infections by *Proteus* species, or microhematuria should all suggest the possibility of stones. Renal colic is less prevalent during pregnancy than at other times.

Table 6.13. Effect of Pregnancy on Common Chronic Renal Diseases

Renal Disease	Effects
Chronic pyelonephritis	No effect on renal lesion
	Increased incidence of symptomatic UTI
Urolithiasis	No direct effect on renal lesion
	UTI more frequent in some cases
Diabetic nephropathy	No effect on renal lesion
	Increased incidence UTI, pre-eclampsia
Chronic glomerulonephritis	No effect on renal lesion in the absence of hypertension
	Increased incidence UTI
Systemic lupus erythematosus	Often no effect on renal lesion, although about 33% of patients show some worsening of renal function
	Prognosis improves if SLE is in remission more than 6 months
Polycystic disease	No effect on renal lesion
Scleroderma	Unusual association with pregnancy, because onset of disease is more common in 4th or 5th decades
	No effect on preexisting renal lesion
	Disease may be fulminant if onset during pregnancy; postpartum exacerbation common
Periarteritis nodosa	Maternal and neonatal mortality rates high, because of frequent association with malignant hypertension; poor prognosis
	Therapeutic abortion should be presented as an option of management

UTI = urinary tract infection; SLE = systemic lups erythematosus.

Chronic renal disease is not a contraindication to pregnancy if creatinine levels are below 2 mg/dL and there is no elevation of diastolic blood pressure above 90 mm Hg. When these criteria are met, there is a minimal increase in the risk of pregnancy complications and long-term renal effects, although there is a slight increase in first trimester losses for these patients. Patients with chronic renal disease are at greater risk of intrauterine growth restriction, necessitating close appraisal of fetal growth and well-being in the later stages of pregnancy. Renal transplants that were placed more than 2 years prior to pregnancy that show no signs of rejection do not alter the normal prognosis for pregnancy.

Proteinuria is found in 50% of patients with renal disease and its level is not predictive of the renal impact of pregnancy. The presence of significant proteinuria in otherwise healthy patients should suggest pathology and requires immediate investigation. The effects of pregnancy on common renal diseases is shown in Table 6.13.

ESTABLISHING THE DIAGNOSIS

Anemias

Because iron-deficiency anemia accounts for approximately 90% of all anemia found during pregnancy, extensive evaluation of any anemia should be delayed until an empiric trial of iron therapy has been instituted and the results noted. Iron-deficiency anemia is characterized by small, pale erythrocytes seen on peripheral smear, along with a reduction in mean corpuscular volume (MCV) and corpuscular hemoglobin concentration (MCHC). Studies of iron dynamics, such as serum iron, iron-binding capacity, and serum ferritin, may be used to confirm the diagnosis. For most patients, the presence of genetically determined anemia will either be known prior to pregnancy or may suspected based on family history or screening tests. Hemoglobin electrophoresis is diagnostic.

Cancer

The evaluation of patients with abnormal cervical cytology proceeds as outlined in Chapter 13, Abnormal Pap Smears, with the exception of endocervical curettage, which is generally omitted during pregnancy. Patients with severe dysplasia or carcinoma in situ may be followed with serial Pap smears and colposcopic examinations. Microinvasive cervical carcinoma must be evaluated by conization performed during the second or third trimesters. This provides vital information about depth of invasion, and may be curative for patients with invasion of 1 mL or less.

The evaluation of patients suspected of breast, ovarian or colorectal cancer, or lymphoma is unchanged by pregnancy, with the exception that exploratory abdominal surgery is generally delayed until after 16 weeks gestation whenever possible.

Cardiac Disease

The diagnosis of cardiac disease in pregnancy is established in the same way as it is for patients who are not pregnant. There are no contraindications to electrocardiography, Holter

Table 6.14. Risk Factors for Gestational Diabetes

Gestational diabetes during a previous pregnancy
Obesity
Persistent glucosuria
Previous infant weighing >4000 g
Repeated spontaneous abortions
Strong family history of diabetes
Unexplained stillbirth

arrhythmia monitoring, or echocardiography. Although excessive exercise in a pregnancy in which cardiac disease is suspected should be discouraged, limited stress testing may be carried out, based on the needs of the individual patient. Although a systolic flow murmur is often found in pregnancy (owing to increased cardiac output), diastolic murmurs, loud or mechanical murmurs, or arrhythmias should suggest the possibility of cardiac disease and warrant further evaluation.

Diabetes

The diagnosis of gestational diabetes is most often made through routine screening tests, although the presence of historical risk factors should increase suspicion (Table 6.14). One half of all patients diagnosed with gestational diabetes have no risk factor identified, underscoring the need for routine screening of all pregnant patients.

The most common screening test for gestational diabetes is a plasma glucose level drawn 1 hour after ingestion of a 50-g glucose load. This is usually performed between 24 and 32 weeks gestation for patients without risk factors and earlier for patients with factors that place them at higher risk. The upper limit of normal for such a test is 140 mg/dL (7.8 mM/L). If a patient's value exceeds this threshold, a formal 3-hour glucose tolerance test is performed. About 15% of patients will have an abnormal screening test and about the same proportion will have an abnormal 3-hour test.

To correctly perform a 3-hour glucose tolerance test, the patient must ingest a minimum of 150 g of glucose per day for the 3 days preceding the test. On the day of the test, a fasting glucose level is drawn, and a 100-g glucose load is consumed. Plasma glucose levels are then determined at 1, 2, and 3 hours after the glucose load was consumed. Upper limits of normal for blood and plasma levels at these times are shown in Table 6.15. If two or more values are greater than these thresholds, the diagnosis of gestational diabetes can be made. If only one value is abnormal, the test is considered equivocal and should be repeated in 4 to 6 weeks.

Table 6.15. Upper Limits of Normal for Oral Glucose Tolerance Tests During Pregnancy

Time	Blood glucose mg/dL (mM/L)	Plasma glucose mg/dL (mM/L)
Fasting	90 (5.0)	105 (5.8)
1 h	165 (9.2)	190 (10.6)
2 h	145 (8.1)	165 (9.2)
3 h	125 (6.9)	145 (8.1)

Gastrointestinal Disease

The diagnosis of gastroesophageal reflux and peptic ulcer disease is suggested by history and confirmed by empiric therapy. Endoscopy is not specifically contraindicated during pregnancy, although it is seldom necessary.

Pancreatitis generally presents with nausea, emesis, and mid-epigastric pain that radiates to the midback. Physical examination of these patients may be unremarkable or may demonstrate left upper quadrant, epigastric, or flank tenderness. Laboratory studies will confirm elevations in serum amylase and lipase levels on the order of 200 U/dL or greater. These levels return to normal within 48 hours of the initial episode. Pregnancy may mask some of the physical findings, but laboratory evidence is unaltered.

Appendicitis is suspected when nausea and vomiting follow anorexia and a periumbilical pain is reported which may migrate toward the right flank or right lower quadrant. Displacement of the appendix upward as the uterus grows often alters the location where pain is described. During the first weeks of pregnancy, appendicitis must be differentiated from ectopic pregnancy, salpingitis, rupture or bleeding in a corpus luteum cyst, or torsion. Because of the complicated clinical course associated with rupture of the appendix, early suspicion and assertive diagnostic evaluation must be pursued.

Hepatobilliary Disease and Cholelithiasis

Hepatitis during pregnancy is diagnosed in the same manner as for nonpregnant patients. Serum chemistry abnormalities indicate active hepatic disease, whereas immunochemistry indicates the presence of infection and the phase of the clinical course. Because of the risk to the fetus posed by vertical transmission, routine screening of all pregnant patients is recommended. Patients who have demonstrated the presence of hepatitis B surface antigen (HBsAg) should be tested for other antibodies and the presence of the envelope antigen. Patients with the envelope antigen have an 80% chance of vertical transmission of the infection.

The diagnosis of cholelithiasis is based on history, physical examination, and laboratory investigation. During pregnancy, the classic complaints of fatty food intolerance, variable right upper quadrant pain with radiation to the back or scapula, nausea, or vomiting, may be masked or misinterpreted. Symptoms are often mistaken for indigestion, "morning sickness," or dyspepsia. Without increased suspicion, the diagnosis is often overlooked.

Laboratory evaluation is supportive, but often not diagnostic. A complete blood count may indicate inflammation by way of leukocytosis. An elevated serum bilirubin may be useful in diagnosing obstruction and serum amylase may indicate the presence of pancreatitis. Determination of serum alkaline phosphatase may indicate obstruction. Alkaline phosphatase is often elevated during pregnancy, compromising the utility of this test in pregnant patients. Elevated serum amino transferase (serum glutamic akalocetic transaminase [SGOT] or serum glutamic pyruvic transaminase [SGPT]) can indicate altered metabolic function of liver cells in cases where obstruction causes damage.

The standard diagnostic tool for cholelithiasis is abdominal ultrasound, which is 96% accurate in making the diagnosis of sludge or stone in the gallbladder. Ultrasonography has surpassed oral cholecystograms as the diagnostic test of choice, even when the patient is not pregnant. The false-negative rate with oral cholecystograms is high and 20% of patients experience nausea, vomiting, or diarrhea from the contrast agent. A flat plate of the abdomen will demonstrate only the 20% of stones that have enough calcium for accurate imaging. The desire to limit x-ray exposure, combined with these shortcomings, supports the use of ultrasonography as the imaging method of choice.

Cholestasis of pregnancy may be suspected based on the history of itching late in pregnancy and confirmed by documenting increased circulating levels of bile acids. Mild elevations of lever enzymes may also be present. Total bilirubin levels are often elevated as well, but are generally less than 86 mmol/L (5 mg/dL).

Human Immunodeficiency Virus (HIV)

The diagnosis of HIV infection is established for pregnant patients in the same way that it is for other patients: Western blot screening, with enzyme-linked immunosorbent assay test (ELISA) confirmation. Based on both the prevalence of HIV in the population served and the potential offered by suppressive therapy during pregnancy, routine screening of all pregnant patients should be considered.

Hypertension

Pregnancy-induced hypertension is defined as a systolic blood pressure of at least 140 mm Hg or a diastolic pressure of at least 90 mm Hg on a minimum of two occasions several hours apart. Pre-eclampsia involves the presence of proteinuria, pathologic swelling, or both. The severity of pre-eclampsia is determined by the indicators shown in Table 6.16.

The vascular constriction of PIH results in a clinical picture suggestive of intravascular volume depletion, with clinical findings such as a rising hematocrit. This impression of volume depletion is spurious and the actual physiology must be borne in mind when treatments are formulated.

Infections

The key to diagnosing infections during pregnancy is suspicion. Cytomegalovirus infections are more common in lower socioeconomic groups, but no group of patients is exempt. There are no reliable serologic tests for CMV, making it a diagnosis of exclusion.

Herpes infections during pregnancy are diagnosed in the same manner as for the non-

Table 6.16. Classification of Pre-eclampsia by Symptoms and Findings

Finding	Mild	Severe
Convulsions	Absent	Present
Diastolic blood pressure (mm Hg)	100	≥100
Fetal growth restriction	Absent	Present
Headache	Absent	Present
Liver function tests	Normal	Abnormal
Oliguria	Absent	Present
Proteinuria	Trace to 1+	≥2+
Serum creatinine level	Normal	Elevated
Thrombocytopenia	Absent	Present
Upper abdominal pain	Absent	Present
Visual changes	Absent	Present

pregnant patient: Clinical findings, cell culture, pap smear, or serologic testing. Patients with a history of herpes infections in the past should be inspected for signs of lesions during the last weeks of pregnancy and when rupture of the membranes occurs. Serial cultures are not cost effective and should be abandoned.

Routine screening for gonorrheal infections should be a part of the first prenatal visit. The high prevalence of this infection in most populations makes this routine screening cost effective. In high-risk populations, a follow-up culture late in gestation should also be considered.

The diagnosis of group B streptococcal colonization is made by cervical culture. Unfortunately, cervical cultures may be positive only intermittently even in the same patient. Routine culture of patients near term has failed to reduce the rate of neonatal infections and is probably unwarranted. Cultures may be reasonable for patients at risk for premature delivery, such as those women with preterm labor or premature rupture of the membranes.

Rubella infection may be suspected clinically and confirmed serologically.

As with rubella, syphilis is suspected clinically and confirmed serologically. Chronic diseases, such as lupus, or some forms of drug addiction can result in false-positive venereal disease research laboratory (VDRL) or rapid plasma reagin (RPR) tests, which should be confirmed by treponemal-specific tests. Dark-field microscopy can identify spirochetes directly in material obtained from primary lesions, although skill in doing so is rapidly being lost.

Infection by toxoplasmosis is generally asymptomatic, so diagnosis is basis on serologic testing. Serologic testing cannot identify the time of infection, making routine testing ineffectual. Fetal blood testing may be done when it is likely that an infection has occurred.

Multiple Gestation

Multiple gestation may be suspected based on the history of use of a fertility agent, a discordance between menstrual dates and uterine size, or an abnormality of gestation-sensitive laboratory tests, such as maternal serum alpha-fetoprotein (MSAFP). A family history of twinning is only a weak indicator. Suspicion may be raised by abdominal palpation or by Doppler ultrasound detection of multiple heart beats. The diagnosis should not be established by these modalities because fetal position, maternal obesity, the presence of hydramnios, or other factors make these techniques unreliable. The diagnosis is best confirmed by ultrasonography. Radiographic studies are generally inadequate to establish the presence or health of a multiple pregnancy, making the routine use of them undesirable. Serial ultrasonographic examinations are necessary to monitor the adequacy and concordance of fetal growth.

Neurologic Disease and Headaches

The diagnosis of seizure disorders and migraine headaches is unchanged by the presence of pregnancy.

Respiratory Disease and Asthma

The diagnosis of asthma is generally established before pregnancy, although new cases of asthma may occasionally become manifest during gestation. In these cases, the diagnosis is established as it would be in any other patient. The physiologic changes induced by pregnancy (decreased residual volume, decreased functional residual capacity, increased total capacity) do not interfere with the most commonly used criterion for asthma—restricted expiratory flow rate.

The degree of compromise induced by a patient's asthma is important to determine and monitor. Patients with severe asthma or frequent attacks must be closely monitored, including aggressive monitoring of maternal oxygenation, electronic fetal monitoring, and biophysical profiles. These patients require collaborative management, with many needing acute or chronic hospitalization.

As with asthma, upper respiratory tract infections are diagnosed using the same criteria during pregnancy that are used when the patient is not pregnant. In severe cases or in patients with pneumonia, blood gas determinations of maternal oxygenation and fetal evaluations may be in order.

Substance Abuse

The only way to establish the diagnosis of substance abuse during pregnancy is to suspect it. Most often, the diagnosis can be confirmed by history, although urine drug screening may be required. Urine toxicology provides objective evidence and may help in identifying the exact substances involved when a history is unavailable or unreliable. Questionnaires that may help to identify alcohol or tobacco abusers are outlined in Chapter 11, Periodic Testing and Health Maintenance.

Surgical Conditions and Trauma

The diagnosis of surgical or traumatic conditions is unaffected by pregnancy. As noted above, radiologic studies and other diagnostic procedures should be performed as needed to protect the health of the mother and, by extension, protect the fetus. Trauma patients who have passed the point of fetal viability should have fetal monitoring performed for several hours after the injury to ensure fetal well-being. Monitoring for vaginal bleeding or uterine tenderness should be maintained for the first 24 hours. The presence and degree of fetal-maternal bleeding that may have occurred can be assessed using a test such as the Kleihauer-Betke test. This can provide guidance regarding the need for, and the amount of, Rh immune globulin that should be offered to Rh-negative mothers.

Thrombophlebitis and Embolism

The diagnosis of thromboembolic processes is little changed by pregnancy and the puerperium. Superficial thrombophlebitis typically presents with redness, tenderness, and tender, palpable veins, usually in the calves. Deep vein thrombophlebitis may be suspected by swelling, tenderness to palpation and manipulation, popliteal tenderness, and fever. Unfortunately, during pregnancy these signs of superficial or deep thrombophlebitis may be absent. Venography, Doppler ultrasonography, or impedance plethysmography may provide confirmation of the diagnosis.

Pulmonary embolism must be suspected even in the face of nonspecific signs and symptoms, such as tachypnea, shortness of breath, diffuse or referred pain, and subtle electrocardiographic changes. Arterial blood gas analysis showing a Pao_2 of less than 80 mm

Hg is suggestive of embolism. Ventilation/perfusion lung scans may be helpful, although pulmonary angiography is sometimes necessary to confirm the diagnosis. In skilled hands, angiography is associated with significantly less than the 0.05 Gy (5 rad) threshold for fetal concern. Because of both the significant mortality rate associated with untreated embolism and the limited fetal risks involved, the benefits of investigation outweigh potential risks.

Septic thrombophlebitis will be manifest by persistent fever spikes despite improvement in other indicators of infection, such as uterine tenderness or elevated white blood count. In some patients, "cords" may be found on palpation of the adnexa. Suspicion provides the best diagnostic ally.

Urinary Tract Infection and Renal Disease

At the first prenatal visit it is usual to obtain a screening urine culture. Growth of a single pathogen at levels of greater than 10^5 colony-forming units (CFU) per milliliter of urine will identify asymptomatic bacteriuria and establish the causative agent. As few as 10^2 to 10^4 CFU/mL of *E. Coli, S. saprophyticus,* or *Proteus* should be considered indicative of infection and warrant treatment.

Screening with dip-stick urine testing at each prenatal visit is not cost effective. Rather, urinalysis or urine culture should be obtained when an infection is suspected based on symptoms.

THERAPEUTIC OPTIONS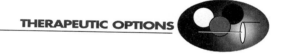

Anemias

The most common forms of anemia, iron or folate-deficiency, respond well to simple dietary supplementation. Supplementation with 30 mg ferrous iron and 1 mg of folate daily is suggested. These iron requirements may be met using 150 mg ferrous sulfate, 300 mg ferrous gluconate, or 100 mg of ferrous fumarate.

Cancer

Cervical dysplasia and carcinoma diagnosed during pregnancy are managed based on the stage of the disease, the stage of the gestation, and the wishes of the patient. Mild, moderate, or severe dysplasia (including carcinoma in situ) may be managed conservatively, with follow-up evaluation at 6 to 8 weeks after delivery. Microinvasive carcinoma of the cervix of less than 1 mm invasion may be cured by the diagnostic conization usually performed to establish the extent of the disease. When invasion of greater than 1 mm is found, postpartum hysterectomy is generally advocated. If a single focus of carcinoma with a depth of invasion of 3 to 5 mm is found, with no lymphatic or vascular involvement, it is often recommended to delay until fetal maturity is attained, followed by abdominal delivery and radical hysterectomy. When vascular or lymphatic invasion is found and the gestation is less than 24 weeks, termination and immediate treatment is thought to be best. If the patient is already beyond 24 weeks, treatment is delayed until fetal lung maturity has been achieved. Clearly, these patients need to be co-managed with, or transferred to the care of, a cancer specialist.

Disseminated or late stage breast cancer is often responsive to hormonal ablation. When diagnosed early in pregnancy, termination followed by chemotherapy is often advised. When the diagnosis is established later in pregnancy, an attempt to delay treatment until fetal maturity is reached may pose acceptable risks. In a few, selected patients, chemotherapy has been given during the second or third trimesters.

The management of melanomas, colorectal cancers, or lymphomas is determined based on the stage of the disease and must be individualized to the needs of the patient and the stage of pregnancy. Consultation or transfer of care will be required for these patients.

Cardiac Disease

The basis of antepartum management of the patient with cardiac disease consists of frequent evaluations of maternal cardiac status and fetal well-being, combined with avoidance of conditions or actions that increase cardiac workload. The latter includes the treatment or avoidance of anemia, prompt treatment of any infection or fever, limitation of strenuous activity, and adherence to appropriate weight gain. Sodium restriction and the use of the lateral decubitus position to promote diuresis may be helpful for some patients. Patients with class I or II heart disease should be encouraged to limit excessive activity and increase home rest wherever possible. More severe cases often require repeated or prolonged hospitalization. Anticoagulation, antibiotic prophylaxis, the use of β-adrenergic receptor blockers, invasive cardiac monitoring, or even surgical correction of cardiac lesions may be required.

Peripartum management of patients with cardiac disease is directed toward lessening the stresses of labor and the physiologic changes of the postpartum period. Labor in the lateral position promotes venous return, facilitating cardiac function. Conduction anesthesia is recommended to reduce the stress of labor, although careful management of fluids and blood pressure must be maintained. Shortening the duration and intensity of the second stage of labor, through the use of forceps or a vacuum-assist device, is often desirable. Vaginal delivery is always preferred over the increased stress of cesarean section.

Careful monitoring during the immediate postpartum period is required because of the rapid hemodynamic changes induced by delivery, blood loss, and the altered size and function of the uterus. Most obstetric cardiac deaths occur following delivery, underscoring the need for increased monitoring during this period.

Diabetes

Optimal management of diabetes begins before pregnancy. Although there is debate whether or not this results in a reduced incidence of congenital anomalies, other maternal and neonatal benefits support the desirability of good glucose control. Optimal diabetic management cannot be attained without patient and family education. For the established diabetic, this teaching is directed toward the need for tighter control and more frequent monitoring. The newly diagnosed diabetic will require general instruction about her disease as well as the unique aspects of diabetes during pregnancy.

Table 6.17. Daily Caloric Recommendations for Women with Gestational Diabetes

Ideal body weight (%)	Daily caloric intake (kcal/kg)*
<80	35–40
80–120	30
120–150	24
>150	12–15

*Present body weight.
Adapted from: Mulford MI, Jovanovic-Peterson L, Peterson CM. Alternative therapies for the management of gestational diabetes. Clin Perinatol 1993;20:630.

For most patients with gestational diabetes, optimal glucose control can be accomplished with diet alone (Table 6.17). Even insulin-dependent diabetics will benefit from nutritional counseling and control. Management, whether by diet, insulin, or a combination, is directed toward maintaining ideal blood sugar values throughout the day (Table 6.18). Patients with type I diabetes are at risk for the development of diabetic ketoacidosis. This is a serious complication that can be avoided by frequent blood glucose determinations and careful education.

Fetal Assessment

Because of the increased risk of fetal anomalies, a determination of maternal serum alpha-fetoprotein and early ultrasonographic studies should be carried out. Maternal alpha-fetoprotein levels may be lower in diabetic pregnancies, requiring care in interpretation.

For patients who do not need insulin therapy, the perinatal outcome is generally good. These patients do require monitoring of fetal growth to detect macrosomia, but delivery plans can remain unaltered.

Patients with poor glucose control or those that require insulin should have close fetal surveillance beginning at about 30 or 32 weeks gestation. Fetal activity counts and weekly biophysical profiles should be instituted. Fetal nonstress testing should be considered as an adjunct to biophysical profiles for many patients and must be considered if the biophysical profile shows signs of fetal compromise. Serial ultrasonographic measurements of fetal weight should be carried out to monitor for the development of either fetal growth restriction or macrosomia.

Delivery Considerations

Because of the prevalence of fetal macrosomia and intrauterine fetal demise in diabetic pregnancies, active management of labor is often undertaken, with labor induced between 38

Table 6.18. Therapeutic Objectives of Plasma Glucose Levels in Pregnancy Complicated by Diabetes

	Plasma glucose (mg/dL)
Fasting	60–90
Before lunch, dinner, evening snack	60–105
After meals: 1 h	<130–140
2 h	<120
Night (2 AM–6 AM)	60–90

and 40 weeks gestation. Induction may have to be considered at an even earlier gestational age based on changes in the biophysical profile, nonstress testing, or maternal status.

Care must be taken to assess fetal lung maturity if induction prior to term is to be considered, which is most often done through amniocentesis. Because the presence of phosphatidylglycerol is not a reliable indicator of fetal maturity in diabetic patients, most clinicians use a combination of two or more indicators of fetal maturity.

Intrapartum glucose control is generally maintained by the infusion of 5% dextrose solution at a rate of 100 mL/h. Frequent measurements of plasma glucose are made and adjustments implemented through the use of short-acting insulin. The use of a constant infusion of insulin has also been advocated. The choice of method should be adjusted for the needs of the patient and the experience of the clinician. Consultation with an experienced maternal-fetal medicine specialist should be considered.

The route of delivery offered to diabetic mothers is predicated on estimated fetal weight. When fetal weight is normal, no change in the normal routes of delivery is needed. When fetal macrosomia is present, cesarean delivery should be considered to avoid birth trauma and shoulder dystocia. Fetuses estimated to weigh more than 4500 to 5000 g should be delivered by cesarean section.

Postpartum Management

In the immediate postpartum period, assessment of vaginal blood loss should be frequent because these patients have a greater incidence of uterine atony and increased blood loss. This uterine atony can be treated as it would with any patient: oxytocin, methylergonovine maleate (Methergine), and fundal massage.

With the loss of the placenta, there is a withdrawal of its antiinsulin factors, resulting in a decreased need for insulin in the first few days following delivery. As a result, many patients require 50% or less of their predelivery levels of insulin. About 95% of gestational diabetic patients will return to normal following delivery. Follow-up glucose tolerance testing 4 to 6 months after delivery should be considered to identify the few patients who remain diabetic and will require further therapy. Barrier contraception is preferred to avoid any potential interaction between steroid contraceptives and diabetes on the maternal vascular system.

Gastrointestinal Disease

The treatment of most gastrointestinal disease is unaltered by pregnancy. Surgical intervention in the treatment of pancreatitis is uncommon, but frequently necessary for the treatment of appendicitis. Fetal monitoring should be maintained and tocolysis must be available should uterine contractions become evident.

Hepatobilliary Disease and Cholelithiasis

Prophylaxis against hepatitis begins with active immunization of those at risk before a pregnancy is planned. Patients exposed to hepatitis A may be given gamma globulin in the same manner as for nonpregnant patients. Patients exposed to hepatitis B or those found to be carriers during routine screening may receive either active immunization with hepatitis vaccine or passive immunization with hepatitis B immune globulin (HBIG). To be effective, HBIG should be given within 48 hours of exposure. The infants of these mothers should receive both forms of immunization soon after birth.

Management of cholelithiasis depends on a number of factors, including patient and physician preference. Variables considered in therapeutic options include the severity and character of symptoms, stone composition and size, and availability of various treatment modalities. For most pregnant patients, expectant and symptomatic therapy carries the least risk. Because of the significant increase in maternal morbidity and fetal mortality associated with surgical therapy, early consultation and co-management of patient with symptomatic stones should be encouraged.

When cholestasis of pregnancy is diagnosed, nonstress testing of the fetus should be implemented and maternal therapy undertaken. Oral cholestyramine therapy can reduce symptoms in about half the patients treated, but takes up to a week to be maximally effective. This therapy is also associated with a high degree of nausea, bloating, and anorexia, making compliance difficult. It should also be recognized that cholestyramine may also absorb fat-soluble vitamins and some medications. Symptomatic therapy with oatmeal or cornstarch baths or antihistamines may be helpful for many patients.

Human Immunodeficiency Virus (HIV)

HIV-infected pregnant women require more careful monitoring of their status because of the slight acceleration in the course of the disease induced by the intercurrent pregnancy. Periodic assessment of the helper lymphocyte (CD4) count can provide an good indication of the patient's status. CD4 counts of $<200/mm^3$ are diagnostic of acquired immune deficiency syndrome (AIDS) and carry a poor prognosis.

Therapy with zidovudine during pregnancy has been shown to reduce the rate of fetal transmission to less than 10%. Published recommendations have been for 500 mg orally each day from 14 weeks gestation onward. This is continued during labor by intravenous loading of 2 mg/kg followed by 1 mg/kg/h until delivery.

Although the route of delivery does not affect the rate of fetal infection, the use of fetal scalp electrodes or fetal scalp blood sampling should be avoided on theoretic grounds to protect those fetuses not already infected. The role of breast feeding in the transmission of HIV is unclear, but current recommendations suggest that it be discouraged.

Hypertension

When pregnancy-induced hypertension is mild, expectant management under the guidance of the primary care team is appropriate (Table 6.19). When PIH is severe, unresponsive to conservative therapy, the fetus is immature, or there is evidence of fetal compromise or impending threat, transfer to the care of an experienced specialist is needed.

Infections

No treatments are available for maternal cytomegalovirus infection. Prevention through personal hygiene and selectivity of personal contacts is important. Unlike herpes, the presence of a CMV infection does not alter obstetric management or route of delivery. When herpes lesions are present on the cervix, in the vagina, or on the vulva at the time of labor

Table 6.19. Management Strategies for Patients with Pregnancy-induced Hypertension (PIH)

Clinical status	Management
Mild PIH, immature fetus	

Compliant patient, improvement documented	Home care
	    Twice weekly visits
	    Weekly fetal assessment*
	    Bed rest (modified)
	    Daily weights
	    Home blood pressure monitoring
	    Serial ultrasonography

Noncompliant patient, failure to improve
       with conservative care
	Hospitalization
	    Bed rest
	    Regular diet
	    Daily weights
	    Blood pressure 4 times/day
	    Daily urine protein test
	    Evaluation of renal function
	    Weekly or biweekly fetal assessment
	    Serial ultrasonography

Mild PIH, mature fetus	Home care
	    Fetal assessment
	    Consider induction of labor

Severe PIH	Hospitalization
	    Prevent convulsions ($MgSO_4$)
	    Consultation/transfer
	    Control blood pressure†
	    Delivery

*Fetal assessment may include fetal activity monitoring, nonstress tests, contraction stress tests, or biophysical profiles based on severity of disease and stage of pregnancy.
†Goal of diastolic pressures of 90–100 mm Hg. Agents: Hydralazine, labetalol, verapamil.

or when the membranes rupture, cesarean delivery is recommended. Despite cesarean delivery, roughly 5% of infants will still develop HSV infection.

Gonococcal ophthalmia in the neonate is effectively prevented by the routine prophylactic treatment of the newborn's eyes with antibiotic ointment (erythromycin or tetracycline) or silver nitrate. Maternal infections should be treated whenever they are found. (See Chapter 26, Sexually Transmitted Disease and "PID.")

Treatment of patients with group B streptococcal colonization of the cervix has been widely debated. Some authors advocate empiric treatment of all patients at increased risk and any patient who is culture positive. The ability of this strategy to reduce morbidity and mortality is uncertain. If treatment is undertaken, penicillin or ampicillin are the agents of choice. Because of the fetal implications of congenital rubella infection, the best strategy to safeguard the health of the fetus is the prevention of rubella itself. Screening for IgG rubella antibody should be performed before pregnancy is contemplated and immunization offered to anyone found to be susceptible. Live virus vaccine provides roughly 95% seroconversion. A follow-up test for immunity should be performed 6 weeks after vaccination to identify the 5% of patients who fail to have an adequate antibody response. Because the vaccine used is a live virus type, most recommend that pregnancy be delayed for 3 months after receiving the injection, although no untoward effects of vaccine exposure have been reported. Patient who lack immunity at the time of delivery should be offered vaccination prior to discharge from the delivery site. Postpartum vaccination does not place others in the family at risk and is not a contraindication to breast feeding.

If a rubella infection does occur during pregnancy, only supportive care can be rendered; there is no effective treatment available. The use of human immune gamma globulin does not prevent or lessen the effect of infection.

The mainstay of syphilis treatment remains benzathine penicillin. Details of treatment and alternatives can be found in Chapter 26, Sexually Transmitted Disease and "PID."

Toxoplasmosis infections can be treated using a combination of sulfadiazine and pyrimethamine; however, pyrimethamine is potentially teratogenic and may not be used in the first trimester. For most patients thought to have become infected during the early phases of pregnancy, management must be limited to careful counseling about the risks of serious congenital infection and the option of pregnancy termination. Prevention of infection, through education, thoroughly cooking meats, and avoidance of exposure to potentially infected waste, is the best option.

Multiple Gestation

Multifetal pregnancies require careful monitoring of both maternal and fetal status. Special attention must be given to nutrition, rest, blood pressure, fetal growth, and fetal activity. Careful observation for the development of complications, such as hypertension, hydramnios, or preterm labor must be sustained, and prompt action taken when complications are detected. Routine preterm hospitalization is not recommended. Management of the patient in labor and the choice of delivery route must be individualized and made in close consultation with someone experienced in the care of these much more complicated cases.

Neurologic Disease and Headaches

Patients with mild seizure disorders, who have been free of seizures for several years, may be tapered off their medications prior to pregnancy. If symptoms recur, therapy can be reinstated with medications less prone to pregnancy complications (e.g., phenobarbital, primidone, or carbamazepine). Patients who remain on antiseizure medications should have frequent monitoring of serum drug levels to ensure the adequacy of the current dosing. Ultrasonography, performed between 18 and 22 weeks, should be directed toward the detection and characterization of fetal anomalies associated with the medical management of seizure disorders. Serial ultrasonographic studies are advised to monitor fetal growth and development.

Supportive therapy for patients with migraine headaches consists of analgesics (including narcotics). Nonsteroidal anti-inflammatory agents can be used early in gestation, but should be avoided late in pregnancy because of the potential for fetal side effects. Some patients will experience improvement with dietary changes or the use of beta blockers and calcium channel blocking agents.

Respiratory Disease and Asthma

The goal of asthma management during pregnancy is to reduce the number and severity of attacks and to alleviate hypoxia and improve ventilation during acute episodes. Patients with mild asthma and infrequent exacerbations can be followed with minimal additional evaluation or treatment. Moderation in exercise, adequate rest and hydration, and the avoidance of allergins are the only suggestions that should be made. More severe asthmatics should be continued on their prepregnancy medical management. Maternal oxygenation (PO_2) must be maintained at levels of greater than 70 to 80 mm Hg through the use of supplemental oxygen or medications. Rapidly acting inhalation agents, such as β-adrenergic receptor stimulants (epinephrine or isoproterenol), or parenteral sympathomimetic agents, may be required for acute management. Long-term management of these patients often includes the use of steroids, further jeopardizing fetal growth. Patients with this degree of asthmatic compromise require aggressive management and monitoring, often by specialists in maternal-fetal medicine. Consultation should be early and unreserved.

Substance Abuse

Active management, in the form of education and support, are often the only interventions possible for the patient who places her pregnancy in jeopardy through substance abuse. Cessation or reduction in the exposure to substances, alcohol, and tobacco products should be the goal. For patients who abuse opiates, the fetal impact may be reduced somewhat by methadone treatment.

Surgical Conditions and Trauma

The management of surgical emergencies and trauma during pregnancy will be dictated by the same principles applied when the patient is not pregnant. Rh immune globulin should be considered for any Rh-negative mother when fetal-maternal bleeding may be suspected to have occurred. Monitoring of both mother and fetus should be dictated by their condition, but the need for fetal assessment is often lost in the urgency of maternal care.

Thrombophlebitis and Embolism

Thromboembolic disorders during pregnancy or following delivery are treated in the same manner as for the nonpregnant patient. Superficial thrombophlebitis is treated with rest, elevation, heat, and mild analgesics. Deep vein thrombophlebitis or pulmonary embolism require anticoagulation with heparin or sodium warfarin (Coumadin), the latter of which is reserved for the postpartum period owing to potential teratogenicity. Patients with pulmonary embolism generally require long-term anticoagulation. Symptoms of deep vein thrombophlebitis should be anticipated to resolve in approximately 1 week. Patients with septic pelvic thrombophlebitis respond rapidly to heparin therapy.

Urinary Tract Infection and Renal Disease

Urinary tract infections found during pregnancy should be treated aggressively using the agents outlined in Chapter 27, Urinary Infection, Incontinence, and Pelvic Relaxation.

Patients diagnosed as having pyelonephritis require hospitalization, parenteral antibiotics, and careful fetal monitoring. During the third trimester, sulfa-based agents should not be used because they compete with bilirubin for albumin-binding sites in the fetus, theoretically producing hyperbilirubinemia in the newborn. Nitrofurantoin should also be avoided during the third trimester because of a risk of hemolysis in the newborn due to a relative lack of erythrocyte phosphate dehydrogenase. Pregnant patients treated for pyelonephritis with an appropriate antibiotic should be expected to become afebrile in 48 to 72 hours in 75% to 95% of cases, respectively. Failure to do so suggests either bacterial resistance or urinary obstruction and endorses the need for consultation.

Patients at risk for stone formation should be encouraged to maintain adequate hydration during the course of pregnancy. Some authors suggest urinary acidification as well, although the value of this during pregnancy is unclear.

HINTS AND COMMON QUESTIONS

When a mixed iron and folate deficiency is responsible for anemia during pregnancy, laboratory red cell indices may be normal because of off-setting changes. Empiric therapy with either iron or folate will not result in a significant rise in red cell production, further compounding the problems of diagnosis.

When maternal cardiac arrhythmias are encountered, mitral stenosis should be suspected. This must be distinguished from paroxysmal atrial tachycardia, which may result from excessive strenuous exercise.

If a patient with gestational diabetes continues to have glucose intolerance after delivery, her diagnosis should be revised to type I or type II diabetes mellitus, depending on her need for insulin.

Urinary tract infections are more common for diabetic patients. Therefore, more frequent screening of these patients is warranted.

Because of the risk of progressive retinopathy, pregnant diabetic patients should have retinal screening early in pregnancy and have periodic reassessment throughout the course of the gestation.

Hemoglobin A_{1c} reflects glucose values over the preceding 6 to 8 weeks. Attempts to use this to predict the likelihood of congenital malformations or other complications of a diabetic pregnancy have been disappointing.

Fetal death may result from maternal ketoacidosis. Although the management of ketoacidosis is no different during pregnancy that for the nonpregnant patient, careful fetal monitoring is required.

Patients with Crohn's disease have a slightly increased risk of early pregnancy loss when their disease is most active and they should consider delaying pregnancy until they are in the remission phase. When trying to differentiate between ulcerative colitis and Crohn's disease, the absence of rectal involvement essentially excludes ulcerative colitis.

Approximately 60% to 70% of adults have evidence of previous CMV infections and 40% to 50% have signs of prior exposure to toxoplasmosis. For this reason, routine serologic testing of patients, either to assess immunity or to attempt to document an acute infection, will be ineffective and is unwarranted except in unusual circumstances.

In the assessment of asthma, expiratory wheezing and the use of accessory muscles of respiration may be misleading during pregnancy and do not reflect the severity of the disease. Simple bedside testing of forced expiratory volume over 1 second or peak expiratory flow, such as blowing out a match held at arm's length, are better indicators for the severity of the disease.

Acrocyanosis is not uncommon during an asthma attack, but central cyanosis warrants immediate aggressive therapy.

Approximately 70% to 75% of cases of pyelonephritis found in pregnancy involve the right side, with 10% to 15% involving the left side, and a similar number involving both kidneys.

SUGGESTED READINGS

General References

Acker DB, Sach BP, Friedman EA. Risk factors for shoulder dystocia. Obstet Gynecol 1985;66:762.

Gabbe SG, Niebyl JR, Simpson JL (eds). Obstetrics: Normal and Problem Pregnancies, 2nd ed. New York: Churchill Livingstone, 1991.

Hypertensive disorders in pregnancy. In Cunningham FG, MacDonald PC, Gant NF, Leneno KJ, Gilstrap III LC (eds). Williams Obstetrics, 19th ed. Norwalk, Conneticut: Appleton and Lange, 1993, p 763.

Pastorek JG. Hepatitis in pregnancy. In Pastorek JG (ed). Obstetrics and Gynecologic Infectious Disease. New York: Raven Press, 1994, p 315.

Specific References

Asthma

Barsky HE. Asthma and pregnancy: a challenge for everyone concerned. Postgrad Med 1991;89:125.

Clark SL. Management of asthma during pregnancy. National Asthma Education Program Working Group in Asthma and Pregnancy. National Institutes of Health, National Heart, Lung and Blood Instituted. Obstet Gynecol 1993;82:1036.

Greenberger PA. Asthma in pregnancy. Clin Chest Med 1992;13:597.

Moore GJ. Asthma in pregnancy. Br J Obstet Gynaecol 1994;101:658.

Schatz M. Asthma during pregnancy: interrelationships and management. Ann Allergy 1992;68:23.

Diabetes

American College of Obstetricians and Gynecologists. Diabetes and pregnancy. ACOG Technical Bulletin 200. Washington, DC: ACOG, 1994.

American Diabetes Association. Position statement: screening for diabetes. Diabetes Care 1989;12:588.

Carpenter MW, Coustan DR. Criteria for screening test for gestational diabetes. Am J Obstet Gynecol 1982;144:768.

Cousins L. Pregnancy complications among diabetic women: review 1965–1985. Obstet Gynecol Surv 1987;42:140.

Dornhorst A, Nicholls JSD, Probst F, et al. Calorie restriction for treatement of gestational diabetes. Diabetes 1991;40(suppl 2):161.

Freinkel N, Dooley SL, Metzger BE. Care of the pregnant woman with insulin-dependent diabetes mellitus. N Engl J Med 1985;313:96.

Girz BA, Divon MY, Merkatz IR. Sudden fetal death in woman with well-controlled, intensively monitored gestational diabetes. J Perinatol 1992;12:229.

Institute of Medicine. Nutrition During Pregnancy. Part I. Weight Gain. Washington, DC: National Academy Press, 1990.

Kitzmiller JL, Gavin LA, Gin GD, Jovanovic-Peterson L, Main EK, Zigrang WD. Preconception care of diabetes. Glycemic control prevents congenital anomalies. JAMA 1991;265:731.

Kjos SL, Walther FJ, Montoro M, Paul RH, Diaz F, Stabler M. Prevalence and etiology of respiratory distress in infants of diabetic mothers: predictive value of fetal lung maturation tests. Am J Obstet Gynecol 1990;163:898.

Klein BEK, Moss SE, Klein R. Effect of pregnancy on progression of diabetic retinopathy. Diabetes Care 1990;13:34.

Landon MB, Gabbe SG. Antepartum fetal surveillance in gestational diabetes melitus. Diabetes 1985;34(suppl 2):50.

Landon MB, Gabbe SG. Antepartum fetal surveillance and delivery timing in diabetic pregnancies. Clin Diabetes 1990;8:33.

Landon MB, Gabbe SG. Diabetes mellitus and pregnancy. Obstet Gynecol Clin North Am 1992;19:633.

Landon MB, Gabbe SG, Piana R, Mennuti MT, Main EK. Neonatal morbidity in pregnancy complicated by diabetes mellitus: predictive value of maternal glycemic profiles. Am J Obstet Gynecol 1987;156:1089.

Langer O, Anyaegbunam A, Brustman L, Divon M. Management of women with one abnormal oral glucose tolerance test value reduces adverse outcome in pregnancy. Am J Obstet Gynecol 1989;161:593.

Lind T. Metabolic changes in pregnancy relavenat to diabetes mellitus. Postgrad Med J 1979;55:353.

Lucas MJ, Leveno KJ, Williams ML, Raskin P, Whalley PJ. Early pregnancy glycosylated hemoglobin, severity of diabetes, and fetal malformations. Am J Obstet Gynecol 1989;161:426.

Martin AO, Dempsey LM, Minogue J, et al. Maternal serum αfetoprotein levels in pregnancies complicated by diabetes: implications for screening programs. Am J Obstet Gynecol 1990;163:1209.

Metzger BE. Summary and recommendations of the Third International Workshop-Conference on Gestational Diabetes Mellitus. Diabetes 1991;40(suppl 2):197.

Mills JL, Knopp RH, Simpson JL, et al. Lack of relation of increased malformation rates in infants of diabetic mothers to glycemic control during organogenesis. N Engl J Med 1988;318:671.

Mulford MI, Jovanovic-Peterson L, Peterson CM. Alternative therapies for the management of gestational diabetes. Clin Perinatol 1993;20:630.

Neiger R, Coustan DR. The role of repeat glucose tolerance tests in the diagnosis of gestational diabetes. Am J Obstet Gynecol 1989;165:787.

Shields LE, Ban EA, Murphy HF, Sahn DJ, Moore TR. The prognostic value of hemoglobin A1c in predicting fetal heart disease in diabetic pregnancies. Obstet Gynecol 1993;81:954.

Sunness JS. The pregnant woman's eye. Surv Ophthalmol 1988;32:219.

HIV and Other Infections

Adler SP. Cytomegalovirus and pregnancy. Curr Opin Obstet Gynecol 1992;4:670.

Alford CA, Stagno S, Pass RF, Britt WJ. Congenital and perinatal cytomegalovirus infections. Rev Infect Dis 1990;12(suppl 7):5745.

American College of Obstetricians and Gynecologists. Perinatal herpes simples virus infections. ACOG Technical Bulletin 122. Washington, DC: ACOG, 1988.

American College of Obstetricians and Gynecologists. Rubella and pregnancy. ACOG Technical Bulletin 171. Washington, DC: ACOG, 1992.

American College of Obstetricians and Gynecologists. Hepatitis in pregnancy. ACOG Technical Bulletin 174. Washington, DC: ACOG, 1992.

American College of Obstetricians and Gynecologists. Perinatal viral and parasitic infections. ACOG Technical Bulletin 177. Washington, DC: ACOG, 1993.

Ayoola EA, Johnson AOD. Hepatitis B vaccine in pregnancy: immunogenicity, safety and transfer of antibodies to infants. Int J Gynaecol Obstet 1987;25:297.

Centers for Disease Control. Rubella vaccination during pregnancy—United States, 1971–1988. MMWR 1989;38:289.

Cochi SL, Edmonds LE, Dyer K, et al. Congenital rubella syndrome in the United States, 1970–1985: On the verge of elimination. Am J Obstet Gynecol 1989;129:349.

Connor EM, Sperling RS, Gelber R, et al. Reduction of maternal-infant transmission of human immunodeficiency virus type 1 with zidovudine treatment. N Engl J Med 1994;331:1173.

Daffos F, Forestier F, Capella-Pavlovsky M, et al. Prenatal management of 746 pregnancies at risk for congenital toxoplasmosis. N Engl J Med 1988;318:271.

Dunn DT, Newell ML, Ades AE, Peckham CS. Risk of human immunodeficiency virus type 1 transmission through breastfeeding. Lancet 1992;340:585.

European Collaborative Study: Mother-to-child transmission of HIV infection. Lancet 1988;2:1039.

Foulon W, Naessens A, Mahler T, de Waele M, de Catte L, de Meuter F. Prenatal diagnosis of congenital toxoplasmosis. Obstet Gynecol 1990;76:769.

Gibbs RS, McDuffie RS JR, McNabb F, Fryer G, Miyoshi T, Merestein G. Neonatal group B streptococcal sepsis during 2 years of a universal screening program. Obstet Gynecol 1994;84:496.

Gibbs RS, Mead PB. Preventing neonatal herpes—current strategies. N Engl J Med 1992;326:946.

Hohlfeld P, Vial Y, Maillard-Brignon C, Vaudaux B, Fawer CL. Cytomegalovirus fetal infection: prenatal diagnosis. Obstet Gynecol 1991;78:615.

Kovelesky RA, Minor JR. Antiretroviral therapy during pregnancy. Am J Hosp Pharm 1994;51:2187.

Lee SH, Ewert DP, Frederick PD, Mascola L. Resurgence of congenital rubella syndrome in the 1990s. JAMA 1992;267:2616.

Lindegren ML, Fehrs LJ, Hadler SC, Hinman AR. Update: Rubella congenital rubella syndrome, 1980–1990. Epidemiol Rev 1990;13:341.

Minkoff HL, Henderson C, Mendez H. Pregnancy outcomes among mothers infected with human immunodeficiency virus and uninfected control subjects. Am J Obstet Gynecol 1990;163:1598.

New York State Department of Health, AIDS Institute. Clinical guidelines for the use of zidovudine therapy in pregnancy to reduce perinatal transmission of HIV. October 1994.

Orenstein WA, Bart KJ, Hinman AR, et al. The opportunity and obligation to eliminate rubella from the United States. JAMA 1984;251:1988.

O'Sullivan MJ, Boyer PJJ, Scott GB, et al. The pharmacokinetics and safety of zidovudine in the third trimester of pregnancy for women infected with human innumodeficiency virus and their infants: Phase I Aquired Immunodeficiency Syndrome Clinical Trials Group Study (Protocol 082). Am J Obstet Gynecol 1993;168:1510.

Pastorek JG, Miller JM, Summers PR. The effect of hepatitis B antigenemia on pregnancy outcome. Am J Obstet Gynecol 1988;158:486.

Roos T, Martius J, Gross U, Schrod L. Systematic serologic screening for toxoplasmosis in pregnancy. Obstet Gynecol 1993;81:243.

Yancey MK, Duff P, Clark P, Kurtzer T, Horn Frentzen B, Kubilis P. Peripartum infection associated with vaginal group B streptococcal colonization. Obstet Gynecol 1994;84:816.

Multiple Gestation

Andrews WW, Leveno KJ, Sherman ML, Mutz J, Gilstrap III LC, Whalley PJ. Elective hospitalization in the management of twin pregnancies. Obstet Gynecol 1991;77:826.

Bebbington MW, Wittmann BK. Fetal transfusion syndrome: antenatal factors predicting outcome. Am J Obstet Gynecol 1989;160:913.

Bejar R, Vigliocco, G, Gramajo H, et al. Antenatal origin of neurologic damage in newborn infants. II. Multiple gestations. Am J Obstet Gynecol 1990;162:1230.

Blickstein I. The twin-twin transfusion syndrome. Obstet Gynecol 1990;76:714.

Bulmer MG. The effect of parental age, parity, and duration of marriage on the twinning rate. Ann Hum Genet 1959;23:454.

Bulmer MG. The familial incidence of twinning. Ann Hum Genet 1960;24:1.

Chervanak FA, Johnson RE, Youcha S, Hobbins JC, Berkowitz RL. Intrapartum management of twin gestation. Obstet Gynecol 1985;65:119.

Crowther C, Chalmers I. Bed rest and hospitalization during pregnancy. In Chalmers I, Enkin M, Keirse MJNC (eds). Effective Care in Pegnancy and Childbirth. Oxford: Oxford University Press, 1989, p 624.

Crowther C, Neilson JP, Ashurst HM, Verkuyl DA, Vannerman C. The effects of hospitalization for rest on fetal growth, neonatal morbidity and length of gestation in twin pregnancy. Br J Obstet Gynaecol 1990;97:872.

D'Alton ME, Mercer BM. Antepartum management of twin gestation: ultrasound. Clin Obstet Gynecol 1990;33:42.

Derom C, Derom R, Vlietinck R, Van den Berghe H, Thiery M. Increased monozygotic twinning rate after ovulation induction. Lancet 1987;1:1237.

Dyson DC, Crites YM, Ray DA, Armstrong MA. Prevention of preterm birth in high-risk patients: the role of education and provider contact versus home uterine monitoring. Am J Obstet Gynecol 1991;164:756.

Jauniauz E, Elkazen N, Leroy F, Wilkin P, Rodesch F, Hustin J. Clinical and morphologic aspects of the vanishing twin phenomenon. Obstet Gynecol 1988;72:577.

Kiely JL, Kleinman JC, Kiely M. Triplets and higher-order multiple births. Am J Dis Child 1992;146:862.

Kovacs BW, Kirschbaum TH, Paul RH. Twin gestations. I. Antenatal care and complications. Obstet Gynecol 1989;74:313.

Long PA, Oats JN. Preeclampsia in twin pregnancy—severity and pathogenesis. Aust NZ J Obstet Gynaecol 1987;27:1.

MacGillivray I. Epidemiology of twin pregnancy. Semin Perinatol 1986;10:4.

MacLennan AH, Green RC, O'Shea R, Brookes C, Morris DE. Routine hospital admission in twin pregnancies between 26 and 30 weeks gestation. Lancet 1990;335:267.

Nageotte MP. Prevention and treatment of preterm labor in twin gestation. Clin Obstet Gynecol 1990;33:61.

Powers WF. Twin pregnancy: complications and treatment. Obstet Gynecol 1973;42:795.

Robinson HP, Caines JS. Sonar evidence of early pregnancy failure in patients with twin conceptions. Br J Obstet Gynaecol 1977;84:22.

Varma TR. Ultrasound evidence of early pregnancy failure in patients with multiple conceptions. Br J Obstet Gynaecol 1979;86:290.

Other

American College of Obstetricians and Gynecologists. Trauma during pregnancy. ACOG Technical Bulletin 161. Washington, DC: ACOG, 1991.

American College of Obstetricians and Gynecologists. Cardiac disease in pregnancy. ACOG Technical Bulletin 168. Washington, DC: ACOG, 1992.

Bag S, Behari M, Ahuja GK, Karmarkar MG. Pregnancy and epilepsy. J Neurol 1989;236:311.

Keirse MJNC. New perspective for the effective treatment of preterm labor. Am J Obstet Gynecol 1995;173:618.

Landon MB, Samuels P. Cardiac and pulmonary disease. In Gabbe SG, Niebyl JR, Simpson JL (eds). Obstetrics: Normal and Problem Pregnancies, 2nd ed. New York: Churchill Livingstone, 1991, p 1057.

McCall ML, Sass D. The action of magnesium sulfate on cerebral circulation and metabolism in toxemia of pregnancy. Am J Obstet Gynecol 1956;71:1089.

Sibai BM, Caritis S, Phillips E, et al. Prevention of preeclampsia: low-dose aspirin in nulliparous women: A multicenter double-blind placebo controlled trial. Am J Obstet Gynecol 1993:168:286.

Sorokin JJ, Levine SM. Pregnancy and inflammatory bowel disease: a review of the literature. Obstet Gynecol 1983;62:247.

Zuspan FP, Rayburn WF. Blood pressure self-monitoring during pregnancy: practical considerations. Am J Obstet Gynecol 1991;164:2.

III

Phases of gynecologic care

7

Pediatric and Adolescent Care

Although gynecologic concerns are rare in neonates, infants, children, and young adolescents, problems do occur. Whereas most of those that arise necessitate referral for specialized evaluation, a basic awareness by the primary care team ensures prompt recognition and appropriate triage.

The challenges presented by adolescent care are very different from those for adults. The many different decisions, concerns, and changes confronting an adolescent are formidable, not the least of which are health issues raised by rapid growth, sexual maturation, and emerging sexuality. Puberty involves physical, emotional, and sexual changes that mark the transition from childhood to adulthood. Despite the potential need for medical education and care, teenagers have the lowest rate of physician office visits of any group. Embarrassment, an inability to pay, a lack of familiarity with health care delivery options, and legal obstructions to care contribute to this lack of care.

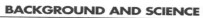 **BACKGROUND AND SCIENCE**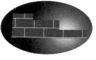

Neonatal and Pediatric Assessment

Newborn Evaluations

In a sense, gynecologic care begins with the initial assessment of the newborn female. Careful appraisal of the infant's genitalia must be an integral part of the physical examination because correct gender assignment carries life-long implications. A rectal examination should also be included to survey the internal structures. The presence of a thin white mucoid vaginal discharge is the normal result of in utero hormone exposure. Similarly, withdrawal vaginal bleeding during the first few days of life is not unusual and should not provoke concern.

In addition to the evaluation of the genitalia, the breast should be checked for budding and the presence of nipple discharge. Both are common and result from maternal hormone stimulation.

Pediatric Patients

The initial evaluation of children with gynecologic problems begins with a history, generally obtained from the parents or care-givers. If the primary care provider performs an examination, it must be preceded by efforts to gain the child's confidence and carried out in the most nonthreatening, atraumatic way possible. For children up to about age 6, this is often best accomplished in a froglike position with the patient sitting on the parent's lap, with the parent supporting the child's legs. This position provides adequate access while affording security and comfort. Often a "show and tell" approach works well. An alternate position for examination of older children is the knee-chest postion. When accompained by a Valsalva maneuver, the vaginal tissues and the lower third of the vagina can be visualized without further instrumentation. A cotton-tipped applicator or calcium calginate swab can be used to obtain samples of secretions for microscopic inspection or culture.

If instrumentation is required, an otoscope, nasal speculum, Cameron-Myers vaginoscope, or a Huffman pediatric speculum may be used (Fig 7.1). Because of the more invasive nature of these instrumented examinations and the more complex problems that may necessitate their use, consideration should be given to referral to someone experienced in pediatric or adolescent gynecology. Imaging with ultrasonography, computed tomography, or magnetic resonance may also be employed, but probably should be reserved for the specialist.

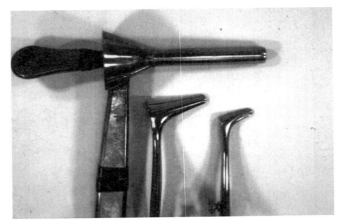

Figure 7.1. Several suitably small specula are available for the examination of adolescents and children. In addition to narrow bladed bivalve specula, nasal specula or a small anoscope/vaginoscope, such as those illustrated here, may be used.

Events of Puberty

Understanding the normal sequence of events involved in sexual maturation is important for counseling young women who may be concerned about "being normal." This understating is also pivotal to the important task of identifying those in whom the progression is not normal so that timely evaluation and intervention can be made. Hormonally, puberty involves a change from negative gonadal feedback to established circadian and ultradian gonadal rhythms and the positive feedback controls that result in monthly cycles and fertility.

In North America, Europe, and Japan the age of sexual maturation underwent a progressive decline during the first third of this century. This has stabilized over the past one to two decades and now appears to be relatively steady. In general, there are many things that affect the onset of puberty (Table 7.1), but the most influential appears to be genetic.

It appears that three broad elements must be present for puberty to progress normally: adequate body mass, adequate sleep, and exposure to light. These factors appear to interact with or allow the complex hypothalamic, pituitary, and ovarian changes that must occur.

The hypothalamus begins to synthesize gonadotropin releasing hormone (GnRH) as early as the 10th week of gestation, reaching a peak at about 20 to 24 weeks with levels approximating or exceeding those found in the adult (Fig 7.2). Negative feedback from placental steroids suppresses this release, but results in a transient rise soon after birth as this suppression is withdrawn. Before puberty, the production of estrogen and progesterone are about one twentieth of that found after puberty. This low level is maintained by the hypothalamus, which is functional but extremely sensitive to suppression by these hormones. This leads to a continuing abatement of follicle-stimulating hormone (FSH) and luteinizing hormone (LH) release from the pituitary. Reduction of this negative feedback is the first step in the transition to maturity.

As the young girl matures, several things begin to change. As body weight increases, the presence of estrogen (even at low levels) causes an increased proportion of body fat. This is important because it is thought that there is a critical body weight and percentage of body fat that is necessary to start menstruation. This is estimated to be between 16% and 24% body fat and a total body weight of 85 to 106 lb. Not all studies have found these relationships and a similar weight requirement for male maturation may not exist.

Table 7.1. Factors Affecting the Onset and Progression of Puberty

Factors that delay puberty
  Anorexia
  Chronic disease
  High altitude
  Poor nutrition
  Severe obesity (>30% over ideal body weight)
  Strenuous exercise
Factors that accelerate puberty
  Exogenous hormone ingestion
  Mild to moderate obesity
  Northern latitudes
  Urban residence

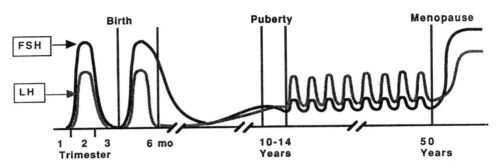

Figure 7.2. Gonadotropin variation by age. The pituitary and hypothalamus begin functional activity early in fetal life, producing adult levels of follicle-stimulating hormone (FSH) and luteinizing hormone (LH) by midgestation. Feedback from estrogen and chorionic gonadotropin suppresses this activity late in pregnancy and withdrawal of suppression causes an early infantile rise. Gonadotropins remain low until approximately 8 to 10 years of age when pubertal changes begin the process of attaining normal reproductive functioning.

As the hypothalamus matures there is a decrease in its sensitivity to estrogen, resulting in an increase in the production and release of GnRH. It is thought that there may also be an increased sensitivity of the pituitary to the effects of GnRH. These two changes allow increased levels of FSH and LH to be released from the pituitary. As a result, FSH levels begin to rise at about the eighth to the tenth year of life, accompanied by a rise in the levels of estrogen.

Luteinizing hormone levels begin to change much later than do the levels of FSH. In addition, the change in LH production also follows a different pattern than the gradual, steady rise seen with FSH. When the LH level first starts to increase it does so through nighttime pulses of LH (Fig 7.3). These pulses are integral to the maturation process; when they are interrupted by inadequate amounts of sleep, delayed or disrupted maturation results. As maturation proceeds, the amount of LH released and the duration of these pulses increase. Eventually these nighttime spurts spill over into the daytime and the day-night cycles disappear, to be replaced by the normal pattern and amount of LH release. Both FSH and LH normally have a pulsatile release pattern in adult life, but the pulses are much smaller and of much shorter duration, so that they are generally imperceptible.

As the sensitivity of the hypothalamus to negative feedback further decreases, FSH and LH levels continue to rise. Eventually these reach a sufficient level that the follicles can respond. Estrogen levels rise and there is an increase in the ovary's ability to respond to FSH and LH, further enhancing the response. The endometrium begins to change in response to the estrogen and eventually bleeding occurs. The average age of first menstruation (menarche) is about 12.8 years, with a normal range of 8 to 16 years of age (Fig 7.4). Menarche generally occurs after a growth spurt and the beginning of breast development, but while changes in the pubic hair and labia are still under way.

The changes of puberty are generally heralded by a growth spurt and the rounding of body curvatures. Breast tissue begins to develop, there is darkening of the nipples, and fat is laid down in the shoulders, hips, buttocks, and in front of the pubic bone (the mons). Body

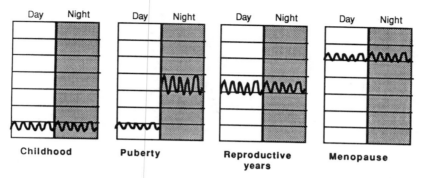

Figure 7.3. Patterns of gonadotropin secretion during different stages of life. During childhood small pulsatile releases of gonadotropin occur but are inadequate to generate an end-organ response. During puberty, nighttime pulsation increases in both frequency and amplitude spilling over to the normal adult patterns as sexual maturation is achieved. These patterns again change in response to the failure of ovarian response that heralds menopause.

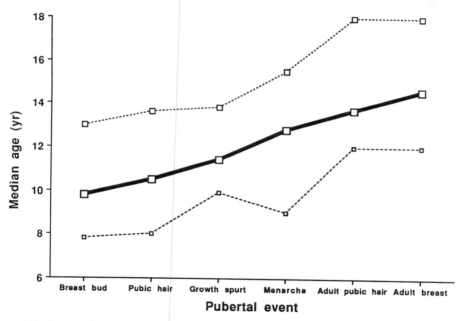

Figure 7.4. Expected sequence of events in puberty. The median age at which six major milestones in the process of puberty occur is shown. Each event may occur over a wide range of "normal" ages, making prediction difficult. When events fall outside these age ranges, however, further evaluation is indicated.

hair begins to appear because of the influence of androgens which are made in small amounts by the ovary and adrenal glands. Height increases owing to accelerated growth in the long bones of the body, capped off by the closure of the growth centers near the end of puberty. This growth spurt generally begins about 2 years before the start of menstruation itself, with growth slowing about the same time menstruation begins. There is some variation in the normal flow of events. Although, for most, thelarche is the indication of pubertal change, fol-

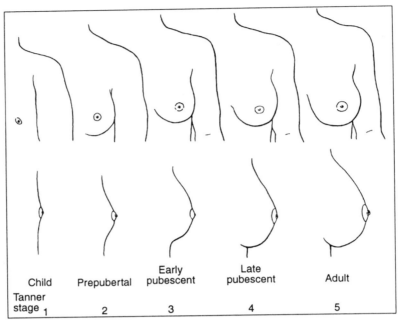

Figure 7.5. Normal progression of breast development. From: Beckman CRB, Ling FW, Barzansky B, et al. Obstetrics and Gynecology, 2nd ed. Baltimore: Williams & Wilkins, 1995, p 368. (From Beckmann RB, Ling FW, Barzansky BM, et al. Obstetrics and gynecology. 2nd ed. Baltimore: Williams & Wilkins, 1995:368.)

lowed by adrenarche, then peak growth velocity, ending with the onset of menstruation. This sequence generally takes 4.5 years to run its course, with a range of from 1.5 to 6 years.

Thelarche

If careful measurements are made, the first indication of puberty is accelerated growth rate. Because this is often not detected, breast budding is generally the first apparent sign of pubertal change. The beginning of breast development occurs under the influence of estrogen. The first signs of breast changes are the elevation of the nipple and the surrounding areola (Fig 7.5). This is followed by the development of a breast bud, which is a small mound of tissue. At this stage the areola enlarges and becomes darker. After moderate growth of the breast, the areola and nipple rise slightly above the contour of the rest of the breast. This secondary rise is lost as the breast finally becomes mature, roughly 3 to 4 years after the onset of change (Table 7.2). Growth and development of the ducts and glands

Table 7.2. Stages of Breast Development

Stage*	Characteristics	Median Age
1	Childlike; no development	
2	Increased diameter of areola; breast bud	9.8
3	Elevation of breast and areola	11.2
4	Secondary mound of areola and papilla above breast	12.1
5	Recession of areola to plane of breast	14.6

*Sexual Maturation Rating (SMR), or Tanner Stage.

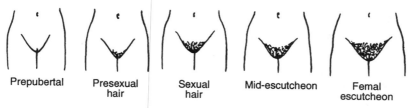

| Prepubertal | Presexual hair | Sexual hair | Mid-escutcheon | Femal escutcheon |

Figure 7.6. Normal progression of pubic hair development. From: Beckman CRB, Ling FW, Barzansky B, et al. Obstetrics and Gynecology, 2nd ed. Baltimore: Williams & Wilkins, 1995, p 8 (From Beckmann RB, Ling FW, Barzansky BM, et al. Obstetrics and gynecology. 2nd ed. Baltimore: Williams & Wilkins, 1995:8.)

within the underlying tissue are also under the control of estrogen. Thelarche is an important indicator that the hypothalamic-pituitary-ovarian axis is intact and functional.

Adrenarche

The development of pubic hair is generally the second event marking the transition to sexual maturity, although it may be the first sign for up to 20% of women. Adrenarche closely follows thelarche, occurring between 11 and 12 years of age. Pubic hair usually appears first and transition to the adult pattern generally becomes complete before axillary hair appears, about 2 years later. The developmental sequence of pubic hair has been classified into stages in much the same way as breast development (Fig 7.6, Table 7.3). Adrenarche comes about as a response to rising levels of dehydroepiandrosterone sulfate (DHEAS); therefore, the onset of adrenarche indicates that the hypothalamic-pituitary-adrenal axis is intact.

Growth Spurt

Small amounts of pubertal estrogen causes a dramatic growth increase in the long bones of the body. It also causes a closure of the growth centers to stop growth. This race between stimulated bone growth and closure of the bone growth centers determines height. Estrogen has a greater effect on growth and epiphyseal closure in women than does testosterone in young men. This is why young women have an earlier (by about 2 years), more marked, but shorter growth spurt, leaving them shorter, on the average, than men. Estrogens also cause the change in shape of the pelvic bones from the narrow, funnel shape of young children and men, into the broader, more oval shape of a mature woman. Exactly how estrogens accomplish this is not known, but it is thought to be the by-product of other more general effects on bone growth.

Table 7.3 Stages of Pubic Hair Development

Stage*	Characteristics	Median Age
1	Childlike; no development	
2	Sparse; long, silky, lightly pigmented hair along labia majora (midline)	10.5
3	Dark, coarse, curly hair sparsely spread over mons	11.4
4	Adult hair; abundant but limited to mons	12.0
5	Adult pattern with spread to thighs	13.7

*Sexual Maturation Rating (SMR), or Tanner Stage.

For women, peak growth velocity approaches 9 cm/y. Peak growth rate is generally achieved about 2 years after breast budding and about 1 year before the first menstrual flow. Growth hormone secretion, which appears to remain at childhood levels during this peak growth, accounts for a velocity of about 4 cm/y. Steroid production, including estrogen, and other growth hormones account for the additional 5 cm/y found at the peak. As with LH, growth hormone is secreted in a pulsatile fashion, with the first indication of increased release occurring in the form of nighttime pulsations.

Menarche

Menarche is more closely tied to level of sexual maturation than it is to chronologic age. There is a close concordance between menarche, body weight, and peak growth velocity, the latter of which occurs about 12 months before the onset of menstruation. For 60% of adolescents, menarche occurs when they reach a sexual maturation level of 4 (Fig 7.7).

Menarche usually does not signify fertility, because ovulation may take 6 to 18 months or longer to arrive, and it may take between 5 and 7 years for a young woman to establish reliably regular ovulatory menstrual cycles. It is for this reason that the highest incidence of anovulatory cycles occur in women below the age of 20 or over the age of 40. The time it takes to become reliably ovulatory may be somewhat predicted based on the age of menarche: those who have earlier menarche achieve regular ovulation more quickly than those whose menarche is delayed. For example, those patients who begin menstruation by age 12 take roughly 1 year until 50% of their cycles are ovulatory; those who start between 12 and 13 require 3 years to reach 50% ovulation rates; and those who begin periods after age 13 take 4.5 years to achieve a 50% ovulation rate.

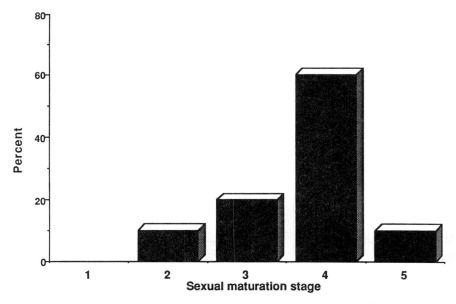

Figure 7.7. Sexual maturation level (Tanner stage) at time of menarche. The majority of adolescent women have reached sexual maturity (Tanner stage 4) at the time of their first menses.

Irregular ovulation means that for most adolescents menstrual periods are unpredictable. Anovulatory periods tend to be lighter, shorter, and less painful than ovulatory cycles, but they tend to arrive at irregular intervals with little prodrome or warning. Ovulatory cycles often provoke breast tenderness, bloating or a sense of fullness, and irritability, which signal their approach. This irregularity of ovulation cannot be equated to fecundity, which is high for teens. Irregular cycles means that predicting the time of fertility within a given cycle is difficult or impossible, leaving those without reliable contraception at risk.

Special Concerns

Emerging Sexuality

Part of adolescence is the emergence of adult sexual drive and sexuality. This begins with interest and flirtation and ends with the evolution of mature sexual relationships. The average age of first intercourse has progressively decreased but is now estimated to be 17.5 years. There are many cultural, gender, and racial differences, with the earliest age of first intercourse for any subgroup occurring at just over age 15 for black men. By age 18, 56% of unmarried urban women have had intercourse and by age 19 rises to over 70%. Despite these statistics, just over one woman in five still has her first experience of intercourse after marriage.

Teens are often confused or worried about their sexual orientation owing to same-sex friends or peer groups, surreptitious peeks in locker rooms, or an interest in the opposite sex that has yet to emerge. This is both common and normal. Unless it presents a source of concern for the patient or her family, no intervention beyond reassurance is warranted. No effort should be made either to hasten the process or to change its direction.

Premature (very young) sexual activity may be a warning sign for more significant psychosocial risks such as abuse, depression, or suicide.

Fertility, Contraception, and Sexually Transmitted Diseases

Teen pregnancy represents a major public health concern. As a group, teens are very fertile (>200 pregnancies per 1000 sexually experienced teens), with 90% of unprotected teens becoming pregnant during the first year of intercourse. Teens in the United States have a pregnancy rate that is double that of all women of reproductive age and double that of most European countries and Canada, despite roughly equal rates of sexual activity. Slight declines in the rate of teen pregnancy in 1992 (60.7 per 1000 women) and 1993 (59.6 per 1000 women) suggest that this may be changing, possibly owing to increased condom use in response to concerns about sexually transmitted disease. In the United States, roughly 1 million teens a year become pregnant. Eighty-five percent of these pregnancies are unplanned and half occur during the first 6 months of sexual activity. (It should be noted, however, that teens account for only about 25% of all unintended pregnancies.) Since the 1960s, adolescent out-of-wedlock birth rate has risen from around 33% to over 80%, owing in part to a later average age of marriage. Roughly 40% of pregnancies occurring to women under the age of 20 are electively terminated.

Despite educational efforts by many sources, teens do not routinely use contraception when they engage in coitus. Only about two thirds of teen use contraception, usually a

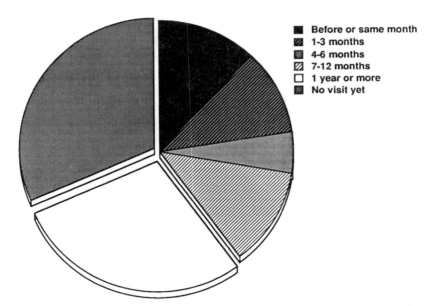

Figure 7.8. Delay in seeking contraception after initiation of sexual activity, U.S. women, age 15–19 years, 1988. Less than 40% of teens have sought medical contraception within one year of becoming sexually active. Data from: The Alan Guttmacher Institute, 1994.

condom (48%), for their first act of intercourse, leaving one third of all first acts unprotected. Studies indicate that most teens do not seek medical contraceptive advice until more than 1 year after their first intercourse (Fig 7.8). It also appears that the younger a woman is when she becomes sexually active, the longer this interval to contraceptive use becomes. Clearly, contraception must occupy an extensive part of any adolescent health care plan or counseling.

About 3 million teens a year become infected by a sexually transmitted disease (STD). This represent 1 of 4 sexually active teens and 25% of all STD cases. Teens are 10 times more likely to develop pelvic inflammatory disease than adults and up to 20% may develop pelvic abscesses. Most teens are aware of the signs and symptoms of STDs, how to prevent them, and the need for treatment, but this does not appear to significantly affect behavior. Discussion of the risks that accompany the serial monogamy common in teen relationships should be a part of routine counseling.

Date Rape and Abuse

Sexual abuse of children and adolescents represent a major health issue. The incidence of childhood sexual abuse has risen more than threefold in recent years and as many as 0.2% to 0.3% of all children are involved in persistent, continuing, incestuous relationships. Girls are the victim in 90% of childhood abuse cases. Some authors report that almost 40% of girls below age 18 have been involved in nonvoluntary sexual activities, including incest, date rape, and other forms of sexual abuse. In 90% of cases, it is a family member who is responsible for the abuse.

Date rape may be the most underreported of all sexual assaults. Recent studies of violence during adolescent dating find 12% to 27% of high school students and 17% to 52% of college students have experienced some form of dating violence. More than 25% of college women report activities that meet the legal definition of rape; 50% of all college campus rapes take place during dates. Women under the age of 24 are at the greatest risk of sexual assault and a frank discussion of the occurrence and prevention should be carried out as a part of both diagnosis and health maintenance.

Suspected sexual assault, whether it involves a child or a young adult, must be reported to police or child welfare authorities. The medical record should only reflect the suspicion or allegation and must not draw conclusions, even when based on concrete observations. It is the province of law enforcement and judicial authorities to render a final decision on the validity of the allegation and legal aspect of each case.

Teen Suicide

Suicide ranks as the third most common cause of death for teens age 15 to 19 years. Some authors report that over 8% of high school students have made at least one suicide attempt in the preceding 12 months. For every successful suicide, there may be between 50 and 200 unsuccessful attempts. Mood changes are prevalent in adolescents. Sudden changes and periods of depression, euphoria, and even violence are common. These are generally self-limited and resolve with the attainment of full sexual maturation. Prolonged depression; withdrawal from activities, school or friends; distribution of prized possessions; expressions of hopelessness or helplessness; self-destructive behaviors including sex, alcohol, or drugs; or suicidal ideation must be taken seriously, with counseling, support, or more aggressive intervention provided as needed. One approach to screening for teen psychosocial problems is the BiHEADS mnemonic that provides a quick structure on which to base a symptom review (Table 7.4). Teenage girls are more likely to use ingestion as a method of suicide but are less likely to carry out a suicide attempt successfully. This means that care must be exercised in the prescription of drugs for teenage patients and other members of the household.

Substance Abuse

As adolescents mature they evolve from self-centered concrete thinkers (ages 12 to 14), to highly peer-driven, risk-taking, invincibility (ages 15 to 17), before acquiring the abstract thinking and planning that characterize adult patterns (by age 18 to 20+). During the mid-

Table 7.4. The BiHEADS Mnemonic of Screening for Psychosocial Problems

Body Image	Internalized conception of attractiveness, evidence of discordance, and actions taken
Home	Home situation, stress, privacy, communications
Education	School success, attitudes, and expectations
Activities	Risk-taking behaviors, idle-time activities, hobbies
Drugs	Experience with or exposure to drugs
Sex/suicide	Sexual activity, abuse, contraception, suicide

Adapted from: Berman HS. Talking HEADS: Interviewing adolescents. HMO Practice 1987;1:3.; Cohall AT, Cohall Rm. Screening for psychosocial health problems. Contempory Adolescent Gynecology 1995;1:11.; Cohen E, Mackenzie RG, Yates GL. HEADSS, a psychosocial risk assessment instrument. J Adolesc Health 1991;12:539.; 2nd Goldenring JM, Cohen E. Getting into adolescent heads. Contempory Pediatrics 1988;5:75.

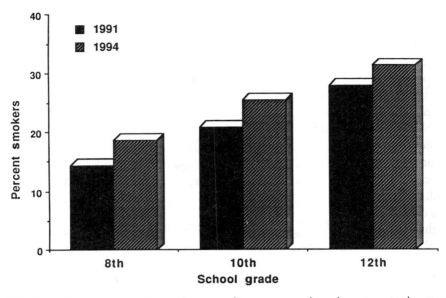

Figure 7.9. Rate of teenage smoking. The rate of teenage smoking has risen in the past several years. From: US News & World Report, 1995;119(June 31):8.

dle phase of development teens are especially vulnerable to experimentation. This may take the form of early sexual expression, drug or alcohol use, fast driving, and other potentially destructive behaviors. Most teens are involved in some risk-taking behaviors; many are involved in multiple ones. The primary care setting is especially suited to watching for and addressing the risks inherent in this period of life.

Teenage smoking has risen rapidly in the recent past. In one University of Michigan study, smoking rose by 30% in 8th graders, 20% for 10th graders, and 12.5% for high school seniors (Fig 7.9). By the 10th grade, 90% of students have used alcohol and almost 10% have tried cocaine at least once. Teenage use of alcohol or tobacco usually precedes experimentation with other illicit substances. Most substance abuse, including alcohol and tobacco, is initiated in the mid- to late teens, with those who have not experimented by age 21 unlikely to do so. Clearly, the probability of use should be sensitively explored with all teens.

Other Concerns

The most common gynecologic complaints of puberty and early adulthood are those of irregular, painful, or heavy menstrual periods. Irregularity of menses is to be expected until regular ovulation is established. Even after some degree of rhythm is present, physical or emotional stress or strain, illness, rapid increases or decreases in weight, or sudden changes in levels of physical activity may result in skipped or irregular cycles. When these factors are present and pregnancy has been ruled out, the patient may be reassured and no further evaluation is needed.

Heavy menstrual flow, which is uncommon during the anovulatory cycles first experienced by adolescents, does occur. When the patient's first menstrual period is heavy, one must consider the possibility of a bleeding disorder or blood dyscrasia, recognizing that leukemia is the fourth most prevalent killer of adolescents. For an adolescent with established periods, a suddenly heavy period should suggest the possibility of a complication of pregnancy. In general, the more severe the bleeding is, the more likely some cause other than anovulatory or dysfunctional bleeding is at fault. Persistent dysmenorrhea or menorrhagia should be evaluated and treated as discussed in Chapter 16 (Heavy Periods and Toxic Shock Syndrome) and Chapter 18 (Menstrual Pain).

Adolescent patients are at high risk for a number of other abnormalities that should be considered as a part of their total health care. Adolescent women are often at risk for eating or self-image disorders that result in anorexia, bulimia, or obesity. Poor hygiene, a lack of exercise, alienation from school or family, and depression are common. If unrecognized, these may lead to sexual or substance experimentation, early pregnancy, injury, disease, or death.

Although teens account for approximately 8% of the United States population, they are involved in almost 20% of fatal traffic accidents. Passengers in vehicles driven by teens comprise almost two thirds of all automotive deaths. Counseling teens about the use of seat belts and designated drivers before they reach driving age should be an important part of any health maintenance program.

ESTABLISHING THE DIAGNOSIS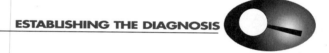

Neonatal and Pediatric Concerns

The most common childhood gynecologic problem is vulvovaginitis. Infection by perineal and anal organisms is much more likely because of the absence of estrogen-induced labial fat and epithelial thickening and the lack of androgen-dependent pubic hair. Infection by nasopharyngeal and other skin organisms arises as a result of poor hygiene practices. Chemical irritation by soaps, bubble bath, or laundry products is also common. The differential diagnosis and therapy vary little from those of adult patients; they are reviewed in Chapter 28, Vulvitis and Vaginal Infections.

Children younger than age 6 may develop labial adhesions or agglutination, which may be found in between 1% and 2% of female children. It is unusual in children younger than age 2, and may occasionally be found up to the age of puberty. Labial agglutination is due to local inflammation and the hypo-estrogen environment of preadolescence. Clinically, this may be recognized by midline adherence that extends from just below the clitoris to the posterior fourchette. Subsequent pooling of urine results in urinary tract infections, vaginal odor, or vaginal infections. Treatment is with topical estrogen (applied nightly for 7 to 10 days), sitz baths, and appropriate cleansing. Spontaneous opening is common. When mechanical separation is required, it should only be done after medical therapy and with minimal traction on the paravaginal tissues.

Lichen sclerosis, lichen planus, seborrheic dermatitis, atopic dermatitis, and contact dermatitis may occur in pediatric patients. Like vaginitis, the diagnosis and treatment is similar to that of adult patients.

Vaginal bleeding and profuse discharge are often the harbingers of a foreign body in the vagina (Table 7.5). The most commonly encountered foreign body is a bit of toilet paper, although almost any small object can innocently (or otherwise) end up in the vagina. Removal of the foreign body is both diagnostic and therapeutic. A malignancy, although rare, should be considered as a source of bloody discharge. Bleeding may also result from a prolapsed urethra, which can be recognized as an exophytic, granular-appearing mass at the external meatus. Irritation and dysuria, which are common, respond well to topical estrogen cream.

Genital trauma is not uncommon in young girls. Most prevalent are the straddle injuries found when learning to ride a bicycle. These may result in vulvar bruising or hematoma formation. Pressure and ice packs will be sufficient for most minor injuries. Because of the atrophic and highly vascular nature of the perineal tissues, large hematomas may form that require surgical intervention. Penetrating trauma involving the perineum or vagina requires immediate consultation because of the possibility of internal injuries and bleeding.

Unfortunately, the possibility of sexual abuse must be considered in any child with vaginal bleeding, suspicious foreign bodies, or recurrent infections. The possibility of sexual abuse must be carefully evaluated and may require special skill or experience available by consultation or referral. (See Chapter 23, Sexual Assault and Abuse.) Sexually transmitted diseases such as trichomonas, gonorrhea, chlamydia, or HIV may easily infect the atrophic preadolescent vagina. Testing for these should be included in any child suspected

Table 7.5. Common Causes of Childhood Vaginal Bleeding or Discharge

ANATOMIC
  Labial agglutination
  Müllerian anomalies
  Urethral prolapse
ENDOCRINOLOGIC
  Exogenous estrogen or steroids
  Neonatal estrogen withdrawal
  Precocious puberty
  Prepubertal discharge (physiologic)
INFECTION
  Condyloma acuminata
  Pinworms
  Sexually transmitted disease
  Vaginitis
  Vulvitis
NEOPLASIA (rare)
  Sarcoma botryoides
  Uterine carcinoma
  Other
TRAUMA
  Accident
  Foreign body
  Sexual abuse
  Other

of sexual molestation. The presence of these infections is supportive, but not diagnostic, of abuse.

Abnormalities of Puberty

Concern should occur anytime there is a significant disturbance in the sequence or timing of sexual maturation milestones. These variations in timing are often difficult to evaluate. For example, the average interval from breast budding to first menstruation is between 2.5 and 3.5 years, but may range from 1.5 to 6 years. For between 10% and 15% of girls, adrenarche may precede thelarche. Despite this range of variability, some general statements may be made.

Precocious Puberty

Pubertal changes before the age of 8 or cyclic menstruation before the age of 10 are generally accepted as indications of precocious puberty. Although precocious puberty is most often heralded by the sequence of increased growth, thelarche, and adrenarche, these events may occur simultaneously, or menarche itself may be the first indication. Precocious puberty is customarily divided into two classifications: true or GnRH-dependent and precocious pseudopuberty, which is independent of GnRH control. Potential causes of precocious puberty are summarized in Table 7.6.

For all patients with precocious puberty, the possibility of a serious process, either central or peripheral, must be evaluated. For most girls over the age of 4, no specific cause is usually discovered for the early development. By contrast, the most common cause of precocious change in girls younger than 4 years is a central nervous system lesion, most often hamartomas of the hypothalamus. Even when the sequence of events appears normal, initially a serious process (such as a slowly progressive brain tumor) must be aggressively sought and watched for with long-term continuing follow-up.

GNRH-DEPENDENT PRECOCIOUS PUBERTY. True precocious puberty, also known as complete, isosexual, or central precocity, is related to early activation of the hypothalamic-pituitary-gonadal axis. In 75% of patients, there is no indication of how or why the normal processes of puberty were accelerated, although up to 50% of these patients may have subtle abnormalities found in their electroencephalograms. In the remaining 25% of patients, a central nervous system abnormality is to blame. A number of central nervous system pathologies may result in activation of GnRH secretion and the early onset of pubertal changes, as also shown in Table 7.6.

GNRH-INDEPENDENT PRECOCIOUS PUBERTY. Precocious pseudopuberty is also referred to as incomplete or peripheral puberty and may be isosexual or heterosexual. In these patients there may be secretion of sex steroids or human chorionic gonadotropin from sources other than the pituitary. These sources are outside the control of the normal GnRH control mechanism and are therefore referred to as GnRH-independent.

Over 10% of girls with precocious puberty have an ovarian tumor. These tumors are palpable in 80% of cases or may be readily detected by ultrasonography or tomographic studies. Bleeding is heavy and irregular, befitting its escape from the normal control mechanisms.

Table 7.6. Causes of Precocious Puberty or Menstruation

ISOSEXUAL PRECOCITY
TRUE PRECOCIOUS PUBERTY
    Congenital adrenal hyperplasia
    Constitutional (idopathic) (74%)
    Organic brain disease (7%)
        Astrocytoma
        Craniopharyngioma
        Encephalitis
        Ependymoma
        Glioma
        Hamartomas of hypothalamus
        Head trauma
        Meningitis, hydrocephalus
        Neurofibroma
        Suprasellar teratoma
        von Recklinghausen's disease
    Long-standing hypothyroidism
PRECOCIOUS PSEUDOPUBERTY
    Adrenal tumors (1%)
    Estrogen ingestion
    McCune-Albright's syndrome (5%)
    Ovarian tumors (11%)
    Peutz-Jeghers syndrome
    Silver's syndrome
INCOMPLETE SEXUAL PRECOCITY
    Premature adrenarche
    Premature pubarche
    Premature thelarche
HETEROSEXUAL PRECOCITY
    Ovarian tumors
    Adrenal tumors
    Congenital adrenal hyperplasia

McCune-Albright syndrome (polyostotic fibrous dysplasia) causes about 5% of precocious puberty cases. This syndrome consists of skin lesions (café au lait spots), disseminated cystic bone lesions that result in easy fractures, and sexual precocity. In this syndrome there is autonomous ovarian production of estrogen.

Evidence of virilization of prepubertal girls should suggest congenital adrenal hyperplasia or androgen secretion by an adrenal or ovarian tumor. Adrenal hyperplasia is often, but not always, associated with genital ambiguity. When this congenital adrenal hyperplasia is a possibility, it must be evaluated rapidly so that steroid therapy can be instituted promptly.

Ingestion of exogenous estrogen must be suspected in any case. Suspicion should be increased by the presence of darkening of the areolae and nipples. Possible sources include oral contraceptives, hormone replacement prescriptions, anabolic steroids, and some cosmetic products and skin creams.

Delayed Puberty

Delayed puberty is a relatively uncommon problem in girls. When it occurs, the possibility of a genetic or hypothalamic-pituitary abnormality must be considered, along with a moderately greater number of other possibilities (Table 7.7). Based on the average age and normal variation of puberty, any girl who has not exhibited breast budding by age 13 requires preliminary investigation. Similarly, girls who do not menstruate by age 15 or 16,

Table 7.7. Causes of Delayed Puberty or Menstruation

Cause	%
Hypergonadotropic hypogonadism (ovarian failure)	43
Ovarian failure, abnormal karyotype	26
Familial gonadal dysgenesis (single gene, autosomal ressessive)	
Chromosomal mosaicism	
Savage syndrome	
Swyer syndrome *(46,XY, testicular feminization)*	
Turner's syndrome	
Ovarian failure, normal karyotype	17
46, XX	15
46, XY	2
Long-arm X chromosomal deletion	
17α-Hydroxylase deficiency	
Alkylating chemotherapy	
Autoimmune disorders (with or without polyglandular immunopathy)	
Galactocemia	
Radiation therapy	
Hypogonadotropic hypogonadism	31
Inadequate gonadotropin-releasing hormone secretion	
Constitutional delayed puberty	10
Craniopharyngioma	
Cushing's disease or syndrome	
Hypothalamic hamartoma	
Marijuana use	
Olfactory tract hypoplasia (Kallmann's syndrome)	
Primary hypothyroidism	1
Inadequate gonadotropin secretion	7
Isolated gonadotropin deficiency	
Inadequate body fat	3
Anorexia nervosa	
Exercise-induced hypothalamic dysfunction	
Gastrointestinal malabsorption	
Pituitary insufficiency	2
Pituitary tumors	
Prolactin-secreting pituitary adenoma	1.5
Eugonadism and genital tract abnormalities	26
Androgen insensitivity syndrome	1
Imperforate hymen	0.5
Inappropriate positive feedback	7
Transverse vaginal septum	3
Vaginal and uterine agenesis (Rokitansky-Küster-Hauser syndrome)	14

regardless of other sexual development, should be evaluated. Patients should also be evaluated anytime there is a disruption in the normal sequence of puberty or patient or parental concern. Patients with significant abnormalities of either height or weight should be evaluated for chromosomal abnormalities or endocrinopathies.

One of the most common chromosomal causes of absent menstruation is the premature ovarian failure found in patients with Turner's syndrome (45, X). The absence of one X chromosome results in accelerated ovarian follicular atresia to the extent that by the age of puberty, no functionally competent follicles remain. These patients are noteworthy for their short stature, webbed neck (pterygium colli), a shieldlike chest with widely spaced nipples, and an increased carrying angle of the arms (cubitus valgus). Buccal smears will not demonstrate Barr bodies and chromosomal analysis will confirm the diagnosis. Because these women will not undergo any secondary sexual maturation, referral to a specialist for counseling and management of replacement hormonal manipulations is advisable. Deletions of only a part of the long arm of the X chromosome have been shown to be associated with premature ovarian failure, the earliest failures with the greatest deletions.

For a more complete discussion of the evaluation and treatment of primary amenorrhea, see Chapter 19, No Periods (Amenorrhea).

CLINICAL IMPLICATIONS

General Health Concerns

The general health care of young and adolescent girls is little different than for boys of the same age (Table 7.8). One exception to this is screening and immunization for rubella. If a young girl enters adolescence and has not recieved immunization for rubella or is uncertain about exposure to the disease, serologic testing for immunity should be strongly considered. If the patient is not immune, immunization should be undertaken before pregnancy (planned or otherwise) occurs.

Once the female adolescent becomes sexually active, screening for sexually transmitted disease (Chlamydia and gonorrhea) should be a part of every pelvic examination. The high prevalence of STDs in adolescents makes this a cost-effective screening measure.

First Examinations

Patients and mothers often ask, "When should a young woman have her first gynecologic examination?" First pelvic examinations should be performed anytime there is a gynecologic problem, when a woman becomes sexually active, or when she reaches age 18, whichever comes first. These are based on specific needs for diagnosis (as in the case of menstrual disorders), screening, or an opportunity to open a dialogue about health issues beyond those affecting reproductive health. Although young women are at low risk for cervical cancer, many predisposing factors, such as human papillomavirus infections or early dysplastic processes, may be identified and either treated or subjected to closer follow-up, as needed. At least a cursory examination is appropriate anytime the adolescent or her parents are concerned. A list of common reasons for first gynecologic examinations is shown in Table 7.9.

Table 7.8. Routine Care for the Adolescent Patient (by Tanner Stage)

	Early (Tanner 2)	Mid (Tanner 3–4)	Late (Tanner 5)
Screening Physical	Hematocrit Urinalysis Tuberculin test	Hematocrit Vision and hearing screening	Hematocrit Tuberculin test
If sexually active		Pap smear VDRL Gonorrhea and Chlamydia cultures	Pap smear VDRL Gonorrhea and Chlamydia cultures HIV Screening if indicated
Psychosocial	Depression Peer relations (including sexuality) School performance Substance abuse (including alcohol & tobacco)	Depression Peer relations (including sexuality) School performance Substance abuse (including alcohol & tobacco) Abuse	Depression Peer relations (including sexuality) School performance Substance abuse (including alcohol & tobacco) Sexual dysfunction Abuse
Prevention	Breast self-examination Nutrition Sports & sports injuries Automobile safety Immunization update	Breast self-examination Nutrition Dental hygiene Sports & sports injuries Automobile safety Immunization update (measles, mumps, rubella, hepatitis B) STD prevention Contraception	Breast self-examination Nutrition & exercise Automobile safety STD prevention Contraception Immunization update (tetanus/diphtheria toxoid)
Physical examination	Blood pressure Weight Height Sexual development Scoliosis Goiter Acne	Blood pressure Weight Height Sexual development Breast masses Vaginal discharge Pregnancy	Blood pressure Weight Height Sexual development Breast masses Adnexal masses Vaginal discharge Pregnancy
Symptomatic treatments	Acne Dysmenorrhea	Vaginal discharge Pregnancy Irregular periods Dysmenorrhea	Vaginal discharge Pregnancy Irregular periods Dysmenorrhea
Guidance	Confidentiality Developmental variation Emerging independence Peer pressure Dating and sexuality First menstruation	Confidentiality Dating and sexuality Menstrual hygiene Vocation or education	Dating and sexuality Marriage Vocation or education Independent living

VDRL = Venereal Disease Research Laboratory; HIV = human immunodeficiency virus; STD = sexually transmitted disease

Table 7.9. Common Indications for First Pelvic Examination

Gynecologic concerns or symptoms
    Amenorrhea
    Disrupted pubertal events
    Dysmenorrhea
    Dysfunctional uterine bleeding
    Menstrual irregularity (significant)
    Pelvic pain
    Suspected pregnancy
    Suspected sexually transmitted disease
    Vulvovaginal discharge or infection
Onset of sexual activity
    Contraceptive counseling
    Sexual abuse or rape
    Sexual dysfunction
    Sexuality counseling
    Sexually transmitted disease screening
    Suspected pregnancy
    Suspected sexually transmitted disease
Age 18

Refusal to undergo a pelvic examination should not, by itself, prevent counseling, pregnancy testing, or the dispensing of limited amounts of contraceptives. Ultrasonography or self-guided insertion of a cotton-tipped applicator or speculum for vaginal evaluations may provide the information required for medical management without producing undue trauma or distress. It is often better to defer the initial pelvic examination until a rapport is established than it is to forever taint the patient's view of gynecologic care.

Diagnosing and Managing Abnormal Puberty

Precocious Changes
Because untimely pubertal changes may be due to potentially life-threatening processes, early and aggressive evaluation must be carried out. This evaluation is directed toward detecting life-threatening diseases and defining the velocity of the process. The evaluation process is summarized in Table 7.10. For most patients, this evaluation is best carried out by referral or close consultation.

When the diagnosis of true precocious puberty is established, generally by exclusion, treatment with GnRH agonists usually halts the progression of change. This therapy is expensive and is only effective if the observed changes are under central control. Suppression of GnRH may also be carried out using medroxyprogesterone acetate (Depo-Provera), in doses of 100 to 200 mg given intramuscularly every 2 to 4 weeks. This therapy is less likely to control bone growth abnormalities than is GnRH agonist treatment. Therapy is worth considering for young children to preserve adult height and to avoid the social and emotional stresses that early maturation can entail.

Delayed Development
The evaluation of patients with delayed pubertal development must begin with a general history, including general health, weight and height records, and family history including

Table 7.10. Diagnostic Elements in Precocious Puberty

PHYSICAL FACTORS
    Percentile evaluation
      Height
      Weight
      Tanner stage
      Growth rate
    Abdominal, pelvic, and neurologic examination
    Status of genitalia (Tanner stage and signs of androgen effect)
    Skin changes (McCune-Albright syndrome)
    Thyroid examination
DIAGNOSTIC STUDIES
    Bone age (left wrist)
    Computed tomography or magnetic imaging of the head
    Computed tomography or ultrasonography of the abdomen
    Serum FSH, LH, and HCG
    Thyroid function tests (sensitive TSH and free T_4)
    Evaluation of steroids (serum DHAS, testosterone, estradiol, progesterone, 17-hydroxprog-
      esterone)
    GnRH testing

FSH = follicle-stimulating hormone; LH = luteinizing hormone; HCG = human chorionic gonadotropin; TSH = thyroid-stimulating hormone; DHAS = dehydroepiandrosterone sulphate; GnRH = gonadotropin-releasing hormone.

the pubertal experience of others in the family. Physical examination should identify the type and degree of sexual development present. The presence of breast changes generally indicates the production of estrogen, whereas the development of pubic or axillary hair indicates the production of androgens.

Laboratory evaluation should include serum FSH, LH, and prolactin measurements, skull x-ray studies, and thyroid function studies. Bone age, chromosomal or cytologic studies, pelvic ultrasonography, or other imagining studies may also be indicated. The complete evaluation is summarized in Chapter 19, No Periods (Amenorrhea). Because of the significance of the potential causes of disordered puberty, most of these patients should be evaluated by or in consultation with a specialist[4].

If hypogonadism is found to be the cause of delayed puberty, hormonal therapy will initiate and sustain the development of normal secondary sex characteristics. Hormonal therapy will also allow for normal height and bone mass deposition to be achieved. Adolescents require much less hormone therapy than do adults or postmenopausal women. Therapy usually begins with unopposed estrogen in the range of 0.3 mg of conjugated estrogen, 0.5 mg estradiol, or their equivalent daily. In 6 to 12 months, this dose is roughly doubled and medroxyprogesterone acetate (10 mg for the first 12 days of the month) is added. This will result in regular menstruation, but is insufficient for contraception. Normal pubertal development will generally proceed when the patient reaches a bone age of 13.

Contraceptive Choices for the Adolescent

The choice of contraceptive methods should be broadly based on the same factors used to select methods for adults (see Chapter 9, Contraception). Concern, however, should be directed to the special needs of the adolescent, which include privacy, reliability, STD protection, and side effect profiles. Many teens have unrealistic impressions of the actions and side effects of various contraceptive methods. Concerns about acne, weight gain, breakthrough bleeding, cancer, and changes in libido may affect the choices made. Although reliability may be paramount in the minds of providers, compliance and STD protection may be of greater importance because of the sporadic nature of teenage sexual behavior. Important factors to consider are those that enhance compliance, such as 28-day oral contraceptive packs or long-acting methods that require only infrequent motivation, and strategies that decrease side effects, such as bedtime oral contraceptive ingestion to reduce nausea. Emotional and physical self-image are often of paramount importance in determining ultimate compliance. The need to combine contraception and STD protection, often in the form of two methods such as oral contraceptives and condoms, should be encouraged.

The most important aspect of any adolescent contraception program or counseling is education. The sexually active, or soon to be active, teen must be extensively counseled about the options available, their actions, use, and side effects. Failure to provide this information invariably results in noncompliance and dissatisfaction, resulting in a high likelihood of the woman using no method at all (Fig 7.10). This is especially true for the long-acting hormonal methods, where some reports cite rates of up to 25% dissatisfaction because of inadequately explained side effects. Because an expanding sense of autonomy is an important part of adolescence, the patient should be allowed maximal latitude in any decision that is to be made. These decisions must be based on information.

Although there are minor variations from one geographic location to another, generally contraceptive counseling and prescribing is permitted for adolescents without either

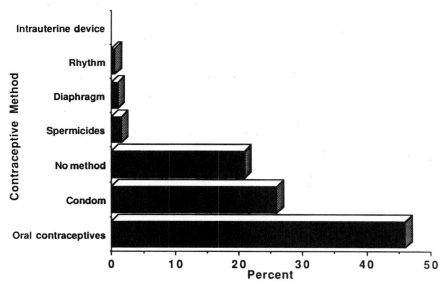

Figure 7.10. Contraceptive methods used by U.S. women age 15–19 years. Although oral contraceptives are the most commonly used adolescent contraceptive method, more than 1 of 5 teenage women use no contraceptive method at all. Data from: Harlap S, Kost K, Forrest JD. Preventing Pregnancy, Protecting Health: a New Look at Birth Control Choices in the United States. New York: The Alan Guttmacher Institute, 1991.

parental approval or notification. It is important that the adolescent be reassured that all communications will be held in confidence and that only information that the teen wishes disclosed will ever be discussed with her parents or guardians. Only in the case of a life-threatening situation should this confidence be violated.

HINTS AND COMMON QUESTIONS

Asymmetric breast development, which is common in pubertal girls, generally is of little significance. Care must be taken not to interpret early unilateral thelarche as a breast tumor, for biopsy may result in the removal of a significant portion of the immature breast tissue.

Absence of axiallary hair can occur, and may be familial. When other pubertal events are normal, this has no clinical significance.

Idiopathic or constitutional precocious puberty is associated with a normal reproductive life and normal age of menopause. The greatest risk for abnormality comes from the early closure of the bony growth plates that often leaves these patients with short stature. (Half are below 5 ft in height at maturity.)

The most common causes of isolated vaginal bleeding in a girl under the age of 8 are foreign bodies or trauma, not precocious puberty. Although the possible implications of advanced puberty are significant, an extensive evaluation should not be undertaken until these two possibilities have been investigated.

Most adolescent menstrual periods, even when ovulatory, tend to be lighter than those experienced later in life. Although heavy flow is less likely, occasional cases of extremely heavy flow do occur. When this happens, consideration must be given to other potential causes such as bleeding abnormalities or complications of early pregnancy. (See also Chapter 16, Heavy Periods and Toxic Shock Syndrome.)

There is often uncertainty about whether to have a parent in the room when interviewing and examining a teenage patient. One middle ground is to have the parent present during the initial phase of the interview to provide medical history and support, and then ask the parent to leave before proceeding with the examination. Before the examination begins, a second opportunity for discussion allows for a sense of independence, the assumption of an adult role, and confidential discussion. It is during this phase that questions about sexuality, contraception, or drug use should be posed.

Both the patient and her parent may be assured that a gynecologic examination will not damage the patient's hymen nor change her virginity.

Questions about how a teen is doing in school are often a useful way to introduce discussions of temperament, peer relations, sexuality, and other behaviors. These may also point out early signs of depression or withdrawal that need to be addressed.

Some clinicians are reluctant to consider oral contraceptives for their teenage patients because of a fear of premature closure of the epiphyses. For most patients this is not a concern because closure has already begun by the time most girls have become ovulatory. Even if closure were not already underway, the impact of an unplanned pregnancy, biologically and otherwise, is far greater.

The period of adolescence is a time of self-assured, inaccurate knowledge, garnered from peers. Anyone who cares for an adolescent must be sensitive to the myths common

Table 7.11. Common Adolescent Myths

A woman can't get pregnant if she has sex only once.	False
A woman can't get pregnant during her period.	Unlikely, but False
A woman can't get pregnant if she doesn't have an orgasm (climax).	False
A woman can't get pregnant if she has sex before her first period.	Unlikely, but False
Birth control pills make you sterile or cause cancer.	False
There is a "morning after pill" that can help prevent pregnancy.	Not a good alternative, but True
You have to be 18 to buy a condom or obtain contraceptives.	False
Condoms provide complete protection from pregnancy and sexually transmitted disease.	False
Only gays and drug addicts get HIV or AIDS.	False
You can't get HIV or AIDS if you have sex with only one person.	False
If a women misses only one birth control pill she still can't get pregnant.	Unlikely, but False
If you take the pill you don't need to use a condom.	False
"Pulling out" before ejaculation is good protection from pregnancy and sexually transmitted disease.	False
"Safer sex" involves more than just using condoms.	True

to this age group, not only to dispel them, but also to appreciate the mind-set under which these young people operate. Some common reproductive myths are listed in Table 7.11.

SUGGESTED READINGS

General References

American College of Obstriticians and Gynecologists. Confidentiality in adolescent health care. ACOG statement of policy. Washington, DC: ACOG, 1988.

American College of Obstetricians and Gynecologists. The Adolesecent Gynecologic Patient. ACOG Technical Bulletin No. 145. Washington, DC: ACOG, 1990.

American Medical Association. AMA Guidelines for Adolescent Preventive Services (GAPS): Recommendations and Rationale. Baltimore: Williams & Wilkins, 1994.

Centers for Disease Control and Prevention/National Center for Health Statistics. Advance report of final natality statistics, 1990. Monthly Vital Statistics Report 1993;41(suppl 9).

Centers for Disease Control and Prevention. Results from the National Adolescnt Student Health Survey. MMWR 1989;38:147.

Lee PA. Neuroendocrinology of puberty. Semin Reprod Endocrinol 1988;6:13.

Marshall WA, Tanner JM. Variation in the pattern of pubertal changes in girls. Arch Dis Child 1969;44:291.

Neinstein LS. Adolescent Health Care. A Practical Guide, 2nd ed. Baltimore: Williams & Wilkins, 1991.

Speroff L, Glass RH, Kase NG. Clinical Gynecologic Endocrinology and Infertility, 5th ed. Baltimore: Williams & Wilkins, 1994, p 361.

Tanner JM. Growth at Adolescence, 2nd ed. Oxford: Blackwell Scientific Publications, 1962.

Specific References

Pediatric Concerns

Bacon JL. Pediatric vulvovaginitis. Adolescent Pediatric Gynecology 1989;2:86.

Paradise JE, Willis ED. Probability of vaginal foreign body in girls with genital complaints. Am J Dis Child 1985;139:472.

Simmons PS. Office pediatric gynecology. Prim Care 1988;15:617.

Williams RS, Callen JP, Owen LG. Vulvar disorders in the prepubertal female. Pediatr Ann 1986;15:588.

Development

deRidder CM, Thijssen JHH, Bruning PF, Van den Brande JL, Zonderland ML, Erich WBM. Body fat mass, body fat distribution, and pubertal development: a longitudinal study of physical and hormonal sexual maturation of girls. J Clin Endocrinol Metab 1992;75:442.

Frisch RE. Body fat, menarche, and reproductive ability. Seminars in Reproductive Endocrinology 1985;3:45.

Frisch RE, McArthur JW. Menstrual cycles: fatness as a determinant of minimum weight for height necessary for their maintenance or onset. Science 1974;185:949.

Knobil E. The neuroendocrine control of the menstrual cycle. Recent Prog Horm Res 1980;36:53.

Lee PA. Normal ages of pubertal events among American males and females. J Adolesc Health 1980;1:26.

Oerter KE, Uriarte MM, Rose SR, Barnes KM, Cutler GB JR. Gonadotropin secretory dynamics during pugerty in normal girls and boys. J Clin Endocrinol Metab 1990;71:1251.

Reindollar RH, Byrd JR, McDonough PG. Delayed sexual development: A study of 252 patients. Am J Obstet Gynecol 1981;140:371.

Reindollar RH, McDonough PG. Pubertal aberrancy: Etiology and clinical approach. J Reprod Med 1984;29:391.

Stein DT. New developments in the diagnosis and treatment of sexual precocity. Am J Med Sci 1992;303:53.

Warren WP. The effect of exercise on pubertal progression and reproductive function in girls. J Clin Endocrinol Metab 1980;51:1150.

Wheeler MD, Styne DM. The treatment of precocious puberty. Endocrinol Metab Clin North Am 1991;20:183.

Zacharias L, Rand WM, Wurtman RJ. A prospective study of sexual development and growth in American girls: the statistics of menarch. Obstet Gynecol Surv 1976;31:325.

Pregnancy and Contraception

Alan Guttmacher Institute. Sex and America's Teenagers. New York, NY: The Alan Guttmacher Institute, 1994.

American Academy of Pedicatrics. Committee on Adolescence: Contraception and adolescents. Pediatrics 1990;86:134.

Berenson AB, Wiemann CM. Patient satisfaction and side effects with levonorgestrel implant (Norplant) use in adolescents 18 years of age or younger. Pediatrics 1993;92:257.

Berenson AB, Wiemann CM. Use of levonorgestrel implants versus oral contraceptives in adolescence: a case-control study. Am J Obstet Gynecol 1995;172:1128.

Carpenter S, Neinstein LS. Weight gain in adolescent and young adult oral contraceptive users. J Adolesc Health 1986;7:342.

Centers for Disease Control and Prevention. Teenage pregnancy and birth rates—United States, 1990. MMWR 1993;42:733.

Cromer BA, Smith RD, Blair JM, Dwyer J, Brown RT. A prospective study of adolescents who choose among levonorgestrel implant (Norplant), medroxyprogesterone acetate (Depo-Provera), or the combined oral contraceptive pill as contraception. Pediatrics 1994;94:687.

Davis AJ. The role of hormonal contraception in adolescents. Am J Obstet Gynecol 1994;170:1581.

Emans SJ, Grace F, Woods ER, et al. Adolescents' compliance with the use of oral contraceptives. JAMA 1987;257:3377.

Harlap S, Kost K, Forrest JD. Preventing Pregnancy, Protecting Health: A New Look at Birth Control Choices in the United States. New York: The Alan Guttmacher Institute, 1991.

Herold ES, Goodwin MS. Perceived side effects of oral contraceptives among adolescent girls. Can Med Assoc J 1980;123:1022.

Jones ES. Teenage Pregnancy in Industrialized Countries. New Haven, CT: Yale University Press, 1986.

Kaunitz AM. Guiding adolescents in proper contraceptive use. Contemp Gynecol Obstet 1992;(May):15.

Khouzam HR. Promotion of sexual abstinence: reducing adolescent sexual activity and pregnancies. South Med J 1995;88:709.

McAnarney ER, Hendee WR. Adolescent pregnancy and its consequences. JAMA 1989;262:74.

Mosher WD, McNally JW. Contraceptive use at first premarital intercourse: United States 1965–1988. Fam Plann Perspect 1991;23:108.

Orr DP, Langefeld CD, Katz BP, et al. Factors associated with condom use among sexually active female adolescents. J Pediatrics 1992;120:311.

Polaneczky M, Slap G, Forke C, Rappaport A, Sondheimer S. The use of levonorgestrel implants (Norplant) for contraception in adolescent mothers. N Engl J Med 1994;331:1201.

Robinson JC, Plichta S, Weisman CS, et al. Dysmenorrhea and use of oral contraceptives in adolescent women attending a family planning clinic. Am J Obstet Gynecol 1992;166:578.

Sabin LS, Kantner JF, Zelnick M. The risk of adolescent pregnancy in the first months of intercourse. Fam Plann Perspect 1979;11:215.

Sexuality, Abuse, Date Rape

American College of Obstetricians and Gynecologists. Adolescent Sexuality: Guides for Physician Involvement. Washington, DC: ACOG, 1992.

American College of Obstetricians and Gynecologists. Adolescent acquaintance rape. ACOG Committee Opinion 122. Washington, DC: ACOG, 1993.

American College of Obstetricians and Gynecologists. Sexual assault. ACOG Technical Bulletin 172. Washington, DC: ACOG, 1992.

Ammerman SD, Perelli E, Adler N, Irwin CE JR. Do adolescents understand what physicians say about sexuality and health? Clin Pediatr (Phila) 1992;31:590.

Berman HS. Talking HEADS: Interviewing adolescents. HMO Practice 1987;1:3.

Braverman PK, Strasburger VC. Adolescent sexual activity. Clin Pediatr (Phila) 1993;32:658.

Braverman PK, Strasburger VC. Adolescent sexuality. Part 4. The practitioner's role. Clin Pediatr (Phila) 1994;33:100.

Centers for Disease Control and Prevention. Sexual behavior among high school students. JAMA 1992;267:28.

Cohall AT, Cohall Rm. Screening for psychosocial health problems. Contemporary Adolescent Gynecology 1995;1:11.

Cohen E, Mackenzie RG, Yates GL. HEADSS, a psychosocial risk assessment instrument. J Adolesc Health 1991;12:539.

Forrest JD, Singh S. The sexual and reproductive behavior of American women, 1982–1988. Fam Plann Persp 1990;22:206.

Goldenring JM, Cohen E. Getting into adolescent heads. Contemporary Pediatrics 1988;5:75.

Khouzam HR. Promotion of sexual abstinence: reducing adolescent sexual activity and pregnancies. South Med J 1995;88:709.

McFarlane J, Parker V, Soeken K, Vullock L. Assessing for abuse during pregnancy. Severity and frequency of injuries and associated entry into prenatal care. JAMA 1992;267:3176.

Morris L, Warren CW, Aral SO. Measuring adolescent sexual behaviors and related health outcomes. Public Health Rep 1993;108:31.

Nagy S, Adcock AG, Nagy MC. A comparison of risky behaviors of sexually active, sexually abused, and abstaining adolescents. Pediatrics 1994;93:570.

Orr DP, Beiter M, Ingersoll G. Premature sexual activity as an indicator of psychosocial risk. Pediatrics 1991;87:141.

Parrot A. Acquaintance rape among adolescents: identifying risk groups and intervention strategies. Journal of Social Work and Human Sexuality 1989;8:47.

Peipert JF, Domagalski LR. Epidemiology of adolescent sexaul assault. Obstet Gynecol 1994;84:867.

Remafedi G, Resnick M, Blum R, Harris L. Demography of sexual orientation in adolescents. Pediatrics 1992;89:714.

Romer D, Black M, Ricardo I, et al. Social influences on the sexual behavior of youth at risk for HIV exposure. Am J Pub Health 1993;83:501.

Springs FE, Friedrich WN. Health risk behaviors and medical sequelae of childhood sexual abuse. Mayo Clin Proc 1992;67:527.

Walch AG, Broadhead WE. Prevalence of lifetime sexual victimization among female patients. J Fam Pract 1992;35:511.

Other

Abrams SA, Silber TJ, Esteban NV, et al. Mineral balance and bone turnover in adolescents with anorexia nervosa. J Petiatr 1993;123:326.

Anderson JW, Brinkman VL, Hamilton CC. Weight loss and 2-year follow-up for 80 morbidly obese patients treated with intensive, very-low calorie diet and an education program. Am J Clin Nutr 1992;56:244S.

Bachrach JK. Decreased bone density in adolescent girls with anorexia nervosa. Pediatrics 1990;86:440.

Chan GM. Dietary calcium and bone mineral status of children and adolescents. Am J Dis Child 1991;145:631.

Claessens E, Cowell CA. Acute adolescent menorrhagia. Am J Obstet Gynecol 1981;139:277.

Colditz GA. Economic costs of obesity. Am J Clin Nutr 1992;55:503S.

Collet ME, Wertenberger GE, Fiske VM. The effect of age upon the pattern of the menstrual cycle. Fertil Steril 1954;5:437.

Felts WM, Mikow VA. Adolescent homicide and suicide. In Wallace HM, Nelson RP, Sweeney PJ (eds). Maternal and Child Health Practices, 4th ed. Oakland: Third Party Publishing Company, 1994, p 657.

Hergenroeder AC. Bone mineralization, hypothalamic amenorrhea and sex steroid therapy in female adolescents and young adults. J Pediatrics 1995;126:683.

Irwin CE, Igra V. Adolescent risk-taking behavior. In Wallace HM, Nelson RP, Sweeney PJ (eds). Maternal and Child Health Practices, 4th ed. Oakland: Third Party Publishing Company, 1994, p 585.

Kurtzman FD, Yager J, Landvesk J, Wiesmeier E, Bodurka DC. Eating disorders among selected female student populations at UCLA. J Am Diet Assoc 1989;89:45.

Lloyd T, Andon MB, Rollings N, et al. Calcium supplementation and bone mineral density in adolescent girls. JAMA 1993;270:841.

Loucks AB, Heath EM, Law T, Verdun M, Watts JR. Dietary restriction reduces luteinizing hormone (LH) pulse frequency during waking hours and increases LH pulse amplitude during sleep in young menstruating women. J Clin Endocrinol Metab 1994;78:910.

Must A, Jacques PF, Dallal GE, Gajema CJ, Dietz WH. Long-term morbidity and mortality of overweight adolescents. N Engl J Med 1992;327:1350.

Robinson JI, Hoerr SL, Strandmark J, Mavis B. Obesity, weight loss, and health. J Am Diet Assoc 1993;93:445.

Sjostrom LV. Mortality of severely obese subjects. Am J Clin Nutr 1992;55:516S.

Treloar AE, Boynton RE, Borghild GB, Brown BW. Variation of the human menstrual cycle through reproductive life. Int J Fertil 1967;12:77.

Wolf AM, Gortmaker SL, Cheung L, Gray HM, Herzog DB, Colditz GA. Activity, inactivity, and obesity: racial, ethnic and age differences among schoolgirls. Am J Pub Health 1993;83:1625.

8

Sexuality

Sexual health is a part of total health. What was referred to in 1925 as "the pervicacious gonadal urge in human beings" has now become the fodder of daytime TV talk shows. It is a field filled with paradoxes. We are all sexual beings, but no one wants to admit to it. It is the only area of life in which professionals are held in lower esteem than amateurs. Sexuality shapes how we dress and move, the kind of car we drive, and even our place in lifeboats and on the dance floor. Clearly, anyone who cares for women must be sensitive to the many special aspects of their sexuality and their sexual concerns.

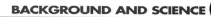 **BACKGROUND AND SCIENCE**

Evolution of Sexuality

At its root, sexuality begins with gender determined at fertilization of the ova with a sperm carrying an X or a Y chromosome. From that point forward, however, the ultimate form and functions that sexuality takes is determined by a myriad of factors, including culture, religion, family values, peer pressures, and individual psychology and variation. Even in adulthood, sexual identity and behaviors remain fluid.

Children

The time from before birth to mid childhood is critical to normal sexual development. Sexual arousal, at a physiologic level, occurs before birth, and continues during infancy and childhood. Studies indicate that chemical effects on the brain may subtly change certain skills and abilities based on the relative abundance of male and female hormones. A sense of maleness or femaleness (gender identity) is imparted to children very early, and becomes an integral part of their self-image. The most critical time for a positive image to be developed is between 18 months and 3 years of age.

Beginning about age 3 to 4 years, children begin to appreciate gender differences. Bodily function, anatomy, gestation, and birth all become topics of interest to children at this age. Basic attitudes about nudity and genital touching (personal and abuse avoidance) become established during this time. During the ages 5 to 9 years greater interest in conception (especially regarding animals and pets) surfaces as does greater mimicking of socially accepted gender roles.

Self-exploration, including the genitals, is a natural part of infancy and childhood. Sexual play, alone or with others, is common, although its degree of acceptance is based on cultural, family, and religious factors. Studies indicate this exploration is normal and those who masturbate early in life and continue through adulthood have the most well-adjusted sex lives. Although arousal may occur as part of this sex play, it is not considered an early form of adult behavior. Adult patterns of sexuality do not emerge until hormonal and physical maturation occurs in adolescence.

By age 9 to 12, most children develop a heightened interest in anatomy, physiology, and the sociologic aspects of sexuality. They take great interest in the physical and emotional changes they are experiencing. The amount, character, and accuracy of information available to the adolescent can have a great impact on self-image and sexual growth.

Adolescents

The physiologic changes that accompany adolescence have been discussed in Chapter 7, Pediatric and Adolescent Care. The factors that shape sexuality are much harder to characterize. Role models in home and media, religious and family values, peer pressure, social norms, self-confidence, and rebellion all play a part. Although gender and sexual identity are established in childhood, the modes of expression an individual chooses for that sexuality evolve during adolescence.

Adolescents receive very mixed messages about sex and sexuality. They are told that "sex is dirty;" however, they are told to "save it for someone you love." The media tells them how to attract another and their parents tell them not to. Despite all these conflicting messages, boys and girls see their sexuality turn from something that served only to identify their gender into a source of power and pleasure.

Sexual identity is independent of sexual orientation. Sexual orientation spans a continuum from heterosexuality through bisexuality to homosexuality. Most studies indicate that few people are purely heterosexual or homosexual, but that most have variable feelings of attraction, the majority of which lie at one end of the scale or the other. The origins of sexual orientation (biologic, social, behavioral) have been debated without resolution. It is common for adolescents to have fears of homosexuality as emerging sexual interest seeks a focus. Studies indicate that it is common for adolescents to have at least one homosexual encounter, ranging from arousal to consummation, during this period. This appears to have little to do with eventual sexual orientation.

Adult patterns of sexuality begin to emerge during adolescence in the form of fantasy, daydreams, and infatuation. Feelings of sexual attraction and attentiveness alter self-image, initiate social interactions, romance, and dating. Erotic dreams, which emerge for both

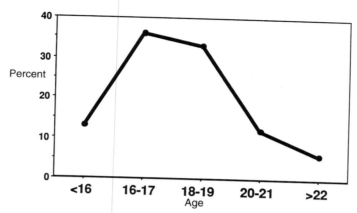

Figure 8.1. Age at first intercourse. (After: Tavris C, Sadd S. The Redbood Report on Female Sexuality. New York: Delacorte Press, 1977.)

boys and girls, may be accompanied by orgasm. These are physiologic, not psychologic, and require reassurance only if they cause concern.

At some point, dating and the search for a mate leads to more intimate expression of sexual pleasure and fulfillment, culminating in adult sex play and intercourse. Figure 8.1 illustrates the age of first intercourse currently found in the United States. About 70% of young women say they wanted intercourse the first time it occurred; 24% felt pressured and 4% were forced against their will into having their first sexual experience. Of those who wanted intercourse, almost half believed themselves to be in love and a quarter expressed a curiosity or readiness for sex as their motivation. Peer pressure or pressure brought by the relationship was a factor in over 60% of those women who had an unwanted first intercourse.

A recent study evaluated the factors related to the loss of virginity in a group of junior high school students in Chicago, Illinois. Among those factors in these 8th graders were gender (male); race (highest for blacks, lowest for whites and Hispanics); pubertal status (having menstruated or ejaculated, a function of age); previous suicide attempt; sibling number; and housing density. Factors that had little or no relation to early sexual activity included church attendance, religious affiliation, grade point average, housing status, marital status of natural parents, self-esteem, sex education knowledge, school attendance, and strict age independent of pubertal status. This study suggests that factors having traditionally been thought to reduce sexual expression may not be effective, and that those considered to increase sexual behavior (such as sexual knowledge) do not have that effect.

Adult Sexual Behavior

Sexual behavior in adults has been the subject of an increasing number of scientific studies and for an unending stream of entertainment vehicles. These studies help to document normative behaviors, but may be of little help in counseling patients except to give limited information when addressing sexual dysfunction (Chapter 24, Sexual Dysfunction).

Some generalities regarding adult sexual behavior may be drawn from recent surveys. These indicate that sexual behavior has changed little over the years and is far more conventional that current media portrayals would indicate. It appears that we are more monogamous, less imaginative, more secretive, and less successful than we once thought.

Although women are more likely to have lived with their spouse before marriage than once was the case (roughly 65% for women born 1963–1974 vs. <10% of women born 1933–1942), we are still a monogamous society, >80% have had one partner or no partner in the past year and over 50% have had only one partner in the past 5 years). The median number of partners since age 18 is only two for women (vs. six for men). Whereas almost half of women believe that sex outside of marriage is acceptable, they do insist that it be part of a serious, faithful, commitment.

The average married woman has intercourse just over six times per month (Fig 8.2), with about one third of women reporting intercourse a few times a year or not at all. Forty percent of married couples (and over half of those living together) have sex twice a week. Marriages are generally happy with almost 90% of spouses reporting great sexual pleasure and 85% experiencing great emotional satisfaction from their marriages. Recent studies indicate that 15% of women have had affairs (vs. 25% of men), but almost 95% were faithful over the past year.

Most couples spend between 15 minutes and 1 hour having sex, with only 15% of women exceeding this time. Unfortunately for many women, married men are five times more likely than single men to spend 15 minuets or less on intercourse. Although intercourse remains the greatest source of sexual pleasure for Americans, watching a mate undress, receiving oral sex, and giving oral sex follow closely behind in popularity (Fig 8.3). (Approxiamately 55% of women and 30% of men say foreplay is better than intercourse or afterplay.) Despite sexual satisfaction, masturbation is still a popular pastime. Overall, 10% of women masturbate at least once a week; roughly 40% of women report masturbating in the past year. This increases to 45% among women living with their partners.

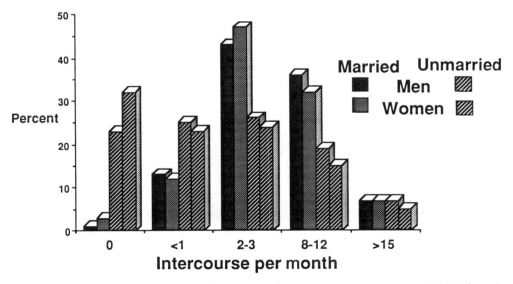

Figure 8.2. Intercourse per Month. (After: Michael RT, Gagnon JH, Laumann EO, Kolata G. Sex in America: a Definitive Survey. Boston: Little, Brown and Company, 1994.)

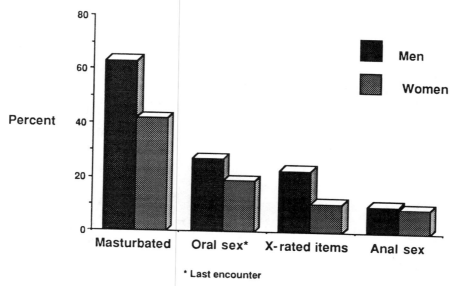

Figure 8.3 Sexual Practices. (After: Michael RT, Gagnon JH, Laumann EO, Kolata G. Sex in America: a Definitive Survey. Boston: Little, Brown and Company, 1994.)

Older Patients

Older women can and should expect to maintain sexual expressiveness even after menopause. For many women, the loss of menstruation, the relative decrease in the estrogen-to-androgen ratio, and the increased availability of their partner after retirement means greater sexual freedom and expressiveness. In one study of women aged 45–69, 41% reported moderate or strong sexual feelings. Unlike 100 years ago, a couple today can expect to have 30 years together after their youngest child is married, and most expect these years to continue to be sexually fulfilling. Indeed, at age 60, 94% of males and 84% of females are still sexually active.

Much of the decline in sexual frequency found in older women is related to the availability and capability of partners. Age and the effects of medications on one or both partners play the greatest role. When the individual or couple is comfortable with noncoital stimulation, sexual activity tends to stay strong. Although coital frequency may change for these couples, the frequency of lovemaking does not. It is sometimes said that sex is like riding a bicycle: The only reasons not to do it are if you have health reasons you cannot, you think it is silly, or you do not have a bicycle. There is no reason, outside of these, that we should not encourage all older patients to remain sexually expressive.

Loss of ovarian steroids at menopause may lead to a loss of vaginal wall thickness and vaginal dryness. If untreated, this can lead to painful intercourse, abrasions, and trauma. Once established, these problems can further inhibit desire and lubrication, create muscle spasms, and begin a cycle that may end in complete abstinence. The addition of a vaginal moisturizer or additional lubrication will provide temporary relief; estrogen replacement can prevent or reverse these changes. If atrophic changes have already occurred, complete reversal with estrogen may take up to 6 months to achieve.

A great deal has been written debating the role of estrogen and androgen in the libidinal function of postmenopausal women. Studies indicate that there is a relationship between serum testosterone levels (in women) and sexual desire and coital frequency. In menopausal women there is a decline in testosterone levels, but the decline is less than that seen in estrogen, resulting in a relative androgen dominance. (This is why older women develop a moustache.) Androgen therapy has been shown to increase sexual motivation, although a change in sexual, coital, or orgasmic frequency has been harder to demonstrate. The doses used in these studies have often exceeded the physiologic range, raising concerns about long-term effects. Until more definitive studies are available, care in the use of testosterone is warranted.

Physiology

Unlike estrus cycles found in many mammals, human sexual response is predominately a volitional phenomenon. As such, factors such as emotion, education, situation, and culture play a greater part in determining receptivity and sexual response than do menstrual phase or hormone levels. At the physiologic level, human sexual response is independent of sexual orientation or the type of sexual activity involved (intercourse, masturbation, fantasy).

Female Sexual Response Cycle

Some authors have divided the sexual response cycle into two broad phases: arousal (characterized by predominately parasympathetic neurologic processes) and orgasmic (characterized by sympathetic processes). This mode of classification is useful in anticipating the sexual impact of medications. More familiar is the four-phase response cycle proposed by Masters and Johnson. This cycle is made up of excitement, plateau, orgasm, and resolution. Many would add a fifth phase—desire—before the other four. This additional phase lies outside the primarily physiologic aspects of sexual activity that Masters and Johnson studied, but it represents an important source of clinical dysfunction. Whether one uses four or five phases, these phases represent an artificial demarcation of a continuum of response that varies from individual to individual and time to time. The changes found in various organs and systems during the four physiologic phases of the sexual response cycle are summarized in Table 8.1.

EXCITEMENT. The duration of both the excitement and plateau phases are quite variable, both from person to person and from one sexual episode to the next. The physiologic changes found are not dependent on the source of the arousal (physical or fantasy), but require only that the source be of an acceptable form of sufficient intensity and duration, provided without distraction, in a supportive setting that allows the couple to enjoy the sensations provided. Although the physiologic response to this stimulation may be stereotyped, the type and character of the stimulus itself is inconsistent and inconstant.

The excitement phase of sexual response (also called arousal) is characterized by diffuse vascular and muscular changes. At the start of arousal heart rate, blood pressure, and respiratory rate and depth all increase. Early in the process vasodilatation causes flushing, engorgement, and a sense of total body warmth. Changes in blood flow to the breast and labia lead to a flushed appearance and swelling. A diffuse increase in cutaneous blood flow to the skin of the chest causes a red rash ("sex flush") to appear and persist until the resolution phase of the cycle. After roughly 10 to 30 seconds of stimulation, increased blood flow

Table 8.1. Physiologic Changes During Sexual Response

Area	Excitement (arousal)	Plateau	Orgasm	Resolution
General	Warmth/erotic feelings (sexual tension)	Voluntary and involuntary muscle contractions	Release of tension; generalized muscle spasms	Feelings of satisfaction and well-being
Cardio-vascular	Increased pulse/blood pressure	Cardiac rate averages 100–175/min; BP rises by 20–60/10–20 mm Hg	Cardiac rate averages 110–180 + /min; BP rises by 30–80/20–40 mm Hg	Return to baseline
Respiratory	Increased depth	Increased rate	Variable, rate as high as 40/min; vocalization; occasional breath holding	Return to baseline
Breast	Engorgement; nipple erection	Marked breast/areolar engorgement; erythematous rash		Involution (may be prolonged)
Skin	Generalized vasocongestion	Marked vasocongestion; erythematous rash on chest/epigastrium spreading to head and shoulders (sex flush)		Resolution of rash in reverse order of appearance; perspiration on palms and soles
Genital				
Clitoris	Erection, tightly applied to clitoral hood; increased diameter/length	Retracts against symphysis		Rapid return to normal position; slower loss of erection
Labia	Engorgement	Marked engorgement; bright red color; Bartholin's gland secretion		Rapid loss of bright color; resolution of engorgement
Perineum		Engorgement with formation of "orgasmic platform"	Muscle contraction around vagina/anus; 0.8-sec interval	Rapid loss of orgasmic platform; full resolution in 10–15 min
Vagina	Transudation	Engorgement of lower 1/3; decreased diameter by 50% upper 2/3 dilates; increased length	Contractions at 0.8-sec intervals; recurring 3–12 times	Full resolution in 10–15 min
Uterus	Tents upward	Further tenting (antiverted uterus only)	Uterine contractions at 0.8-sec intervals	Gaping of os for 20–30 min; cervical descent

to the vaginal walls results in vaginal lubrication. This process of lubrication last only as long as stimulation persists, stopping abruptly if distraction intervenes. A small amount of fluid is also released by the Bartholin's glands. The clitoris becomes erect, increasing both in length and diameter, and becomes tightly applied to the clitoral hood (foreskin). The erection is slower and less dramatic than that of the penis. Studies indicate that there is no correlation between clitoral size or degree of erection and sexual performance or enjoyment.

Diffuse muscular changes are also a part of the excitement phase of sexual response. Nipple erection and a diffuse increase in muscle tone (sexual tension) are prominent parts of early arousal. The uterus tents upward in the pelvis, possibly owing to deep breathing combined with increased muscle tone.

PLATEAU. The plateau phase represents a continuation of the changes started during excitement. As the name suggests, this phase may be either a launching place for orgasm or an end by itself. Vasocongestion throughout the body increases with the most noticeable changes found in the breasts, areolas, labia, and vaginal walls. The area that is flushed expands in size and intensity. The areolas and labia become coral red and engorged. In the vagina, vasocongestion results in a thickening and narrowing of the lower one third of the vaginal canal. This thickening may narrow the vaginal barrel by as much as 50%. This is referred to as the orgasmic platform, and serves to increase pressure and friction on and by the penis during intravaginal thrusting. This narrowing of the vagina may also facilitate sperm retention following ejaculation. At the same time the outer third of the vagina is narrowing, the upper portion elongates and widens as the uterus tents further upward, producing an expansion of about 40% in length and up to 6 cm in width. During the plateau phase, the clitoris retracts tightly against the symphysis.

Increased muscle tension leads to voluntary and involuntary muscle spasms, especially in the hands and feet. Increased muscle tone in the perineal muscles adds to the formation of the orgasmic platform by constricting the vaginal opening. Heart rate, respiratory rate, and blood pressure continue to rise as the plateau phase continues to orgasmic release.

ORGASM. Orgasm brings to a peak all the changes that have gone before and culminates in the release of the sexual tensions built up throughout the body. Generalized muscular spasms, typically including the neck, face, hands, and feet are common and may be as extreme as to mimic the spasms of seizures. Muscular contractions of the perineum, anal sphincter, and uterus occur in a rhythmic fashion with a period of 0.8 seconds. These rhythmic contractions begin 2 to 4 seconds after the sensation of orgasm begins and typically last for 3 to 15 contractions (3 to 12 seconds). Although a hallmark of orgasm, these contractions are not always consciously felt.

Although the orgasm provides relief of sexual tension, re-establishing that tension with multiple or prolonged orgasms is possible and common. The likelihood of this is based on the type and degree of stimulation provided. The most intense muscular contractions tend to be those induced through masturbation or vibrator stimulation. Although orgasmic intensity is usually related to the strength of these contractions, many women report that orgasms obtained through intercourse are more satisfying.

A great deal of debate has centered around both the source of orgasms and the existence of a "G-spot." Current theory holds that there are no differences between orgasms caused by clitoral or vulvar stimulation and those from vaginal, cervical, uterine, or psychological stimulation. Many authors feel that most, if not all, orgasms arise from direct or indirect stimulation of the neural bundles in and around the clitoris, although orgasm secondary to other forms of stimulation may occur even in paraplegia. Efforts to duplicate the original work suggesting the existence of a sensitive area on the anterior vaginal wall under the urethra (the G-spot) have been unsuccessful, raising doubts about its existence and significance.

RESOLUTION. During the resolution phase there is a reversal of the changes that led to orgasm. Heart and respiratory rates return to normal, the sex flush fades (in the reverse order it appeared), and vasocongestion resolves, resulting in loss of engorgement of the breasts, areolas, labia, and vagina. The orgasmic platform is lost and the uterus returns to its normal position. The resolution phase is longer for women than it is for men and, unlike men, women have no refractory period, and thus may re-enter the excitement or plateau phase if appropriate stimulation is available.

Beyond Intercourse

Autoerotic practices can either be a true celebration of nature, personally or mutually, or a furtive, clandestine act of defiance or maladaptation. Some of the most physically intense orgasms come from self-stimulation. There is no evidence that the orgasms obtained through masturbation are better or worse, although they may be "different" owing to circumstances, expectation, or intensity. Despite the prevalence of masturbation (to orgasm; 60% to 80% of women and 70% to 95% or more of men; during the last year; 40% of women and 60% of men) it is estimated that 20% of women learn to masturbate from their partners. Although self-exploration and pleasuring provide very valuable sources of information and sexual education, roughly half of adults view it as undesirable or objectionable. In a study of 105 male and 123 female college students asked to select pictures of women most likely to masturbate, the least attractive women were consistently selected.

During rapid eye movement (REM) sleep, episodic erections or nocturnal penile tumescence (NPT) occur. In women, the analogous process results in vaginal lubrication and vulvar engorgement. Although orgasms (wet dreams) are far less common for women than for men, they do occur and can be the source of considerable distress for some patients. Both arousal and occasional orgasmic release are physiologic and require no more than reassurance.

Pregnancy, a common outcome of sexual expression, may itself further modify sexuality. During pregnancy most couples experience a decline in the frequency of intercourse and a change in the forms of sexual expression used. Intercourse declines by about 50% by the end of pregnancy, while pleasuring, holding, cuddling, and other forms of closeness increase. Discomfort, fear, and declining interest are the most common reasons for this change. Except in unusual circumstances (e.g., previous premature labor, premature rupture of the membranes, placenta previa) there is no need to restrict sexual expression during pregnancy. Many couples may benefit, however, from reassurance that the normal changes they experience are natural and not a cause for concern.

Psychology

The conscious control of biologic urges sets humans apart. Sexual expression is a complex process that may be broken down into three phases: proximation, preparation, and consummation. Most of the physiology of sex occurs in the preparation and consummation phases, whereas the psychology of sex plays the greatest role in proximation (and to a lesser extent preparation as well).

Proximation, which involves courting, flirting, and desire, begins the progress toward physical sexual expression. This may be influenced by many factors including expectation, experience, setting, mood, fatigue, and others. Seeing a long-separated lover has a different effect than seeing a stranger.

Erotic arousal, or the preparation phase, is due to a variety of stimuli that vary widely from person to person and time to time. Although much has been ascribed to the role of romance and courtship, studies indicate that there are very few differences in what causes arousal for men and women.

In a broad sense, sexuality is fundamentally different for women and for men. For women, sexual expression is an internalized phenomenon. It requires invasion, figuratively and literally; it demands psychological and physical vulnerability. For men, it is external and peninsular; from toilet training on, boys take pride in their genitals and what can be done with them. For girls, there is a void, physically and socially, that may leave them without even the instruction to wipe from front to back. It is little wonder then that in one study of 800 women they listed their genitalia as the "ugliest" part of their body.

CLINICAL IMPLICATIONS

Effects of Medical Care

It is relatively easy to understand that many commonly prescribed medications (e.g., antihypertensives, anticholinergics, antihistamines, sedatives, tranquilizers, and so forth) can markedly interfere with sexual function. Less obvious is the general role that medical care can play in sexuality.

From counseling to contraceptive advice, from assessing developmental milestones to lending a listening ear, the inclusion of sexuality and sexual matters in the day-to-day practice of medical care is essential. In addition to the immediate benefit, opening the door to this aspect of patients' lives ensures an avenue of discussion should problems occur at a later date. We have a profound effect on our patients' lives and we should employ that effect in all areas, including sexuality. This has become even more pressing owing to concerns over sexually transmitted diseases. A discussion about sexuality can also open a discussion of safer sex, contraception, and abstinence.

Effects of Surgical Conditions

Any surgical procedure that leaves a scar or alters bodily function simultaneously alters body image. Although the sexual impact of a procedure (e.g., a mastectomy) may be obvious, it is often overlooked in pre- and postoperative discussions. It is easy to dismiss or see as an advantage the loss of a symptomatic uterus, but for many women this loss goes to the very core of being feminine. Despite the ability to restore hormonal normality (when the ovaries are removed), hysterectomy may profoundly alter sexuality if the patient herself believes it will. The negative impact of surgery is discussed in Chapter 24, Sexual Dysfunction. For some women, the change in sexuality is a positive one, freeing them from menstruation, pain, or the fear of pregnancy so they can be completely expressive sexually, which also represents a change that should be explored with the patient.

SPECIAL CONSIDERATIONS

The Lesbian Patient

Everyone craves personal warmth and affection. Between 1% and 3% of women seek it from members of their own sex. When viewed in the context of human needs, discussions about whether this represents a personal preference or a disease seem moot. Although somewhat more labile in women, it appears that sexual orientation is relatively fixed, making efforts to "change" these patients misdirected and futile. More germane are the special medical concerns presented by these patients.

Vaginitis and sexually transmitted diseases are not solely the province of heterosexual women. All forms of vaginitis, including trichomonas, may affect women who are exclusively homosexual. Transmission of syphilis, gonorrhea, and Chlamydia are less common in exclusively homosexual women and, as a result, diagnoses such as pelvic inflammatory disease should be suspect in these women. The same cannot be said of genital herpes infections, which can easily be transmitted by oral-genital contact. Although data are sparse, there is good reason to believe that in the absence of drug abuse, exclusively homosexual women should be at very low risk for acquiring human immunodeficiency virus (HIV). Unfortunately, there are no methods available to reduce the homosexual spread of HIV if one partner is infected. Although the risk is low, vaginal and menstrual fluids are known to contain the virus in amounts sufficient to constitute a risk. Homosexual women are at slightly lower risk of cervical dysplasia, although cases do still occur, especially if these women have had heterosexual intercourse in the past. The prevalence of menstrual disorders appears to be unchanged for these women.

Between 25% and 50% of lesbians either have been pregnant or are raising children, most by previous heterosexual liaisons. Options for having children include adoption, surrogacy, artificial insemination, and natural insemination with or without the knowledge and cooperation of the man. Once a pregnancy occurs, no differences are required in the care of these patients. Most studies indicate no differences in the development, behavior, or sexual orientation of children raised in homosexual homes.

Society places strong stresses on these patients because of their life-style choices. Despite this, lesbian women do not appear to have any greater or lesser frequency of sexual dysfunction. When sexual dysfunction does occur, it is treated with the same techniques used for heterosexual sexual difficulties. Although data are sparse, it appears that lesbian couples are as stable as heterosexual couples (or more so), and the total number of lifetime sexual partners is comparable between the two groups.

There is one area where lesbian patients do require special care: alcohol abuse. Studies indicate that these patients are more likely to abuse alcohol at a rate that is five to seven times higher that the rate found in heterosexual women, which translates to an incidence of 25% to 35%. This high rate has been attributed to the importance of gay bars as a part of the lesbian life-style, societal repression, and a disinterest on the part of alcohol treatment centers in providing care for this segment of the population. Whatever the reason for the higher incidence of alcoholism, clearly anyone who cares for these patients must be alert for the possibility and institute support and therapy as needed.

The Seductive Patient

An infrequently encountered aspect of sexuality that deserves special mention is the seductive patient. These rare individuals behave seductively during the medical encounter. This may take the form of remarks, unnecessary nudity, or trivial concerns for which the patient insists on excessively intimate discussion or examinations. These patients do this for many reasons. They may do it to exercise power or control in an uncomfortable situation, to embarrass the interviewer, to entrap or entice impropriety, or to obtain sexual satisfaction through the process (even without consummation). It may be part of a personality disorder, an innocent infatuation, or a way to initiate a relationship that they desire. No matter what the source of the behavior, it can be very insidious and disquieting.

Both ethics and good medical judgment dictate that this situation be handled directly, but tactfully. Most authors recommend that this be addressed in a straight forward manner. When the intent is obvious, statement such as "I am flattered that you are interested in me, but I believe I can be of more help to you medically than I can through any other type of relationship" or "I think it would be better if we kept this on a more professional level" may be appropriate. If the behavior is less clear cut, it may be lightly dismissed ("let's keep you covered up so you don't catch cold") wthout offending an innocent patient.

Sexual liaisons are strongly discouraged between provider and patient. These two roles must remain separate at all times, even to the point of a written termination of the medical relationship, followed by a period of no contact, before any relationship is pursued.

HINTS AND COMMON QUESTIONS

Questions about sexuality may be raised by patients as a form of testing. Even when this is the suspected motivation, this topic should be dealt with using the same nonjudgmental, matter-of-fact manner that any other medical topic would elicit. Your correct perception will defuse the process. If you are wrong, a professional attitude validates the topic and facilitates further communication on this important subject.

To help with counseling, a group of common myths and the truths associated with them are shown in Table 8.2. These may present clinically as specific questions or may be apparent as background misinformation behind other questions or behaviors.

Table 8.2. Common Sexual Myths

Myth	Facts
Orgasms are different for men and women.	Studies indicate organisms are subjectively and objectively the same.
Men are more aroused by pornography and fantasy than women.	Generally accepted to be the same and is culturally and situationally determined for both sexes.
Men are faster to arouse than women.	Culturally and situationally determined for both sexes.
Men and women reach sexual peaks at different ages. (Women wear well, men wear out.)	Some physiologic differences, but mostly culturally and situationally determined for both sexes.
You are allowed only so many orgasms—don't use them up.	Wrong.
It is dangerous to have sex during menstruation.	Usually not. Acceptability determined by culture and personal preference.
Sex during pregnancy can "mark" a child and should be avoided.	Wrong. Sex is usually O.K.
Oral-genital sex indicates homosexual tendencies.	A popular practice among all couples, regardless of sexual orientation.
There is a difference between "vaginal" and "clitoral" orgasms.	There is no difference. No "right" way to have an orgasm; by the way, there is no "G-spot" either.
Menopause or hysterectomy ends a woman's sex life.	Should have no deleterious effect, especially with estrogen replacement. It improves for some couples.
There are racial differences in genital size and sexual ability.	Cultural bias without actual basis.
Male genital size is important. (Bigger is better.)	Function of expectation and expertise.
Today's youth are going wild.	More openness. Small change.
Simultaneous orgasm is required for conception.	Wrong.
You must be 18 to by a condom.	False.

SUGGESTED READINGS

General References

The Allan Guttmacher Institute. Sex and America's Teenagers. New York: Allan Guttmacher Institute, 1994.

The America College of Obstetricians and Gynecologists. Adolescent Sexuality: Guides for Physician Involvement, 2nd ed. Washington DC: ACOG, 1992.

American Medical Association. Guidelines for Adolescent Preventive Services. Chicago: AMA, 1994.

D'Emilio J, Freedman EB. Intimate matters: a history of sexuality in America. New York: Harper & Row, 1988.

Fogel CI, Lauver D, eds. Sexual Health Promotion. Philadelphia: WB Saunders, 1990.

Friedman RC, Downey JI. Homosexuality. N Engl J Med 1994;331:923.

Gilman SL. Sexuality: An Illustrated History Representing the Sexual in Medicine and Culture from the Middle Ages to the Age of AIDS. New York: John Wiley, 1989.

Greydanus DE, Shearin RB. Adolescent Sexuality and Gynecology. Philadelphia: Lea & Febiger, 1990.

Hollender MH. A rejected landmark paper on sexuality. JAMA 1983;250:228.

Janus SS, Janus CL. The Janus Report on Sexual Behavior. New York: John Wiley, 1993.

Jones RE. Human Reproductive Biology. San Diego: Academic Press, 1991.

Kenyon FE. Homosexuality in gynaecologic practice. Clin Obstet Gynaecol 1980;7:363.

Ladas AK, Whipple B, Perry JD. The G Spot and Other Recent Discoveries about Human Sexuality. New York: Holt, Rinehart and Winston, 1982.

Lewis D. The gynecologic considerations of the sexual act. JAMA 1983;250:222.

Levine SB. Sexual Life: A Clinician's Guide. New York: Plenum Press, 1992.

Lief HI, ed. Medical Aspects of Human Sexuality: 750 Questions Answered by 500 Authorities. Baltimore: Williams & Wilkins, 1975.

Masters W, Johnson V. Human Sexual Response. Boston: Little Brown, 1966.

Michael RT, Gagnon JH, Laumann EO, Kolata G. Sex in America: A Definitive Survey. Boston: Little Brown, 1994.

Rossi AS, ed. Sexuality Across the Life Course. Chicago: University of Chicago Press, 1994.

Russo RM, ed. Sexual Development and Disorders in Childhood and Adolescence: An Advanced Textbook. New Hyde Park, NY: Medical Examination Publishing Co., 1983.

Sanger M. Happiness in Marriage. New York: Brentano's, 1926 (reprinted by Applewood Books, 1993).

Sprecher S, McKinney K. Sexuality. Newbury Park: Sage Publications, 1993.

Tavris C, Sadd S. The Redbook Report on Female Sexuality. New York: Delacorte Press, 1977.

Woods NF, ed. Human Sexuality in Health and Illness. St. Louis: CV Mosby, 1984.

Specific References

Abel G, Murphy W, Becker J, Bitar A. Women's vaginal responses during REM sleep. J Sex Marital Ther 1979;5:5.

Bachmann GA, Leiblum SR, Kemmann E, et al. Sexual expression and its determinants in the post-menopausal woman. Maturitas 1984;6:19.

Benson MD, Torpy EJ. Sexual behavior in junior high school students. Obstet Gynecol 1995;85:279.

Bray P, Myers RAM, Cowley RA. Orogenital sex as a cause of nonfatal air embolism in pregnancy. Obstet Gynecol 1983;61:653.

Butler RN, Lewis MI, Hoffman E, Whitehead ED. Love and sex after 60: how to evaluate and treat the sexually active woman. Geriatrics 1994;49:33.

Butler RN, Lewis MI, Hoffman E, Whitehead ED. Love and sex after 60: how physical changes affect intimate expression. A roundtable discussion: Part 1. Geriatrics. 1994;49:20.

Butler RN. Love and sex after 60 [editorial; comment]. Geriatrics. 1994;49:10.

Chilman CS, ed. Adolescent Sexuality in a Changing American Society: Social and Psychological Perspectives for the Human Services Professions. New York: John Wiley, 1983.

Cohen R, Rosen R, Goldstein L. Human EEG laterality changes during human sexual orgasm. Arch Sex Behav 1976;5:189.

Dameron GW JR. Helping couples cope with sexual changes pregnancy brings. Contemp OB/GYN 1983;21:23.

Dickinson RL, Pierson HH. The average sex life of American women. JAMA 1925;85:1113.

Fisher C, Cohen H, Schiavi R, et al. Patterns of female sexual arousal during sleep and waking: vaginal thermo-conductive studies. Arch Sex Behav 1983;12:97.

Goldberg DC, Whipple B, Fishkin RE, et al. The Gräfenberg spot and female ejaculation: a review of initial hypothesis. J Sex Marital Ther 1983;1:27.

Good RS. The gynecologist and the lesbian. Clin Obstet Gynecol 1976;19:473.

Goodlin RC, Keller DW, Raffin M. Orgasm during late pregnancy: possible deleterious effects. Obstet Gynecol 1971;38:916.

Goodlin RC. Orgasm and premature labour. Lancet 1969;2:646.

Gräfenberg E. The role of the urethra in female orgasm. International Journal of Sexology 1950;3:145.

Heiman J. Female sexual response patterns: interaction of physiological, affective, and contextual cues. Arch Gen Psychiatry 1980;37:1311.

Heiman J. Sexuality in older women. In Stenchever MA (ed). Care of the Aging Woman. Washington, DC: Association of Professors of Gynecology and Obstetrics, 1994, p 11–1.

Helstrom L, Lundberg PO, Sorbom D, Backstrom T. Sexuality after hysterectomy: a factor analysis of women's sexual lives before and after subtotal hysterectomy. Obstet Gynecol 1993;81:357.

Hensen D, Rubin H, Henson C. Labial and vaginal blood volume responses to visual and tactile stimuli. Arch Sex Behav 1982;11:23.

Hoon P, Bruce K, Kinchelow G. Does the menstrual cycle affect erotic arousal? Psycholphysiology 1982;19:21.

Levin R. The physiology of sexual function in women. Clin Obstet Gynaecol 1980;7:213.

Maypole J. Medical students learn about sexuality and sensitivity. JAMA 1994;272:1069.

McCoy N, Davidson JM. A longitudinal study of the effects of menopause on sexuality. Maturitas 1985;7:203.

Mills JL, Harlap S, Harley EE. Should coitus late in pregnancy be discouraged? Lancet 1981;2:136.

Naeye RL. Coitus and antepartum hemorrhage. Br J Obstet Gynaecol 1981;88:765.

Perkins RP. Sexuality in pregnancy: what determines behavior? Obstet Gynecol 1982;59:189.

Reamy K, White SE, Daniell WC, LeVine ES. Sexuality and pregnancy: a prospective study. J Reprod Med 1982;27:321.

Robertson P, Schachter J. Failure to identify veneral disease in a lesbian population. Sex Transm Dis 1981;8:75.

Rubenstein C. Sex generation. Mademoiselle 1993;(June):129.

Schreiner-Engel P, Schiavi R, Smith H, White D. Sexual arousability and the menstrual cycle. Psychosom Med 1981;43:199.

Sipski ML, Alexander CJ. Sexual activities, response and satisfaction in women pre- and post-spinal cord injury. Arch Phys Med Rehabil 1993;74:1025.

Solberg DA, Butler J, Wagner NN. Sexual behavior in pregnancy. N Engl J Med 1973;288:1098.

Stock W, Greer J. A study of fantasy based sexual arousal in women. Arch Sex Behav 1982;11:33.

Wagner NN, Butler JC, Sanders JP. Prematurity and orgasmic coitus during pregnancy: data on a small sample. Fertil Steril 1976;27:911.

Patient Education Materials

These sources may be of help to adolescent patients or parents trying to address emerging sexuality.

The America College of Obstetricians and Gynecologists. Patient information series: Teaching Your Children About Sexuality (AP-016); Growing Up (about puberty, for ages 9–14, AP-041); Being a Teenager: You and Your Sexuality (understanding adolescence, ages 11–19, AP-042); and Menstruation and the Menstrual Cycle (AP-049)

Boston Women's Health Book Collective. Our Bodies, Ourselves, 2nd ed. New York: Simon & Schuster, 1976.

Calderone M, Johnson E. The Family Book About Sexuality. New York: Harper & Row 1981.

Kelly G. Learning About Sex: The Contemporary Guide for Young Adults. Barron's Educational Series, 1976.

Madaras A, Madaras L. The What's Happening to My Body? Book for Girls. Newmarket, 1983.

Madaras A, Madaras L. The What's Happening to My Body? Book for Boys. Newmarket, 1984.

Nilsson L. A Child is Born. New York: Delacorte 1977.

9

Contraception

The desire (and now the ability) to control fertility, whether to induce fields to grow or to allow women to pursue careers, has shaped us as individuals and cultures more than almost any other force. Changing patterns of sexual expression, new technologies, increased consumerism, and heightened cost pressures are all affecting the choices patients make in their search for fertility control. The very nature of the topic gives contraception personal, religious, and political overtones that often lead to conflict, emotionality, and confusion. Each of these aspects must be considered in counseling patients about their options and helping them arrive at the best choice for their individual needs.

BACKGROUND AND SCIENCE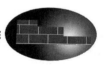

In the United States, over half (56%) of all pregnancies are unplanned, despite the fact that 90% of women at risk (fertile, sexually active, and neither pregnant nor seeking pregnancy) are using some form of contraception (Table 9.1). The 10% or so of women not using contraception account for over half of these unintended pregnancies. The remaining unplanned pregnancies occur because of the failure of the contraceptive method used or the improper or inconsistent use of the method (Table 9.2). Roughly half of the unintended pregnancies in the United States end in abortion.

History and Basic Mechanisms of Fertility Control

Documented historical attempts to control fertility date to the beginning of written history. Some of the methods (e.g., vaginal plugs and early penile sheaths) may have been marginally effective, whereas most others (e.g., jumping backwards, having intercourse

Table 9.1. Contraceptive Use in the United States*

Method	Estimated use (%)
Oral contraceptives	28
Female sterilization	25
Condom	13
Male sterilization	11
Spermicides	3
Withdrawal	2
Periodic abstinence (Rhythm method)	2
Intrauterine device	2
No method	10

*Estimated percentage of all women.

Table 9.2. Contraceptive Failure Rates

Method	Estimated pregnancy rates (%)*
Implantable rod (Norplant)	0.05–1.5
Male sterilization	0.1
Injectable (DMPA†)	0.1–0.4
Female sterilization	0.4
Oral Contraceptives	0.5–8.7
Intrauterine Device	1.8–4.5
Condom	
Male	4–36
Female	5–25
Diaphragm (with spermicide)	10–39
Spermicide	
Suppositories	0.6–21.1
Foam	0.6–30
Jelly, cream	0.6–35
Rhythm	
Calendar	15–45
Temperature	6–20
Temperature + intercourse only after ovulation	1–10
Cervical mucus	6–25
Not Recommended:	
Withdrawal	6–27+
Postcoital douche	40+
No method	85–90

*During the first year of use. Variations represent the difference between method failure and user failure (inconsistent or incorrect usage).
†Depot-medroxyprogesterone acetate.

standing up, or forcibly yelling or coughing after intercourse to expel the semen) were based on folk lore or myth and probably had little effect. Only in recent years has a selection of effective, safe, and widely available methods been available.

Currently available contraceptive methods seek to prevent pregnancy by preventing the sperm and egg from uniting or by preventing implantation and growth. These goals are accomplished by preventing the development and release of the egg (oral contraceptives, long-acting hormonal methods); preventing union of sperm and egg by imposing a mechanical, chemical, or temporal barrier between sperm and egg (condom, diaphragm, foam, rhythm, withdrawal); or altering the likelihood of implantation or growth (intrauterine devices, postcoital oral contraception, RU-486). Each approach has its own singular advantages and disadvantages, which gives unique properties to individual contraceptive methods. For this reason, it is often much more than the pregnancy (failure) rate that determines the final choice of a contraceptive method.

Temporary (Reversible) Methods

Periodic abstinence (rhythm)

Periodic abstinence (rhythm or "natural" family planning) is based on determining the time of ovulation, then using this information either to avoid intercourse during the fertile period or to augment other methods such as barriers or spermicides. It presumes that the egg can be fertilized only during the first 24 hours after ovulation, that sperm can survive no more than 4 days in the female genital tract, and that ovulation always occurs 14 days before the start of the next menses. Determining the fertile period may be based on calendar calculations, variations in basal body temperature (thermal method), or changes in cervical mucus (Billings method), singly or in combination.

In the calendar method, menstrual intervals are recorded for a minimum of 1 year and the fertile period is calculated to be from 18 days before the time of shortest cycle to 11 days before the longest cycle. For a woman with absolutely regular 28-day cycles, this would be from days 10 through 17. Failures are twice as likely if data on menstrual intervals from only 9 months are used, and three to seven times more likely if only 6 months of cycles are recorded. When basal body temperatures are used, abstinence is maintained from the first day of menses until the third consecutive day of elevated basal body temperatures (one half to one degree Fahrenheit). When changes in cervical mucus are used to detect ovulation, abstinence is maintained until 4 days after the last day of wet, slippery cervical mucus. Ovulation may also be inferred by monitoring daily luteinizing hormone (LH) levels using home urine dipsticks. Expense, motivation, and a certain amount of skill needed to carry out and interpret the test limits its use.

For couples who are highly motivated and have regular menstrual cycles, these methods may provide acceptable contraception. Periodic abstinence is safe, costs little, and requires no drugs, devices, or surgery. The high motivation and cycle regularity required, the restrictions and loss of spontaneity, debate about some of the principles on which it is founded, and a natural tendency to "cheat" reduce the effectiveness of these methods, making them less than ideal. In one study, less than 10% of couples continued to use the method after 1 year. A summary of advantages and disadvantages of periodic abstinence that may be used in counseling are listed in Table 9.3.

Table 9.3. Attributes of Periodic Abstinence (for Counseling Purposes)

Advantages	Disadvantages
Safe (free of side effects)	Moderate failure rate
Inexpensive	Requires regular cycles
"Natural" (no devices or drugs)	Requires high motivation
May be combined with other methods	Long periods of abstinence required
Improved communication between partners	Interferes with spontaneity
Enhanced libido during abstinence	Libidinal dysfunction

Spermicides

Most of the spermicides marketed today rely on one of two agents to immobilize or kill sperm—nonoxynol-9 and octoxynol-3. These compounds are delivered in a variety of vehicles including creams, jellies, foams, films, and suppositories. These agents must be placed in the vagina from 15 to 30 minutes prior to each act of intercourse. (Some suggest up to an hour may be acceptable, although lower failure rates are associated with shorter insertion intervals.) Postcoital douching should be avoided for at least 8 hours. A spermicidal sponge (polyurethane plus nonoxynol-9) was introduced to allow up to 24 hours of protection with a single application, but a failure rate higher than that of other spermicides, reports of toxic shock, and manufacturing problems resulted in the withdrawal of this delivery system.

Failure rates for spermicides are difficult to evaluate but range from less than 1% to as high as 35%. For a greater certainty of protection, spermicides are often combined with condoms to achieve lower failure rates. The greatest effectiveness rate is found among well-motivated older couples.

Spermicides are inexpensive, well-tolerated, and provide acceptable protection from pregnancy, especially when pregnancy spacing is the primary goal. Spermicide use may decrease the likelihood of some bacterial and viral sexually transmitted diseases; they are also associated with a reduced risk of cervical cancer. A summary of advantages and disadvantages of spermicides that may be used in counseling are listed in Table 9.4.

Barriers

The oldest and most widely used contraceptive methods are based on providing a physical barrier between sperm and egg. What was once limited to penile condoms now includes condoms for both partners, diaphragms, and cervical caps. Each is dependent on proper use before or at the time of intercourse, which exposes the user to a higher failure rate from inconsistent or incorrect use.

DIAPHRAGM. Diaphragms (a rubber dome with a springy ring) are used with a contraceptive jelly or cream to provide contraception by both barrier and spermicidal actions. In use, spermicidal jelly or cream is applied to the cervical side of the diaphragm, providing a spermicidal barrier to fertilization. The diaphragm is inserted into the vagina, beyond the

Table 9.4. Attributes of Spermicides (for Counseling Purposes)

Advantages	Disadvantages
Safe (infrequent side effects)	Moderate failure rate
Inexpensive	Messy
Widely available	Requires advance planning (to buy)
May be combined with other methods	Interferes with spontaneity
Provides some additional lubrication	Interferes with oral sex
May provide some measure of protection from sexually transmitted diseases and cervical cancer	Occasional local irritation (either partner)
	Does not protect from STD such as herpes, HPV, trichomonas, and others

STD = sexually transmitted diseases; HPV = human papilloma virus.

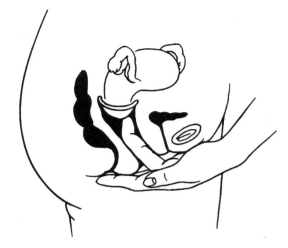

Figure 9.1 Correct positioning of a diaphram in the vagina. (From Beckmann RB, Ling FW, Barzansky BM, et al. Obstetrics and gynecology. 2nd ed. Baltimore: Williams & Wilkins, 1995:257.)

cervix and behind the symphysis. In this position, the diaphragm covers the anterior vaginal wall and cervix, providing a mechanical barrier to sperm passage and positioning the spermicide against the cervix to optimize its effect. The diaphragm must be inserted before intercourse commences and it must be left in place for 6 to 8 hours after. It is then removed, washed, and stored. Should additional intercourse be desired before the 6 to 8 hours have passed, additional spermicide is applied to the vaginal side of the diaphragm and the waiting time to removal restarted. Postcoital douching is not recommended.

The patient must understand the proper position of the diaphragm and how to verify its correct insertion. (If the cervix can be felt through the dome of the diaphragm, the positioning is correct.) The correct position of a diaphragm in the vagina is shown in Figure 9.1. When correctly positioned, the diaphragm should not be noticeable by either partner.

Diaphragms must be fitted to the individual patient, choosing the largest size that may be comfortably accommodated by the vagina. Diaphragms come in sizes that range from 50 to 105 mm in diameter, graduated in 5-mm increments. The most common size prescribed is 75 mm. The optimal size may change with significant weight change (10–15 lbs or more), vaginal birth, or pelvic surgery. Following delivery, diaphragms may be fitted at the 6- to 8-week postpartum visit. Diaphragms are made with a coiled spring, or with a flat or arching rim that somewhat alters the fit. The flat type is better suited to those women with a less well-defined subpubic arch.

Some women who use the diaphragm for contraception will insert the diaphragm each evening before bed, leave it in place until the following evening, when it is removed, washed, and reinserted. This removes contraception with the diaphragm from the act of intercourse. The potentially prolonged interval from insertion to coitus, which increases contraceptive failure, may lead to the possibility of vaginal or urinary tract infections or to pressure damage to the vaginal wall, making this approach less desirable and it should be discouraged.

Diaphragm users have a lower rate of gonorrheal infections, tubal disease and infertility, and cervical neoplasia. Urinary tract infections, however, are more common in these patients. A summary of advantages and disadvantages of diaphragms that may be used in counseling are listed in Table 9.5.

Table 9.5. Attributes of Diaphragms (for Counseling Purposes)

Advantages	Disadvantages
Safe (infrequent side effects)	Must be fitted
Inexpensive	May be slippery or messy (insertion)
Widely available	Requires advance planning (to place)
May be used for several years before replacement	Interferes with spontaneity
Does not affect sexual sensation (either partner)	May interfere with oral sex (less than spermicides above)
May provide some measure of protection from sexually transmitted diseases and cervical cancer	Occasional local irritation from spermicide (either partner), rare latex allergy
	Does not protect from STD such as herpes, HPV, trichomonas, and others

STD = sexually transmitted diseases; HPV = human papilloma virus.

CERVICAL CAP. The cervical cap was originally intended to allow virtually continuous wear (except during menstruation). Concerns about toxic shock and a high prevalence of malodorous discharge (60% after 5 days) have prevented this goal from being realized. Currently available cervical caps should be left in place no less than 6 to 8 hours and removed no later than 48 hours after intercourse. The cervical cap is approved for use, but not widely available in the United States. For counseling purposes, cervical caps may be considered as comparable to diaphragms.

CONDOMS. Condoms are sheaths worn over the erect penis or inside the vagina to physically prevent sperm from reaching the cervix and upper genital tract and, hence, prevent fertilization. Condoms may be made of latex, polyurethane, or less commonly, animal membrane (usually lamb intestine, accounting for about 1% of sales). Male (penile) condoms are available with or without lubricants or spermicides. They may be plain or have reservoir tips; are available in colors and flavors; and may have ridges or other attributes (including the ability to glow in the dark). Whereas the latter choices are a matter of personal preference only, both spermicidal lubrication and a reservoir tip reduce the likelihood of breakage and increase contraceptive reliability. Although roughly half of all penile condoms sold are sold to women, the condom is the only reliable male contraceptive method available.

The condom is well tolerated with only rare reports of skin irritation and even rarer reports of latex allergy. Some reports indicate that the male condom, backed up by pregnancy termination when failure occurs, carries the lowest morbidity and mortality figures for any contraceptive method. Breakage is uncommon, with most pregnancies occurring because of inconsistent use, intercourse before donning the condom, and careless or late withdrawal following ejaculation that results in spillage. Some men complain of reduced coital sensation with condom use, although this may be an advantage in cases of premature ejaculation.

The female condom is a polyurethane sheath with an inner and outer ring that is inserted into the vagina prior to intercourse. The inner ring facilitates insertion while the outer ring prevents the sheath from being pushed inward during intercourse. The outer ring also provides some coverage of the vulvar skin, further reducing skin-to-skin contact and the risk of sexual disease transmission. As with the male condom, motivation and

Table 9.6. Attributes of Male Condoms (for Counseling Purposes)

Advantages	Disadvantages
Safe (infrequent side effects)	Moderate failure rate
Inexpensive, portable, small	Requires advance planning (to buy)
Widely available	Interferes with spontaneity
May be combined with other methods	May reduce male sensation
May provide some measure of protection from STD, including HIV	Occasional local irritation (either partner)
May retard premature ejaculation	Does not protect from STD, such as herpes, HPV and others
May be used during fellatio to reduce risk of sexually transmitted diseases	Requires cooperation of male partner
Effectiveness and compliance may be verified	Requires erection, linking use to intercourse
Gives male an active part in contraception	

STD = sexually transmitted diseases; HIV = human immunodeficiency virus; HPV = human papilloma virus.

proper use are required with each episode of intercourse. Unlike the male condom, which requires erection, the female condom can be inserted up to several hours before intercourse. Cost, availability, possibile penetration outside of the condom, and noise during use have so far limited the use of the female condom.

Both male and female condoms provide some protection against sexually transmitted diseases, including viruses such as human immunodeficiency virus (HIV). Animal membrane condoms, however, do not decrease the risk of viral (HIV) transmission. Because of ready availability, low cost, reliability, and the reduced risk of sexually transmitted disease, condoms are an excellent choice for casual sexual encounters. Neither male nor female condom provides complete protection, so couples should still be cautioned about high-risk behaviors. A summary of advantages and disadvantages of male and female condoms that may be used in counseling are listed in Tables 9.6 and 9.7.

Intrauterine Devices

Internationally used by more than 60 million women, intrauterine contraceptive devices (IUCDs) have the highest continuation rates of all reversible contracetpive methods. First

Table 9.7. Attributes of Female Condoms (for Counseling Purposes)

Advantages	Disadvantages
Safe (infrequent side effects)	Moderate failure rate
Inexpensive, portable	Requires advance planning (to buy)
May be combined with other methods	Interferes with spontaneity
May provide some measure of protection from STD, including HIV	Not widely available
Theoretical reduced risk of HPV, herpes, and so forth	Expensive ($\sim$ $2.50 per use)
Gives female more control than male condom	Noisy
Effectiveness and compliance may be verified	Appearance
May be inserted in advance of sexual activity improving spontaneity	Penile insertion outside of the device possible

STD = sexually transmitted diseases; HIV = human immunodeficiency virus; HPV = human papilloma virus.

introduced over 50 years ago, IUCDs have been made of various materials and configurations. As a group, they generally consist of plastic objects which are inserted into the endometrial cavity and can remain for several years. The IUCDs currently available in the United States augment their actions through the addition of hormones (Progestasert) or copper wire (ParaGard). These additions increase the efficacy of the IUCD, although they also limit the duration of use (1 to 10 years, respectively).

Intrauterine contraceptive devices are associated with a relatively low failure rate (2% to 4.5% overall) but do have a moderate complication rate. Intermenstrual bleeding, menorrhagia, and dysmenorrhea are more prevalent in IUCD wearers. These complications are one to five times more common for women who are nulliparous. There is slight variation in the occurrence of these side effects based on the type of IUCD. For example, copper-bearing IUCDs are associated with a 50% increase in menstrual blood loss, whereas there is no change, or a slight reduction, in blood loss for wearers of progesterone-containing devices. Dysmenorrhea and menorrhagia may respond to nonsteroidal anti-inflammatory drug therapy, allowing the patient to continue using the IUCD.

Intrauterine contraceptive device wearers, especially those using copper-bearing devices, have an increased risk of upper genital tract infections and a 50% increase in subsequent fertility. Pelvic infections (gonococcal and nongonoccal) are 1.9 to 6.5 times more likely in IUCD users compared with nonusers. Most of these infections occur in the first 2 weeks after insertion or in nulliparous women with multiple sexual partners. As a result, many authors suggest limiting the use of IUCDs to those at low risk for sexually transmitted disease and those who are less likely to desire further children. Other contraindications to IUCD use are listed in Table 9.8.

Even IUCD users who are at low risk for upper genital tract infections have an increased risk of infection with *Actinomyces israelii*. If evidence of these organisms is found (e.g., sulfur granules found on Pap smear), antibiotic therapy (penicillin or tetracycline) is generally successful without removing the device; it need only be removed when the infection fails to clear or signs of other infection is present.

Table 9.8. Contraindication to Intrauterine Contraceptive Device Use

ABSOLUTE CONTRAINDICATIONS
  Current pelvic inflammatory disease
  History of prior ectopic pregnancy
  Known or suspected pregnancy
  Suspected genital tract malignancy
  Undiagnosed uterine pregnancy
  Uterine anomalies
RELATIVE CONTRAINDICATIONS
  Anemia
  Cervical stenosis
  Coagulopathies
  Dysmenorrhea
  Menorrhagia
  Nulliparity
  Wilson's disease (copper storage disease)

Intrauterine contraceptive devices act primarily to prevent implantation and growth of a fertilized egg. This aspect of their action may make them less acceptable to some patients. There is evidence that IUCDs may also alter tubal transport and the sperm's ability to fertilize the egg. These additional actions may provide reassurance for some couples. Because IUCDs are most effective at preventing intrauterine pregnancies (97% to 99.5%) compared with tubal or ovarian implantation (90% to 95%), ectopic pregnancies are five to ten times more common for women who wear IUCDs. Because of an overall lower rate of pregnancies, women who use IUCDs have only 40% of the risk of ectopic pregnancy experienced by women who use no contraception. The increased risk of ectopic pregnancy among those who become pregnant may be owing to the higher rate of pelvic (tubal and ovarian) infections found in IUCD users. Because of the increased risk of ectopic pregnancies, the location of the pregnancy should be investigated for any woman who conceives with an IUCD in place. This investigation is best accomplished with transvaginal ultrasonography. When an intrauterine gestation is identified (the most likely situation), a coexisting ectopic pregnancy is unlikely. The absence of an identifiable intrauterine gestation does not confirm ectopic implantation, whereas adnexal cardiac activity is pathognomonic.

Women who conceive with an IUCD in place have a threefold increase in the risk of spontaneous and septic abortion. If the patient wishes to continue the pregnancy and the strings of the device are visible, the IUCD should be removed by gentle traction. When the strings are no longer visible, the IUCD can be removed under ultrasound guidance, although most would leave the device in place. Signs of sepsis must be aggressively treated, as with any other suspected septic miscarriage. Other than the increased risk to the early pregnancy, no adverse effects later in pregnancy are likely.

Intrauterine contraceptive devices are generally placed in the uterus at the time of menstruation. This reduces the likelihood of an ongoing pregnancy, obscures the small amount of bleeding caused by placement, and may be technically easier owing to slight cervical dilatation at the time of menstrual flow. Postpartum placement can be carried out at the time of a routine 6- or 8-week check-up. Perforation of the cervix or uterus occurs in 1 of every 600 to 2,000 insertions. Perforation may occur in any patient but is more likely in patients with an unrecognized retroverted uterus.

Most IUCDs have one or two filaments (strings) attached which protrude from the cervix and serve to facilitate removal and to allow the patient to confirm its presence. This ability to check for the IUCD reduces the chance of undetected expulsion or migration. Expulsion of IUCDs occurs in roughly 10% of patients during the first year of use and about one fifth of these go unnoticed by the patient. About one third of IUCD-related pregnancies occur following unnoticed expulsion. Should the IUCD become "lost," a pregnancy test and ultrasonography may be able to identify the presence of the IUCD in the uterine cavity or the possibility of a pregnancy moving the IUCD upward as the uterus enlarges. When ultrasonography cannot confirm the presence of the IUCD in the uterus, x-ray study (involving anteroposterior and lateral pelvic views, often with sound placed in the uterine cavity for identification), hysteroscopy, or laparoscopy may be required to localize and retrieve the device.

A summary of advantages and disadvantages of intrauterine contraceptive devices that may be used in counseling are listed in Table 9.9.

Table 9.9. Attributes of Intrauterine Contraceptive Devices (for Counseling Purposes)

Advantages	Disadvantages
Reliable	Risk of upper genital tract infection
Convenient	Decreased long-term fertility
No systemic metabolic effects	Requires medical intervention
Requires only one act of motivation	Moderate initial expense (device and insertion)
May be used for a prolonged period	Risk of menorrhagia and dysmenorrhea
High compliance and continuation	
Low cost of use when used for a prolonged period	

Oral Contraceptives

In the United States, birth control is almost synonymous with the oral contraceptive pill. Approximately 80% of American women of reproductive age are using or have used oral contraceptives. Between one quarter and one third of sexually active, fertile women in the United States currently use these agents. Despite this wide exposure and extensive world-wide experience, the "pill" is often mistrusted or misunderstood. In a 1985 Gallup poll, two thirds of those surveyed said that they thought the pill was more dangerous than pregnancy and up to one third thought that oral contraceptives caused cancer.

TYPES. Combination contraceptive formulations contain an estrogen (generally ethinyl estradiol) and a progestin. Progestin-only oral contraceptives are also available, but have higher rates of failure and complication. Currently there are almost 30 estrogen-progesterone products on the market in the United States (Table 9.10). The most frequently used estrogen is ethinyl estradiol, although a few products contain mestranol. Most oral contraceptives contain a fixed ratio of estrogen and progestin. "Phasic" pills vary this ratio two or three times over the course of the month. This results in a slight decrease in the total dose of hormones (mainly the progestin) used per month but is associated with a slightly higher rate of intermenstrual bleeding.

Oral contraceptive agents prevent pregnancy through several mechanisms: ovulation suppression, altered cervical mucus, and endometrial changes. The main action confering protection from pregnancy is ovulation suppression brought on by abating pulsatile release of follicle-stimulating hormone (FSH) and luteinizing hormone (LH) from the pituitary. Oral contraceptives also alter cervical mucus, making it thicker and resistant to sperm penetration. Atrophic change in the endometrium may also assist in preventing successful pregnancy, but the role of these effects remains conjectural. Failure rates of oral contraceptives are in the range of 1% or less and are generally related to missed pills.

Fertility rates after using oral contraceptives appear to be no different than those for the barrier method once a slight delay in the return of ovulation is taken into account. Most patients will resume ovulatory cycles within 4 to 6 weeks of discontinuing the pill. The incidence of prolonged amenorrhea (postpill amenorrhea) is between 0.2% and 0.8%, which roughly matches the background rate of secondary amenorrhea. Rates of fetal loss, congenital anomalies, and chromosomal abnormalities appear no different in women who have used oral contraceptives.

Table 9.10. Current Oral Contraceptives

Product	μg	Progestin	mg
COMBINED MONOPHASIC*			
Brevicon	35	Norethindrone	0.5
Demulen 1/35	35	Ethynodiol diacetate	1
Demulen 1/50	50	Ethynodiol diacetate	1
Desogen	30	Desogestrel	0.15
Genora 0.5/35	35	Norethindrone	0.5
Genora 1/35	35	Norethindrone	1
Genora 1/50	50†	Norethindrone	1
Jenest	35	Norethindrone	0.5
Levelen	30	Levonorgestrel	0.15
Lo/Ovral	30	Norgestrel	0.3
Loestrin 1/20	20	Norethindrone acetate	1
Loestrin 1.5/30	30	Norethindrone acetate	1.5
Modicon	35	Norethindrone	0.5
N.E.E. 1/35	35	Norethindrone	1
Nelova 0.5/35	35	Norethindrone	0.5
Nelova 1/50	50†	Norethindrone	1
Nordette	30	Levonorgestrel	0.15
Norethin 1/35	35	Norethindrone	1
Norethin 1/50	50†	Norethindrone	1
Norinyl 1 + 35	35	Norethindrone	1
Norinyl 1 + 50	50†	Norethindrone	1
Ortho-cept	30	Desogestrel	0.15
Ortho-Cyclen	35	Norgestimate	0.25
Ortho-Novum 1/35	35	Norethindrone	1
Ortho-Novum 1/50	50†	Norethindrone	1
Ovcon 35	35	Norethindrone	0.4
Ovcon 50	50	Norethindrone	1
Ovral	50	Norgestrel	0.5
BIPHASIC			
Nelova 10/11	35	Norethindrone (1–10)	0.5
Ortho-Novum 10/11		(11–21)	1.0
TRIPHASIC			
Ortho Tri-Cyclen	35	Norgestimate (1–7)	0.18
		(8–14)	0.215
		(15–21)	0.25
Ortho-Novum 7/7/7	35	Norethindrone (1–7)	0.5
		(8–14)	0.75
		(15–21)	1.0
Tri-Norinyl	35	Norethindrone (1–7)	0.5
		(8–16)	1.0
		(17–21)	0.5
Tri-Levlen	30 × 6	Levonorgestrel (1–6)	0.05
Triphasil	40 × 5	(7–11)	0.075
	30 × 10	(12–21)	0.125

*Estrogen content is ethiny/estradiol except as noted.
†Mestranol.

EFFECTS. Oral contraception has widespread systemic effects. The estrogen used can cause alterations in glucose tolerance, affect lipid metabolism, potentiate sodium and water retention, increase renin substrate, and reduce antithrombin III. The progestin component can increase sebum and facial and body hair, induce smooth muscle relaxation, and increase the risk of cholestatic jaundice. Newer progestational agents (desogestrel and gestodene) have less androgenic impact, but are not free of other effects. The effects of oral contraceptives on the cardiovascular system, the breasts, and the liver and billiary system, and the potential impact on processes, such as migraine headache, and dermatologic conditions are of concern.

The first, high-dose oral contraceptive formulations were associated with an increased risk of thromboembolism, stroke, and heart disease. The subsequent dramatic decline in the dose of hormones used (three- to fourfold for estrogen and roughly tenfold for progestins) has reduced these risks to the point that now factors such as smoking, hypertension, obesity, lack of physical activity, and others have a greater impact than does the use of oral contraceptives. Women who do not smoke appear to have no increase in their risk of myocardial infarction regardless of age, although there is an increase for women over the age of 35 who do smoke. For this reason, while nonsmokers may continue the use of oral contraceptive after the age of 35, smokers should not. Similarly, low-dose oral contraceptives appear to cause little or no increase in the risk of thromboembolism, even in those who undergo surgery. Low-dose combination oral contraceptives are not associated with an increased risk of hypertension.

Debate continues regarding the relationship between oral contraceptive use and breast cancer. Most studies show no difference in the prevalence of breast cancer between users and nonusers, although some studies have suggested that women who begin use early (before age 25) and continue for prolonged periods may have a transient increase in the frequency of breast cancer during their 30s and early 40s. This risk returns to that of nonusers after this period. The most extensive American studies to date have failed to find an increased risk in this group, in women with family histories of breast cancer, or in those with benign breast disease.

Women who use oral contraceptives experience a twofold increase in the risk of cholelithiasis during the first several years of use. This risk appears to decline with time, suggesting an acceleration of the background rate of disease, rather than an independent risk factor. Although oral contraceptives are extensively metabolized by the liver, a past history of hepatic disease, including hepatitis, is not a contraindication to their use as long as liver function tests are normal. Benign liver tumors (adenomas), a rare occurrence thought to be linked to long-term oral contraceptive use, have been most closely associated with mestranol-containing formulations. The incidence of these tumors is about 1 in 50,000 users, or less.

Oral contraceptives have been linked in earlier studies to an increase in the risk of cervical cancer. Recent studies have shown that factors such as age of first intercourse, number of sexual partners, sexually transmitted diseases (especially human papillomavirus), smoking, and others may be more significant cofactors than oral contraceptive use. The supplemental use of barrier methods (associated with lower risk) and periodic Pap smear screening should be encouraged for all women at risk, independent of oral contraceptive use.

The effects of oral contraceptives on the central nervous system are debated. The nausea and vomiting occasionally seen in oral contraceptive users is thought to be mediated through the central nervous system and is related to the level of estrogen in the formulation chosen. Migraine headaches are more common in women who use oral contraceptives. Those women who suffer from migraine headaches may experience a worsening of their symptoms if they choose this method. Severe migraines, visual loss, or the development of other neurologic signs require immediate cessation of oral contraceptive use and further evaluation. Depression is occasionally found as a side effect of higher estrogen formulations. This is thought to be related to alterations in tryptophan metabolism, sometimes responding to vitamin B_6 therapy, although discontinuation of the oral contraceptive is generally recommended.

Patients with acne may note a worsening of their symptoms (or the emergence of acne in those without it) with progestin-dominant oral contraceptives. This is due to the androgenic character of many of the progestins used and should be diminished with a less androgenic progestin such as gestodene and desogestrel. Some patients, especially those who are exposed to the sun, may note a darkening of the skin (chloasma) similar to that seen in pregnancy. This is less likely with low estrogen formulations.

SIDE EFFECTS. In general, side effects of oral contraceptive use are infrequent and mild. The type of side effect encountered is related to the estrogen content of the preparation. High-dose oral contraceptives are associated with a greater, although still infrequent, risk of serious complications. The risk of death due to a complication of oral contraceptive use is estimated to be between 0.3 and 3 per 100,000 woman-years. This compares with a risk of 3.2 deaths per 100,000 abortions, 22.8 deaths per 100,000 pregnancies, and 27 automobile deaths per 100,000 person-years.

Use of low-dose oral contraceptives is associated with a greater likelihood of breakthrough bleeding or contraceptive failure. Breakthrough bleeding usually disappears with continued use or with a switch to a higher dose product. Estrogen may cause a sense of bloating and weight gain, breast tenderness, nausea, fatigue, or headache. The estrogen in oral contraceptives may cause changes in the curvature of the lens of the eye, necessitating re-refraction, or a change in prescription for corrective lenses. Progestins may cause symptoms of acne or depression. Most of these side effects will improve by altering the dose or composition of the agent used.

NONCONTRACEPTIVE HEALTH BENEFITS. Oral contraceptive use is associated with a substantial number of noncontraceptive health benefits. It has been estimated that as many as 1 of 750 women, or some 50,000 women a year in the United States, avoid hospitalization because of the beneficial effects of these medications. Oral contraceptive users have a lower incidence of ovarian cancer (40% reduction), pelvic infection, and benign breast (50% reduction) and ovarian disease. In one study, oral contraceptive users were found to have a 64% reduction in the incidence of benign ovarian neoplasms. Menstrual blood loss and endometrial cancer rates are reduced by 50%. Anemia is reduced, yielding an estimated 27,000 cases of iron-deficiency anemia prevented annually. The beneficial effects of oral contraceptives in reducing ovarian and endometrial cancer appear to persist for up to 10 years after the medications have been discontinued. Ectopic pregnancy is prevented along with the complications of intrauterine pregnancies. Fewer cases of toxic shock are reported. There

Table 9.11. Attributes of Oral Contraceptives (for Counseling Purposes)

Advantages	Disadvantages
Reliable	Risk of systemic side effects
Convenient	Requires medical intervention
Multiple noncontraceptive benefits	Moderate expense
Improved regularity and character of periods	Harmful interactions with smoking and other drugs
May be used for a prolonged period	Requires continuing use for even infrequent intercourse
High compliance and continuation	May alter some laboratory tests
Does not interfere with spontaneity	May cause intermenstrual bleeding
	May increase the risk of some types of vaginitis ("yeast")
	May stimulate fibroid growth

even appears to be a 50% reduction in the rate of rheumatoid arthritis among oral contraceptive users.

A summary of advantages and disadvantages of oral contraceptives that may be used in counseling are listed in Table 9.11.

Long-Acting Agents

Long-acting hormonal contraception by injectable or implantable progestins offer long-term reversible contraception without estrogen effects. These agents offer efficacy rates comparable or superior to sterilization methods. Although generally well tolerated, they are associated with a moderate incidence of random vaginal bleeding, amenorrhea, and progesterone-related side effects. For the duration of their action, these methods do not rely on compliance, but they may not be reversed rapidly or without medical assistance (in the case of implantable methods). None the less, these methods offer an attractive alternative for many women.

DEPOT MEDROXYPROGESTERONE ACETATE. Depot medroxyprogesterone acetate (DMPA) (Depo-Provera) 150 mg intramuscularly (IM) every 12 weeks (3 months) provides reversible contraception that is comparable in efficacy to sterilization. DMPA provides contraception by suppressing the midcycle luteinizing hormone surge and ovulation, the formation of viscous cervical mucus that reduces sperm penetration, and a thinned, atrophic endometrium that discourages implantation. DMPA is generally given within the first 5 days of the menstrual cycle. When given in this time interval, it provides immediate contraceptive protection. DMPA may also be given immediately after a pregnancy loss or immediately postpartum to nonlactating mothers. Women who wish to breastfeed should wait until lactation is firmly established before receiving treatment. A single injection of DMPA provides contraception for at least 14 weeks, but ovulation may not reliably return for 7 to 9 months or more after the injection. The median time to conception following discontinuation of DMPA is 10 months.

The most common side effect of DMPA is menstrual cycle disruption. Roughly one third of users experience irregular or intermenstrual bleeding. This usually subsides during the first 3 to 6 months; by 1 year of use roughly half of all users become amenorrheic. By 2 years of use, this rate rises to 70%. Headaches, abdominal discomfort, and nervousness are reported by more than 10% of users. DMPA is associated with a weight gain of 3 to 5 lb in the first year of use.

DMPA offers a number of advantages over other agents. It can be used in patients in whom estrogen-containing hormonal contraception would not be considered (e.g., sickle-cell disease). DMPA has no neoplastic effects and provides some protection against endometrial cancer. Inadvertent in utero exposure to DMPA is not associated with an adverse pregnancy outcome. A summary of advantages and disadvantages of DMPA contraception that may be used in counseling are listed in Table 9.12.

LEVONORGESTREL (IMPLANTABLE CONTRACEPTIVE RODS). Levonorgestrel delivered via implantable contraceptive rods (Norplant) provides excellent long-term contraception that requires no additional motivation or action on the part of the patient for a 5-year period. As with DMPA, contraceptive rods gain most of their contraceptive effect from ovulation inhibition, with the addition of cervical mucus changes and endometrial atrophy. Unlike DMPA, ovulation appears to become more common as use continues, although contraceptive efficacy is not compromised. The 5-year cumulative pregnancy rate is reported as 1.1 to 1.5 per 100 users. As with DMPA, the most common side effects are menstrual cycle disruption, although patients using the rod system are more likely to have regular cycles as time passes.

The high degree of reliability of this system is partially offset by concerns specific to this method, which carries a high initial expense for the system and its insertion. This is partially offset by the possibility of 5 years of use, although 20% of users stop after 1 year and 50% stop after 3 years, with 3.8 years reported as the average duration of use, blunting these calculations. Although levonorgestrel implantable rods may not be discontinued by the patient without medical intervention (to remove them), ovulation usually occurs within 2 to 4 weeks of their removal. Care in the placement and removal of this contraceptive system is required and specific training in the techniques of both is strongly recommended.

A summary of advantages and disadvantages of levonorgestrel implantable rods that may be used in counseling are listed in Table 9.13.

Table 9.12. Attributes of Depot Medroxyprogesterone Acetate Contraception (for Counseling Purposes)

Advantages	Disadvantages
Extremely reliable (comparable to sterilization)	May not be rapidly stopped
Convenient	High degree of cycle disruption
No systemic estrogen effects	Requires medical intervention
Requires only periodic motivation	Potential for progesterone side effects
May be used for a prolonged period	
High compliance and continuation	
Low cost of use when used for a prolonged period	
May be used while breast feeding	

Table 9.13. Attributes of Levonorgestrel Implantable Rod (Norplant) Contraception (for Counseling Purposes)

Advantages	Disadvantages
Extremely reliable (comparable to sterilization)	May not be rapidly stopped
Convenient	High degree of cycle disruption
No systemic estrogen effects	Requires medical intervention
Requires only single act of motivation	Potential for progesterone side effects
May be used for a prolonged period	Requires surgical implantation and removal
High compliance and continuation	High initial and removal costs
Acceptable cost of use when used for a prolonged period	
May be used while breast feeding	

Ineffective Methods

Although any contraception is better than none, it is important to counsel against the routine use of less than effective contraceptive techniques at the time we provide access to reliable methods. Techniques including postcoital douching, withdrawal, makeshift barriers (e.g., food wrap or a dental dam), and the use of coital positions reputed to prevent pregnancy (e.g., standing) are associated with failure rates that range from 6% to over 40%. Postcoital douching is not only a medical example of too little, too late, but some have argued that douching could even facilitate the movement of sperm into the upper genital tract.

Withdrawal (coitus interruptus) can be used when no other method is available, but significant release of sperm prior to ejaculation and the very high degree of motivation, self-awareness, and self-control required limit both the applicability and reliability of this method. Some authors suggest that fewer than 50% of men are able to use this method. Use of any of these methods should be discouraged in favor of more reliable techniques.

Permanent (Sterilization)

Sterilization provides effective birth control without continuing expense, effort, or motivation, accounting for roughly a million procedures annually. It is the leading contraceptive choice for couples where the wife is over 30 years of age or for couples who have been married more than 10 years. In one third of married couples in the United States one or the other partner has undergone a sterilization procedure. The choice of which partner undergoes sterilization is generally a personal one. Although considerations of individual medical factors may affect this choice, the decision is most often based on the motivation of the individuals involved. Surprisingly, twice as many women as men choose sterilization, despite the greater operative hazards involved, underscoring the need for accurate counseling of both members of the couple.

Current methods of sterilization are less invasive, less expensive, safer, and as effective as procedures used in the past. Despite this, and the complacency it engenders, sterilization remains an invasive procedure. Counseling of patients must include the operative risks and chance of failure (less than 1%), as well as the permanent nature of the procedure. Although it is possible to reverse some forms of sterilization, the difficulty of doing so and the generally poor rate of success, demands that patients understand the permanent nature of the decision. Despite counseling, approximately 1% of patients undergoing sterilization subsequently request reversal of the procedure because of a change in marital status, loss of a child, or desire for more children. Successful reversal occurs in only 40% to 60% of cases.

Female Sterilization

Surgical sterilization methods for women may be carried out as postpartum or interval (nonpregnant) procedures, although most techniques can be performed at either time. Factors such as parity, obesity, previous surgery or pelvic infections; and medical conditions, such as hypertension or respiratory diseases, affect the timing and specific method chosen. The final choice of method is probably best left to the patient and her surgeon.

Failure of surgical sterilization occurs in 1% or less of all procedures but the rate depends on the method chosen and operator experience. Infection, bleeding, injury to surrounding structures, or anesthetic complications may occur with any surgical technique. Laparoscopic and hysterscopic techniques carry risks that are unique to their instrumentation, such as complications of trocar insertion or cervical damage, respectively.

Debate continues about the existence of a "posttubal ligation syndrome," consisting of irregular bleeding patterns and pelvic pain. It has been postulated that disruption of blood flow in the area of the fallopian tubes may influence ovarian function, leading to menstrual dysfunction or dysmenorrhea. Efforts to document such an effect have not been successful and the existence of this syndrome remains conjectural.

The oldest methods of female sterilization use laparotomy. Laparotomy provides excellent access to the uterine tubes either in the postpartum period or as an interval procedure. Permanent obstruction or interruption of the fallopian tubes can be accomplished by a variety of surgical techniques or by means of clips, rings, or cautery. Laparotomy techniques do not require special tools or training, which makes them attractive to a wider number of physicians and smaller hospitals.

The development of efficient light sources, fiberoptic light guides, and smaller instruments has led to an increase in the use of laparoscopy for female sterilization. Performed as an outpatient interval procedure, laparoscopic techniques can be carried out under either local or general anesthesia. Small incisions, a relatively low rate of complications, and a degree of flexibility possible in the procedures have led to high physician and patient acceptance.

The posterior cul-de-sac offers a convenient port of entry into the peritoneal cavity for sterilization procedures. All of the techniques used in laparoscopy, and many used via laparotomy, can be applied to the fallopian tubes through this route. Vaginal tubal procedures carry a moderate rate of infection to the vaginal incision site or ovaries if prophylactic antibiotics are not used. Vaginal tubal procedures require that the patient refrain from intercourse and the use of tampons or douches for 2 weeks while the vaginal incision heals. Some physicians place these same restrictions on patients following laparoscopic sterilization procedures as well, minimizing the differences between the two approaches.

The possibility of transcervical obstruction of the fallopian tube is attractive because it avoids penetration of the peritoneal cavity. Methods proposed include formed-in-place silicon plugs, chemical cautery, or occlusive agents such as methyl cyanoacrylate. Endometrial ablation by cautery or laser, which can be done for other purposes, has also been proposed as a sterilization method. These procedures remain in the developmental stage at the present time.

Male Sterilization

Roughly one third of surgical sterilization procedures are performed on men. Because the vas deferens is located outside the abdominal cavity, vasectomy is safer and generally less expensive than female sterilization. Vasectomy is also more easily reversed than female sterilization. Vasectomy is routinely performed as a outpatient procedure, under local anesthesia. Potential complications include bleeding, hematomas, and local skin infections, but these are infrequent ($<3\%$ of cases). Some authors report a greater incidence of depression and change in body image following vasectomy than with female sterilization, although this may be minimized with preoperative counseling and education. Concern has been raised about the formation of sperm antibodies in approximately 50% of patients, but no adverse long-term effects of vasectomy have been identified.

Pregnancy after vasectomy occurs in about 1% of cases. Because vasectomy is not immediately effective, many of these pregnancies result from intercourse too soon after the procedure, rather than recanalization. Multiple ejaculations are required before the proximal collecting system is emptied of sperm produced prior to the procedure. Therefore, couples must use another method of contraception for 4 to 6 weeks or until azoospermia is confirmed by semen analysis. Similar follow-up confirmation of efficacy is not easily accomplished with female sterilization methods.

Pregnancy Interdiction

Postcoital interdiction of pregnancy is not a substitute for planning and effective contraception. In instances of rape, unintended intercourse, IUCD expulsion, or barrier failure (e.g., condom breakage or diaphragm displacement), these methods may have merit. High-dose estrogen, such as diethylstilbestrol (25–50 mg/d for 5 days), conjugated estrogen (Premarin; 30 mg/d), estradiol (5 mg/d), or oral contraceptives (Ovral; 2 tablets followed by 2 more tablets 12 h later, continued for 2 to 10 days) may be effective if begun within 48 hours after intercourse and continued for 5 days. Efficacy is markedly reduced after 72 hours following intercourse, or with multiple episodes of intercourse. Failure of hormonal interdiction is reported to be as low as 0.2 to 0.4 per 100 women treated. Insertion of a copper-bearing IUCD up to 5 days after unprotected intercourse may offer some protection. The patient must be warned not to have additional unprotected intercourse during the rest of the current cycle, as these techniques will not provide continuing contraception later in the cycle.

These methods should not be used on a routine basis because they are associated with numerous side effects and a moderate risk of failure. When pregnancy continues, intrauterine exposure to high-dose steroids or an IUCD can have significant consequences, warranting recommending termination of these pregnancies. Because of this risk, these therapies are often reserved for those who would consider a pregnancy termination should failure occur. There may be a slight increase in the risk of ectopic pregnancy in these patients, but this increase appears to minimal.

The antiprogesterone RU-486 holds promise as an effective "menstrual induction" agent. Studies from outside the United States show that this agent is safe and effective in inducing withdrawal bleeding (menstruation) when taken at the time of anticipated menstruation or in the face of documented early pregnancy. Currently this therapy is only available outside of the United States. Clinical trials in the United States are underway, which may lead to the availability of RU-486 in the United States in the future.

Future Technologies

New Spermicides

Spermicidal contraception offers use-based, reversible contraception with some protection from sexually transmitted diseases. Products containing nonoxynol-9 are undergoing re-evaluation and reformulation, including one product under development that combines nonoxynol-9 with an agent that promotes adherence to the vaginal tissues. This is hoped to enhance protection against sexually transmitted disease and provide up to 24 hours of contraception. Other agents currently under study are spermicides containing polyanionic polysaccharides (dextran sulfate), benzalkonium chloride, chlorhexidine, propranolol, acrosin inhibitors, and seminal liquefaction inhibitors. Although one contraceptive sponge has been removed from the market, a new sponge incorporating three spermicides and a dispersing agent is currently under testing.

New Barrier Methods

At least two disposable diaphragms are in clinical trials. These devices are made of silicone or polyurethane and contain a spermicide, eliminating the need for additional spermicidal agents, even with multiple acts of intercourse. These devices may be used for up to 24 hours without removal.

A new cervical cap incorporating a valve to allow passage of cervical secretions is currently under development. It is hoped that this device will permit longer wear than currently available devices.

The Evloving Intrauterine Device

Several IUCDs, now available outside the Unites States, may be introduced for use in this country in the next few years. Most of these devices use either copper or levonorgestrel much like the currently marketed IUCDs, differing mainly in their shape. Pregnancy rates and the type and frequency of side effects are similar to the currently marketed models.

Improved Hormonal Technologies

Progress in hormonal contraception has centered around improving delivery systems, mainly through modification of currently available technologies. One example is a two-rod version of the currently available levonorgestrel rod system (Norplant) that will last for 3 to 5 years. These rods are longer than those in the six-rod system currently used, giving them sufficient surface area to be used for longer durations. Single-rod systems employing nomegestrol acetate, 3-keto-desogestrel, or the synthetic progesterone ST-1435 are also under evaluation. These single-rods systems will probably be used for 1- to 2-year periods before they need to be replaced.

Biodegradable implants containing levonorgestrel or norethindrone in rods or pellets, respectively, are currently under development. Moderate failure rates and concerns about the ability to remove a degenerating rod prematurely, if necessary, may delay the availability of the biodegradable rod. Norethindrone pellets, which are about the size of a grain of rice, are made up of a mixture of hormone and cholesterol that degrade over a period of 12 to 18 months. Microspheres containing norethindrone or norgestimate that may be injected to provide contraception for 1 to 6 months are being developed. Menstrual irregularities remain the most common side effects of progesterone-based long-acting contraception.

Hormone delivery via vaginal rings, containing either a progesterone or estrogen and progesterone, are being investigated. These rings are approximately 50 to 60 mm in diameter and are worn continuously, except for 1 week a month, when it is removed to induce withdrawal bleeding. These rings do not require specific fitting or exact placement in the vagina. They may be left in place during intercourse or removed briefly without compromising contraceptive efficacy. In preliminary trials, progesterone-only rings are associated with a discontinuation rate of almost 20% because of menstrual irregularity.

Once a month injectable combinations of estrogen (estradiol cypionate or estradiol enanthate) and progesterone (hydroxyprogesterone or dihydroxyprogesterone acetophenide) are under investigation in China and Latin America. These agents are used on a monthly basis and have the advantage of improved menstrual cycle control. Preliminary results of these studies suggest excellent contraceptive efficacy.

Permanent Methods

Efforts to develop less invasive permanent sterilization and long-term methods that may be reversed are under way at many locations around the world. For women, smaller occlusive clips that cause less damage to the fallopian tube while still producing acceptable success rates, may allow a greater likelihood of reversibility. Fimbrial caps or hoods have been explored, but have not proved to be more reversible than other methods.

For men, sclerosing agents and formed-in-place silastic plugs are under evaluation. Plugs or implantable valves were hoped to provide reversibility, but trials to date have been disappointing. Research continues and may yet provide useful alternatives.

New Technologies

FEMALE CONTRACEPTION. Transdermal delivery of a synthetic progesterone (ST-1435) is being evaluated as a possible contraceptive. Preliminary results suggest effective suppression of ovulation, but full-scale clinical trials have not yet been carried out.

Early studies of gonatropin-releasing hormone (GnRH) agonists and antagonists as contraceptive agents are promising. These agents give good ovulation suppression, but they may not be given orally and supplemental estrogen is often required. High cost may limit acceptance.

Currently under development is permanent contraception based on nonsurgical methods. One approach is the development of an antipregnancy vaccine. Based on immunization to progesterone, human chorionic gonadotrophin (HCG), sperm-binding glycoprotein, or the sperm itself, these experimental techniques may hold promise.

MALE CONTRACEPTION. In the past, little success has been achieved in developing new male contraceptive methods. On the horizon are some new approaches that may change this situation. Testosterone (testosterone enanthate) injections given weekly have been successful in producing azoospermia in a 1-year preliminary trial. A once-a-month injection combining medroxyprogesterone acetate and testosterone has also been evaluated, but both the single and double agent techniques appear to be more reliable in causing azoospermia in Asian men than in Caucasians. This racial difference has yet to be explained, but the answer may provide insight leading to additional methods of contraception. Peptides, such as GnRH agonists and inhibin, can inhibit spermatogenesis, but their cost will probably limit the widespread use of these agents.

Condoms made of polyurethane will be available shortly. Polyurethane provides more rapid heat transfer, improving sensation. These condoms provide protection against sexually transmitted disease to the same degree that latex condoms do, but without the possibility of latex allergy and irritation.

Plant extracts (such as gossypol, from cottonseed oil) may provide agents that can affect sperm in the epididymis, resulting in inhibited sperm motility and reduced sperm counts. To date, significant side effects such as hypokalemia, alterations in blood pressure, and concerns about reversibility have limited progress with these drugs. (Gossypol may prove to be an effective intravaginal agent with fewer side effects.)

Preliminary studies on a small number of subjects suggest that nifedipine may have a contraceptive effect that may be exploited. Nifedipine appears to inhibit the acrosome reaction and to alter surface proteins on the heads of the sperm, both of which reduce the likelihood of fertilization even in the presence of adequate numbers.

Contraception based on testicular heating has been investigated. Raising the temperature of the testes slightly, through warming or microwave heating, results in a reversible azoospermia. It remains to be seen if this will become a viable contraceptive technology.

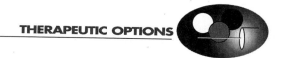

THERAPEUTIC OPTIONS

Assisting with Contraceptive Choices

There is no "ideal" contraceptive method. While efficacy and an acceptable risk of side effects are important in the choice of contraceptive methods, these are often not the factors on which the final choice is made. Motivation to use or continue to use a contraceptive method is based on education, cultural background, cost, and individual needs, preferences, and prejudices. Factors such as availability, cost, coital dependence, personal acceptability, and the patient's perception of risk play a role in the final choice of methods.

For a couple to use a contraceptive method, it must be accessible, immediately available (especially in coitally dependent or use-oriented methods), and of reasonable cost. The impact of a method on spontaneity or the modes of sexual expression preferred by the patient and her partner may also be important considerations. A decision tree based on these concepts is presented in Figure 9.2.

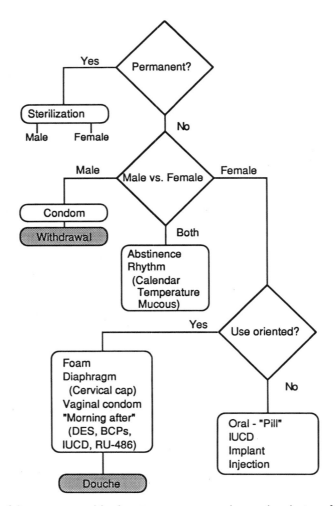

Figure 9.2 One of the many possible decision tree approaches to the choice of contraceptive methods. (Methods shown in gray have a relatively higher failure rate and should not be used if pregnancy prevention is a high priority.) (Modified from Beckmann RB, Ling FW, Barzansky BM, et al. Obstetrics and gynecology. 2nd ed. Baltimore: Williams & Wilkins, 1995:250.)

Before prescribing oral contraceptives, a careful evaluation is required. The pill is relatively or absolutely contraindicated for some patients (Table 9.14); however, even factors such as menstrual history may have an impact on the choice of these agents. For example, less than 1% or 2% of patients experience problems with amenorrhea after prolonged oral contraceptive use ("postpill amenorrhea"). Young women, and those with a history of irregular periods, are more likely to experience this problem. These patients should be alerted to this possibility. Oral contraceptive agents may interact with other medications, reducing the efficacy of either the oral contraceptive or the other medications involved. Medications with known or suspected interactions are shown in Table 9.15. These factors are not contraindications to the use of the pill, but they may prompt both the patient and provider to include other options in their considerations.

Table 9.14. Contraindications to the Use of Oral Contraceptives

ABSOLUTE

  Cardiovascular disease (severe)
  Cerebrovascular disease (stroke)
  Congenital hyperlipidemia
  Hepatic disease (with abnormal liver function)
  Hepatic tumor
  Malignancy (current): breast, endometrium, ovary
  Obstructive jaundice of pregnancy (history)
  Ongoing pregnancy
  Pulmonary embolism
  Vaginal bleeding (of unknown source)
  Venous thrombosis

RELATIVE

  Acne (severe)?
  Age 35+ with smoking
  Age over 40?
  Depression?
  Diabetes mellitus
  Epilepsy
  Galactorrhea (of unknown cause)
  Gallbladder disease
  Gestational diabetes?
  History of anovulation or oligo-ovulation
  Lactation
  Moderate uterine fibroids
  Obesity?
  Sickle-cell disease
  Vaginal adenosis
  Varicose veins (severe)
  Vascular headaches (migraine, cluster)

Special Considerations

Anyone who counsels couples in contraceptive choices must be aware of the special needs of adolescents, breast feeding mothers, older patients, those who have recently delivered or lost an early pregnancy, and others.

Adolescent patients require reliable contraception, but often have problems with compliance. Careful counseling about options (including abstinence), the risks of pregnancy and sexually transmitted disease, as well as the need for both contraception and disease protection must be provided. Barrier contraception addresses several of these needs, but irregular compliance suggests at least consideration of methods not based on time of use implementation. Patients who have normal development and established menstruation (at least two or three spontaneous periods) may be considered for oral contraception or long-acting progesterone agents, in addition to condoms for disease protection.

Contraception for breast feeding mothers may include oral contraceptives if milk flow is well established. Combination oral contraceptives may slightly reduce the volume or duration of lactation, whereas progestin-only oral contraceptives or long-acting progestins do not have this effect. There is some evidence that use of long-acting progesterone con-

Table 9.15. Oral Contraceptive Drug Interactions

Drugs that may decrease the effectiveness of oral contraceptives
  Ampicillin
  Barbiturates
  Benzodiazepines
  Chloral hydrate
  Clofibrate
  Cyclophosphamide
  Ethosuximide
  Ibuprofen
  Indomethacin
  Penicillin V
  Phenobarbital
  Phenylbutazone
  Phenytoin
  Primidone
  Rifampin
  Sulfonamides
  Tetracycline
Drugs potentially affected by oral contraceptives (retarded biotransformation)
  Anticoagulants
  Guanethidine monosulfate
  Insulin
  Meperidine hydrochloride
  Methyldopa
  Oral hypoglycemics
  Phenazone
  Phenothiazines
  Reserpine
  Tricyclic antidepressants

traceptives may actually result in a slight increase in breast milk production. Barrier contraceptives are not contraindicated in these patients. Intrauterine devices, copper or hormone containing, may also be placed once the uterus has returned to normal.

Patients over the age of 35 may continue to use low-dose oral contraceptives if they have no other risk factors and do not smoke. (Although the risk of serious complication of oral contraceptives increases with age, the risks of pregnancy rise faster.) Compliance concerns are generally less in these patients, making use-oriented methods more acceptable and reliable. Long-term methods such as IUCDs, long-acting progesterone contraception, or sterilization procedures may also be appropriate. Until menopause is confirmed by clinical or laboratory methods (see chapter 12, Menopause) contraception must be continued if pregnancy is to be avoided.

Because the return of fertility is often early, but unpredictable, contraceptive options should be discussed with patients immediately following delivery or abortion. Following abortion (spontaneous or induced) ovulation may occur as soon as 2 weeks after the loss. If oral contraceptives are chosen, they should be started immediately after the loss. Counseling regarding the risk of endometritis in the immediate period and sexually transmitted disease, in general, should be provided.

Patients with uterine leiomyomata (fibroids) are not good candidates for IUCD use but may still be considered for hormonal contraceptives. Oral contraceptives may cause the fibroids to grow, but with care may still be used. Long-acting progestin contraception does not appear to carry the same risk. Barrier methods are not affected by the presence of fibroids. A possible exception would be the use of a diaphragm in patients with significant distortion of the vaginal canal due to large or unusually placed fibroids.

Common Concerns and Their Management

Menstrual irregularities are very common in the first few months of long- acting progesterone contraceptive use. Reassurance and watchful waiting is appropriate, as most of these problems spontaneously resolve during the first 6 months of therapy. When intermenstrual or random bleeding is troublesome, supplemental estrogen (such as Premarin 0.625, Estraderm 0.05, or their equivalents) for a single month often stabilizes the endometrium and improves symptoms. Intermenstrual spotting may also be a problem for IUCD users. Like long-acting progestin users, this generally improves with time, but supplemental hormone administration may be used to improve troublesome or persistent problems. When simple interventions are unsuccessful, consideration should be given to terminating the current method.

Two common problems for low-dose oral contraceptive pill users are breakthrough bleeding and amenorrhea. Although these side effects may occur with any oral contraceptive, they are most common with the low-dose and polyphasic preparations. When mild breakthrough bleeding occurs in the first 3 months of use, reassurance is all that is required. Most cases will resolve spontaneously within the first 6 months of use. When bleeding is heavy it may be reduced or stopped by the addition of supplemental estrogen for a month. A change to a monophasic preparation, or a slightly more estrogen-dominant agent, is probably warranted for these patients.

The absence of withdrawal bleeding while taking oral contraceptives does not indicate an increased risk of pregnancy, and there is no medical intervention beyond reassurance required. Patients who fail to have withdrawal bleeding should be questioned about the possibility of missed pills and thus pregnancy, with pregnancy tests performed often for these women. Because many patients view the presence of withdrawal bleeding as desirable to confirm effectiveness, a change to a more estrogen-dominant formulation may be desirable. When menstrual bleeding has gradually diminished to the point of amenorrhea, switching to a formulation with more estrogen for two to three cycles usually returns regular withdrawal bleeding. Estrogen supplementation of low-dose formulations also accomplishes the same end, although total estrogen dose is higher and convenience is less than when the formulation alone is altered.

HINTS AND COMMON QUESTIONS

Intrauterine contraceptive devices date only to Graafenberg's work early in the 20th century, not to nomadic camel drivers. It appears that this myth dates to approximately 1964 and an off-hand comment made by Dr. Anna L. Southam, then at the College of Physicains and

Surgeons of Columbia University. An excellent review of this historic detective story is found in the article by Thomsen shown in the references.

If a patient experiences excessive bleeding with a copper-bearing IUCD but would like to continue intrauterine contraception, removal with reinsertion a month later of a progesterone IUCD may allow continued use.

For patients who do not have withdrawal bleeding on oral contraceptives but do not want to alter their pill or repeatedly perform pregnancy tests, basal body temperatures taken during the last 5 days of the pill-free interval may be used to provide reassurance. Temperatures below 98°F are unlikely to occur in the presence of a pregnancy.

The injection site should not be massaged after giving depot medroxyprogesterone acetate (DMPA) for contraception. Massaging the site increases the absorption and may decrease the effectiveness of the agent.

Patients who experience random bleeding while using long-acting progesterone-based contraception (DMPA, Norplant) may be treated with low- dose supplemental estrogen (e.g., Premarin 0.625 mg/d, Estraderm 0.05) for 3 to 4 weeks with generally good resolution of symptoms. This may be repeated later if needed.

A common myth among young patients is that a woman cannot conceive during her first act of intercourse. This is clearly wrong. Young women are most fertile, and a significant number of pregnancies occur with only one act of unprotected intercourse. Every effort should be made to combat such misinformation and provide correct contraceptive facts.

SUGGESTED READINGS

General References

American College of Obstetricians and Gyneologists. The intrauterine device. ACOG Technical bulletin 164. Washington, DC: ACOG, 1992.

Grimes DA. Reversible contraception for the 1980s. JAMA 1986;255:69.

Hatcher RA, Trussell J, Stewart F, et al. Contraceptive technology, 16th ed. New York: Irvington Publishers, 1994.

Ory HW. Mortality asssociated with fertility and fertility control 1983. Fam Plann Perspect 1983;15:57.

Powell MG, Mears BJ, Deber RB, Ferguson D. Contraception with the cervical cap: effectiveness, safety, continuity of use, and user satisfaction. Contraception 1986;33:215.

Prentice RL, Thomas DB. On the epidemiology of oral contraceptives and disease. Adv Cancer Res 1987;49:285.

Robertson WH. An illustrated history of contraception. Park Ridge, New Jersey: Parthenon Publishing Group, 1990.

Rothman KJ, Louik C. Oral contraceptives and birth defects. N Engl J Med 1978;299:522.

Service RF. Contraceptive methods go back to the basics. Science 1994;266:1480.

Shoupe ED, Haseltine FP (eds). Contraception. New York: Springer-Verlag, 1993.

Speroff L, Darney PD. A clinical guide for contraception. Baltimore: Williams & Wilkins, 1992.

Specific References

Spermicides

Faich G, Pearson K, Fleming D, et al. Toxic shock syndrome and the vaginal contraceptive sponge. JAMA 1986;255:216.

Louik C, Mitchell AA, Werler MM, et al. Maternal exposure to spermicides in relation to certain birth defects. N Engl J Med 1987;317:474.

Mills JL, Reed GF, Nugent RP, Harley EE, Berendes HW. Are there adverse effects of periconceptional spermicide use? Fertil Steril 1985;43:442.

Barriers

Cagen R. The cervical cap as a barrier contraceptive. Contraception 1986;33:487.

Intrauterine device

Alvarez F, Guiloff E, Brache V, et al. New insights on the mode of action of intrauterine contraceptive devices in women. Fertil Steril 1988;49:768.

Curtis EM, Pine L. Actinomyces in the vaginas of women with and without intrauterine contraceptive devices. Am J Obstet Gynecol 1981;140:880.

Daling JR, Weiss NS, Metch BJ, et al. Primary tubal infertility in relation to use of an intrauterine device. N Engl J Med 1985;312:937.

Farley TMM, Rosenberg MJ, Fowe PJ, Chen J, Meirik O. Intrauterine devices and pelvic inflammatory disease: an international perspective. Lancet 1992;339:785.

Lee NC, Rubin GL, Borucki R. The intrauterine device and pelivc inflammatory disease revisited: new results from the Women's Health Study. Obstet Gynecol 1988;72:1.

Sivin I. Dose- and age-dependent ectopic pregnancy risks with intrauterine contraception. Obstet Gynecol 1991;78:291.

Thomsen RJ. Camels and the IUD: It was a good story. Contemporary Ob/Gyn 1988;(March):152.

Oral Contraceptive

Bacon JF, Shenfield GM. Pregnancy attrbutable to interaction between tetracycline and oral contraceptives. BMJ 1980;280:293.

Beller FK, Ebert C. Effects of oral contraceptives on blood coagulation. A Review. Obstet Gynecol Surv 1985;40:425.

Goldbaum GM, Kendrick JS, Hogelin GC, et al. The relative impact of smoking and oral contraceptive use on women in the United States. JAMA 1987;258:1339.

Mishell DR JR, Shoupe D. Oral contraceptives for women over the age of 35. In Shoupe ED, Haseltine FP (eds). Contraception. New York: Springer-Verlag, 1993:85.

Notelovitz M, Levenson I, McKenzie L, Lane D, Kitchens CS. The effects of low-dose oral contraceptives on coagulation and fibrinolysis in two high-risk populations: young female smokers and older premenopausal women. Am J Obstet Gynecol 1985;152:995.

Ory HW. The noncontraceptive health benefits from oral contraceptive use. Fam Plann Perspect 1982;14:182.

Pititti DB, Wingerg J, Pellegrin F Ramcharan S. Risk of vascular disease in women: smoking, oral contraceptives, noncontraceptive estrogens, and other factors. JAMA 1979;242:1150.

Ramcharan S, Pellegrin FA, Ray R, Hsu JP. Mortality. In The Walnut Creek Contraceptive Drug Study: A Prospective Study of the Side Effects of Oral Contraceptives, vol 3. An Interim Report—A Comparison of Disease Occurrence Leading to Hospitalization or Death in Users and Nonusers of Oral Contraceptives. Bethesda, MD: Center for Population Research, 1982.

Royal College of General Practitioners' Oral Contraceptive Study: Oral contraceptives, venous thrombosis, and varicose veins. J R Coll Gen Pract [Occas Pap] 1978;28:393.

Shoupe D. Effects of desogestrel on carbohydrate metabolism. Am J Obstet Gynecol 1993;168:1041.

Spellacy WN, Buhi WC, Birk SA. Carbohydrate metabolism prospectively studied in women using a low-estrogen oral contraceptive for six months. Contraception 1979;20:137.

Stampfer MF, Willett WC, Colditz GA, Speizer, FE, Hennekens CH. A prospective study of past use of oral contraceptive agents and risk of cardiovascular disease. N Engl J Med 1988;319:1313.

The Cancer and Steriod Hormone Study of the Centers for Disease Control and the National Institute of Chile Health and Human Development. The reduction in risk of ovarian cancer associated with oral contraceptive use. N Engl J Med 1987;316:650.

Tri-Norinyl and Ortho-Novum 7/7/7: Two triphasic oral contraceptives. Med Lett 1984;26:93.

Wiseman RA. Absence of correlation between oral contraceptive usage and cardiovascular mortality. Int J Fertil 1984;29:198.

Long-Acting Agents

Berenson AB, Wiemann CM. Use of levonorgestrel implants versus oral contraceptives in adolescence: a case-control study. Am J Obstet Gynecol 1995;172:1128.

Brache V, Alvarez-Sanchez F, Faundes A, Tejada AS, Cochon L. Ovarian endocrine function through five years of continuous treatment with Norplant subdermal contraceptive implants. Contraception 1990;41:169.

Fraser IS. A survey of different approaches to management of menstrual disturbances in women using injectable contraceptives. Contraception 1983;28:385.

Huovinen K, Tikkanen MJ, Autio S, et al. Serum lipids and lipoproteins during therapeutic amenorrhea induced by lynestrenol and depot-medroxyprogesterone acetate. Acta Obstet Gynecol Scand 1991;70:349.

Liang AP, Levenson AG, Layde PM, et al. Risk of breast, uterine corpus, and ovarian cancer in women receiving medroxyprogesterone injections. JAMA 1983;249:2909.

Konje JC, Otolorin EO, Ladipo OA. Changes in carbohydrate metabolism during 30 months on Norplant. Contraception 1991;44:163.

Singh K, Viegas OA, Loke DF, Ratnam SS. Effect of Norplant implants on liver, lipid and carbohydrate metabolism. Contraception 1992;45:141.

Other Methods

Johnson JH. Contraception: the morning after. Fam Plann Perspect 1984;16:266.

Van Santen MR, Haspels AA. A comparison of high-dose estrogens versus low-dose ethinylestradiol and norgestrel combination in postcoital interception: a study in 493 women. Fertil Steril 1985;43:206.

Wade ME, McCarthy P, Abernathy JR, et al. A randomized perspective study of the use effectiveness of two methods of natural family planning: An interim report. Am J Obstet Gynecol 1979;134:628.

Sterilization

Massey FJ, Bernstein GS, O'Fallon WM, et al. Vasectomy and health: results from a large cohort study. JAMA 1984;252:1023.

Future Directions

Beck L, Pope V. Long-acting injectable norethisterone contraceptive system: review of clinical studies. Research Frontiers in Fertility Regulation 1984;3:1.

Comhaire FH. Male contraception: hormonal, mechanical and other. Hum Reprod 1994;9:586.

Coutinho EM. One year contraception with a single subdermal implant containing nomegestrol acetate (Uniplant). Contraception 1993;47:97.

Coutinho EM, Melo JF, Barbosa I, Segal SJ. Antispermatogenic action of gossypol in men. Fertil Steril 1984;42:424.

Cunningham GR, Silverman VE, Thornby J, Kohler PO. The potential for an androgen male contraceptive. J Clin Endocrinol Metab 1979;49:520.

Darney PD. Hormonal implants: contraception for a new century. Am J Obstet Gynecol 1994;170:1536.

Darney PD, Klaisle CM, Monroe SE, et al. Evaluation of a 1-year levonorgestrel-releasing contraceptive implant: side effect, release rates, and biodegradability. Fertil Steril 1992;58:137.

Fraser IS. Vaginal bleeding patterns in women using once-a-month injectable contraceptives. Contraception 1994;49:399.

Jones WR, Bradley J, Judd SJ, et al. Phase I clinical trial of a World Health Organization birth control vaccine. Lancet 1988;1:1295.

Laurikka-Routtie M, Haukkamaa M, Lahteenmaki P. Suppression of ovarian function with the transdermally given synthetic progestin ST-1435. Fertil Steril 1992;58:680.

Mishell DR JR. Vaginal contraceptive rings. Ann Med 1993;25:191.

Singh M, Saxena BB, Graver R, et al. Contraception efficacy of norethindrone encapsulated in injectable biodegradable poly-dl-lactide-coglycolide microspheres: Phase II clinical study. Fertil Steril 1989;52:973.

Sujuan G, Mingkun D, Linde Z, et al. A five-year evaluation of Norplant II implants in China. Contraception 1994;50:27.

Waites GMH. Male fertility regulation: the challenges for the year 2000. Br Med Bull 1993;49:210.

Wang C, Yeung RTT. Gossypol and hypokalemia. Contraception 1985;32:237.

WHO Task Force on Methods for the Regulation of Male Fertility. Contraceptive efficacy of testosterone-induced azoospermia in normal men. Lancet 1990;336:955.

10

Cancer Screening

An important part of preventative care for all patients, not just women, is screening for malignant disease. Cancer represents a significant medical and economic threat to the well-being of our patients. Fear of cancer is universal. Despite this deserved reputation for devastation, many cancers have attributes that make early detection and, therefore, early effective therapy both possible and practical. Cancer screening, tailored to the needs of the individual patient, must be an integral part of the preventative primary care we provide.

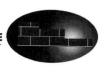

BACKGROUND AND SCIENCE

Cancer screening works best with a knowledge of historical factors that identify individuals at high risk and an understanding of the technologies at our disposal. The best screening programs can be directed toward moderately prevalent conditions that have identifiable antecedents or a long prodromal phase and for which effective early treatment and reliable screening technology exist. Diseases that may be cured when detected late in their course do not lend themselves to cost-effective early screening programs. The screening technology applied must have a high sensitivity and an acceptable positive predictive value. The negative predictive value of the test must be high.

Risk Factors

To some degree, all patients are at risk for cancer (Table 10.1). For most this risk is small, making screening ineffective and cost prohibitive. There are, however, risk factors that may be identified that can make screening more effective. The most common of these is age.

Table 10.1. Cancer in Women (1995 Estimates)

Cancer	Cancers	Deaths	Cases/y	Death/y
Lung	13%	24%	73,900	62,000
Breast	32%	18%	182,000	46,000
Colon/rectum	12%	11%	51,000	24,500
Ovary	5%	6%	26,600	14,500
Pancreas	2%	5%	13,000	13,800
Uterus	8%	4%	48,600	10,700
Cervical			15,800	4,800
Corpus			32,800	5,900
Lymphoma			30,100	16,330
}	6%	8%		
Leukemia			11,000	9,300
All sites			575,000	258,000

Source: Wingo PA, Tong T, Bolden S. Cancer statistics 1995. CA Cancer J Clin 1995;45:8.

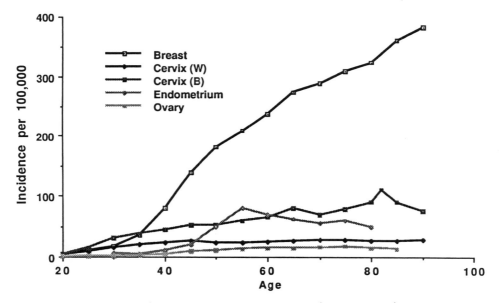

Figure 10.1. Cancer Rates by Age. Cervix (W) = cervical cancer in white women, cervix (B) = cervical cancer in black women.

For many cancers, the incidence rate increases predictably with age (Fig 10.1). Founded on this changing risk, screening strategies for cancers, such as breast or colon, change according to the age of the patient.

Diet and lifestyle choices made by patients may increase their risk for some cancers, suggesting a need for specific or altered screening programs for these women. Women who maintain diets high in fats, meat protein, or calories are at greater risk of colon cancer, whereas those who maintain high-fiber diets have a decreased risk. Obese patients have a higher incidence of endometrial cancer. Smoking is clearly associated with an increased risk of lung cancer, but it is also associated with a 3.5 times increased risk of cervical and bladder cancer. When risk factors are present, the timing of, and emphasis on, periodic screening may have to be re-evaluated to provide maximal protection for the individual patient.

Racial and ethnic background may also be risk factors for some tumors. An example of this differential risk for women is choriocarcinoma and its higher incidence among Southeast Asian women. One recent report found that cervical cancer is higher among Asians and blacks, suggesting a need for increased vigilance for these women. This same study discovered that Southeast Asian women were less likely than white and black women to comply with recommended follow-up diagnostic and treatment procedures for cervical disease, which also places them at higher risk.

A growing number of tumors have been related to specific genetic markers that appear to be associated with either an increased risk of disease or the actual source of that risk. Gene markers, such as the BRCA gene (associated with breast cancer) or chromosome 5 deletions (colon cancer), are beginning to provide indicators of risk, prompting increased vigilance with currently available screening tools. Currently, this technology is limited to families with a high prevalence of very specific tumors or disease processes. As the list of diseases for which a genetic link has been established grows, biochemical and genetic markers may soon become screening tools in their own right.

Technology of Screening

Not all diagnostic methods are well suited as screening tests. Screening tests must have a high validity with a clear distinction between positive and negative endpoints. An ideal method should be simple, inexpensive, and easy to perform. It should be noninvasive, carry no side effects, and cause little or no discomfort or risk.

The technology of screening is based on specifics of tumor behavior or evolution that provide clues to the existence of the tumor and allow detection. In the case of superficial tumors, such as cervical cancer, exfoliation of cells and a well-defined progression from normal to abnormal, allows early detection. Biochemical markers may herald the presence of some tumors, facilitating detection or providing a means to monitor the results of therapy. Examples of this are the use of beta-human chorionic gonadotrophin (β-HCG) in choriocarcinoma or CA-125 in ovarian cancer. Other tumors can produce physical signs of their presence, such as subclinical bleeding (colorectal cancer) or microcalcification (breast cancer), which may be used in detection strategies.

The cytologic detection of cancer and precancerous lesions is based on the prototypic example of the Papanicolaou (Pap) smear. Although the idea of cytologic detection of cancer was first published in 1928, by the Rumanian pathologist, Aureli Babes, it was the work of George N. Papanicolaou in the early 1940s that popularized the test in this country. What Dr. Papanicolaou showed was that cancer of the cervix or endometrium could be detected by careful examination of cells obtained from the vaginal pool. The Canadian gynecologist, J. Ernest Ayre, improved the process by demonstrating that examining cells obtained directly from the cervix was easier and more efficient.

Most often associated with the uterine cervix, a Pap smear can be obtained from any site in the body where cells can be exfoliated or removed by other means (e.g., a Pap smear of the under side of the diaphragm in pelvic cancer staging or examinations of peritoneal washing or cyst fluids). The predictable changes in cellular morphology that occur as cells evolve from normal to dysplastic to cancerous are sufficiently universal that the organ or tissue involved does not prevent the use of cytology as a detection tool. As cells evolve toward cancer, the relative size and activity of the cell's nucleus increases and the degree of normal cellular maturation decreases.

The presence of occult blood is often used as an early marker for the possibility of malignancy. Although most often associated with fecal testing for possible colorectal disease, the presence of blood in urine, sputum, or semen generally signifies a significant pathologic process that requires further investigation. The most common form of occult blood testing is the guaiac test. The sample to be tested is applied to guaiac-impregnated filter paper and a developing solution (hydrogen peroxide and denatured alcohol-stabilizing mixture) is applied. The formation of a pink ring at 30 seconds indicates the present of hemoglobin. The false-positive rate for the guaiac test is approximately 10% with false-negative rates as high as 50% often reported.

SCREENING STRATEGIES

By definition, screening is directed toward detecting a condition in asymptomatic patients. Often the distinction between screening and detection is blurred. Screening and detection strategies are best based on a combination of identified risk factors, knowledge of tumor behavior, and available technology. For a screening program to be effective, the condition being tested for must be sufficiently prevalent to make identification practical and must carry the risk of significant adverse outcome that may be averted by early identification and intervention. If the condition fails any of these criteria, effective screening will not be possible. It is for these reasons that most clinical screening programs are based on factors such as age and prevalence of disease.

Gynecologic Cancers

Breast Cancer

Breast cancer represents the largest cancer risk female patients face throughout their lives, with lifetime risk estimates that run as high as 1 in 10. Effective screening is based on mammography, breast self-examination, and careful clinical examinations, all performed on a regular basis.

Despite a false-negative rate as high as 10%, mammography is the best screening tool currently available for breast cancer. Routine mammography should be started with a baseline study around age 35 and progress to annual examinations for women over the age of 50. Current guidelines for mammographic screening are shown in Table 14.2 (Chapter 14, Breast Disease). Mammographic examinations may be begun at an earlier age based on the presence of specific risk factors, even though these risk factors will identify less than 25% of cancer patients.

While mammography can detect cancer below 5 mm in size, mammography often leads to an increase in breast biopsies for benign disease, increasing cost and anxiety. The increased cost must be balanced against early detection. It is for this reason that routine screening should be based on risk factors, such as age or family history, and not applied to all young women. A more complete discussion of breast cancer screening is presented in Chapter 14, Breast Disease.

Cervical Cancer

Screening for cervical cancer has been one of the great successes of preventive medicine. The development of the Papanicolaou (Pap) smear has significantly contributed to the decline in deaths due to cervical cancer. Routine screening for cervical cancer has become well accepted by the majority of American women, with an estimated 50 million Pap smears performed annually. Despite this success, false-negative rates of up to 15% are common (although the specificity of Pap smears remains almost 100%). With repetition of the Pap smear or the additional information provided by colposcopy, the early detection of premalignant cervical change should be routine.

Despite the progress made, the Pap smear has not fulfilled its potential. Much of the failure to make cervical cancer a preventable disease lies in factors over which the clinician has a degree of control: education, correct technique, appropriate follow-up, and effective therapy. (The latter two aspects of this problem are discussed in Chapter 13, Abnormal Pap Smears.)

PAPANICOLAOU SMEARS. The most common source for false-negative cytologic examinations is a sampling error. A cytologic examination is only as good as the sample of cellular material submitted. Therefore, care in how a Pap smear is obtained is as important as its periodicity.

A reliable Pap smear of the cervix must include cellular material obtained from the endocervical canal and from the entire transformation zone. Endocervical cells can be obtained using either a cotton (or Dacron) tipped applicator or an endocervical brush. Theoretic arguments over the relative merits of these two methods abound, but definitive studies are limited. Some improvement in cell transfer rate may be found with the use of the endocervical brush. For patients who have had a series of smears, the differences are probably inconsequential. Both techniques can be used in pregnancy, although spotting is more likely with the use of the endocervical brush.

Material from the endocervical canal and the ectocervix (transformation zone) can be combined on one slide or separated onto two separate slides, at the discretion of the clinician or cytology laboratory involved. Rapid fixation, with either a fixative spray or immersion in a fixing liquid, is imperative. Cells from the cervix, and especially the endocervix, will air-dry extremely rapidly, producing artifacts or making the smear unreadable. Other sources for error are summarized in Table 10.2 and discussed at length in the paper by Koss listed in the references at the end of this chapter.

Based on the recommendations of the first and second Bethesda conferences sponsored by the National Cancer Institute, most cervical (or vaginal) cytology reports now follow the "Bethesda system." The previous five-class system of reporting had perceived shortcomings that these workshops attempted to resolve with the new reporting system. The new system provides standardized terminology that addresses the adequacy of the sample and the presence of benign changes or epithelial cell abnormalities. This system is designed to be more descriptive and to provide more information about the abnormalities found. The Bethesda system is not without its own problems and a number of concerns

Table 10.2. Dos and Don'ts of Pap Smears

Do

    Obtain smears prior to bimanual examination

    Visualize the entire cervix prior to sampling

    Obtain the ectocervical sample prior to sampling the endocervix

    Obtain cultures (if any) after taking cells for cytology

    Cleanse (gently) the cervix of excessive vaginal discharge prior to sampling

    Spread the sample uniformly on the slide

    Fix the slide promptly

Don't

    Contaminate the smear with lubricant or glove powder

    Rotate brush or applicator excessively

    Allow the smear to air-dry

    Use a spray fixative closer than 10 in from the slide

    Obscure cellular material by clumping or excessive blood

about its widespread implementation without further discussion or testing. Despite these concerns, over 80% of cytology laboratories now use this system. A more complete discussion of the Bethesda reporting system and the management of abnormal Pap smears is found in Chapter 13, Abnormal Pap Smears.

COLPOSCOPY AND CERVICOGRAPHY. Although not a true screening tool in its own right, colposcopy is an important addition to the screening process. Colposcopic evaluation of the cervix allows adjunctive information and directed biopsies to be obtained to amplify and clarify the abnormalities detected by cytologic testing. It is not adequate by itself to detect premalignant changes, but must supplement and be supplemented by cytologic or histologic evaluations. The techniques and typical findings of colposcopy lie beyond the scope of this discussion, but may be easily found in a number of currently available texts.

Cervicography is a photographic variant of colposcopy in which stereoscopic photographs of the cervix are obtained and sent for independent interpretation. This technique has received little popular support and currently plays little or no role in clinical practice.

Endometrial Cancer

Endometrial cancer is nearly twice as prevalent as cervical cancer. It is thought to progress through hyperplasia to adenomatous hyperplasia, atypia, and early carcinoma. This progression is neither uniform nor invariant, for only about 10% of women with adenomatous hyperplasia progress to frank cancer. Obesity, hypertension, diabetes, nulliparity and infertility, menstrual irregularities, cirrhosis, tamoxifen citrate use, late menopause or early menarche, and unopposed estrogen stimulation have all been implicated as risk factors for endometrial cancer. Although these factors increase a woman's risk of endometrial cancer by factors that vary from four- to eightfold, the incidence of cancer in these women is still sufficiently low that large scale screening is not practical. Fortunately, a high percentage of women with endometrial malignancies or premalignant conditions experience intermenstrual bleeding, suggesting their presence. In these patients, the application of diagnostic techniques such as endometrial suction biopsy or focused transvaginal ultrasonography will often suggest or establish the diagnosis.

Office endometrial suction biopsy has greatly simplified the process of histologic sampling relegated in the past to dilatation and curettage. A number of sampling devices are available and have been shown to provide reliable tissue diagnosis in 90% to 100% of cases. This office diagnostic technique is valuable in evaluating patients suspected of having endometrial cancer based on irregular perimenopausal or postmenopausal bleeding. This procedure is best suited for diagnosis, not screening, because it is associated with some discomfort, a small but not insignificant risk of perforation or infections, and carries the cost of both the procedure and the histologic diagnosis.

Pretreatment, follow-up, or periodic endometrial sampling for women taking estrogen replacement is not indicated. Similarly, routine sampling of climacteric women with no menstrual abnormality cannot be recommended. Indications for diagnostic endometrial sampling are discussed in Chapter 12, Menopause.

Ultrasonography, especially transvaginal imaging and Doppler flow studies, has been proposed as a screening modality for endometrial cancer. Most of the studies to date indicate a high degree of dependence on the expertise of the person performing the study and a poor degree of correlation with the pathology found. As technology evolves, this may prove to be a useful diagnostic tool; for the moment, its utility in diagnosis is debated and it has no place as a screening tool.

Ovarian Cancer

Ovarian cancer is the fourth most common cause of cancer deaths in women and carries a 5-year survival rate of only 40% (all stages). Seventy percent of patients have International Federation of Gynecology and Obstetrics (FIGO) stage III or IV at the time of diagnosis. These patients have only a 15% to 20% 5-year survival.

Despite the desirability of having a screening test to identify early ovarian cancer, by its nature ovarian cancer is not well suited to mass screening: Its incidence is low (13–15/100,000 women) as is the life-time risk (1 in 70); it has an uncertain pathogenesis; a number of distinct histologic cancers are grouped under the heading of "ovarian cancer;" and many nonmalignant conditions may mimic early cancers, resulting in unacceptable levels of false-positive examinations.

Pelvic examination is the most widespread method for ovarian cancer detection despite a lack of studies documenting its efficacy and concerns about its poor sensitivity. Ultrasonography, computed tomography (CT), magnetic resonance imaging (MRI), radioimmunoscintography, and positron-emission tomography (PET) scanning are all more precise diagnostic tests; however, expense, limited availability, and the high level of expertise required for performance and interpretation make them unsuitable for mass screening. Transvaginal ultrasonography has been proposed for screening because it is the least expensive of these and carries a high specificity (up to 97.7%). The low incidence of ovarian cancer in the general population means that a positive ultrasound finding is 50 times more likely due to benign disease than it is to cancer. Doppler imaging of adnexal vascular flow is an emerging diagnostic examination, but does not lend itself to mass screening. False-positive ultrasound and Doppler tests lead to unnecessary anguish, expense, and risk as more invasive modalities are used to establish a diagnosis.

A number of proteins and cell-surface antigens associated with ovarian cancer may now be detected. Biochemical markers such as CA-125 are useful for monitoring the response of some ovarian cancers to therapy or to detect early recurrences. Most of these markers are not unique to ovarian cancer and even the most extensively studied and widely used (CA-125) is elevated in 80% of cancer cases and in less than 50% of those with early disease. Benign conditions such as endometriosis, pelvic inflammatory disease, pregnancy, and uterine fibroids are all associated with elevated levels of this marker. A number of national laboratories now market screening panels that include several biochemical markers, which are combined in an effort to improve specificity. These may include combinations of CA-125, lipid-associated sialic acid (LASA), carcinoembryonic antigen (CEA), TAG-72, CA15–3, or OVX1. Because of a lack of controlled studies of these panels as screening tools, use should limited to those familiar with their limitations and applied only to patients suspected of, or confirmed to have, a malignancy.

A careful family history may suggest patients who are at higher risk for developing an ovarian neoplasm, and for whom some form of screening may be cost effective. Several familial cancer syndromes exist (Table 10.3) that are associated with risks of cancer as high as 82% by age 70. Regrettably, 95% of cases of ovarian cancer are sporadic and carry no identifiable pattern of risk. Unless a specific familial cancer syndrome is identified, patients with relatives diagnosed with ovarian cancer should only undergo increased surveillance. Prophylactic oophorectomy has been advocated, but is probably not warranted except for those with familial syndromes, and even then reservations about effectiveness persist.

Less Common Cancers

Cancers of the vulva, vagina, Bartholin's, or Skene's glands are relatively rare. These cancers account for less than 5000 combined cases annually in the United States, with vulvar cancer far and away the most common. The best and only screening available for these lesions are genital self-examination and careful physical examination. Itching, irritation, cracking, or bleeding of the vulva may be present in vulvar cancer or premalignant lesions and should increase clinical suspicion of its presence. Early skin changes can be overlooked if careful inspection is not made a part of the clinician's routine pelvic examination.

Patients who were exposed to diethylstilbestrol (DES) while in utero are at increased risk for vaginal adenosis or cancer. These women should have cytologic samples obtained from the upper two thirds of the vaginal canal at the time of cervical Pap smear. The samples should be taken from the entire circumference of the vaginal barrel. Serial colposcopic

Table 10.3. Syndromes Associated with Ovarian Neoplasia

Syndrome	Associated Ovarian Neoplasm
Gonadal dysgenesis	Gonadoblastoma, dysgerminoma
Hereditary breast/ovarian cancer syndrome	Breast and epithelial ovarian cancer
Hereditary site-specific ovarian cancer	Epithelial ovarian cancer
Lynch II (hereditary nonpolyposis colorectal cancer)	Colorectal, endometrial, breast, and epithelial ovarian cancer
Multiple nevoid basal cell carcinoma	Ovarian fibroma
Peutz-Jeghers syndrome	Granulosa theca cell tumor

examinations for these patients have been advocated, although many now feel that after two or three normal examinations periodic Pap smears may suffice. For many patients, this decision will be made as much by their level of comfort or concern as it is by true medical risk.

Nongynecologic Cancer

Lung Cancer

The American Cancer Society estimates that 73,900 new cases of lung cancer will have occurred in women during the course of 1995. While the incidence of lung cancer has declined for men, it is steadily increasing for women. Most authors agree that almost 90% of these cancers are attributable to active or passive smoking. Lung cancer does not produce symptoms until well advanced, making early detection desirable. Unfortunately, no cost-effective mass screening is currently available. Studies indicate that lung cancer screening by chest x-ray study and sputum cytology is not effective in reducing cancer mortality. Clearly, any patient who smokes should be counseled about the risks and aggressive evaluation carried out of any symptoms that might present. Routine chest x-ray study is not cost effective in the absence of other indications.

Gastrointestinal Tract Cancer

Colorectal cancer is the third most common cancer in the United States. The American Cancer Society estimates for 1995 predicted that 51,000 new cases would occur to women in the United States. Mortality rates for this cancer have changed little in the past 40 years, although a slight decline for women may be occurring. Although about 90% of colorectal cancers occur after the age of 50, approximately 8% of cases are found before the age of 40. Bowel cancer is notable for its absence of specific symptoms or signs that correlate with the presence or stage of the disease. Only late in the disease are symptoms of obstruction, tenesmus, or narrowing of the stool found. Rectal bleeding, either microscopic or gross bleeding, is often the first sign of a tumor, but it is not always associated with early lesions. Left-sided lesions are more likely to be associated with bright rectal bleeding, whereas right-sided lesions often have occult bleeding due to mixing of the blood with the fecal stream. Large-scale screening for colon tumors is based on detecting this fecal bleeding.

The risk of colon or rectal cancer increases with age, low-fiber and high-fat diets, sedentary lifestyle, obesity, and increased alcohol consumption. A family history of adenomatous polyps or colorectal cancer is also associated with an increased risk. A genetic marker associated with colon cancer has recently been identified, but it will not play a significant role in screening because it is present in only about 1% of colon cancer patients.

Other Cancers

The American Cancer Society currently recommends that asymptomatic low-risk women undergo examinations directed toward the detection of thyroid, mouth, skin, and lymph node cancer every 3 years. In addition to these examinations, education about cancer-related behaviors (e.g., smoking and diet), as well as the merits of cancer self-examination, should be a part of all routine encounters.

CLINICAL IMPLEMENTATION

Although not all malignancies can be effectively screened for, it is incumbent on those who care for women to encourage regular participation in the screening programs that are available (Table 10.4). No screening test will have an impact if it is not used effectively. Education, provided in the office or to lay and profession groups, is often pivotal to gaining participation. The need for this encouragement may be seen in data reflecting the use of current Pap smear and mammography programs (Table 10.5). In one study, almost one quarter of women reported that they did not receive preventive services because their physician never suggested it or discussed it with them. Clearly, such counseling and information should be a priority.

Gynecologic Screening

One quarter of all breast cancers are found during routine examination. Therefore, a careful breast examination should be a part of every general examination of women after the age of puberty. While American Cancer Society guidelines suggest that this may be performed every 3 years up to age 40, it is a test involving minimal time, little or no morbidity, and no added expense to a general examination. Clinical breast examination provides an opportunity to discuss the value of breast self-examination (BSE), reinforce the value and timing of mammography, and identify breast health as a topic of importance and open communication. For these reasons, there is little reason not to recommend breast examination as a part of more frequent examinations.

All patients should be questioned about breast self-examination and encouraged to perform it on a monthly basis. Monthly breast self-examination should be begun by age 18 and continue throughout the woman's lifetime. It should be noted that despite widespread popular support for breast self-examination, it has not been shown to be an effective screening technique for early breast cancer. Consensus groups, including the Canadian

Table 10.4. Summary of Cancer Screening Recommendations for Asymptomatic Women*

Test	Age	Periodicity
Sigmoidoscopy	>50	3 to 5 y
Occult stool blood	>40	Yearly
Rectal examination	>40 (many suggest should be part of all pelvic examinations)	Yearly
Pap/pelvic	>18	Yearly
Breast self-examination	>20	Monthly
Clinical breast examination	20–39	3 y
	≥40	Yearly
Mammography	35–39	Baseline
	40–49	1 to 2 y
	≥50	yearly

*Based on American Cancer Society Guidelines. Holleb AI, Fink DJ, Murphy GP. American Cancer Society Textbook of Clinical Oncology. Atlanta, Georgia: The American Cancer Society, Inc, 1991.

Table 10.5. Participation in Cancer Screening Programs

Race	Pap test*		Mammography†	
	Never heard of test (%)	Heard of but never had test (%)	Never heard of test (%)	Heard of but never had test (%)
All races	4	7	16	48
Whites	2	7	12	49
Blacks	4	8	29	41
Hispanics	15	10	32	42

*Percent of women age 18 and over.
†Percent of women age 40 and over.
Source: National Health Interview Survey, National Center for Health Statistics, 1987. Statistical Bulletin of Metlife 1991;72:17.

Task Force and the U.S. Preventive Service Task Force have not endorsed its use. As noted in Chapter 14 (Breast Disease), a lack of cost, the evaluation of benign disease, and other benefits make breast self-examination still worthy of recommendation.

Vulvar self-examination is often overlooked as a valuable screening modality. The infrequent occurrence of malignant disease make this an ineffective cancer screening test but, as with breast self-examination, other benefits can be sufficient to advocate practicing this simple test.

Routine cervical Pap smears should be begun once a woman become sexually active or reaches the age of 18. The optimal frequency of cervical cytologic screening has been strongly debated in the recent past. Organizations like the American Cancer Society have proposed that low-risk women, who have had two or more negative (annual) studies, may reduce their rate of Pap smears to every 3 years. Other groups, such as The American College of Obstetricians and Gynecologists, suggest that annual examinations should continue for most patients. This is based on the poor predictive value of risk factors and the role of the Pap smear as only a part of other health maintenance and prevention aspects of the annual examination. In addition, some studies have shown an almost fourfold increase in the risk of cervical cancer in women whose Pap smear interval exceeds 3 years. All groups agree that patients who are at increased risk for cervical abnormalities should be screened annually or more often. Factors that make a woman at high risk for change are shown in Table 10.6. Whatever frequency is chosen for a particular patient, Pap smear screening programs will be most successful if at least two sequentially negative tests are obtained before an assumption of normality is made.

Less clear is the optimal role of cytologic smears in women who have had a hysterectomy. If the hysterectomy was performed for malignant or invasive disease, Pap smears from the vaginal vault should be obtained every 3 to 4 months for a year, and then every 6 months for an additional 2 to 3 years. Annual smears should then be considered. Patients who have hysterectomies for benign disease should still be monitored for vaginal abnormalities but the frequency of cytologic smears may be reduced to every 2 to 5 years. Remember that one of the most important aspects of the annual pelvic examination is the assessment of the adenexa. Therefore, for patients who still have one or both ovaries, annual examinations should still be encouraged even if no cytologic examination is performed.

Table 10.6. Factors that Increase the Risk of Cervical Abnormalities

Cigarette smoking (including passive smoking)
Early age of first intercourse
Human immunodeficiency virus (HIV) infections
Human papillomavirus (HPV) infection
In utero exposure to diethylstilbestrol (DES)?
Multiple sexual partners

Despite the diagnostic promise of combined panels of biochemical markers for ovarian cancer, a meta-analysis of published studies estimated that the use of CA-125 and ultrasonography would detect 1 cancer (stage I) for every 2153 women tested. If this were applied to all women over the age of 45, it has been estimated that 20,000 new cases could be found, but at a cost of roughly $700,000 per case. Until prospective, randomized trials are available, the use of currently available tests and modalities for the detection of early ovarian cancer remains investigational and should not be used for routine clinical screening of low-risk women.

Nongynecologic Screening

Colon cancer detection is based on the triad of rectal examination, stool blood test, and sigmoidoscopy. Screening for colon cancer by rectovaginal examination and modified guaiac test should be a part of routine care of all women over the age of 40. Before this age, the high occurrence of false-positive guaiac tests makes routine screening (without specific suspicion) impractical. After the age of 40, the false-positive rate is roughly 5% to 6%, but the false-negative rate may be as high as 50%. For this reason, any patient deemed to be at higher risk should undergo multiple stool sampling while on a meat-free diet. Other precautions recommended by the American Cancer Society prior to stool sampling are shown in Table 10.7. Positive tests require follow-up by radiologic imaging (barium enema or air contrast studies) and flexible sigmoidoscopy. Current recommendations for low-risk women over the age of 50 include flexible sigmoidoscopy every 3 to 5 years regardless of the results of rectovaginal and guaiac testing.

Nongynecologic cancers should be considered and tested for above and beyond normal screening when subtle symptoms suggest a higher risk. Symptoms of anemia, malaise, or vague abdominal complaints should suggest the possibility of a gastrointestinal process. Chronic cough, hoarseness, or shortness of breath in a tobacco user should prompt a consideration of pulmonary neoplasia. A skin lesion that fails to heal, or undergoes change, should provoke consideration of dermatologic malignancy.

A time-line summary of recommended cancer screening tests based on the patient's age is shown in Figure 10.2.

HINTS AND COMMON QUESTIONS

Small amounts of blood on a Pap smear, such as that caused by endocervical sampling, should cause no problems with the interpretation of the sample.

Table 10.7. American Cancer Society Dietary Preparations for Stool Blood Testing*

Do not take vitamin C supplements
Do not take oral iron supplements
Do not take multivitamins with vitamin C or iron
Avoid foods with high peroxidase activity (broccoli, turnips, cantaloupes, radishes, horseradish, parsnips)
Do not eat red meat—fish or poultry are acceptable
Do not take aspirin or nonsteroidal anti-inflammatory medications
(Increase dietary fiber—value unproved)

*To be implemented 48 h prior to first stool sample and continued until last sample is obtained.
After: Holleb Al, Fink DJ, Murphy GP. American Cancer Society Textbook of Clinical Oncology. Atlanta, Georgia: The American Cancer Society, Inc, 1991.

Unless great concerns for a cervical abnormality are present, patients with vaginitis should be treated prior to cytologic sampling. A healing period of 3 to 6 weeks is usually sufficient for the inflammatory changes engendered by the vaginitis to abate.

Pregnant patients should be warned that endocervical sampling often causes a small amount of "spotting" or "staining," which is not a cause for alarm. Failing to provide this information can result in unnecessary anguish and late-night telephone calls.

To increase the sensitivity of guaiac testing for fecal blood, three or more stool samples should be tested. This is best carried out after 48 to 72 hours of a high-residue, low-meat diet.

If mail-in guaiac test cards are used, test development more than 4 days after the specimen is applied to the card is associated with an increased false-negative rate. If delivery to the office or laboratory in under this time is unlikely, consideration should be given to teaching the patient to develop the test herself or limiting the test to office visits.

False-positive stool guaiac tests may occur owing to bleeding from hemorrhoids, dietary red meat, or inflammatory disease of the bowel. Although the standard recommendations advocate a meat-free diet for 3 days before the test, for most patients this is unnecessary, but the possibility of a false-positive must be borne in mind.

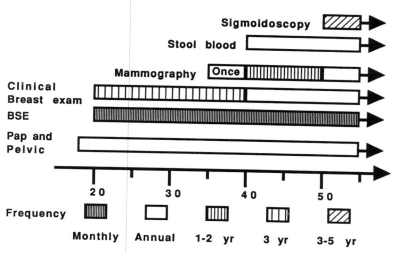

Figure 10.2. Recommended Cancer Screening by Age

SUGGESTED READINGS

General References

American Cancer Society. Cancer facts and figures—1994. Atlanta: ACS, 1994.

Broder S. Rapid communication—the Bethesda System for reporting cervical/vaginal cytological diagnoses—report of the 1991 Bethesda Workshop. JAMA 1992;267:1892.

Campion MJ, Reid R. Screening for gynecologic cancer. Obstet Gynecol Clin North Am 1990;17:695.

Canadian Task Force. Cervical cancer screening programs. I. Epidemiology and natural history of carcinoma of the cervix, 1976. Can Med Assoc J 1976;114:1003.

The Commonwealth Fund. The Commonwealth Fund survey of women's health. New York: The Commonwealth Fund, 1993.

Grimes DA, Economy KE. Primary prevention of gynecologic cancers. Am J Obstet Gynecol 1995;172:227.

Holleb AI, Fink DJ, Murphy GP. American Cancer Society Textbook of Clinical Oncology. Atlanta: The American Cancer Society, Inc, 1991.

Horton JA. The Women's Health Data Book, 2nd ed. Washington, D.C.: The Jacobs Institute of Women's Health, 1995.

Kurman RJ, Malkasian GD JR, Sedlis A, Solomon D. From Papanicolaou to Bethesda: the rational for a new cervical cytologic classification. Obstet Gynecol 1991;77:779.

Kurman RJ, Solomon D. The Bethesda System for Reporting Cervical/Vaginal Cytologic Diagnoses: Definitions, Criteria and Explanatory Notes for Terminology and Specimen Adequacy. New York: Springer-Verlag, 1994.

Lawhead RA JR. Vulvar self-examination: What your patient should know. The Female Patient 1990;15:33.

Miller AB, Anderson G, Brisson J, et al. Report of a national workshop on screening for cancer of the cervix. Can Med Assoc J 1991;145(suppl):1301.

National Cancer Institute Workshop. The 1988 Bethesda system for reporting cervical/vaginal cytological diagnoses. JAMA 1989;262:931.

National Cancer Institute Workshop. National Health Interview Survey Supplement on Cancer Control. Bethesda, MD: National Center for Health Statistics, 1989.

U.S. Preventive Services Task Force. Guide to clinical preventive services: An assessment of the effectiveness of 169 interventions. Baltimore: Williams & Wilkins, 1989.

Wilson JMG, Jungner G. Principles and practice of screening for disease. Public Health Paper No. 34. Geneva: World Health Organization, 1968.

Wingo PA, Tong T, Bolden S. Cancer statistics 1995. CA Cancer J Clin 1995;45:8.

Specific References

Breast Cancer

Eddy DM. Screening for breast cancer. Ann Intern Med 1989;111:389.

Eddy DM, Hasselblad V, McGivney W, et al. The value of mammography screening in women under age 50 years. JAMA 1988;259:1512.

Fletcher SW, Black W, Harris R, Rimer BK, Shapiro S. Report of the International Workshop on screening for breast cancer. Bethesda, MD: National Cancer Institute, 1993.

Foster RS, Costanza MC. Breast self-examination practices and breast cancer survival. Cancer 1984;53:999.

Freig SA. Decreased breast cancer mortality through mammography screening: results of clinical trials. Radiology 1988;167:659.

Medical News and Perspectives: Breast cancer screening guidelines agreed on by AMA, other medically related organizations. JAMA 1989;262:1155.

Moskowitz M. Predictive value, sensitivity, and specificity in breast cancer screening. Radiology 1988;167:576.

Smart CR. The role of mammography in the prevention of mortality from breast cancer. Cancer Prevention 1990;June:1.

Cervical Cancer

Ayre JE. Selective cytology smear for diagnosis of cancer. Am J Obstet Gynecol 1947;53:609.

Babes A. Diagnostique du cancer utérine pâr les frottis. Presse Med 1928;36:451.

Beilby JOW, Bourne R, Guillebaud J, et al. Paired cervical smears: a method of reducing the false-negative rate in population screening. Obstet Gynecol 1982;60:46.

Brinton LA, Hamman RF, Huggins GH, et al. Sexual and reproductive risk factors for invasive squamous cell cervical cancer. J Natl Cancer Inst 1987;79:23.

Douglass LE. A further comment on the contributions of Aurel Babes to cytology and pathology. Acta Cytol 1967;11:217.

Eddy DM. Screening for cervical cancer. Ann Intern Med 1990;113:214.

Hellberg D, Nilsson S, Haley NJ, Hoffman D, Wynder E. Smoking and cervical intraepithelial neoplasia: nicotine and cotinine in serum and cervical mucus in smokers and nonsmokers. Am J Obstet Gynecol 1988;158:910.

Herbst AL. The Bethesda System for cervical/vaginal cytologic diagnoses. Clin Obstet Gynecol 1992;35:22.

International Agency for Research on Cancer Working Group on Evaluation of Cervical Cancer Screening Programmes: Screening for squamous cervical cancer. Duration of low risk after negative results of cervical cytology and its implication for screening policies. BMJ 1986;293:659.

Johannesson G, Geirsson G, Day N. The effect of mass screening in Iceland, 1965–1974, on the incidence of mortality of cervical carcinoma. Int J Cancer 1978;21:418.

Kirk S, Chu J, Mandelson M, Greer B, Figge D. Papanicolaou smear screening interval and risk of cervical cancer. Obstet Gynecol 1989;74:838.

Koss LG. The Papanicolaou test for cervical cancer detection. A triumph and a tragedy. JAMA 1989;261:737.

Orr JW JR, Barrett JM, Orr PF, Holloway RW, Holimon JL. The efficacy and safety of the cytobruch during pregnancy. Obstet Gynecol 1992;44:260.

Taylor PR JR, Andersen WA, Barber SR, Covell JL, Smith EB, Underwood PB JR. The screening Papanicolaou smear: Contribution of the endocervical brush. Obstet Gynecol 1987;70:734.

Weintraub NT, Nicoli E, Freedman ML. Cervical cancer screening in women age 65 and over. J Am Geriatr Soc 1987;35:870.

Winklesten W JR. Smoking and cervical cancer—current status: A review. Am J Epidemiol 1990;131:945.

Endometrial Cancer

Cramer DW, Knapp NC. Review of epidemiologic studies of endometrial cancer and exogenous estrogen. Obstet Gynecol 1979;54:521.

Goldstein SR. Use of ultrasonohysterography for triage of perimenopausal patients with unexplained uterine bleeding. Am J Obstet Gynecol 1994;170:565.

Holbert TR. Screening transvaginal ultrasonography of postmenopausal women in a private office setting. Am J Obstet Gynecol 1994;170:1699.

Kaunitz AM, Masciello A, Ostrowski M, Rovira EZ. Comparison of endometrial biopsy with the endometrial pipelle and Vabra aspirator. J Reprod Med 1988;33:428.

Koonings PP, Moyer DL, Grimes DA. A randomized clinical trial comparing Pipelle and Tis-u-trap for endometrial biopsy. Obstet Gynecol 1990;75:293.

Kurjak A, Shalan H, Sosic A, et al. Endometrial carcinoma in postmenopausal women: evaluation by transvaginal color Doppler ultrasonography. Am J Obstet Gynecol 1993;169:1597.

Nolan TE, Smith RP, Smith MT, Gallup DC. A prospective evaluation of an endometrial suction curette. J Gynecol Surg 1992;8:231.

Rubin GL, Peterson HB, Lee NC, Maes EF, Wingo FA, Becker S. Estrogen replacement therapy and the risk of endometrial cancer: remaining controversies. Am J Obstet Gynecol 1990;162:148.

Sladkevicius P, Valentin L, Marsal K. Endometrial thickness and Doppler velocimetry of the uterine arteries as discriminators of endometrial status in women with postmenopausal bleeding: a comparative study. Am J Obstet Gynecol 1994;171:722.

Stovall TG, Ling FW, Morgan PL. Prospective, randomized comparison of the Pipelle endometrial sampling device with the Novak curette. Am J Obstet Gynecol 1991;165:1287.

Ovarian Cancer

Andolf E. Ultrasound screening in women at risk for ovarian cancer. Clin Obstet Gynecol 1993;36:423.

Barber H. Prophylaxis in ovarina cancer. Cancer 1993;71:1529.

Boente MP, Godwin AK, Hogan WM. Screening, imaging and early diagnosis of ovarian cancer. Clin Obstet Gynecol 1994;37:377.

Bourne T, Campbell S, Steer C, Whitehead M, Collins W. Transvaginal colour flow imaging: a possible new screening technique for ovarian cancer. BMJ 1989;299:1367.

Campbell S, Bhan V, Royston P, Whitehead MI, Collins WP. Transabdominal ultrasound screening for early ovarian cancer. BMJ 1989;299:1363.

Creasman WT, DiSaia PJ. Screening in ovarian cancer. Am J Obstet Gynecol 1991;165:7.

DePriest PD, Shenson D, Fried A, et al. A morphology index based on sonographic findings in ovarian cancer. Gynecol Oncol 1993;51:7.

Einhorn N, Sjövall K, Knapp RC, et al. Prospective evaluation of serum CA 125 levels for the early detection of ovarian cancer. Obstet Gynecol 1992;80:14.

Herbst AL. The epidemiology of ovarian carcinoma and the current status of tumor markers to detect disease. Am J Obstet Gynecol 1994;170:1099.

Holbert TR. Screening transvaginal ultrasonography of postmenopausal women in a private office setting. Am J Obstet Gynecol 1994;170:1699; discussion 1703.

Jacobs I, Bast RC JR. The CA 125 tumour-associated antigen: A review of the literature. Hum Reprod 1989;4:1.

Jacobs I, Davies AP, Bridges J, et al. Prevalence screening for ovarian cancer in postmenopausal women by CA 125 measurement and ultrasonography. BMJ 1993;306:1030.

Jacobs IJ, Oram DH, Bast RC JR. Strategies for improving the specificity of screening for ovarian cancer with tumor-associated antigens CA 125, CA 15–3, and TAG 72.3. Obstet Gynecol 1992;80:396.

Jacobs I, Stabile I, Bridges J, et al. Multimodal approach to screening for ovarian cancer. Lancet 1988;1:268.

Kerlikowske K, Brown JS, Grady DG. Should women with familial ovarian cancer undergo prophylactic oophorectomy? Obstet Gynecol 1992;80:700.

NIH Consensus Development Panel on Ovarian Cancer. Ovarian cancer: Screening, treatment, and follow-up. JAMA 1995;273:491.

Piver M, Recio F. Issues in ovarian cancer screening. Contemporary Oncology 1992;2:26.

Rubin SC. Monoclonal antibodies in the management of ovarian cancer: a clinical perspective. Cancer 1993;71:1602.

Schwartz PE. The role of tumor markers in the preoperative diagnosis of ovarian cysts. Clin Obstet Gynecol 1993;36:384.

Teneriello MG, Park RC. Early detection of ovarian cancer. CA Cancer J Clin 1995;45:71.

Tobacman JK, Greene MH, Tucker MA, et al. Intra-abdominal carcinomatosis after prophylactic oophorectomy in ovarian-cancer-prone families. Lancet 1982;2:795.

Woolas RP, Xu F, Jacobs IJ, et al. Elevation of multiple serum markers in patients with stage I ovarian cancer. J Natl Cancer Inst 1993;85:1748.

Lung Cancer

Berlin NI, Buncher CR, Fontana RS, et al. The National Cancer Institute Cooperative Early Lung Cancer Detection Program: Results of the initial screen (prevalence): Early lung cancer detection: Introduction. Am Rev Respir Dis 1984;130:S45.

Centers for Disease Control. Trends in lung cancer incidence and mortality—United States, 1980–1987. MMWR 1990;39:875.

Eddy DM. Screening for lung cancer. Ann Intern Med 1989;111:232.

Melamed MR, Flehinger BJ, Zaman MB, et al. Detection of true pathologic stage I lung cancer in a screening program and the effect on survival. Cancer 1981;47:1182.

National Cancer Institute. SEER cancer statistics review 1973–90. Bethesda,MD: U.S. Department of Health and Human Services, 1993.

Risch HA, Howe GR, Jain M, Burch JD, Holowaty EJ, Miller AB. Are female smokers at higher risk for lung cancer than male smokers? Am J Epidemiol 1993;321:281.

Stitik FP, Tockman MS. Radiographic screening in the early detection of lung cancer. Radiol Clin North Am 1978;16:347.

Colorectal Cancer

Ahlquist DA, McGill DB, Schwartz S, et al. Fecal blood levels in health and disease: a study using Hemoquant. N Engl J Med 1985;312:1412.

American Cancer Society. Cancer of the colon and rectum: A summary of a public attitude survey. CA Cancer J Clin 1983;33:31.

DeCosse JJ, Tsioulias GJ, Jacobson JS. Colorectal cancer: detection, treatment and rehabilitation. CA Cancer J Clin 1994;44:27.

Eddy DM. Screening for colorectal cancer. Ann Intern Med 1990;111:373.

11

Periodic Testing and Health Maintenance

The care of women entails more than just the diagnosis and treatment of gynecologic problems. It must also address disease prevention, risk reduction, and promotion of beneficial activities or behaviors. The primary care setting is ideal for addressing these global concerns.

In many respects, the periodic testing and health maintenance strategies appropriate for women are little different from those for men. Despite their potential benefits, preventive services must be tailored to the needs of the individual and population served, to ensure that those benefits derived exceed the potential for harm. This harm may be in the form of physical risk, emotional stress, or economic costs. For these reasons, sometimes the most cost-effective impact we have on a patient's health is through counseling, augmented by carefully chosen testing.

In establishing programs of periodic testing and health maintenance, there are several areas that pose unique problems for women that should be addressed: weight and exercise, substance abuse (including alcohol and tobacco), prophylaxis and risk reduction (including immunizations that impact on reproductive function), and the emerging concerns about cardiovascular disease in women. Cancer is also a natural concern to patients and an important part of any screening program. It is of sufficient concern to warrant its separate coverage (see Chapter 10, Cancer Screening).

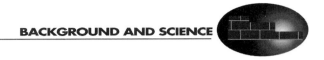

The purpose of screening is to use readily applied tests, examinations, or procedures to identify unrecognized disease at a stage when intervention can significantly alter the eventual outcome. Preventive medicine is based on the application of selective screening and the encouragement of healthy behaviors that reduce adverse health risk. These two goals demand a familiarity with the prevalence of both disease and risk (Table 11.1), as well as the tools available for screening and risk reduction. In addition, effective screening requires that several other conditions be met (Table 11.2). Based on these principles, it is possible to construct an effective plan for screening and risk reduction, which incorporates prophylaxis and counseling. An overview of screening strategies based on age is shown in Table 11.3. Although many screening and risk reduction programs applicable to women are sufficiently universal or obvious that little additional discussion is warranted, several areas of specific concern do deserve further discussion.

Screening and Counseling

Diet and Exercise

EATING DISORDERS AND OBESITY. Obesity is an American problem. With affluence and increased leisure time have come corpulence and inactivity. On the whole, two thirds of American women feel they have a weight problem, with almost 30% of women meeting objective criteria for obesity. Americans spend uncounted millions of dollars annually on diet and exercise programs to control weight, often with little or no success.

Table 11.1. Leading Causes of Death for Women in the United States, by Age

Cause of death	Age 12–18	19–39	40–64	>65
Motor vehicle accidents	√	√		
Homicide	√	√		
Suicide	√			
Leukemia	√			
Cardiovascular/coronary disease		√	√	√
Breast cancer		√	√	√
Obstructive lung disease		√	√	√
AIDS		√		
Uterine cancer		√		
Lung cancer			√	√
Stroke			√	√
Colorectal cancer			√	√
Ovarian cancer			√	
Falls/accidents				√
Pneumonia/influenza				√

After: Beckmann & Ling 2nd ed. table 1.2, p2.
(From Beckmann RB, Ling FW, Barzansky BM, et al. Obstetrics and gynecology. 2nd ed. Baltimore: Williams & Wilkins, 1995; p 2.)

Table 11.2. Criteria for Effective Screening

Characteristic	Attribute
Disease or condition	Must cause significant morbidity or mortality
	Prevalent enough to justify screening
Natural history	Asymptomatic period during which diagnosis is possible
	Early treatment superior to later intervention
Test	Specific and sensitive
	Clear endpoint
	Ease of application
	Reasonable cost
	Good patient acceptance
Patient	Sufficient life expectancy to warrant intervention
	Willing to undergo screening and possible treatment

Table 11.3. An Overview of Preventive Health Care for Women

Age	Recommended screening and care	Frequency
Newborn	Genital and breast examination	Once
Prepubertal (<12)	Height, weight, blood pressure, external genitalia, Tanner staging	Annual
Adolescent (12–17) (18 or sexually active)	Basic examination*, height, Tanner staging	Annual
	Basic examination, Pap smear	Annual
	Chlamydia screening if sexually active	As needed
	Total cholesterol (repeat in 6 mo if on oral contraceptives) consider triglycerides/lipids	Baseline
Reproductive (20–39)	Basic examination, Pap smear, dipstick urine test	Annual
	Sexually transmitted disease screening	As needed
	Visual acuity, tonometry, hearing check	1–5 y
	Total cholesterol, triglycerides/lipids	5 y
	Baseline mammography	Age 35
Climacteric (40–49)	Basic examination, Pap smear, fecal occult blood, dipstick urine test	Annual
	Sexually transmitted disease screening	As needed
	Mammography	Biannually
	Visual acuity, tonometry, hearing check	1–5 y
	Total cholesterol, triglycerides/lipids	5 y
	Thyroid-stimulating hormone baseline	Age 45
Menopausal (50–60)	Basic examination, Pap smear, fecal occult blood, mammography	Annual
	Sexually transmitted disease screening	As needed
	Visual acuity, tonometry, hearing check	1–5 y
	Total cholesterol, triglycerides/lipids, hematocrit	5 y
	Sigmoidoscopy	3–5 y
(>60)	Basic examination, Pap smear, fecal occult blood, mammography	Annual
	Thyroid-stimulating hormone	Biannual
	Visual acuity, tonometry, hearing check	1–5 y
	Sigmoidoscopy	3–5 y

*Basic examination: History update, weight, blood pressure, breast, abdomen, pelvic, and rectal examinations.

Obesity is associated with a number of health risks that make it an appropriate priority for periodic assessment and intervention. Obesity contributes directly to mortality; it also contributes indirectly through increased risks of hypertension, diabetes, coronary heart disease, hyperlipidemia, stroke, digestive disease, and cancer (Fig 11.1). Overweight patients are three times more likely to develop diabetes, hypertension, and uterine cancer. Patients who are 6 kg to 8 kg (15–20 lb) overweight are twice as likely to develop gallstones. This increases to a sixfold risk if the patient is 27 kg to 34 kg (50–75 lb) above ideal weight. Obese patients are more likely to have cardiovascular disease, respiratory problems, sleep apnea, circulatory complications, arthritis, and psychological problems. Some studies indicate that the cardiovascular risks of obesity are magnified in women. Clearly, assessment and intervention are warranted.

Although it is well established that our body composition changes with age (Fig 11.2) and that women have an age-related weight gain that is one third above that of men, this cannot be used as an excuse for frank obesity nor is this change in composition the same as excessive weight. The evaluation of obesity and the quantization of its risk is based on the body mass index. The body mass index (BMI) is calculated by the formula:

$$BMI = \text{Body weight (kg)}/\text{Height (m)}^2$$

$$\text{or}$$

$$BMI = \text{Body weight (lb)}/\text{Height (in)}^2 \times 703.1$$

This measure correlates well with other indexes of obesity. Based on life tables, the average BMI for women in the United States is 22.5 kg/m². For overweight patients, the degree of obesity can be established by comparing the patient's calculated BMI to standardized tables

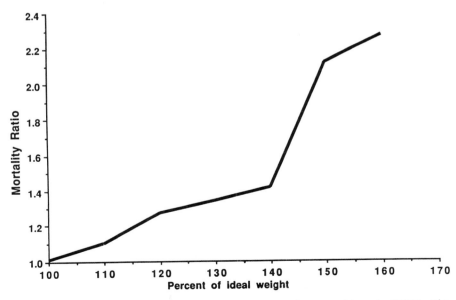

Figure 11.1. Effect of obesity on mortality. Based on data from: Build study 1979. Chicago: Society of Actuaries and Association of Life Insurance Medical Directors of America, 1980.

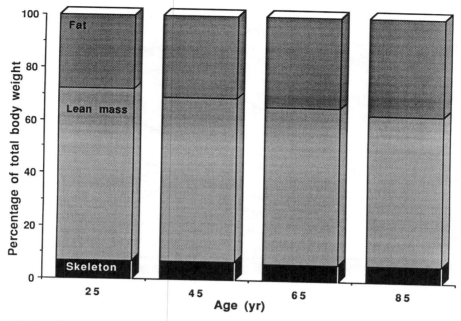

Figure 11.2. Change in body composition with age (60-kg woman). Proportion of body mass that is fat rises gradually with age.

or graphs (Fig 11.3). Measurement of skinfold thickness, in four locations, can also be used, but for most clinical situations it does not provide any more information than the more easily measured BMI. For research purposes, body fat can be estimated by inference from measures of total body water, calculation of body density by underwater weighing, or estimates of body potassium. These are neither practical nor necessary for routine clinical care.

At the opposite end of the spectrum of eating disorders lies anorexia nervosa and bulimia. In these two disorders there is a disturbed body image and morbid fear of obesity. Approximately 90% to 95% of all cases occur in young women, usually adolescents from middle to upper income families. These two conditions may vary from mild to life-threatening, with mortality rates of between 2% and 20% reported in the current literature. Both the etiology and true incidence remain unknown.

In anorexia the patient's appetite remains unchanged, but a preoccupation with food results in obsessive-compulsive behaviors. This preoccupation persists even in the face of cachexia. Binge eating, followed by induced vomiting, purgatives, or diuretic use, is found in 50% of anorectics. Amenorrhea is universal, with loss of libido, hirsutism, bradycardia, and hypotension common. The patients tend to be depressed and are manipulative. They often hide or conceal their behaviors, including their induced vomiting.

Bulimia is now recognized as a separate disorder. It is characterized by episodic binge-purge eating patterns that occur at least twice a week over a 3-month period. Unlike anorectics, bulimia patients do not become emaciated, but rather fluctuate 10% to 15% above and below their normal weight. Episodes of bulimia are often precipitated by psychological or social stress. Bulimic patients tend to have more awareness of their condition, even though they persist in their behavior.

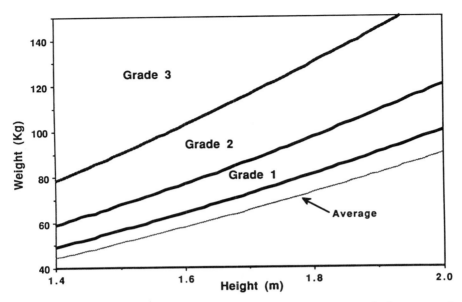

Figure 11.3. Obesity grading based on height and weight. Degree of obesity can be defined based on body mass index (BMI). Grade 1: BMI of 25–29.9; Grade 2: BMI of 30–40; Grade 3: BMI of > 40.

EXERCISE. Exercise is an important supplement to weight reduction programs, active management of diabetes, cardiac hardening and rehabilitation, achieving improved strength and flexibility, and enhancing general fitness and well-being. Reduced bone loss, alterations in lipid profile, and a reduced rate of cardiovascular disease also derive from regular exercise. Any program of primary care for women must include prescriptions for exercise as a part of periodic testing and health maintenance.

Weight-bearing or resistance-based exercise programs have been shown to have a beneficial effect on bone mass. This change appears to be independent of calcium intake or estrogen status. This benefit does not accrue unless sufficient stress is placed on the bones by the actions of gravity or large muscle groups. Walking or swimming does not provide sufficient force to significantly influence bone health, whereas impact aerobics and resistance training does result in increased bone mass. Moderation and the consequences of other medical conditions such as cardiovascular disease or arthritis are better guides in determining the place of exercise in the care of perimenopausal and menopausal women. For many, a program that provides well-rounded exercise, such as swimming, may result in greater overall benefits than one aimed at only bone health.

Exercise can have adverse menstrual and reproductive impact. This is almost always associated with extremes of activity, such as Olympic athletes, elite runners, and competitive sports figures. Delayed menarche, irregular menstrual periods, amenorrhea, dysmenorrhea, and infertility are more prevalent in this group. The mechanism by which this occurs remains uncertain; most, if not all, reproductive changes related to exercise will reverse if the level of activity is reduced.

THE IMPACT OF PREGNANCY. Exercise during pregnancy and the postnatal period presents special concerns. The physiologic changes brought about by pregnancy and the postnatal state, as well as the needs of the individual, must be considered when exercise is prescribed. During pregnancy there is an increased laxity of connective tissue, placing pregnant women at greater risk for strains and sprains. The enlarging uterus and increased breast mass contribute to the change in the body's center of gravity. (This is what causes the back-leaning, lordotic 'duck waddle' of late pregnancy.) This can result in balance problems and increased strain in the lumbosacral area and hips, resulting in possible injury.

During pregnancy, maternal blood volume is increased by approximately 30%; there is a drop in hematocrit and a rise in heart rate and cardiac output. These changes persist for 3 to 4 weeks after delivery and result in reduced cardiac reserve, which must be considered when calculating target heart rates for activities. In general, target heart rates for pregnant women should be set 25% to 30% lower than would otherwise be appropriate.

Substance Abuse

Alcohol and tobacco use are ubiquitous in our society. In 1990, $136 billion was spent on alcohol-related health problems. Nearly two thirds of Americans over the age of 14 drink alcoholic beverages. Cigarette smoking has been labeled as the largest preventable public health hazard in the United States. It has been estimated that one sixth of all deaths in the United States (almost 400,000 deaths per year) can be directly or indirectly attributed to cigarette and tobacco use. As primary care providers, we cannot ignore health risks of this magnitude and must make questions about alcohol and tobacco use a part of periodic testing and health maintenance.

ALCOHOL. Consumption of alcoholic beverages in the United States is almost universal. Per capita annual consumption is equal to 9.7 gallons of whiskey, 89 gallons of beer, or 31 gallons of wine. Half of all the alcohol consumption is by only 10% of drinkers (about 7% of the overall adult population). It is also this group of heavy or abusive drinkers that account for nearly all of the social and medical complications of alcohol use. It has been estimated that the prevalence of alcohol-related problems among hospitalized patients may be as high as 25%. In 1990, two thirds of women of childbearing age reported being current drinkers. Of this group, 5% to 9% reported consuming two or more drinks per day, with approximately one third of all women continuing some level of alcohol consumption during pregnancy. Some authors estimate that 7% to 10% of women seeking prenatal care are alcohol abusers.

Although we often presume that alcoholics are men, women are not immune to alcoholism, which occurs in 3.5% of all adult women. Alcohol has different effects for women than for men: In women, serum alcohol concentrations rise faster and higher following a given dose of alcohol, even when adjusted for body weight. Women are more prone to alcohol-related medical complications than are men. Women also suffer from unique alcohol-related effects, including reduced fertility, and increased rates of pregnancy complications, sexually transmitted diseases, and abuse.

Alcohol is rapidly absorbed from the stomach and small intestines and circulated within the body. Because there is no blood-brain barrier for alcohol, neurologic symptoms appear rapidly and can persist for long periods. These symptoms can be found with blood levels of 50–150 mg/dL, and are most noticeable when the levels are rising. Both short- and long-term tolerance develops rapidly, leading to progressively larger intakes of alcohol to obtain the same effects. Typical effects of alcohol are shown in Table 11.4.

For both men and women, alcohol has deleterious effects throughout the body, ranging from nutritional deficiencies such as reduced folate and thiamin to hepatic and cerebral damage. Women who abuse alcohol are prone to menstrual irregularities and amenorrhea, reduced fertility, and increased pregnancy losses. They also suffer the consequences of alcohol-associated problems such as depression, sexually transmitted diseases, abuse, and assault.

Alcohol is both a morphologic and behavioral teratogen, with an estimated 5,000 births per year affected by fetal alcohol syndrome. Fetal alcohol syndrome is a collections of recognized morphologic and behavioral sequellae that result from in utero exposure to chronic alcohol intake (Table 11.5). Alcohol use is the most commonly identifiable cause of mental retardation in the United States. Although fetal alcohol syndrome is usually seen in children of women who consume 3 oz or more of alcohol per day during pregnancy, there does not appear to be a threshold below which alcohol is completely safe. Lower levels of alcohol intake are associated with less severe manifestations, often referred to as fetal alcohol effects.

TOBACCO. Annual cigarette consumption has declined somewhat from its peak of 4336 cigarettes per capita in 1963 (the year before the Surgeon General's landmark report), but current rates still represent a dramatic increase from the 54 cigarettes per capita consumed in 1900. The rise in the popularity of smoking has been followed by an equally dramatic rise in the incidence of lung cancer deaths. Increased health awareness in general, a greater appreciation of the health risks of cigarettes specifically, and a growing social trend to restrict locations that permit smoking has resulted in a decline in cigarette use from the 1963 high. Despite this general trend, there are more than 50 million smokers in the United States. In 1990, 27% of white women between the ages of 18 and 44 still smoked. This number is up by 2% from just 5 years earlier. Roughly 1 million teenagers begin smoking each year. This number is important because roughly 90% of smokers begin smoking before the age of 20.

The onetime image of a macho-male smoker has given way to equality of the sexes and with it equality of health problems due to smoking. Roughly 26% of all American women

Table 11.4. Clinical Impact and Blood Ethanol Level

mg/dL	Sporadic drinker	Chronic drinker
50–100	Euphoria Gregariousness Incoordination	Minimal or no effect
100–200	Slurred speech Ataxia Drowsiness Nausea	Sobriety or incoordination Euphoria
200–300	Lethargy Combative Stuporous Incoherent speech Vomiting	Mild emotional/motor changes
300–400	Coma	Drowsiness
>500	Death	Lethargy, coma

Table 11.5. Characteristics Found in Fetal Alcohol Syndrome

Growth retardation (before and/or after birth)
Facial anomalies
    Absent or hypoplastic philtrum
    Broad, thin upper lip
    Epicanthic folds
    Flattened nasal bridge
    Low set, often unparallel ears
    Micrognathia
    Microphthalmia
    Retarded midfacial development
    Short nose
    Small palpebral fissures
Central nervous system anomalies
    Attention-deficit disorders
    Hyperactivity
    Mental retardation, varying degrees
    Microcephaly
Other
    Cardiac defects
    Genitourinary defects
    Limb defects
    Spinal defects (including spina bifida)

of reproductive age smoke, and about 35% of women between age 18 and 25 smoke. Somewhere between 19% and 30% of pregnant women continue to smoke during pregnancy.

It is well documented that smoking is associated with large increases in the risks of heart disease, lung cancer, and other cancers. Smoking contributes greatly to chronic lung disease, peptic ulcer, esophageal reflux, and bladder cancer. Smoking is associated with a less-favorable course in patients with Crohn's disease. Paradoxically, smoking cessation is associated with the onset or worsening of ulcerative colitis. The risk of smoking increases with the number of cigarettes smoked, depth of inhalation, and the duration of the smoking habit. There is evidence that these risks are magnified when smoking begins at an early age. Risks do return to roughly normal if a person can stop smoking for 10 years or longer.

Women who smoke have lower fertility rates, more frequent ovulatory dysfunction, earlier menopause, and increased rates of tubal pregnancy and spontaneous abortion. Once pregnancy is established, smokers have higher rates of pregnancy complications including premature rupture of the membranes, prematurity, and low birth weight infants.

Cardiovascular Disease and Hypertension

There is a growing awareness of the impact of cardiovascular disease on the overall health of women. It is often overlooked that more women die of heart disease every year than do men. Coronary heart disease accounts for 35% of deaths among women. As a part of periodic screening and health maintenance it is important to seek those factors that can influence or reduce a patient's risk of cardiac disease: smoking, physical inactivity, hypercholesterolemia, and hypertension.

Table 11.6. Classification of Hypertension

Diastolic blood pressure (mm Hg)

<85	Normal
85–90	High Normal
90–104	Mild hypertension
105–114	Moderate hypertension
>115	Severe hypertension

Systolic blood pressure (normal diastolic)

<140	Normal
140–159	Borderline
>160	Isolated systolic hypertension

Hypertension represents a significant risk factor for cardiovascular disease. The identification and treatment of patients with hypertension can significantly reduce the risk of long-term sequelae; therefore, the diagnosis and treatment of mild essential hypertension is an appropriate part of preventative health care. Approximately 60 million patients in the United States are affected by hypertension to some degree. Because there is a bias that hypertension and cardiovascular disease, in general, are the province of men, many women are not evaluated, counseled, or treated for hypertension. However, more women over the age of 50 are affected than men. Although not exclusively the province of older patients, 65% of hypertensive patients are between 65 and 74 years of age.

The strict definition of hypertension is a blood pressure of greater than 140/90 mm Hg on two separate occasions. Some extend this to require elevated pressures on three separate visits, with measures taken at least twice at each visit. Despite the clarity of the diagnosis, it is uncertain when intervention is warranted. Some suggest that diastolic pressures below 100 mm Hg require no therapy, whereas others suggest diastolic pressures above 85 mm HG may be grounds for therapeutic intervention. A generally agreed-on classification is shown in Table 11.6. This classification is unchanged by gender.

The role of hypercholesterolemia in women is less clear. Evidence has been found of a moderate relationship of risk in older women who are not receiving hormone replacement. Current guidelines suggest that screening should be limited to every 5 years except for women with known coronary heart disease or peripheral vascular disease, and for those with multiple risk factors such as age, diabetes, smoking, or a family history of premature coronary heart disease.

Sexually Transmitted Disease and HIV

There has been a new upsurge in the prevalence of sexually transmitted infections. In the last few years, there has been an increase of approximately 75% in the number of cases of syphilis reported, with steady or increased rates of gonococcal infections, herpes vulvitis, and other sexually transmitted diseases (STDs). With approximately 13 million cases of STD, excluding human immunodeficiency virus (HIV) infections, reported annually in the United States, it is clear that screening for STDs must be a part of periodic testing and health maintenance.

Although more than 85% of sexually transmitted infections occur to young people age 15 to 29, patients older and younger than this are not exempt from risk. Any sexually active women should be questioned about high-risk behaviors, number of partners, use of condoms, and the presence of symptoms that suggest elevated risk. Cervical, anal, and oropharyngeal cultures should be a part of every routine examination for high prevalence or high-risk groups.

Immunization and Prophylaxis

Immunization of girls and women follows the same guidelines as those for men and boys. Of particular importance are those diseases that carry reproductive significance: chiefly, measles, rubella, hepatitis B, and erythroblastosis fetalis. Women at special risk should also be considered for immunization against influenza or pneumococcal infections. Ideally, all women of reproductive age should be immune to measles, mumps, rubella, tetanus, diphtheria, and poliomyelitis through either natural infection or vaccination. A summary of general immunization considerations for women is shown in Table 11.7. Erythroblastosis fetalis prevention represents an unusual, but important example of passive immunization.

CLINICAL APPLICATION

Clinical application of the principles of screening and risk reduction must be done with responsibility toward the dual masters of responsible cost and patient advocacy. The clinician who provides primary care for women is in an ideal position to provide this balance.

Table 11.7. Recommended Immunizations for Adolescent and Adult Women

Immunization	Timing	Special considerations
Hepatitis B	Series of three: second at 1 month, third at 6 months	Intravenous drug users, recipients of blood products, health workers, contacts of hepatitis B patients, prostitutes, patients with multiple sexual partners in preceding 6 months
Influenza	Annually over age 65, Every 10 y	High risk: chronic disease, immunosuppression, cardiopulmonary disease, diabetes, hemoglobinopathies, renal disease
Measles, mumps, rubella (MMR)	Once Second immunization	Women lacking immunity Those unable to show proof of immunity
Pneumococcus	Every 10 y	High risk: chronic disease, immunosuppression, cardiopulmonary disease, diabetes, hemoglobinopathies, renal disease, alcoholism, cirrhosis, asplenia, Hodgkin's disease, multiple myeloma
Tetanus-diphtheria booster	Once, age 14 to 16 Every 10 y Booster	Initial immunization Periodic update Anytime risk occurs and uncertain of last booster

History

Clinical screening and health maintenance often begins with those aspects of the "routine" history and review of systems that are not directly related to the patient's presenting complaint. The early detection of disease is the essence of the review of systems performed by most clinicians. Areas of special inquiry should be based on increased risk. This increase may be based on changing patterns of disease due to age, behavior, genetics, population prevalence, or concomitant factors such as interrelated disease. Of special concern are those aspects of health care for women, such as reproductive function and unique risk, outlined earlier. Techniques for reviewing these factors is covered in Chapter 3, Secrets of the Gynecologic History and Physical Examination.

As a part of the routine interview, women should be questioned about their dietary and exercise routines. This is especially important for adolescents. These patients are more likely to exhibit behaviors that place them at risk. They are also forming patterns that will become life-long. A few moments spent detecting or modifying diet and exercise habits may be repaid in life-time benefits.

In a similar way, a review of sexual practices, immunization history, past screening, and risk reduction or health-promoting activities (e.g., smoking cessation, automobile seat-belt use, and breast self-examination) should be explored. Reviewing a patient's current medications, their use, and the patient's understanding of their action provides not only factual information, but may detect a potential problem before complications develop.

Although it would seem easy to spot the patient who is abusing alcohol or tobacco, it is often well hidden because of the stigma that is more and more placed on the use of these substances. When we realize that the greatest impact we can have with those patients who have not yet reached the extremes of use, some form of strategy for diagnosis is in order.

Alcohol

Detecting a pattern of alcohol abuse or dependence is not as simple as asking the amount of alcohol consumed per day or month (e.g., greater than 45 drinks per month or 5 per day). Although these amounts are indications of drinking problems, the diagnosis of true alcohol abuse requires evidence of craving, tolerance, and physical dependence (Table 11.8). To protect the health of our patients, we should also be seeking indications of alcohol misuse that fall short of abuse or dependency. Screening for alcohol-related problems may be based on intake measures, such as the Single Screening Question, the Ten Question Drinking History, or outcome measures, such as the NET, TWEAK, CAGE, TACE, or SMAST questionnaires. Examples of these questionnaires are shown in Tables 11.9 through 11.15. For complete information on the use and scoring of these tools, please consult the relevant references provided. Depression, anxiety, bipolar personality disorders, diabetes, gastritis, and solar skin damage may all mimic alcohol abuse and must be considered before a diagnosis is rendered.

Cigarettes

Unlike alcohol abuse, cigarette use and abuse are more likely to be accurately reported. To assess the risk from tobacco, the amount and duration of use is established. For cigarettes, this is expressed as the number of 'pack-years' (packs per day times years of use). The depth

Table 11.8. Criteria for Alcohol Abuse and Dependence

Abuse (at least 1)
    Use despite awareness of harm
    Recurrent hazardous use
    Symptoms >1 month or recurrence
Dependence (any three)
    Larger amounts or over a longer time than intended
    Persistent desire or failed attempts to quit
    Larger amount of time spent to obtain or recover from alcohol
    Intoxication or withdrawal that affects life obligations (school, work, family)
    Social changes to accommodate alcohol
    Continued use in face of adverse impact
    Tolerance leading to increased use
    Has experienced symptoms of withdrawal
    Use of alcohol to avoid withdrawal

Table 11.9. Intake-Based Screening Questionnaires for Alcohol Abuse

Single Screening Question
    Which describes your use?
        • drink regularly now (unchanged)
        • drink regularly now, but less
        • drink once in a while
        • have quit drinking
        • wasn't drinking (still not)

Table 11.10. Intake-Based Screening Questionnaires for Alcohol Abuse

Ten Question Drinking History
    For beer, wine, and liquor:
        How often?
        How much?
        Ever more?
    Any change in the past year?

Table 11.11. Outcome-Based Screening Questionnaires for Alcohol Abuse

The NET Questionnaire
    Do you consider yourself a **N**ormal drinker?
    Do you ever have an **E**ye-opener?
    How many drinks does it **T**ake to get high?

of inhalation, the age at which smoking began, and the presence of other risk factors all play a part in the medical impact of the smoking habit. Potentially just as dangerous is environmental exposure to cigarette smoke. It has been estimated that between 500 and 5000 cancer deaths a year are due to second-hand smoke exposure. (Some studies have found that wives of one-pack-per-day smokers have a twofold increase in their risk of lung can-

Table 11.12. Outcome-Based Screening Questionnaires for Alcohol Abuse

The "TWEAK" Test

Tolerance: How many drinks does it take to feel the first effects?

Have friends or relatives **W**orried or complained about your drinking?

Eye-opener: Do you sometimes take a drink in the morning when you first get up?

Amnesia: Are there times when you drink and can't remember afterward what you said or did?

Do you sometimes feel the need to **K**(c)ut down on your drinking?

Table 11.13. Outcome-Based Screening Questionnaires for Alcohol Abuse

The CAGE Questionnaire

Have you ever felt the need to **C**ut down on drinking? What was it like? Were you successful? Why did you decide to cut down?

Have you ever felt **A**nnoyed by criticism of your drinking? What caused the worry or concern? Do you ever get irritated by their worry? Have you ever limited what you drink to please someone?

Have you ever felt **G**uilty about your drinking, or about something you said or did while you were drinking? Have you ever been bothered by anything you said or did while you were drinking? Have you ever regretted anything that has happened while you were drinking?

Have you ever taken a morning "**E**ye-opener" drink? Have you ever felt shaky or tremulous after a night of heavy drinking? What did you do to relieve the shakiness? Have you ever had trouble getting back to sleep early in the morning after a night of heavy drinking?

Table 11.14. Outcome-Based Screening Questionnaires for Alcohol Abuse

The TACE Questionnaire

How many drinks does it take to make you feel "high"? (**T**olerance).

Have people **A**nnoyed you by criticizing your drinking?

Have you ever felt you ought to **C**ut down on your drinking?

Have you ever had a drink first thing in the morning to steady your nerves or to get rid of a hangover? (**E**ye-opener).

cer.) Questions that can help assess the degree of cigarette dependence are listed in Table 11.16.

Physical

In much the same way as the history, the physical examination itself is a screening test in that it seeks signs of covert, asymptomatic disease which may be manifest by physical findings. Area of focus specifically amenable to screening during a physical examination will be based on prevalence of disease, which in turn is most closely related to age. These areas are summarized in Table 11.3. It should be noted that not all authors agree about the utility of an annual physical examination. For example, the clinical breast examination and periodic evaluations of serum cholesterol have come under fire as routine screening tests.

Table 11.15. Outcome-Based Screening Questionnaires for Alcohol Abuse

The SMAST Questionnaire

Do you feel you are a normal drinker—that is, do you drink less than or as much as most other people?

Does your partner, a parent, or other close relative ever worry or complain about your drinking?

Do you ever feel guilty about your drinking?

Do friends or relatives think you are a normal drinker?

Are you able to stop drinking when you want to?

Have you ever attended a meeting of Alcoholics Anonymous?

Has drinking ever created problems between you and your partner, a parent, or other close relative?

Have you ever gotten in trouble at work because of drinking?

Have you ever neglected your obligations, your family, or your work for 2 days or more in a row because you were drinking?

Have you ever gone to anyone for help about your drinking?

Have you ever been in a hospital because of drinking?

Have you ever been arrested for drunken driving, driving while intoxicated, or driving under the influence of alcohol?

Have you ever been arrested, even for a few hours, because of other drunken behavior?

Table 11.16. Indications of Cigarette Addiction

1. Do you smoke your first cigarette within 30 minutes of waking up in the morning?
2. Do you smoke 20 cigarettes (one pack) or more each day?
3. At times when you can't smoke or haven't got any cigarettes, do you feel a craving for one?
4. Is it tough for you to keep from smoking for more than a few minutes?
5. When you are sick enough to stay in bed, do you still smoke?

Two or more "yes" answers may mean addiction

There is little doubt about the value of these examinations for high-risk individuals, but there is controversy about what constitutes high risk and what value may be derived from these tests for low-risk individuals.

Extremes of weight will be apparent on first meeting the patient. Assessments of the degree of variance from ideal weight are easily made and should prompt appropriate intervention. A record of the patient's weight should be made at most visits so that trends may be identified and progress toward goals tracked when necessary. Young patients who are 25% or more underweight should be suspected of having anorexia nervosa.

The value of routine blood pressure measurement has been well established. It is critical to recognize that hypertension is most often an asymptomatic condition. Headaches are not generally a sign of hypertension and only in the presence of vascular disease will symptoms such as angina, visual disturbances, vertigo, or fatigue be present. It is therefore incumbent on all practitioners to be vigilant. The need for early diagnosis and intervention is pointed out by life insurance studies, which indicate that if blood pressure is controlled to below 140/90, normal life expectancy may be maintained.

The assessment of hypertension begins with the initial screening. If the diastolic pressure is below 100 mm HG, and the systolic pressure is greater than 150 mm HG, re-evaluation in approximately 2 months is appropriate. Roughly one third of these patients will have spontaneous return to normal pressures. If the diastolic blood pressure is greater than 115 mm HG, secondary hypertension must be considered and a referral is appropriate. Patients with systolic blood pressure above 160 mm Hg and normal diastolic pressures deserve additional assessment and intervention. Physical examination in these patients is directed toward detecting signs of processes that could yield secondary hypertension. These include cushingoid changes, evidence of coarctation of the aorta, or vascular bruits. A funduscopic examination is appropriate to check for arterial narrowing, arterial-venous crossing defects, or for the presence of hemorrhages, exudates, or papilledema.

Laboratory

Screening laboratory studies should be limited to periodic assessments of cholesterol, triglycerides, lipids, and thyroid function. Other studies, including the common practice of office urinalysis or periodic assessment of hemoglobin, have not been proved to be cost-effective without clinical indications or suspicion.

Laboratory studies are of limited help in assessing alcohol use or abuse. A blood ethanol level of greater than 0.1 mg/mL on a random sample, greater than 0.15 mg/mL without signs of intoxication, or a level greater than 0.3 mg/mL at any time, are indications of abuse. Suggestive of abuse are elevated liver enzymes, bilirubin, amylase, or prothrombin times. Similarly, decreased blood urea nitrogen (BUN) or serum protein are suggestive, but not diagnostic.

Patients with mild essential hypertension should have an initial urinalysis for protein, blood, and glucose. They should have a baseline hemoglobin or hematocrit, an electrocardiogram, serum creatinine evaluation, or BUN, potassium, and fasting blood glucose level. Additional laboratory studies, including lipid screening, serum calcium, phosphate and uric acid values, chest roentgenogram, and others, should be based on the needs of the individual patient. Abnormalities in these latter areas warrant immediate consultation.

Imaging

The only imaging study that should be performed on a routine basis is mammography, and even this should be performed only on the basis of advancing age, as outlined in published guidelines, or in response to a specific clinical indication. Other imaging, such as chest x-rays for smokers, have not been proved to be cost-effective. Other forms of imaging, such as ultrasonography, color Doppler flow studies, computerized tomography, or bone density studies, should also be reserved for specifically indicated investigations.

Other Tests

Because of a rising incidence of tuberculosis, skin testing should be considered for anyone at increased risk because of occupation, living conditions, behavior patterns, or immunocompromise.

Immunization and Prophylaxis

Rubella vaccine is recommended for adults without a prior history of rubella, those not vaccined on or after the first birthday, or patients without laboratory evidence of immunity. Many authors suggest eliminating a history of rubella from this list because of its unreliability as a marker for immunity. A single dose of vaccine is 95% effective in providing immunity, although many patients will receive a second dose as part of the two-dose schedule of measles, mumps, rubella (MMR) vaccine. Because this is a live vaccine, it should not be given within 3 months before a planned pregnancy or to those who are pregnant, even though no adverse effects have been reported. For the same reason, yellow fever and polio vaccines should not be given during pregnancy unless there is substantial risk of disease.

Protection from Rh sensitization is based on passive immunity provided by the administration of Rh immune globulin. This should be given to all Rh-negative mothers prophylactically during the last trimester of pregnancy, following the birth of an Rh-positive infant, after procedures such as amniocentesis or chorionic villus sampling, or following a miscarriage or abortion.

Prophylaxis against influenza should be offered to any women who is at high risk. This should include women in the third trimester of pregnancy, the very young, those with chronic disease such as chronic heart or pulmonary disease, and those with immunosuppression (iatrogenic or otherwise). The most important group to offer immunization to is the elderly, because there is a rapid rise in the mortality rate as age increases (Fig 11.4). For those at high risk who contract influenza, therapy with amantadine (100 mg orally twice daily for adults) can reduce the duration of symptoms by about one third, but only if therapy is begun during the first 48 hours of an infection.

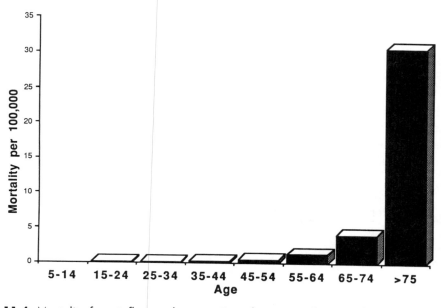

Figure 11.4. Mortality from influenza by age. Data from: Wiselka M. Influenza: Diagnosis, management and prophylaxis. BMJ 1994;308:1341.

Pneumococcal vaccine should be offered to older women and to those with chronic disease. This vaccine should be given once with a follow-up booster 6 or more years after the initial vaccination.

There is roughly a 5% lifetime risk of contracting hepatitis B, unless the patient is at increased risk owing to occupation or family situation. Hepatitis B vaccine is 85% to 90% effective in preventing clinical infection. Vaccination for those at increased risk, with a follow-up test of immunity, should be seriously considered. Many public health authorities are now advising routine hepatitis B vaccination for newborns and women in the third trimester of pregnancy. The cost-effectiveness of global vaccination of young adults is being evaluated and recommendations for routine prophylaxis may well be forthcoming.

The idea of chemoprophylaxis (the use of medications or other agents to reduce the risk of disease) has begun to enjoy wider acceptance. This has ranged from dietary calcium supplementation to support bone mass to low-dose aspirin therapy to reduce the risk of myocardial infarction. One of the most commonly used forms of prophylaxis is the protective effects gained through estrogen replacement therapy. It is estimated that in the United States, only 20% to 30% of eligible patients ever begin estrogen replacement therapy. Encouraging use, when appropriate, and maintaining compliance once therapy has begun are important parts of preventive medicine.

Counseling for Healthy Behaviors and Clinical Intervention

The general goal of any counseling program is to improve health by modifying behaviors to reduce risk or enhance benefits. This may take a general form (Table 11.17) or be adjusted to the circumstances of the patient.

Diet and Exercise

Weight reduction and good nutrition are generally a matter of common sense. While the genetics of obesity are being explored, it remains an immutable truth that weight will be lost as long as calories expended exceed calories consumed, with the rate of loss proportional to the magnitude of the difference. It does not matter which of the two caloric values are altered or their absolute values as long as the relationship between the two is maintained in a negative balance. These truths are independent of gender. The only allowance in diet counseling that should be made for women is a slight increase in caloric intake for pregnant or breastfeeding mothers. This additional allowance is in the range of 200 kcal/d for nursing mothers and 300 kcal/d during pregnancy.

Table 11.17. Recommended Habits to Improve Health

Avoid smoking
Eat breakfast
Eat moderately
Eat regularly
Exercise regularly
Sleep 7 to 8 h per night
Use alcohol in moderation or not at all

In prescribing any diet, care must be taken that adequate amounts of vitamins and minerals are provided and balance is maintained. It is unlikely that these goals will be reached with any diet consisting of less than 1000 kcal/d. To protect lean body mass, any diet should contain 0.8 to 1.2 g of protein per kilogram of desirable body weight. This level of protein intake provides nitrogen-sparing while losing fat mass.

Exercise may be prescribed for most patients, except for those with obvious medical contraindications. Exercise provides cardiac conditioning, enhances carbohydrate metabolism as a part of weight or diabetes control programs, decreases the risk of osteoporosis, and improves mood. Exercise must be begun gradually and should be tailored to the needs of the individual. General guidelines for exercise prescriptions are shown in Table 11.18. The type of activities recommended should be based on the preferences of the patient, degree of motivation, and the specific goals of the exercise program. Some activities are better suited to muscle building or endurance training, whereas others provide greater caloric demands (Table 11.19). A balanced program that provides both variety and conditioning may improve long-term compliance. For most programs, including those for the postpartum patient, activities should be designed to generate heart rates that approximate 75% of the maximal rate (Fig 11.5). This maximal heart rate is calculated by the formula:

$$\text{Maximal Heart Rate (MHR)} = 220 - \text{age in years}$$

Table 11.18. Exercise Guidelines

Types
    Aerobic
    Stretching/flexibility
    Muscle building (isometrics, resistance)
Frequency
    Daily (<30 min and <65% of maximum heart rate)
    Alternate days (>30 min and >65% of maximum heart rate)
Duration
    20 to 45 min per session based on activity
Intensity
    Target caloric expenditure—300 Kcal
    50% to 75% of capacity or 65% to 80% of maximal heart rate
Pattern of exercise
    Warm-up, 3–5 min
    Activity, 15–40 min (keep pulse in target range)
    Cool-down, 2–5 min
Warning signs
    Chest pressure, pain, or discomfort
    Claudication
    Dizziness
    Excessive or persistent fatigue
    Excessive or prolonged muscle pain
    Faintness
    Irregular heartbeat
    Nausea or vomiting
    Severe muscle or skeletal pain
    Unusual or exaggerated shortness of breath

Table 11.19. Energy Use for Selected Activitie (approximate kilocalories per 30 minutes)

Activity	Weight (lb)		
	110	150	190
Running			
5.5 min/mile	435	591	747
7 min/mile	366	468	573
9 min/mile	291	393	498
11.5 min/mile	204	276	351
Judo	294	399	504
Swimming			
Competetive	315	420	525
Backstroke	255	345	435
Crawl	192	261	330
Stair climbing	189	252	315
Cross country skiing	216	291	369
Aerobics			
"Running" pace	204	276	351
"Jogging" pace	159	213	270
"Walking" pace	99	132	168
Tennis	165	222	282
Disco dancing	156	210	267
(Ballroom dancing)	78	105	132
Gardening	150	204	258
Cycling			
9–10 miles/h (mph)	150	204	258
5–6 mph	96	132	165
Golf	129	174	219
Walking			
4 mph	120	162	207
3 mph	102	126	153
Mopping floor	96	120	153
Standing	39	51	66
Sitting down	33	45	57

Adapted from: American College of Obstetricians and Gynecologists. Women and exercise. ACOG Technical Bulletin 1992; No. 173; and Pi-Sunyer FX. Obesity. In Wyngaarden JB, Smith LH, JR., Bennett JC (eds). Cecil Textbook of Medicine, 19th ed. Philadelphia: WB Saunders, 1992, p 1162.

Patients should be encouraged to keep an exercise log and to periodically evaluate progress and goals. Gradual increases in the intensity and duration of activity are appropriate until the desired level is reached. For daily activity this should consist of those that last less than 30 minutes and achieves heart rates of less than 65% of MHR. If the patient wishes to go above these levels for individual sessions, the frequency of activity should be reduced to every other day. A cool-down period of from 5 to 10 minutes after exercise is important to allow the gradual return of diverted blood flow to the central circulation. The average woman will take 10 to 12 weeks to attain significant fitness even at these rates, so patience must be counseled.

When developing an exercise program for a pregnant patient, it is best to err on the side of conservatism. It is not possible to maintain cardiovascular fitness nor attain maxi-

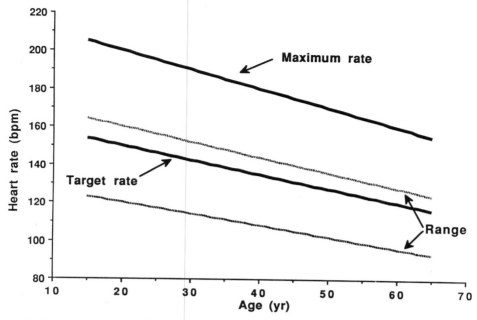

Figure 11.5. Heart rate guidelines for exercise. Target rate is 75% of maximal rate for age. Aerobic conditioning seeks to have heart rates in the range of 60% to 80% of maximal, as shown. Higher rates may be allowable for short periods or under supervision. Pregnant patients and those in the immediate postnatal period should reduce their target heart rate by 25% to 30%.

mal strength-training during pregnancy. Activity should be limited to less than 15 minutes and the maternal heart rate should be maintained below 140 beats per minute during pregnancy. Because of thermal and cardiovascular changes, pregnant patients should be warned to avoid overheating (> 38°C) and dehydration. They should drink a lot of fluids before, during, and after exercise. Exercise that employs the Valsalva maneuver or must be performed in the supine position should be avoided after the fourth month of pregnancy. Additional guidelines for exercise programs targeted toward pregnant and postnatal patients is shown in Table 11.20. Specific relative and absolute contraindications to exercise programs in pregnancy are shown in Table 11.21.

Of special concern during the postnatal period are exercises for the back. The combination of joint laxity, altered pregnancy posture, the forces of labor, and the bending inherent in the care of a newborn, all set the stage for significant back complaints in the postnatal period. Back strengthening exercises are not recommended during pregnancy because they require supine positioning or the Valsalva maneuver. During pregnancy and thereafter, pelvic tilt exercises will help to reduce lumbar lordosis and improve abdominal strength. In these, the patient contracts the muscles of the abdomen and buttocks to gently thrust the pelvis forward, rotating the pubis upward. This position is held for 10 seconds and then released. This should be performed as many times throughout the day as practical. Once the patient has delivered, back strengthening programs may be tailored to the patient's needs.

Table 11.20. Pregnancy and Postnatal Exercise Dos and Don'ts

Do
  Exercise regularly (three times a week)
  Use warm-up and cool-down periods
  Exercise on a shock-absorbing surface
  Wear good shoes designed for the specific activity
  Monitor heart rate and set conservative limits
  Maintain fluids before, during, and after activity

Don't
  Participate in competitive activities
  Exercise in hot humid weather or during febrile illness
  Use jerky, bouncy motions or rapid changes in direction
  Over flex or extend joints
  Change position rapidly
  Become overheated or dehydrated

Table 11.21. Contraindication to Vigorous Activity During Pregnancy

Absolute contraindications
  Bleeding
  Incompetent cervix
  Maternal cardiac disease
  Multiple gestation
  Placenta previa
  Premature labor (current or previous pregnancies)
  Ruptured membranes
  Three or more spontaneous abortions
Relative contraindications
  Anemia
  Breech presentation in last trimester
  Cardiac arrhythmia or palpitations
  Diabetes
  Extremes of weight (over- or underweight)
  History of bleeding during current pregnancy
  History of extremely sedentary lifestyle
  History of precipitous labor
  Hypertension
  Intrauterine growth restriction (current or past)
  Thyroid disease

Substance Use and Abuse

Two areas in which all providers can have a positive impact are alcohol and tobacco use. Many studies indicate that interest, support, and counseling (with referral when needed) by a physician greatly increases the chances of a patient changing risky behaviors.

Counseling directed toward substance use and abuse is at once both simple and complex. Simplistic approaches such as 'just say no' do not work, yet are clearly well intentioned and hold the essence of the desired behavior. All women should be asked about substance abuse (including alcohol and tobacco) and counseling or support should be made available, through other providers if necessary. This may include specialized providers or community resources such as Alcoholics Anonymous.

ALCOHOL INTERVENTIONS. The cornerstone of intervention designed to decrease alcohol use is nonjudgmental support. Care must be taken to safeguard the medical condition of the patient during the process of withdrawal. Because of the potential severity of alcohol withdrawal, including the possibility of death in up to 15% of cases, withdrawal is best managed by those experienced with the process. Nutritional support, through multivitamins and thiamin (100 mg intramuscular), is appropriate for most patients regardless of the setting. The best success rates for long-term alcohol withdrawal comes through trained personnel in detoxification centers and will involve the help of the patient's friends and family.

SMOKING CESSATION. Of people who have ever smoked, 45% have quit. Despite this number, two thirds of current smokers are not ready to take any action to quit. Because 65% of those who quite smoking will relapse in 3 months, continuing support is required. Often all that can realistically be accomplished in any one encounter is to move the patient gradually along toward eventual cessation: For those who have never considered quitting, we can get them to start considering it; for those who have thought about it, get them to try; and for those who have failed in the past, get them to try again.

Most successful smoking cessation plans advocate stopping smoking all at once ("cold turkey"), rather than tapering the amount smoked or switching to lower tar cigarettes. Unlike other types of addiction, nicotine withdrawal is only prolonged and not eased by tapering the dose. Most smokers who switch to cigarettes that are lower in tar or nicotine will, unconsciously, increase their use to deliver the same net dose of nicotine. In addition to addressing nicotine withdrawal, modification of the patient's habits and environment is required.

Any smoking cessation program must take into consideration the patient's fears of weight gain and oral cravings. These fears, which are especially common among women, are best addressed early and in a positive way. Increasing fluid intake (not alcohol), the use of chewing gum or raw vegetables, and avoiding skipping meals help to decrease these problems.

Cardiovascular Disease and Hypertension

The most likely source of treatment failure in hypertensive patients is poor compliance. Therefore, education, reinforcement, and periodic re-evaluation are of paramount importance. It is also important to watch for weight gain, changes in sodium intake, and the use of concurrent medications, such as diet pills and cold preparations, which might interfere with therapy.

Sexually Transmitted Disease and HIV

Unless both partners were virginal and remain monogamous, any patient who is sexually active may be at risk for sexually transmitted disease, including HIV. Counseling regarding high-risk behaviors, avoidance of blood or body fluid exchange, and regular condom use is appropriate for all women. If both partners are known to be free of disease, those in mutually monogamous relations may take comfort in reduced risk. Liberal availability of testing and a free exchange of confidential information, are critical to reducing the risk of sexually transmitted disease.

Other Healthy Behaviors

An overlooked area where the clinician can positively influence reducing risk is through encouraging of the use of automobile passenger restraint systems (seat belts), which have been well documented to reduce the likelihood of death and severe injury, when consistently and correctly used. Use should be encouraged for all patients, including pregnant women. The use of approved child restraints and motorcycle helmets must also be strongly supported.

HINTS AND COMMON QUESTIONS

Healthy, women have an erythrocyte sedimentation rate (ESR) that is higher than men (20 mm/h vs. 15 mm/h). This value is even greater for women over the age of 50 (30 mm/h). For these reasons, care must be taken in evaluating the significance of "borderline" elevations in ESR.

At the present time, aspirin prophylaxis to prevent myocardial infarction in women remains unproved. The decision to take prophylactic aspirin should be made on an individual basis.

The use of patient-maintained immunization records, especially for children and young adults, increases awareness and compliance with immunization schedules.

Any involuntary weight gain or loss of greater than 10 lb over a period of 6 months should suggest the possibility of disease. This may range from wasting processes, such as malignancy, to depression and eating disorders.

Women are prone to fad and crash diets perceived to yield quick or easy solutions to long-standing problems. At worst, these may be dangerous and at best are associated with a high probability of failure. Gradual weight loss, on the order of 1 to 2 lb/mo, combined with lifestyle changes, and a diet that can be maintained for long periods, offer the best chance of lasting weight loss.

One pound of fat is approximately equal to 3500 to 4000 kcal. Therefore, if a patient can maintain a calorie deficit of 400 kcal/d, it will take 10 days to loose a pound of body fat. Including this information in a program of diet education can be helpful in providing encouragement and realistic goal setting.

Studies indicate that nibbling or grazing patterns of eating are more effective in reducing serum cholesterol and lipids compared with the traditional three-meals-a-day pattern. Care must be used in recommending this pattern so that total calories and nutrition balance are maintained.

Muscle is twice the weight of fat per unit volume. As a result, a patient may loose fat without a change in body weight. Patient should be reassured that this is the case and it is desirable. The best indication that this type of loss is ongoing is the fit of clothing.

Extreme weight loss is associated with an increased risk of gallstone formation and symptoms. Therefore, when assisting patients with weight loss programs, additional vigilance is warranted.

Success in an exercise program is predicated on a knowledge of what must be done and why, a positive sense of confidence that those goals may be achieved, and a willingness to wait an appropriate amount of time while those goals are met. Each of these three aspects depend on time spent in education and counseling.

Indoor exercise or fitness machines offer no more conditioning or calorie consumption than a comparable outdoor activity. They do offer security, privacy, and climate control, but at the expense of boredom. If used, care should be taken to follow the manufacturer's operating instructions carefully.

Women may be assured that even with prolonged weight training they will not take on a male musculature appearance. The only exception is the use of anabolic steroids, which are associated with significant known and theoretic risks and should not be condoned.

There are no contraindications to any currently available contraceptive method based on exercise or activity.

There are no reports of serious adverse effects on the breast due to exercise or normal sports activities. Contusions and nipple abrasions may occur, however, and the use of a well-fitting, supportive sports bra is recommended.

Despite popular claims, there is no evidence that regular exercise will result in shorter or easier labor, or improve the eventual outcome of pregnancy. There are some reports that suggest that increased occupational activity may be related to a slight decrease in the average duration of gestation, although the significance of this finding is debatable.

After exercise, hot tub baths, showers, and saunas should be avoided until well after the heart rate has returned to normal. Failure to do so causes peripheral pooling of blood, which may be sufficient to result in significant cardiac or central nervous system ischemia.

Patients with either anorexia nervosa or bulimia often have scars on the knuckles of the hand (from induced vomiting) or dental erosion from exposure to stomach acid. These are not diagnostic, but should arouse suspicion.

Oral cravings caused by smoking and nicotine withdrawal may be partially addressed by consuming carrot sticks. These are easily portable, keep well, contain few calories, and are socially acceptable.

It is important to counsel patients that the use of condoms does not result in completely "safe sex." Although condoms reduce the risk of acquiring most STDs, including HIV, they do not reduce the risk to zero or absolve irresponsible behaviors. Studies indicate that condoms may only reduce the risk of HIV transmission by 70%.

SUGGESTED READINGS

General References

American College of Obstetricians and Gynecologists. Health maintenance for perimenopausal women. ACOG Technical bulletin 210. Washington, DC: ACOG, 1995.

Belloc NB. Relationship of health practices and mortality. Prev Med 1973;2:67.

Canadian Task Force on the Periodic Health Examination: Report of the task force. Can Med Assoc J 1979;121:1193.

Canadian Task Force on the Periodic Health Examination: Report of the task force, 1984 update. Can Med Assoc J 1986;134:724.

Canadian Task Force on the Periodic Health Examination: The periodic health examination. 2. 1987 update. Can Med Assoc J 1988;138:618.

Canadian Task Force on the Periodic Health Examination: The periodic health examination, 1991 update. 6. Acetylsalicylic acid and the primary prevention of cardiovascular disease. Can Med Assoc J 1991;145:1091.

Canadian Task Force on the Periodic Health Examination: The periodic health examination, 1993 update. 2. Lowering the total cholesterol level to prevent coronary heart disease. Can Med Assoc J 1993;148:521.

Hayward RSA, Steinberg EP, Ford DE, Roizen MF, Roach KW. Preventive care guidelines: 1991. Ann Intern Med 1991;114:758.

Joint National Committee on Detection, Evaluation, and Treatment of High Blood Pressure: The fifth report of the Joint National Committee on Detection, Evaluation, and Treatment of High Blood Pressure. Arch Intern Med 1993;153:154.

Mully AG. Screening tests for the healthy patient. Med Clin North Am 1987;71:625.

Oboler SK, LaForce FM. The periodic physical examination in asymptomatic adults. Ann Intern Med 1989;110:214.

Peipert JF, Sweeney PJ. Diagnostic testing in obstetrics and gynecology: a clinicians guide. Obstet Gynecol 1994; 82:619.

Rosen M. Health maintenance strategies for women of different ages. Obstet Gynecol Clin North Am 1990; 17:673.

Simmons PS. Office pediatric gynecology. Prim Care 1988;15:617.

Sox HC JR. Preventive health services in adults. N Engl J Med 1994;330:1589.

Task Force on Adult Immunization. Adult immunizations 1994. Ann Intern Med 1994;121:540.

Task Force on Primary and Preventive Health Care of the American College of Obstetricians and Gynecologists. The Obstetrician-Gynecologist and Primary-Preventive Health Care. Washington, DC: ACOG, 1993.

Update on adult immunization: Recommendations of the Immunization Practices Advisory Committee. MMWR 1991;40(No. RR-12):Table 7.

U.S. Preventive Services Task Force. Guide to Clinical Preventive Services, 2nd ed. Baltimore: Williams & Wilkins, 1995.

Wilson JR. The older woman: what are the physician's concerns? Prim Care 1995;2:35.

Specific References

Diet and Exercise

Aloia JF. Premenopausal bone mass is related to physical activity. Arch Int Med 1988;148:121.

American College of Obstetricians and Gynecologists. Women and exercise. ACOG Technical bulletin 173. Washington, DC: ACOG, 1992.

American College of Obstetricians and Gynecologists. Exercise during pregnancy and the postnatal period. Washington, DC: ACOG, 1985.

American College of Sports Medicine. Guidelines for Graded Exercise Prescription, 4th ed. Philadelphia: Lea & Febiger, 1990.

Arnaud CD. Role of dietary calcium in osteoporosis. Adv Intern Med 1990;35:93.

Avtal R, Wiswell RA, Drinkwater BL. Exercise in Pregnancy, 2nd ed. Baltimore: Williams & Wilkins, 1991.

Bachrach JK. Decreased bone density in adolescent girls with anorexia nervosa. Pediatrics 1990;86:440.

Ballard JE. The effect of high level of physical activity (8.5 METs or greater) and estrogen replacement therapy upon bone mass in postmenopausal females, aged 50–68 years. Int J Sports Med 1990;11:208.

Birfge SJ, Dalsky G. The role of exercise in preventing osteoporosis. Public Health Rep 1989;104(suppl):54.

Chestnut CH III. Bone mass and exercise. Am J Med 1993;95:34S.

Dilsen G. The role of physical exercise in prevention and management of osteoporosis. Clin Rheumatol 1989; 8(suppl 2):70.

Drinkwater BL. Menstrual history as a determinant of current bone density in young athletes. JAMA 1990;263:545.

Hergenroeder AC. Bone mineralization, hypothalamic amenorrhea and sex steroid therapy in female adolescents and young adults. J Pediatrics 1995;126:683.

Howat PM. The influence of diet, body fat, menstrual cycling & activity upon the bone density of females. J Am Diet Assoc 1989;89:1305.

Hubert HB, Feinleib M, McNamara PM, et al. Obesity as an independent risk factor for cardiovascular disease: a 26-year follow-up of participants in the Framingham Heart Study. Circulation 1983;67:968.

Kanis JA. Calcium supplementation of the diet II: not justified by present evidence. BMJ 1989;298:205.

Lew EA, Garfinkle L. Variations in mortality by weight among 750,000 men and women. Chronic Diseases 1979;32:563.

Metheny WP, Smith RP. The relationship between exercise, stress, and primary dysmenorrhea. J Behav Med 1989;12:569.

McCulloch RG, Bailey DA, Houston CS, Dodd BL. Effects of physical activity, dietary calcium intake and selected lifestyle factors on bone density in young women. Can Med Assoc J 1990;142:221.

National Institutes of Health Consensus Development Panel on the Health Implications of Obesity: Health implications of obesity. Ann Intern Med 1985;103:147.

Nordin BEC. Calcium supplementation of the diet: justified by the present evidence. BMJ 1990;300:1056.

Pi-Sunyer FX. Obesity. In Wyngaarden JB, Smith LH JR, Bennett JC (eds). Cecil Textbook of Medicine, 19th ed. Philadelphia: WB Saunders, 1992, p 1162.

Posner BM. Diet, menopause and serum cholesterol levels in women: the Framingham Study. Am Heart J 1993;125:483.

Smith CW JR. Exercise: A practical guide for helping the patient achieve a healthy lifestyle. J Am Board Fam Pract 1989;2:238.

Sjostrom LV. Mortality of severely obese subjects. Am J Clin Nutr 1992;55:516S.

Van Itallie TB, Yang MU. Diet and weight loss. N Engl J Med 1977;297:1158.

Alcohol and Tobacco

American College of Obstetricians and Gynecologists. Smoking and reproductive health. ACOG Technical Bulletin 180. Washington, DC: ACOG, 1993.

American College of Obstetricians and Gynecologists. Substance abuse in pregnancy. ACOG Technical Bulletin 195. Washington, DC: ACOG, 1994.

Anokute CC. Epidemiology of spontaneous abortions: the effects of alcohol consumption and cigarette smoking. J Natl Med Assoc 1986;78:771–775.

Autti-Rämö I, Korkman M, Hilakivi-Clark L, Lehtonen M, Halmesmäki E, Granström ML. Mental development of 2-year-old children exposed to alcohol in utero. J Pediatr 1992;120:740.

Bottoms SF, Martier SS, Sokol RJ. Refinements in screening for risk drinking in reproductive-aged women: the "net" results. Alcoholism 1989;13:339.

Burns DM. Tobacco and health. In Wyngaarden JB, Smith LH JR, Bennett JC (eds). Cecil Textbook of Medicine, 19th ed. Philadelphia: WB Saunders, 1992, pp 34–37.

Campbell OM, Gray RH. Smoking and ectopic pregnancy: A multinational case-control study. In Rosenberg MJ (ed). Smoking and Reproductive Health. Littleton, Massachusetts: PSG Publishing Co, 1987, pp 70–75.

Centers for Disease Control and Prevention. Cigarette smoking among reproductive-aged women—Behavioral risk factor surveillance system, 1989. MMWR 1991;40:719–723.

Chan AWK, Pristach EA, Welte JW, Russell M. Use of the TWEAK test in screening for alcoholism/heavy drinking in three populations. Alcohol Clin Exp Res 1993;17:1188–1192.

Diamond I. Alcoholism and alcohol abuse. In Wyngaarden JB, Smith LH JR, Bennett JC (eds). Cecil Textbook of Medicine, 19th ed. Philadelphia: WB Saunders, 1992, pp 44–47.

Ewing JA. Detecting alcoholism: the CAGE questionnaire. JAMA 1984;252:1905.

Hammond EC. Smoking in relation to physical complaints. Arch Environ Health 1961;3:28–46.

Hanauer SB. Nicotine for colitis—The smoke has not yet cleared. N Eng J Med 1994;330:856–857.

Hill SY. Vulnerability to the biomedical consequences of alcoholism and alcohol-related problems among women. In Wilsnack SC, Beckman LJ (eds). Alcohol Problems in Women: Antecedents, Consequences and Intervention. New York: The Guilford Press, 1984, pp 121–154.

Howe G, Westhoff C, Vessey M, Yeates D. Effects of age, cigarette smoking, and other factors on fertility: findings in a large prospective study. BMJ 1985;290:1697.

Kitchens JM. Does this patient have an alcohol problem? JAMA 1994;272:1782.

Mattison DR, Plowchalk DR, Meadows MJ, Miller MM, Malek A, London S. The effect of smoking on oogenesis, fertilization, and implantation. Semin Reprod Endocrinol 1989;7:291–294.

McKinlay SM, Bifano NL, McKinlay JB. Smoking and age at menopause in women. Ann Intern Med 1985;103:350–356.

Midanik LT, Room R. The epidemiology of alcohol consumption. Alcohol Health Res World 1993;16:183–190.

Mullen PD, Carbonari JP, Glenday MC. Identifying pregnant women who drink alcoholic beverages. Am J Obstet Gynecol 1991;165:1429–1430.

Nelson HD, Nevitt MC, Scott JC, Stone KL, Cummings SR. Smoking, alcohol, and neuromuscular and physical function of older women. JAMA 1994;272:1825.

Pattinson HA, Taylor PJ, Pattinson MH. The effect of cigarette smoking on ovarian function and early pregnancy outcome of in vitro fertilization treatment. Fertil Steril 1991;55:780–783.

Seizer ML, Vinokur, A, Van Rooijen L. A self-administered Short Michigan Alcoholism Screening Test (SMAST). J Stud Alcohol 1975;36:117.

Serdula M, Williamson DF, Kendrick JS, et al. Trends in alcohol consumption by pregnant women: 1985 through 1988. JAMA 1991;265:876–879.

Sexton M. Hebel JR. A clinical trial of change in maternal smoking and its effect on birth weight. JAMA 1984;251:911–915.

Sokol RJ, Martier SS, Ager JW. The TACE questions: practical prenatal detection of risk-drinking. Am J Obstet Gynecol 1989;160:863.

Stokes EJ. Alcohol abuse screening. What to ask your female patient. Female Patient 1989;14:17–24.

Streissguth AP, Clarren Sk, Jones KL. Natural history of the fetal alcohol syndrome: a 10-year follow-up of eleven patients. Lancet 1985;2:85.

Transdermal Nicotine Study Group. Transdermal nicotine for smoking cessation. JAMA 1991;266:3133–3138.

Weiner L, Rosett HL, Mason EA. Training professionals to identify and treat pregnant women who drink heavily. Alcohol Health Res World 1985;9:32–36.

Cardiovascular Health

Burkman RT. Strategies for reducing cardiovascular risk in women. J Reprod Med 1991;36(suppl):238.

Clarke WR, Lauer RM. The predictive value of childhood cholesterol screening: a response. JAMA 1992;267: 1101.

Dalen JE, Goldberg RJ. Prophylactic aspirin and the elderly population. Clin Geriatr Med 1992;8:119.

Grady D, Rubin SM, Petitti DB, et al. Hormone therapy to prevent disease and prolong life in postmenopausal women. Ann Intern Med 1992;117:1016.

Manson JE, Stampfer MJ, Colditz GA, et al. A prospective study of aspirin use and primary prevention of cardiovascular disease in women. JAMA 1991;266:521.

Manson JE, Tosteson H, Ridker PM, et al. The primary prevention of myocardial infarction. N Engl J Med 1992;326:1406.

Steering Committee of the Physician's Health Study Research Group. Final report on the aspirin component of the ongoing physician's health study. N Engl J Med 1989;321:129.

Writing Group for the PEPI Trial. Effects of estrogen or estrogen/progestin regimens on heart disease risk factors in postmenopausal women. The Postmenopausal Estrogen/Progestin Interventions (PEPI) Trial. JAMA 1995;273:199.

Other Concerns

American College of Obstetricians and Gynecologists. Immunization during pregnancy. ACOG Technical Bulletin 160. Washington, DC: ACOG, 1991.

Anderson JW, Brinkman VL, Hamilton CC. Weight loss and 2-year follow-up for 80 morbidly obese patients treated with intensive, very-low calorie diet and an education program. Am J Clin Nutr 1992;56:244S.

Centers for Disease Control and Prevention. Prevention and control of influenza recommendations of the Advisory Committee on Immunization Practices (ACIP). MMWR 1995;44(RR-3):1.

Centers for Disease Control and Prevention. Update: Barrier protection against HIV infection and other sexually transmitted diseases. MMWR 1993;42:589.

Colditz GA. Economic costs of obesity. Am J Clin Nutr 1992;55:503S.

Eddy DM. Screening for cervical cancer. Ann Intern Med 1990;113:214.

Felicetta JV. Thyroid changes with aging: significance and management. Geriatrics 1987;42:86.

Kiel DP, Moskowity MA. The urinalysis: a critical appraisal. Med Clin North Am 1987;71:607.

Phillips RS, Aronson MD, Taylor WC, et al. Should tests for Chlamydia trachomatis cervical infection be done during routine gynecologic visits? Ann Intern Med 1987;107:188.

Raisz LG (ed). Clinical indications for bone mass measurements: a report from the Scientific Advisory Board of the National Osteoporosis Foundation. J Bone Miner Res 1989;4(suppl 2):1.

Robinson JI, Hoerr SL, Strandmark J, Mavis B. Obesity, weight loss, and health. J Am Diet Assoc 1993;93:445.

Washington EA, Katz P. Cost of a payment source for pelvic inflammatory disease. JAMA 1991;266:2565.

Waller SC. A meta-analysis of condom effectiveness in reducing sexually transmitted HIV. Soc Sci Med 1993;36:1635.

Weintraub NT, Nicoli E, Freedman ML. Cervical cancer screening in women age 65 and over. J Am Geriatr Soc 1987;35:870.

Wiselka M. Influenza: Diagnosis, management and prophylaxis. BMJ 1994;308:1341.

12

Menopause

More and more, we are coming to view menopause as not the "natural process" we once considered it, but rather as organ failure. Strong evidence has accumulated to show that the loss of ovarian steroids is detrimental to overall health through its impact on tissues throughout the body. These adverse effects may be reversed or prevented through the use of estrogen replacement. The quality of life is improved, short-term memory enhanced, and even the youthful qualities of the skin restored through estrogen replacement. As our population ages, the impact and special problems menopause presents become greater. Everyone who cares for women must be aware of this aspect of their needs.

BACKGROUND AND SCIENCE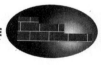

At around the turn of the century, the United States had about 3.1 million people over the age of 65, and the average life expectancy of a woman was almost exactly the same as the average age of menopause. By 1980, 16% of the population was over the age of 60, 25 million people were over the age of 65, and 10 million over the age of 75. In 1980, the average woman could expect to live 30 years beyond the average age of menopause, or roughly one third of her entire life expectancy. By the year 2000, it is predicted that there will be 50 million Americans over the age of 65. What once was a problem for only a few women—menopause—is now a national health concern.

Where once menopause was considered a natural event that a woman "went through" or passed, somewhat like a stop sign, it is now recognized that the loss of ovarian steroids bring about a cascade of events, the full impact of which may not be appreciated until many years later when osteoporotic fractures, premature heart disease, or other sequella become

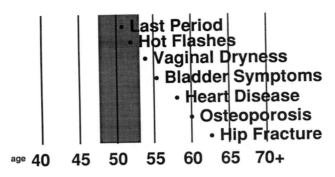

Figure 12.1. Impact of estrogen Loss. The loss of ovarian steroids brings about a cascade of events, the full impact of which may not be appreciated for many years.

evident (Fig. 12.1). This change in focus means that we now view menopause as an endocrinopathy (the loss of the function of an endocrine gland with adverse consequences). Once reserved for only those with intractable symptoms, now routine replacement of ovarian hormones is considered for almost all older patients. Several changes have taken place to induce this altered view: a better understanding of the pathophysiology of menopause, a greater appreciation of the role of estrogen in osteoporosis and cardiovascular disease, and enhanced awareness of the risk and benefits of estrogen replacement therapy.

Beginning at approximately age 40 for most women, there is a decline in the sensitivity of the follicles remaining in the ovary. There are also fewer follicles (a few thousand) available owing to attrition and ovulation. This results in declining estrogen production and gradually rising levels of follicle-stimulating hormone (FSH), as the pituitary attempts to compensate. Irregular ovulation, a shortened follicular phase, and an inadequate luteal phase all contribute to the unpredictable character of menses during this period, which is often referred to as dysfunctional uterine bleeding (DUB). As estrogen ebbs, the ability of the few remaining follicles to respond to FSH also declines, hastening the spiral of effects, until estrogen production is inadequate to support endometrial withdrawal and menopause occurs.

The average age for menopause in the United States is between 50 and 52 years of age (median 51.5), with 95% of women experiencing this event between the ages of 44 and 55. The age of menopause is not influenced by the age of menarche, number of ovulations or pregnancies, lactation, or the use of oral contraceptives. Race, socioeconomic status, education, and height also have no effect on the age of menopause. Undernourished women and smokers do tend to have an earlier menopause, although the effect is slight. About 1% of women undergo menopause before the age of 40. This is generally referred to as "premature ovarian failure" rather than menopause because of the social implications inherent in the latter.

Estrogen levels do not fall to zero after the menopause. A small amount of estrogen is still made by the ovary, and estrogen (mainly estrone) is made through extraglandular aromatization of androstenedione produced by the adrenal gland. This process is a function of age and weight, with most of the aromatization taking place in peripheral fat deposits. Testosterone, made by the ovarian stroma, does not undergo an appreciable drop during natural menopause, although it is reduced by bilateral oophorectomy as might be expected. The continued production of testosterone and androstenedione reduces the estrogen-to-androgen ratio, often leading to a relative androgen excess, resulting in phenomena such as beard growth and darkening and breast regression.

Hot Flashes, REM Sleep, and Sexuality

Approximately 75% to 85% of menopausal women experience the most common complaint of menopause: hot flashes. Hot flashes, flushes, and night sweats are a source of very real disruption and inconvenience for these women, with up to a third requiring medical assistance for their symptoms. More than 50% of women will experience hot flashes within 3 months of natural or surgical menopause. Between 25% and 50% of women will experience these symptoms for 5 or more years. Hot flashes may occur even before the loss of regular menses signals the onset of menopause. These symptoms are most closely related to the loss of estrogen, but less education, increased weight, stress, and smoking are also factors that increase the risk of hot flashes.

Hot flashes are the symptoms of a group of physiologic phenomena associated with luteinizing hormone (LH) surges (mediated by the hypothalamus); a rise in circulating norepinephrine levels; and changes in blood pressure, heart rate, skin, and core temperature. These changes may occur as often as every 20 to 30 minutes, last for about 4 minutes, and are thought to arise because of disruptions in the thermoregulatory centers of the hypothalamus. These centers appear to be suppressed by estrogen. With the loss of estrogen from the ovary, they become hyperactive and prone to wide swings similar to that seen by engineers in undamped oscillators. The result is periods of elevated core temperature, followed by increased cutaneous blood flow (resulting in the flushed feeling and look) that radiates excess heat away from the body. Temperature loss may overshoot, resulting in chills or a sensation of cold. When this cycle happens at night, in the form of night sweats, it can be very disruptive to normal sleeping patterns for both the patient and her bedmate. In addition, menopausal women experience an increase in sleep latency and a decrease in rapid eye movement (REM) sleep patterns, further disrupting restful sleep. This can quickly give rise to fatigue, irritability, depression, and somatic complaints if not corrected.

With the loss of ovarian steroids, vaginal atrophy generally occurs over the course of 3 to 6 months. This results in vaginal dryness, vulvar itching and burning, dyspareunia, and cracking or bleeding from the thinned tissues of the genital tract. Changes in the urinary tract may result in dysuria, urgency and urgency incontinence, urinary frequency, nocturia, and an increased incidence of stress incontinence. These symptoms are reduced by greater than 50% with estrogen replacement therapy.

For some women, there is a decrease in libido that occurs with menopause. As noted in Chapter 8, Sexuality, some of this decline is owing to a drop in serum testosterone levels, but much of the change may also be related to decreased availability or capability of partners, and dyspareunia brought on by vaginal atrophy. Most studies indicate improvement in libidinal function, although not always coital frequency, with estrogen and testosterone therapy.

Bleeding Abnormalities

Although the hallmark of menopause is the loss of cyclic menstruation, irregular bleeding that occurs during the period of transition (perimenopause) and random bleeding that occurs after menstruation has stopped deserve special mention because of the possibility of genital tract malignancy, endometrial disease (hyperplasia, endometritis), a complication of an unexpected pregnancy, or bleeding from sources other than the uterus. The most common reason for this irregular bleeding is the loss of ovulation leading to loss of cyclic progesterone stimulation. Without periodic progestin stimulation the endometrium may initially become hyperplastic and, later as estrogen levels fall, hypoplastic (atrophic). Under either condition, irregular shedding of the endometrium may occur.

When noncyclic bleeding occurs in these patients, endometrial biopsy should be strongly considered to evaluate the cause and to check for the possibility of a malignancy masquerading as simple climacteric irregularity. The advent of simple office endometrial sampling systems (e.g., Accurette, Explora, Gynocheck, Pipelle, Z-Sampler, and others) makes sampling quick, easy, inexpensive, and safer than the traditional dilation and curettage. Because of an increased incidence of hyperplasia in women who continue to have regular menstruation after the age of 55, these women should be considered for sampling in the office as well.

Osteoporosis

Osteoporosis (decreased bone density) and the fractures engendered by it are responsible for the expenditure of between $7 and $9 billion for acute and chronic care each year in the United States. Women have a higher rate of osteoporosis and, therefore, account for almost two thirds of the roughly 1.2 million annual osteoporotic fractures in the United States. The rate of Colles' fractures for women rises tenfold between the age of 35 and age 60, but stays stable for men over the same period. It is estimated that 80% of hip fractures are associated with osteoporosis. Following hip fracture, half of patients require assistance walking and 15% to 25% will be institutionalized, often for the rest of their lives. Roughly one of five hip fracture patients dies within 6 months of the fracture. Fracture of the hip is the 12th leading cause of death for women. A greater understanding of the role of estrogen loss in this process has contributed to the current view of menopause as an endocrinopathy.

Bone is a dynamic tissue, constantly undergoing destruction and reconstruction throughout our lives. As we age, both constructive and destructive processes slow, but there is a greater decrease in constructive activities. This yields a net loss of bone mass that begins in our 40s and continues for the rest of our lives. There is a further increase in bone loss that happens once we reach our 70s and beyond. Bone can also be lost through medical therapy with anticonvulsants, corticosteroids, excess thyroid hormone replacement, long-term heparin or tetracycline use, loop diuretics, chemotherapy, and radiation therapy. Factors that increase the risk of bone loss for women are shown in Table 12.1.

Women suffer roughly a tenfold increase in the normal rate of bone loss for a period of about 10 years beginning with the loss of ovarian function. This results in an average lifetime loss of approximately 35% of cortical bone mass and 50% of the more metabolically active trabecular bone. (By comparison, men lose only about two thirds this amount.) This increased loss, combined with less total bone mass than men and the effects of pregnancy-induced calcium loss, put women at greater risk for osteoporotic fractures. As a result, one third of women over the age of 65 will have vertebral fractures and by age 90 one third will suffer a hip fracture (vs. 17% of men).

Table 12.1. Factors that Increase Bone Loss In Older Women

Alcohol use
Chronic illness
Diabetes mellitus
Estrogen loss, especially early menopause
Excessive caffeine use
Family history of osteoporosis
High parity
High protein intake
Inactivity/sedentary lifestyle
Inadequate vitamin D intake
Low body weight
Poor diet/inadequate calcium intake (<1000 mg/d)
Race: white or Asian
Smoking
Steroid therapy (e.g., arthritis)

Strong evidence supports the contention that the accelerated bone loss women experience is a direct effect of the loss of ovarian steroids and that it is prevented by estrogen replacement. This effect is independent of age, and it may be seen in premature ovarian failure or surgical menopause, or in hypoestrogenic conditions such as anorexia nervosa or hyperprolactinemic amenorrhea. The mechanism by which this occurs is complex and still being mapped, but it has been well documented that bone has estrogen receptors present and when estrogen is lacking, there is an increased loss of calcium from preformed bone. There is evidence that estrogen encourages the deposition of new bone and calcium through stimulation of osteoblast and osteoblastlike cells. This leads to an increase in the deposition of collagen and encourages the formation of new bone. Estrogen appears to block the action of parathyroid hormone, thereby reducing bone resorption. The loss of estrogen leads to decreased levels of calcitonin, which return to normal with estrogen replacement therapy. Estrogen may increase intestinal absorption of calcium. Estrogen alters prostaglandin production and may have a controlling effect on growth factors such as fibroblast growth factor, transforming growth factor, or β_2-microglobulin, all of which stimulate bone metabolism and may act in a protective way to hold calcium in place.

Cardiovascular Disease

Heart disease is the most common cause of death for women, resulting in ten times the number of deaths per year as are caused by breast cancer. Studies show an increased risk of heart disease for women after menopause. The ratio of heart disease for men and women is roughly 2:1 at age 65 and 1:1 by age 80. By contrast, prior to menopause, the rate is only one third that for men, suggesting a protective role for estrogen. Patients who undergo premature or surgical menopause have about a twofold increase in their risk of heart disease compared with their peers and later in life have an even greater risk than those who go through natural menopause (possibly because of the longer time spent after hormone loss). Although large, controlled, randomized studies are lacking, epidemiologic studies investigating the use of estrogen (with controls matched for age and smoking) have found that this apparent increase can be reversed (and in some cases actually decreased below the rate for the controls).

Most prospective studies suggest that there is a 40% to 60% reduction in the rate of heart disease for women placed on estrogen replacement. The exact mechanism for this change is unknown, although studies do indicate some possible explanations. The improved risk of heart disease may, in part, be owing to a decrease in low-density lipoproteins (LDL) and increase in high-density lipoproteins (HDL) found in patients before menopause and on hormonal therapy. Although the use of progestins tends to push HDL levels down and LDL levels up, there is no evidence that concomitant treatment with progestins will negate these beneficial effects. Studies suggest that only about a quarter of the beneficial effects of estrogen therapy can be explained by lipid changes. Direct effects of estrogen on blood pressure, vessel walls, cyclooxygenase, insulin metabolism, altered platelet function, and changes in the rate of atheroma development may all contribute as much or more to this protective effect.

Other Concerns

Many aspects of a patient's life change at or around the time of menopause, which can be the source of major disruptions or stress but which have little to do with the hormonal changes occurring in the woman's body. These include both psychosocial and physical changes (Table 12.2) that the health care provider must be aware of and should be addressed when present.

Many patients (and their families) express concern over emotional aspects of "the change." Most studies indicate that the rate of psychiatric disorders, for both men and women, drops sharply after the age of 45. Anecdotal reports of depression, nervousness, irritability, and insomnia are common, but studies that have attempted to remove confounding factors have failed to support estrogen as an exclusive cause. Trials of estrogen re-

Table 12.2. Problems Common to Menopausal Women

Psychosocial problems
    Dependence
    Depression
    Financial stress
    Grieving (loss of friends and family)
    Institutionalization
    Loneliness
    Loss of autonomy
    Substance abuse
Physical problems
    Altered sexuality
    Arthritis
    Chronic illness
    Dental problems
    Hearing loss
    Osteoperosis
    Thyroid dysfunction
    Visual acuity loss

placement have indicated cognitive and affective improvements with therapy, as well as increases (back to normal levels) of β-endorphin and β-lipotropin. In these studies, memory was enhanced and anxiety and irritability were decreased for these patients, although a role for other factors, such as improved sleep, has not been resolved. Modest improvement on estrogen therapy does not establish proof of a worsening of these parameters with menopause, but does suggest that for those who have a change, estrogen therapy may be of help.

Following menopause, there is a loss of dermal collagen leading to a thinning of the skin. Although this is most marked in the genital tissues and breast, it occurs throughout the body, resulting in wrinkling and loss of skin tone. Definitive studies are lacking, but anecdotal studies suggest that estrogen therapy can prevent or possibly reverse these changes. Well-controlled, randomized studies are needed to answer this question.

ESTABLISHING THE DIAGNOSIS

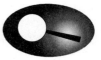

The diagnosis of menopause is established on the permanent absence of menstrual bleeding due to ovarian failure (or removal) in the presence of adequate gonadotrophin stimulation. The period of perimenopause encompasses the 4 to 5 years immediately surrounding the time of the last period. The climacteric period (Greek, meaning turning point) is a more general term for the period of waning ovarian function, changing self-image, and new life roles.

Laboratory Testing

When the diagnosis of ovarian failure must be confirmed, measurement of serum FSH is sufficient. Levels of greater than 100 mIU/mL are diagnostic, although lower levels (40–50 mIU/mL) may be sufficient to establish a diagnosis when symptoms are also present. The loss of circulating inhibin (made by the ovary) tends to keep FSH levels elevated even in the face of estrogen replacement, although the most reliable values will be obtained after a week off from therapy. Serum estradiol levels may be determined (generally less than 15 pg/mL) but are less reliable as a marker of ovarian failure. The perimenopausal period often presents an opportunity to perform other routine screening evaluations appropriate to the older patient. These include thyroid function, cholesterol, lipid profiles, and others.

Specialized Concerns

There are several areas of special concern in the care of the perimenopausal and postmenopausal woman: the roles of osteoporosis screening, endometrial sampling, and surveillance for ovarian cancer.

Osteoporosis Screening

Bone densitometry is an important tool for research on bone health and the impact of estrogen replacement, but has little clinical value in managing postmenopausal osteoporosis. Routine radiographic studies (e.g., chest x-ray) will not detect changes until almost 30% of bone has been lost. This level of loss is about the level at which fractures occur, making routine studies of little clinical value in osteoporosis prevention. Bone scans may show increased uptake at the sites of previous fractures but will not indicate areas of lost bone mass prior to the occurrence of the fractures.

Most office-based devices for measuring bone density lack sensitivity, reliability, repeatability, and measure the less metabolically active appendicular bone. Dual-photon densitometry or quantitate computed tomography (QCT) are required if accurate, reproducible measures are to be obtained. The role of even this screening in therapy is controversial, however. Notelovitz has published a review of screening, prevention, and management that concludes that aggressive prevention and individualized treatment plans are best. These general recommendations could be applied to all peri- and postmenopausal patients regardless of the results of screening, making the test moot. Until more studies are available, pretreatment measurements or follow-up evaluations while on therapy appear to be neither indicated nor helpful clinically.

Endometrial Sampling

As noted, when patients experience unanticipated perimenopausal or postmenopausal bleeding (not associated with cyclic estrogen and progesterone therapy), careful assessment is required. Endometrial biopsy should be considered for any climacteric patient with unusual bleeding (even if immediate estrogen replacement is not considered). There is no need to biopsy every patient prior to estrogen therapy or to periodically evaluate patients. Cyclic withdrawal bleeding in conjunction with adequate cyclic progesterone therapy may safely be ignored. Any bleeding that occurs outside of the period of progesterone withdrawal or in patients on continuous progestins, requires biopsy. The cost-effectiveness of currently available techniques for evaluating postmenopausal bleeding was studied by Feldman who suggested that for low-risk patients with a single episode of bleeding, biopsy may be delayed and carried out if a second episode occurs. Should this happen, office biopsy is the most cost-effective method of sampling. Good endometrial samples may be obtained with a variety of sampling devices.

Some authors have suggested ultrasound to augment the traditional pelvic examination, reducing the need for endometrial sampling. The exact role of this technology is yet to be established. The cost-effectiveness of this option has not been studied and probably remains inappropriate for large scale screening. For the moment, the clinician must continue to rely on histologic evaluations in patients with suspected carcinoma.

Evaluation of the Postmenopausal Ovary

In the absence of good screening tools for ovarian cancer, patients with postmenopausal ovarian enlargement have been a special concern. Improved ultrasound screening may help decrease the need for exploratory surgery, but it is not a cost-effective modality for mass screening. For a patient with suspected pathology or one who is at high risk for cancer (such as those with a strong family history), ultrasound evaluations may provide some benefit. Currently, there is no serum test for ovarian cancer. CA 125 and other markers are used to monitor cancer chemotherapy, but these markers are not specific to cancer and have little or no value in screening or in the evaluation of a pelvic mass. (See also Chapter 10, Cancer Screening and Chapter 21, Pelvic Masses.)

THERAPEUTIC OPTIONS

In choosing the best therapy for a given patient, one must consider the impact and risks of therapy. Along with the options for therapy, there are many clinical considerations to be made about who should start, when, how, and for how long. The short-term goal of therapy is the relief of symptoms, whereas the long-term intent is protection from osteoporosis and cardiovascular disease.

Impact of Therapy

Hot Flashes, REM Sleep, and Sexuality

Therapy with estrogen or progesterone can prevent hot flashes, flushes, night sweats, improve REM sleep, and decrease sleep latency. A number of studies have indicated dose-dependent changes in the frequency and severity of hot flashes with estrogen replacement therapy. Most studies indicate a 95% or greater success rate after 3 to 4 weeks of therapy. Progestins such as medroxyprogesterone (Provera) and megestrol acetate (Megace) effect similar improvement in hot flash symptoms (70% effectiveness rate), but do not have the same effect on sleep patterns or sexual performance. Clonidine, alpha-methyldopa, naloxone, and veralipride have also been used with some success. These agent lack the other benefits of estrogen replacement, limiting their use. An often prescribed mixture of ergotamine tartrate, levorotatory alkaloids, and phenobarbital (Bellergal) appears to provide transitory relief from hot flashes, but this effect wears off after roughly 8 weeks of therapy.

Enhanced libido, sexual function, and vaginal lubrication are also obtained through the use of hormone therapy. Vaginal moisture can be supplemented through the use of water-based lubricants (e.g., KY-Jelly) or vaginal moisturizers (e.g., Replens, Lubrin). Estrogen therapy is also associated with 60% to 70% improvement rates in urologic symptoms, including genuine stress incontinence. Because of a high prevalence of mixed (stress and detrusor-based) incontinence, complete resolution of symptoms cannot be promised. (See also Chapter 27, Urinary Infection, Incontinence, and Pelvic Relaxation.)

Care must be exercised with patients who request hormones for changes in sexuality, libido, depression, mood swings, interpersonal problems, and the like. Most often these are not due to a metabolic or hormonal factors, but rather to other causes that will be unchanged by any hormonal therapy.

Osteoporosis

The most effective treatment of osteoporosis is prevention. For this reason, risk avoidance and good bone health should be encouraged from adolescence, when maximal bone is deposited, on to old age. For older women, osteoporosis prevention is predicated on adequate dietary intake of calcium (1000 to 1500 mg/d) and vitamin D (400 to 800 IU/d), weight-bearing exercise, cessation of smoking, alcohol and caffeine in moderation, and replacement of estrogen. The American diet tends to supply only about 500 mg of calcium daily. This may be improved through increased consumption of calcium-rich foods (Table 12.3). Calcium supplements should be reserved for those with inadequate intake or food intoler-

Table 12.3. Calcium Content of Common Foods

Food	Serving Size	Calcium (mg)
Almonds, dried	100 gm	254
Apricots (dried)	100 gm	86
Beans, kidney	1/2 cup	40
	100 gm	163
Beets (peeled, fresh)	100 gm	30
(tops)	100 gm	118
Broccoli, cooked	1/2 cup	70
Carrots (fresh)	1–6"	20
Caviar, pressed	100 gm	140
Cheese, American	1 oz	163
Blue	1 oz	150
Camembert	100 gm	680
Cheddar	1 oz	200
	100 gm	725
Cottage	1/2 cup	60
	100 gm	96
Parmesan	100 gm	1220
Swiss	1 oz	275
	100 gm	1090
Chicory and endives	100 gm	104
Chocolate (sweetened, milk)	100 gm	216
Dandelion greens (fresh)	100 gm	187
Dates (dried)	100 gm	65
Figs (dried)	100 gm	162
Hazelnuts	100 gm	290
Ice cream	1/2 cup	90
Kale (fresh)	100 gm	225
Lobster	100 gm	60
Milk, (cows) whole	100 gm	125
	1 cup	300
Buttermilk	1 cup	285
Chocolate	1 cup	284
Condensed (sweetened)	100 gm	273
Dried whole	100 gm	949
Dried nonfat	100 gm	1300
Molasses	100 gm	273
Olives (green)	100 gm	87
Parsley (fresh)	100 gm	190
Peanut butter	100 gm	74
Potato chips	100 gm	30
Raisins	100 gm	78
Sardines (with bones)	3 oz	350
Soy beans (dried)	100 gm	227
Spinach (fresh)*	100 gm	87
Turnip greens	100 gm	260
Water cress	100 gm	187
Yogurt, low-fat	1/2 cup	400

*Some high calcium food such as spinach, Swiss chard, and other "greens" contain high levels of oxalic acid which bind calcium, reducing its absorption by the gastrointestinal tract.

ance that prevents achieving sufficient dietary levels. Calcium carbonate provides the greatest percent of elemental calcium and calcium citrate is highly absorbable, making either acceptable supplements. When used, these should be taken in divided doses over the course of the day. Excessive intake of calcium supplements has been associated with an increased risk of stone formation and should be discouraged. Most individuals receive adequate amounts of vitamin D through diet or exposure to light. Supplementation significantly increases the risk of renal stones and has had little proven value in preventing osteoporosis.

Weight-bearing exercise (such as walking 1 mile twice a day) has been established as valuable in maintaining bone and cardiovascular health. Trials of calcium supplementation in combination with exercise have demonstrated a synergy between these two therapies. When not contraindicated, a program of exercise should be advocated for all patients.

As important as diet and exercise are, they are not sufficient to prevent osteoporosis by themselves. When combined with estrogen, however, bone mass can be maintained or even increased. Estrogen replacement will not significantly affect the normal (background) rate of bone loss due to aging. Therefore, optimal response will only be obtained when replacement therapy is begun at the time of estrogen loss or soon after. Estrogen's effect on bone protection appears to be dependent on obtaining a relatively normal (premenopausal) blood level (40–60 pg/mL) and is not affected by the route of administration. Estrogen replacement is associated with a reduction by about 50% in the rate of hip and arm fractures in postmenopausal women. This value has been reported to rise to over 90% reduction in fracture rates when estrogen is used for more than 5 years. Vertebral fractures may be reduced by as much as 80% for these same women.

These improvements in bone health are predicated on obtaining a serum estrogen level comparable to that of premenopausal women. This may be accomplished using 0.625 mg of conjugated equine estrogen or estrone sulfate, 1.0 mg of micronized estradiol, a 0.05-mg estradiol patch, or their equivalent. Dosages below these levels generally will not give adequate bone protection.

Several studies indicate that progesterone therapy can also decrease bone loss. This effect may be less than that found with estrogen and may have only slight or no additive effect when both estrogen and progesterone are used. Progesterone-only therapy does not provide any cardiovascular protection.

When estrogen or progesterone replacement is contraindicated or unacceptable, the use of biphosphonates may also inhibit bone resorption. This therapy lacks the additional cardiovascular and other benefits of estrogen, relegating it to a second-line therapy.

Cardiovascular Disease

Although estrogen therapy appears to have a significant effect on cardiovascular health for postmenopausal women, it cannot substitute for a healthy lifestyle or reverse the effects of high-risk behaviors such as smoking. When other factors are controlled for, estrogen replacement may reduce cardiovascular disease and strokes by roughly one half. Concern has been raised in the past over the use of estrogen in the presence of hypertension. Most published studies suggest no worsening and, in some cases, an improvement in hypertension with estrogen replacement. It appears that hypertension, by itself, is not the absolute contraindication to replacement therapy that it once was.

Risks of Therapy

No medical therapy is without risk and not all patients are candidates for estrogen replacement. Absolute and relative contraindications for estrogen replacement are shown in Table 12.4. Concerns about the risks of estrogen replacement therapy have generally centered around three areas: cancer, metabolic effects of steroids, and side effects.

Concerns about estrogen possibly inducing cancer have generally focused on the area of breast and uterine malignancies. Most studies suggest that there is no effect or a small, but probably not significant, decrease in the risk of breast cancer for patients on estrogen replacement therapy. The relatively small effects seen mean that any definitive study would have to be prohibitively large. Even less clear is the impact, if any, that may be associated with progestin or androgen therapy. The absence of definitive proof and the relatively high prevalence of breast cancer require that vigilance be maintained for all women. (See also Chapter 14, Breast Disease.)

One area of controversy has been the role of hormone replacement in patients with known (treated) breast cancer. Some help with this question is provided by a committee opinion on the subject from the American College of Obstetricians and Gynecologists. Based on an extensive review of the literature, they conclude that there are no data indicating an increased risk of breast cancer recurrence in patients receiving estrogen replacement therapy. There is even one study in the literature that suggests a better survival for women with breast cancer when estrogen replacement is used. Other risk factors, short- and long-term benefits, as well as the desires of the patient must all be balanced against an uncertain role for hormones in recurrent breast cancer. As in most such instances, the best approach is one tailored to the specifics of the individual patient and agreed on by both physician and patient after an informed discussion.

Less controversial is the role of estrogen in endometrial pathology. Unopposed estrogen therapy is associated with a three to twelve times increase in the risk of endometrial cancer (from a rate of roughly 1/1000 women). This increase in risk is dependent on the dose

Table 12.4. Contraindications to Estrogen Replacement Therapy

Contraindications
> Active liver disease
> Carcinoma of the breast (current)
> Chronic liver damage (impaired function)
> Endometrial carcinoma (current)
> Recent thrombosis (with or without emboli)
> Unexplained vaginal bleeding

Relative contraindications/special considerations
> Endometriosis
> Familial hyperlipidemia
> Gallbladder disease
> Hypertension (uncontrolled)
> Migraine headaches
> Seizure disorders
> Thrombophlebitis (unknown risk)
> Uterine leiomyomas

and duration of therapy, but not the manner in which the estrogen is given. (Cyclic administration offers no protection.) When unopposed estrogen therapy is used, the rate of endometrial hyperplasia approaches 30%. The risk of endometrial cancer appears to return to the background rate roughly 6 months after therapy is discontinued. In women who continue therapy, the risk may be reduced to below that of untreated women through the addition of progestins to the therapeutic plan. The exact duration of progestin therapy each month required to confer this protection is not known. Treatment with 7 days of progestin per month is associated with an annual incidence of hyperplasia of about 3%. Most authors suggest a minimum of 12 days of progestin therapy, which is also dose-dependent. Common agents are medroxyprogesterone acetate (5–10 mg), norethindrone (0.35–1.0 mg), and norgestrel (0.15 mg). Continuous therapy with 2.5 mg of medroxyprogesterone acetate daily appears to give adequate protection, but unpredictable bleeding and possible adverse effects on lipids limits this therapy. Current evidence suggests that estrogen replacement is not contraindicated in patients with successful surgical treatment of endometrial cancer.

The metabolism of steroids by the liver induces enzymatic changes that may be both beneficial and harmful. Liver metabolism, especially the first pass metabolism of orally administered steroids, causes the lipid changes noted above as well as changes in renin-angiotensin and antithrombin III. It is these latter changes that were thought to be responsible for the elevations of blood pressure and increased risk of thromboembolism seen in early, high-dose, oral contraceptive pills. At the doses used for estrogen replacement, these changes are minimal and do not represent a problem therapeutically, except in patients at high risk. Estrogen given through non-oral routes (e.g., transdermal) is associated with less change in hepatic clotting factors and theoretically poses less risk because of a lower metabolic load.

Hepatic metabolism of orally administered estrogen also leads to an increase in bile cholesterol and biliary stasis. As a result, the risk of gall stone formation is increased more than 2.5 times with oral therapy. (This is also true for oral contraceptives.) Nonoral estrogen therapy does not appear to carry these risks even though serum lipid changes (after 3–6 months of therapy) are the same.

The side effects generally associated with estrogen administration are weight gain, bloating, breast soreness, and mood swings. These are the effects that were also associated with the early high-dose oral contraceptive pills. Once again, in the dosage range usually used for replacement, these effects are uncommon and mild. Changes in dosage, route, or compound usually correct problems encountered.

Clinical Choices

As with most other areas of medicine, the best course of therapy is one decided by a collaborative effort with the patient, based both on the needs and circumstances of the individual and on a thorough understanding of the involved pathophysiology and pharmacology.

Who

Should all women be started on estrogen replacement? Only thin women, smokers, or those with a bad family history? Although there is considerable variation from patient to patient, most would agree that all patients should be considered for estrogen replacement. Replacement is most important for those with premature menopause (natural or surgical), a family history of osteoporosis or heart disease, and those with symptoms.

When

When should therapy be considered or started? When hot flashes or other symptoms appear but before the loss of periods? At an arbitrary age? After 6 months of amenorrhea? Each option could be defended, but many feel that an early start on replacement minimizes bone loss and increases compliance (especially when the presence of a uterus demands a progesterone and periodic withdrawal bleeding).

Before any estrogen therapy is instituted, a careful history and physical examination (including breast and pelvic examinations) is required. Possible sources of caution or contraindication are sought. Routine health maintenance issues such as blood pressure, mammography, Pap smear, and periodic laboratory evaluations should also be addressed.

What

What route is most appropriate? Oral? Patch? Vaginal? What role should progesterone play? The route of estrogen delivery is a source of continuing debate. The most common routes are oral, transdermal, and topical. The use of injectable estrogen and subdermal pellets has fallen out of favor. Injectable estrogen tends to give excessive levels initially, declining to subtherapeutic values just before the next treatment is due. Subdermal estradiol implants are available in some parts of the world. Like injectable methods, these eliminate concerns about compliance, although unpredictable absorption patterns have caused their withdrawal from use in the United States.

Oral estrogen is inexpensive and generally well tolerated. The need for gastrointestinal absorption and initial liver metabolism results in higher doses needed to obtain the desired serum levels. The induction of liver enzymes help to push HDL levels up and LDL levels down, but non-oral estrogen gives the same effect, although only after 3 to 6 months of therapy. Oral estrogen is associated with a greater risk of hypertension, clotting abnormalities, and gallstones.

Many clinicians like the more physiologic approach to estrogen replacement offered by the transdermal patch (β-estradiol delivered directly to the blood stream), but skin irritation and adherence of the patch is a problem in 5% to 10% of patients. This has been of special concern in hot, humid climates, although recent reports suggest this is less of a problem than anticipated. Many patients experience fewer gastrointestinal side effects with transdermal estrogen.

Topical estrogen is useful as a local adjunct, but up to 25% of the dose is absorbed systemically. Therefore, topical estrogen does not eliminate systemic side effects; it also does not provide cost-effective systemic therapy.

If the patient still has her uterus, a progesterone is always indicated to reduce the risk of hyperplasia and malignancy. Less clear is the role of testosterone, which should probably be reserved for carefully selected patients only.

A list of currently available estrogen and progesterone preparations are shown in Tables 12.5 and 12.6.

Table 12.5. Currently Available Estrogens (noncontraceptive)

Generic name	Available doses (mg)	Brand name(s)
Oral		
Conjugated equine estrogens	0.3, 0.625, 0.9, 1.25, 2.5	Premarin, PMB (Premarin + meprobamate)
Diethylstilbestrol	0.1, 0.25, 0.5, 1, 5	(generic)
Esterified estrogens	0.3, 0.625, 1.25, 2.5	Estratab, Menest, Estratest/ Estratest HS (+ methyltestosterone)
Ethinyl estradiol	0.02, 0.05, 0.5	Estinyl
Micronized estradiol	0.5, 1, 2	Estrace
Piperazine estrone sulfate, estropipate	0.3, 0.625, 1.25, 2.5, 5	Ogen, Ortho-est, (generic)
Quinestrol	0.1	Estrovis
Injectable		
Conjugated equine estrogens	25 mg/mL	Premarin (IV)
Estradiol benzoate	0.5 mg/mL	(generic)
Estradiol cypionate	1, 5 mg/mL	Depo-estradiol, Depo-Gynogen, Depogen, Estra-D, Estacyp, Estroject, (generic)
Estradiol valerate (oil)	2 mg/mL	Deladiol, Diaval, Duragen, Estra-L, Gynogen, Menaval, (generic)
Estradiol valerate (oil)	10, 20, 40 mg/mL	Delestrogen, Valergen
Estrone (aqueous)	2, 5	Estrone, Thelin
Ethinyl estradiol	1 g (powder)	(generic)
Polyestradiol phosphate	20 mg/mL	Estradurin
Topical		
17β-estradiol	0.05, 0.1 mg/d	Estraderm (patch)
Conjugated equine estrogens	0.625 mg/g	Premarin
Estradiol	0.1 mg/g	Estrace
Estropipate	1.5 mg/g	Ogen

Table 12.6. Currently Available Progestins (Noncontraceptive)

Generic name	Available doses (mg)	Brand name(s)
Oral		
Medroxyprogesterone acetate	2.5, 5, 10	Amen, Cycrin, Curretab, Provera
Megestrol acetate	20, 40	Megace
Norethindrone (norethisterone)	0.35, 5	Norlutin, Nor-Q-D, Micronor
Norethindrone acetate	5	Agestin, Norlutate
Injectable		
Medroxyprogesterone acetate	100, 150, 400 mg/mL	Depo-provera
Hydroxyprogesterone caproate	125, 250 mg/mL	Delalutin, Gesteval LA, Hilutin, (generic)
Progesterone	50, 100 mg/mL	Gesterol, Progestaject

How

How much is enough, too much, or just right? Oral: 0.625 mg or 1.25 mg conjugated estrogens? Patch: 0.05 mg or 0.1 mg? The objective of estrogen replacement is to approximate physiologic levels found during the reproductive years. This may be accomplished by a level at or above 0.625 mg of conjugated estrogen, 0.05 mg transdermal estrogen, 1 mg of micronized estradiol, 1.25 mg of estrone sulfate, or their equivalent. This dose may have to be raised in patients who continue to have symptoms or in those where a lower resulting blood level might be anticipated (smokers). For osteoporosis prevention, the addition of calcium supplements may be appropriate for most patients, which it appears cannot substitute for, or allow a reduction in, estrogen replacement. This level of estrogen replacement provides good symptom relief and appears to be adequate to obtain the proposed cardiovascular benefits as well.

How should it be given? Three weeks on, one week off? Continuously? The most commonly used estrogen replacement strategy (for women who still have their uterus) is a combination of estrogen and cyclic progestin that results in periodic withdrawal bleeding (Fig. 12.2). This provides protection from unopposed estrogen-mediated hyperplasia and reduces the risk of cancer, but at a cost of convenience that many patients find objectionable. While there are many approaches to this therapy, many are shifting to continuous estrogen with progestins once a month. Continuous estrogen is easier to remember and provides better hormone levels for bone and heart protection.

The use of continuous progesterone to prevent withdrawal bleeding has been disappointing in its degree of success (about 30% of women actually remain amenorrheic) and concerns about the long-term adverse effects of currently available progestins have been raised. Alternative regimens using continuous estrogen and progestin have been proposed, but random or continuous bleeding is still often encountered, necessitating biopsy. In one published study of 1724 women at 99 sites studied for 1 year, only half of the patients remained amenorrheic. An alternative pattern of replacement has been suggested based on experience with a group of 40 women placed on continuous estrogen with alternating

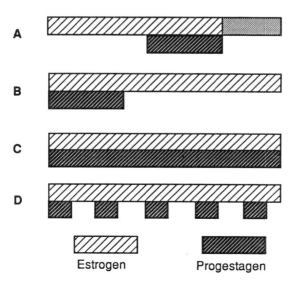

Figure 12.2. Common patterns of estrogen and progestin administration. The three most common patterns of estrogen replacement for women with a uterus are shown. One of the oldest patterns is a 3 weeks on, 1 week off approach that mimics oral contraceptives (**A**). For a variety of reasons, many physicians have moved to continuous estrogen with progestin added for a period of 12 to 14 days at the beginning of the calendar month (**B**). For some selected patients, a continuous estrogen and low-dose progestin pattern (**C**) may be appropriate. A new method has been proposed (**D**) using alternating 3-day periods of progestin (see text).

Estrogen   Progestagen

3-day segments of progestin and rest. Most patients in this study had resolution of hot flashes (76%) and 80% had no vaginal bleeding by 6 months of therapy. No endometrial hyperplasia was found in 33 patients who continued this therapy for 24 months. A smaller series of women given progesterone withdrawal on a quarterly basis found it to be a safe alternative as well. Although only pilot studies, alternate therapeutic methods hold the promise of greater compliance and patient satisfaction. These alternative therapies must still be considered investigational until more data are accumulated.

Compliance

The issue of compliance deserves mentioning. Many reports indicate that compliance with hormonal replacement therapy is poor. Often quoted figures indicate that 20% to 30% of women do not fill their prescriptions and 20% of women stop taking their medication within 9 months. Roughly 10% of patients take their hormones sporadically. It has been estimated that only 15% to 25% of eligible women take replacement hormones. Clearly, the medical benefits of estrogen replacement will only have an impact if we can motivate our patients to start and stay with therapy. A few minutes of education may make a big difference. Periodic follow-up visits should be scheduled to encourage compliance and to check for both therapeutic effects and the possibility of unwanted side effects. This should include a menstrual and sexual history and blood pressure measurement.

HINTS AND COMMON QUESTIONS

Although it is obvious, there is always the possibility of a pregnancy as the source for lost periods or irregular bleeding, even in the older patient with "hot flashes."

Often debated is the role of progesterone in patients without a uterus. There have been several reports that suggest an added benefit in osteoporosis and cardiovascular protection, and reduced risks of breast cancer for patients given progestins in addition to estrogen replacement. Unfortunately, this effect has been small and most other studies have failed to support these reports. Progestin therapy is often associated with bloating, breast tenderness, premenstural syndrome (PMS), and adverse lipid changes. In the absence of proved benefit, most now recommend that patients without a uterus receive estrogen replacement only.

The role of oral contraceptives in older patients is changing (see Chapter 9, Contraception), but we may now face the problem of when to declare fertility ended and begin estrogen replacement for the older woman having artificially regular menses on oral contraception. The most effective way to evaluate the status of these patients is to obtain a serum FSH just prior to the first pill of a patient's contraceptive pack. If the FSH is elevated, ovarian failure is likely and a transition to replacement estrogen may be made. (The use of adjunctive contraception such as condom for a period of 6 months or a year may still be prudent if for no other reason than peace of mind.) If the FSH level is normal or only slightly elevated, continued contraceptive coverage is warranted.

Whichever route is selected for estrogen replacement, there is evidence that patients who smoke should be considered for a higher dose of estrogen. While this is being discussed with the patient, it is often a good time to address smoking and other health issues. Patients are more aware of health issues as their bodies are changing. As a result, counseling about smoking cessation, weight reduction, exercise programs, routine screening (e.g., mammography, breast self-examination, cholesterol, thyroid), and other health protection strategies is often better received and more successful.

Occasionally, one will encounter a patient who requires increased, or increasing, doses of estrogen to control symptoms. When moderate doses are required, some consideration should be given to changing the type or route of estrogen use. Agents that give higher levels of estradiol (micronized estradiol, transdermal estradiol) will give better symptom relief owing to the greater biologic activity of estradiol over estrone. If continuing night sweats are the problem, have the patient take her estrogen just before bedtime.

Some women experience thinning or loss of hair during the climacteric period or with the start of estrogen replacement. To determine whether this is physiologic or owing to scalp pathology, look at the base of a few shed hairs. If the hair shaft tapers or ends abruptly, the loss is due to the normal resting phase of the follicle and the hair loss will not be permanent. If the base is bulbous with adherent white or gelatinous material (a portion of the follicle itself), the loss may be due to scalp disease and a dermatologic referral is in order.

Many patient express concern about the possibility of weight gain due to estrogen therapy. There is at least one study in the literature that suggests that estrogen replacement therapy avoids a 1 kg to 2 kg increase in body fat found in untreated women.

"How long will I have to take my estrogen?" is a common question posed by patients when they are started on replacement therapy. The same changes that take place when the ovaries cease their production will occur when estrogen ceases to be supplied by the pharmacy. Until something better comes along, estrogen therapy is a life-long process.

It is important to reassure patients that the change of life is no longer the milestone marking the end of something (reproduction, vitality, sexuality, activity, health, and so forth). While it does signal the loss of reproductive function, there is no reason that one should expect disability, inactivity, loss of sexuality, family conflicts or estrangement, depression, and the like to be a part of this period of life. Just as adolescence, marriage, job change, or a death in the family represent a change of life, menopause is just another stage in its evolution; no less, no more. For many patients, this phase of their life may be even more rewarding with the opportunity for retirement, travel, pursuit of hobbies, and sexuality freed from the worries of pregnancy.

SUGGESTED READINGS

General References

American College of Obstetricians and Gynecologists. Hormone Replacement Therapy. ACOG Technical Bulletin 166. Washington, DC: ACOG, 1992.

American College of Obstetricians and Gynecologists. Osteoporosis. ACOG Technical Bulletin 167. Washington, DC: ACOG, 1992.

Awwad JT, Toth TL, Schiff I. Abnormal uterine bleeding in the perimenopause. Int J Fertil 1993;38:261.

Committee on Gynecologic Practice. Estrogen replacement in women with previously treated breast cancer. Washington, DC: American College of Obstetricians and Gynecologists Committee Opinion No. 135, April 1994.

Henderson BE, Paganini-Hill A, Ross RK. Decreased mortality in users of estrogen replacement therapy. Arch Intern Med 1991;151:75.

Jones KP (ed). Estrogen replacement therapy. Clin Obstet Gynecol 1992;35:854.

Kaplan FS. Osteoporosis. Pathophysiology and prevention. Clin Symp 1987;39:1.

Lorrain J, Plouffe L JR, Ravnikar V, Speroff L, Watts N, eds. Comprehensive Management of Menopause. New York: Springer-Verlag, 1993.

Mishell DR. Menopause Physiology and Pharmacology. Chicago: Year Book Medical Publishers, 1987.

National Institutes of Health, Consensus Conference. Osteoporosis. JAMA 1984;252:799–802.

Notelovitz M. Osteoporosis: screening, prevention, and management. Fertil Steril 1993; 59:707.

Spencer G. Population estimates and projections. In: Projections of the Populations of the United States, by Age, Sex and Race: 1988–2080. Series P-25, No. 1018. Washington, DC: US Department of Commerce, Bureau of the Census, 1989.

Yen SSC, Jaffe RB. Reproductive Endocrinology. Philadelphia: WB Saunders, 1986.

Specific References

General

Bonilla-Musoles F, Ballester MJ, Simon C, Serra V, Raga F. Is avoidance of surgery possible in patients with perimenopausal ovarian tumors using transvaginal ultrasound and duplex color doppler sonography? J Ultrasound Med 1993;12:33.

Butler RN, Lewis MI, Hoffman E, Whitehead ED. Love and sex after 60: how to evaluate and treat the sexually active woman. Geriatrics 1994;49:33.

Byrjalsen I, Haarbo J, Christianses C. Role of cigarette smoking on the postmenopausal endometrium during sequential estrogen and progesterone therapy. Obstet Gynecol 1993;81:1016.

Committee on Gynecologic Practice. Contraception for women in their later reproductive years. Washington, DC: American College of Obstetricians and Gynecologists Committee Opinion No. 41, April 1985.

Fleischer AC, Rodgers WH, Kepple DM, Williams LL, Jones HW III. Color doppler sonography of ovarian masses: a multiparameter analysis. J Ultrasound Med 1993;12:41.

Grady D, Rubin SM, Petitti DB, et al. Hormone therapy to prevent disease and prolong life in postmenopausal women. Ann Intern Med 1992;117:1016.

Hassanger C, Christiansen C. Estrogen/gestagen therapy changes soft tissue body composition in postmenopausal women. Metabolism 1989;38:662.

Heiman J. Sexuality in older women. In Stenchever MA (ed). Care of the Aging Woman. Washington, DC: Association of Professors of Gynecology and Obstetrics 1994, p 11–1.

Kampen DL, Sherwin BB. Estrogen use and verbal memory in healthy postmenopausal women. Obstet Gynecol 199;83:979.

Kronenberg F. Hot flashes: epidemiology and physiology. Ann NY Acad Sci 1990;592:52.

LaRosa J. Metabolic effects of estrogens and progestins. Fertil Steril 1994;62(suppl):140s.

Limousiz-Lamothe M-A, Mairon N, Joyce CRB, Le Gal M. Quality of life after the menopause: influence of hormonal replacement therapy. Am J Obstet Gynecol 1994;170:618.

Maheux R, Naud F, Rioux M, Grenier R, Lemay A, et al. A randomized, double-blind, placebo-controlled study on the effect of conjugated estrogens on skin thickness. Am J Obstet Gynecol 1994;170:642.

Schwingl PJ, Hulka BS, Harlow SD. Risk factors for menopausal hot flashes. Obstet Gynecol 1994;84:29.

Tatryn IV, Lomax P, Bajorek JD, et al. Postmenopausal hot flashes: a disorder of thermoregulation. Maturitas 1980;2:101.

Weber AM, Walters MD, Schover LR, Mitchinson A. Sexual function in women with uterovaginal prolapse and urinary incontinence. Obstet Gynecol 1995;85:483.

Weiner Z, Beck D, Sheiner M, et al. Screening for ovarian cancer in women with breast cancer with transvaginal sonography and color flow imaging. J Ultrasound Med 1993;12:387.

Cardiovascular

Avila MH, Walker AM, Jick H. Use of replacement estrogens and the risk of myocardial infarction. Epidemiology 1990;1:128.

Cook D, Stevenson JC. Progestins, lipid metabolism and hormone replacement therapy. Br J Obstet Gynaecol 1991;98:749.

Crook D, Cust MP, Gantger KF, et al. Comparison of transdermal and oral estrogen-progestin replacement therapy: effects on serum lipids and lipoproteins. Am J Obstet Gynecol 1992;166:950.

Gordon T, Kannel WB, Hjortland MC, McNamara FM. Menopause and coronary heart disease: the Framingham study. Ann Int Med 1978;89:157.

Hazzard WR. Estrogen replacement and cardiovascular disease: serum lipids and blood pressure effects. Am J Obstet Gynecol 1989;161:1847.

Henderson BE, Ross RK, Paganini-Hill A. Estrogen use and cardiovascular disease. J Reprod Med 1985;30(10 suppl):814.

Julius U, Fritsch H, Rehak E, Fucker K, Leonhardt MH. Impact of hormone replacement therapy on postprandial lipoproteins and lipoprotein (a) in normolipemid postmenopausal women. Clin Invest 1994;72:502.

Kuhn FE, Rackley CE. Coronary artery disease in women: risk factors, evaluation, treatment, and prevention. Arch Intern Med 1993;153:2626.

Lindheim SR, Notelovitz M, Feldman EB, Larsen S, Khan FY, Lobo RA. The independent effects of exercise and estrogen on lipids and lipoproteins in postmenopausal women. Obstet Gynecol 1994;83:167.

Lobo RA, Speroff L. International consensus conference on postmenopausal hormone therapy and the cardiovascular system. Fertil Steril 1994;62(suppl):176s.

Manson JE. Postmenopausal hormone therapy and atherosclerotic disease. Am Heart J 1994;128:1337.

Petitti DB, Perlman JA, Sidney S. Noncontraceptive etrogens and mortality: long-term follow-up of women in the Walnut Creek Study. Obstet Gynecol 1987;70:289.

Posner BM. Diet, menopause and serum cholesterol levels in women: the Framingham Study. Am Heart J 1993;125:483.

Stampfer MJ, Graham A, Colditz A. Estrogen replacement therapy and coronary heart disease: a quantitative assessment of the epidemiologic evidence. Prev Med 1991;20:47.

Stampfer MJ, Willett WC, Colditz GA, Rosner B, Speizer FE, Hennekens CH. A prospective study of postmenopausal estrogen therapy and coronary heart disease. The Framingham Study. N Engl J Med 1985;313:1044.

Wilson PWF, Garrison RJ, Castelli WP. Postmenopausal estrogen use, cigarette smoking and cardiovascular morbidity in women over 50. The Framingham Study. N Engl J Med 1985;313:1038.

Wren BG, Routledge AD. The effect of type and dose of estrogen on the blood pressure of post-menopausal women. Maturitas 1983;5:135.

Writing Group for the PEPI Trial. Effects of estrogen or estrogen/progestin regimens on heart disease risk factors in postmenopausal women. The Postmenopausal Estrogen/Progestin Interventions (PEPI) Trial. JAMA 1995;273:199.

Osteoporosis

Cavanaugh DJ, Cann CE. Brisk walking does not stop bone loss in postmenopausal women. Bone 1988;9:201.

Davis MR. Screening for postmenopausal osteoporosis. Fertil Steril 1987;1:156.

Eriksen EF, Colvard DS, Berg NJ, et al. Evidence of estrogen receptors in normal human osteoblast-like cells. Science 1988;241:81.

Ettinger B, Genant HK, Cann CE. Postmenopausal bone loss is prevented by treatment with low-dosage estrogen with calcium. Ann Int Med 1987;106:40.

Gamgacciani M, Spinetti A, Taponeco F, et al. Longitudinal evaluation of perimenopausal vertebral bone loss: effects of a low-dose oral contraceptive preparation on bone mineral density and metabolism. Obstet Gynecol 1994;83:392.

Holland EFN, Chow JWM, Studd JWW, Leather AT, Chambers TJ. Histomorphometric changes in the skeleton of postmenopausal women with low bone mineral density treated with percutaneous estradiol implants. Obstet Gynecol 1994;83:387.

Lindsay R, Hart DM, Clark DM. The minimum effective dose of estrogen for prevention of postmenopausal bone loss. Obstet Gynecol 1984;63:759.

Paganini-Hill A, Ross RK, Gerkins VR, et al. A case control study of menopausal estrogen therapy and hip fractures. Ann Intern Med 1981;95:28.

Quigley MET, Martin PL, Burnier AM, Brooks P. Estrogen therapy arrests bone loss in elderly women. Am J Obstet Gyencol 1987;156:1516.

Raisz LG (ed). Clinical indications for bone mass measurements: a report from the Scientific Advisory Board of the National Osteoporosis Foundation. J Bone Miner Res 1989;4(suppl 2):1.

Riis B, Thomsen K, Christiansen C. Does calcium supplementation prevent postmenopausal bone loss? A double-blind, controlled clinical study. N Engl J Med 1987;316:173.

Stevenson JC, Cust MP, Gangar KF, Hillard TC, Lees B, Whitehead MI. Effects of transdermal versus oral hormone replacement therapy on bone density in spine and proximal femur in postmenopausal women. Lancet 1990;335:265.

Toteson AN, Rosenthal DI, Melton LJ III, Weinstein MC. Cost-effectiveness of screening perimenopausal white women for osteoporosis: bone densitometry and hormone replacement therapy. Ann Intern Med 1990;113:594.

Weiss NS, Ure CL, Ballard JH, et al. Decreased risk of fractures of the hip and lower forearm with postmenopausal use of estrogen. N Engl J Med 1980;303:1195.

Postmenopausal bleeding

Cohen I, Rosen DJD, Tepper R, et al. Ultrasonographic evaluation of the endometrium and correlation with endometrial sampling in postmenopausal patients treated with tamoxifen. J Ultrasound Med 1993;5:275.

Feldman S, Berkowitz RS, Tosteson ANA. Cost-effectiveness of strategies to evaluate postmenopausal bleeding. Obstet Gynecol 1993;81:968.

Ferry J, Farnsworth A, Webster M, Wren B. The efficacy of the pipelle endometrial biopsy in detecting endometrial carcinoma. Aust NZ J Obstet Gynaecol 1993;33:76.

Goldchmit R, Katz Z, Blickstein I, Caspi B, Dgani R. The accuracy of endometrial pipelle sampling with and without sonographic measurement of endometrial thickness. Obstet Gynecol 1993;82:727.

Goldstein SR. Use of ultrasonohysterography for triage of perimenoapusal patients with unexplained uterine bleeding. Am J Obstet Gynecol 1994;170:565.

Law J. Histological sampling of the endometrium—a comparison between formal curettage and the pipelle sampler. Br J Obstet Gynaecol 1993;100:503.

Lipscomb GH, Lopatine SM, Stovall TG, Ling FW. A randomized comparison of the pipelle, accurette, and explora endometrial sampling devices. Am J Obstet Gynecol 1994;170:591.

Reid PC, Brown VA, Fothergill DJ. Outpatient investigation of postmenopausal bleeding. Br J Obstet Gynaecol 1993;100:498.

Warwick A, Ferryman S, Musgrove C, Redman C. An evaluation of the gynecheck for endometrial sampling. J Obstet Gynaecol 1993;13:198.

Weiner Z, Beck D, Rottem S, Brandes JM, Thaler I. Uterine artery flow velocity waveforms and color flow imaging in women with perimenopausal and postmenopausal bleeding. Acta Obstet Gynecol Scand 1993;72:162.

Therapy

Archer DF, Pickar JH, Bottiglioni F, Menopause study group. Bleeding patterns in postmenopausal women taking continuous combined or sequential regimens of conjugated estrogens with medroxyprogesterone acetate. Obstet Gynecol 1994;83:686.

Casper RF, Chapdelaine A. Estrogen and interrupted progestin: a new concept for menopausal hormone replacement therapy. Am J Obstet Gynecol 1993;168:1188.

Ettinger B, Selby J, Citron JT, VanGessel A, et al. Cyclic hormone replacement therapy using quarterly progestin. Obstet Gynecol 1994;83:6693.

Kainz C, Gitsch G, Stani J, Breitenecker G, et al. When applied to facial skin, does estrogen ointment have systemic effects? Arch Gynecol Obstet 1993;253:71.

Notelovitz M. Estrogen replacement therapy: indications, contraindications, and agent selection. Am J Obstet Gynecol 1989;161:1832.

O'Neill S, Kirkegard Y. An Australian experience of transdermal oestradiol patches in a subtropical climate. Aust NZ J Obstet Gynecol 1993;33:327.

Ravnikar VA. Compliance with hormone therapy. Am J Obstet Gynecol 1987;156:1332.

Seleh AA, Dorey LG, Dombrowski MP, et al. Thrombosis and hormone replacement therapy in postmenopausal women. Am J Obstet Gynecol 1993;169:1554.

Suhonen SP, Allonen HO, Lähteenmäki P. Sustained-release subdermal estradiol implants: a new alternative in estrogen replacement therapy. Am J Obstet Gynecol 1993;169:1248.

Estrogens and Cancer

Bergkvist L, Adami HO, Persson I, Hoover R, Schairer C. The risk of breast cancer after estrogen and estrogen-progestin replacement. N Engl J Med 1989;321:293.

Bergkvist L, Adami HO, Persson I, et al. Prognosis after breast cancer diagnosis in women exposed to oestrogens and progesterone replacement therapy. Am J Epidemiol 1989;130:221.

Butler WJ. Hormone-replacement therapy in patients with estrogen-sensitive malignancies. Female Patient 1995; 20:43.

Campbell S, Whitehead M. Oestrogen therapy and the menopausal syndrome. Br J Obstet Gynaecol 1987;4:31.

Colditz GA, Egan KM, Stampfer MJ. Hormone replacement therapy and risk of breast cancer: results from epidemiologic studies. Am J Obstet Gynecol 1993;168:1473.

Colditz GA, Hankinson SE, Hunter DJ, et al. The use of estrogens and progestins and the risk of breast cancer in postmenopausal women. N Engl J Med 1995;332:1589.

Colditz GA, Stampfer MJ, Willet WC, et al. Prospective study of estrogen replacement therapy and risk of breast cancer in post-menopausal women. JAMA 1990;264:2648.

Dupont WD, Page DL. Menopausal estrogen replacement therapy and breast cancer. Arch Intern Med 1991;151:67.

Gambrell RD Jr, Massey FM, Castaneda TA, et al. The use of the progestogen challenge test to reduce the risk of endometrial cancer. Obstet Gynecol 1980;55:732.

Henderson BE. The cancer question: An overview of recent epidemiologic and retrospective data. Am J Obstet Gynecol 1989;161:1859.

Henderson BE, Ross RK, Lobo RA, Pike MC, Mack TM. Re-evaluating the role of progesterone therapy after menopause. Fertil Steril 1988;49(suppl 5):9s.

Steinberg KK, Thacker SB, Smith SJ, et al. A meta-analysis of the effect of estrogen replacement on the risk of breast cancer. JAMA 1991;265:1985.

World Health Organization. Research on the menopause. World Health Organization Technical Report Series 670. Geneva: WHO, 1981.

IV

Specific gynecologic problems

13

Abnormal Pap Smears

The Papanicolaou "Pap" smear represents one of the most outstanding examples of a simple screening test that can alter the impact of a disease. The incidence of and mortality from cervical cancer has steadily and dramatically declined over the years since the widespread use of Pap smears has become routine. Recent changes in the way these smears are interpreted and reported have made the management of patients with abnormalities at once both easier and more difficult.

No modality in medicine, be it screening, diagnostic, or therapeutic, is perfect. Therefore, is must be recognized that despite adherence to screening protocols, careful execution of the collection technique, and experienced interpretation of the findings a few women will still develop cervical cancer. We should, however, make every attempt to aggressively identify, treat, and follow those patients identified by Pap smear as having abnormalities.

BACKGROUND AND SCIENCE

The Pap smear that began as a way of assessing the endocrinology of the menstrual cycle, has become a major tool in the detection of cancer that can be applied to many diverse sites throughout the body. The cytologic detection of malignant and premalignant change is based on the well-recognized progression of cellular changes that normal cells undergo as they mature. Abnormalities of this progression are the hallmark of dysplastic and malignant cells. These cellular changes may be related to the underlying histologic changes responsible, allowing clinical decisions to be rendered (Table 13.1).

Table 13.1. Histologic Changes Detected by Cytologic Testing

Descriptive convention					
Class system	Class I (normal)	Class II inflammation	Class III Mild dysplasia or Moderate dysplasia	Class IV Severe dysplasia CIS	Class V Suggestive of cancer
CIN system	Normal	Inflammatory	CIN I or / CIN II	CIN III	Suggestive of cancer
Bethesda system	Within normal limits	Inflammatory a) Without atypia b) With atypia	Low-grade SIL	High-grade SIL	Squamous cell cancer
Histology					

Histology diagram labels: Basal cells, Basement membrane, WBCs, Cervical Cancer, Invasive.

CIN = cervical intraepithelial neoplasia. SIL = squamous intraepithelial lesion; CIS = carcinoma in situ; WBC = white blood cells. (From Beckmann RB, Ling FW, Barzansky BM, et al. Obstetrics and gynecology. 2nd ed. Baltimore: Williams & Wilkins, 1995:386.)

Cytologic testing's promise to detect and prevent malignancy is blunted by a number of potential sources of error inherent in the test. False-negative rates as high as 15% may occur. Errors may be introduced by the way the sample is obtained, the fixation and processing of the sample, and the subjective interpretation of the microscopic findings encountered. (Correct techniques for obtaining cellular material and its fixation are discussed

Table 13.2. The Bethesda System for Reporting Cervical Cytology Findings

Adequacy of Smear
    Satisfactory for interpretation
    Satisfactory but limited by
      Inflammation
      Blood
      Absence of endocervical component
    Unsatisfactory due to
      Low cellularity
      Drying artifact
      Other
Diagnosis/Comment
    Within normal limits
    Benign cellular changes
      Infection
        Trichomonas vaginalis
        Fungi consistent with Candida
        Coccobacilli consistent with shift in flora
        Cellular changes associated with herpes simplex virus
        Other (see comments)
      Reactive Changes
        Inflammatory changes (includes repair)
        Changes consistent with radiation
        Atrophic with inflammation (atrophic vaginitis)
        Radiation changes
        Other (see comments)
    Epithelial Cell Abnormality
      Squamous cell
      ASCUS
      LSIL including CIN I, mild dysplasia, and HPV changes
      HSIL including CIN II, CIN III, moderate and severe dysplasia
      Squamous cell carcinoma
      Glandular cell
      AGUS
      Endometrial cells, cytologically benign, in a postmenopausal woman
      Endocervical adenocarcinoma
      Endometrial adenocarcinoma
      Extrauterine adenocarcinoma
      Adenocarcinoma, not otherwise specified
      Hormonal evaluation
        Compatible with age and history
        Incompatible with age and history
        Evaluation not possible due to (specify)

LSIL = low-grade squamous intraepithelial lesion; HSIL = high-grade squamous intraepithelial lesion; CIN = cervical intraepithelial neoplasia; HPV = human papillomavirus; ASCUS = atypical cells of undetermined significance; AGUS = abnormal glandular cells of undetermined significance.

in Chapter 10, Cancer Screening.) Although most cervical cancers make their presence known by superficial cellular changes, cancers that predominately infiltrate and grow below the visible surface may escape detection by cytologic techniques.

Critical to the interpretation of abnormal cytologic smears is an understanding of the pathophysiology of cervical metaplasia, dysplasia, and malignancy. The management of cytologic findings is predicated on an understanding of the natural history of the processes involved. One overlooked aspect of this natural history is the fact that the ratio of precancerous lesions to invasive cancer is on the order of 10:1. That is, probably less than 10% of precancerous lesions progress to frank malignancy. This should not engender complacency, but rather indicates the opportunity that long latency and low progression rates offer for therapeutic intervention.

Papanicolaou's original five-class system for reporting smear results has been supplanted by a system developed by a conference committee, held in Bethesda, Maryland (hence, the "Bethesda system"). This reporting protocol is designed to encompass three elements: the adequacy of the specimen for interpretation, a general categorization of the findings (normal or abnormal), and a descriptive diagnosis. The elements making up these three areas, as well as the type of findings that may be reported, are shown in Table 13.2.

The intent of the Bethesda system was to make the report of cytologic findings more like a clinical consultation. New terms and the lack of a preintroduction trial of the system have caused clinical confusion. It is currently estimated that in the United States almost $6 billion are spent annually on colposcopy and interventional therapy prompted by abnormal cervical smears. If these costs are to be spent appropriately, care must be taken to understand both the system and the underlying pathophysiology. Not all patients with an abnormality require either colposcopy or aggressive treatment.

ESTABLISHING THE DIAGNOSIS

Fundamental to the establishment of a diagnosis for a patient with an abnormal Pap smear is a familiarity with the Bethesda system for reporting cytologic findings. As noted in Chapter 10, the Bethesda system has been advocated to provide a formalized structure for diagnosis and reporting of cytologic changes found on cervical or vaginal smears. Although some aspects of the system provide clarification, others have led to confusion and reservation about the universal adoption of this system without further evaluation. Central to this new system is a modified report that addresses the adequacy of the specimen and the presence of benign changes or epithelial cell abnormalities. The structure of the report is shown in Table 13.2.

Less than 10% of cervical cytologic smears will show an abnormality, the most common of which are the atypical squamous cells of undetermined significance (ASCUS) and low-grade squamous intraepithelial lesion (LSIL) diagnoses. Uncertainty surround these changes because of the unpredictable behavior of low-grade cervical lesions. (Up to 60% of LSIL Pap smears will undergo spontaneous return to normal.) As we try to balance the opposing needs of cancer vigilance and responsible expenditure of health care resources, uncertainty has resulted. For some patients, conservative follow-up may be appropriate, whereas for others colposcopy and biopsy may be required to establish a firm diagnosis.

Diagnostic Procedures

Whereas the first line in the evaluation of abnormal Pap smears is the repeat smear itself, colposcopy, colposcopically directed biopsy, and endocervical curettage represent the second level. Colposcopy allows inspection of the cervix to establish the origin of the abnormal cells found on the cytologic smear. For a colposcopy to be considered "adequate," the entire transformation zone must be visualized. The full extent of any lesion present must also be visible. If the colposcopy is "inadequate," diagnostic conization will be required. The presence of vascular abnormalities or acetowhite areas (through the use of dilute acetic acid [3% to 5%]) can help to direct the biopsy site for histologic diagnosis.

Based on the size and type of abnormality suspected at the time of colposcopy, generous biopsy of the lesion, combined with close follow-up, may be appropriate for some patients. Because of the high costs associated with routine colposcopic evaluation of every patient with an abnormal Pap smear, there is more and more pressure to use less intensive management for selected patients. One recently published study suggests that close follow-up consisting of Pap smears only may provide roughly equal protection from cervical cancer to that provided by routine colposcopy, reserving colposcopy for only those with persistent or progressive abnormalities. Conservative management such as biopsy and observation must be restricted to only those with relatively minimal changes, who lack significant risk factors, and who will be compliant with the follow-up required. Any biopsies taken should include the margin of the visible lesion.

Curettage of the endocervical canal must be included in colposcopic examination to exclude the possibility of endocervical lesions above the limits of visibility. Endocervical curettage (ECC) helps to identify lesions that are located beyond the transformation zone. The ECC is especially helpful as a first stage in the evaluation of atypical glandular cells. The ECC should be performed under direct vision to avoid inadvertent contamination with ectocervical material. ECC should not be performed during pregnancy.

Cervicography (a photographic form of colposcopy) has been advocated as an alternative or adjunct to other forms of cervical evaluation. With this technique, a photographic record of the cervix is obtained and sent to a reference source for interpretation. This technique has yet to attain a significant following and should be restricted to those familiar with its use and limitations.

Human papillomavirus (HPV) detection and serotyping has been advocated by some as an aid to assessing the risk of cervical cancer. Although up to 70% of invasive cervical cancers have HPV serotypes 16 or 18 present, these types may be detected in patients with LSIL as well. Normal patients have HPV prevalence rates that vary from 10% to 50% depending on the study technique and population evaluated. It has been estimated that 10 to 20 million women between the ages of 18 and 50 have HPV DNA detectable in their cervix. This is in contrast to the roughly 16,000 cases of cervical cancer that occur yearly. High prevalence, a poor correlation with later risk, and the cost of screening have resulted in the general recommendation that routine HPV screening or serotyping not be carried out.

Table 13.3. Indications for Diagnostic Conization

Intraepithelial lesion or microinvasive carcinoma in endocervical curettings (abnormal ECC)
Incongruity between Pap smear and colposcopic findings
Incomplete visualization of transformation zone (inadequate colposcopy)
Microinvasive carcinoma found in colposcopically directed biopsies
Glandular malignant or premalignant disease

ECC = endocervical curettage.

Cervical Conization

Conization can be performed for either diagnosis or therapeutic indications. The tissue plug removed should encompass the entire cervical transformation zone and extend up the endocervical canal. Conization is vital for the evaluation of early neoplasms where the entire transformation zone is not visualized on colposcopy or where the extent of a lesion cannot be determined. It is also required for the definitive evaluation of patients with abnormal Pap smears where the colposcopic findings are inconsistent with that expected from Pap smear data. Conization is not required for the evaluation of grossly cancerous lesions; biopsy alone will suffice. Indications for diagnostic conization are summarized in Table 13.3.

Conization can be performed using a variety of techniques including sharp dissection ("cold knife cone"), laser excision or vaporization, or in modified form, by loop electrosurgical excision of the transformation zone (LEETZ) or loop electrosurgical excision procedure (LEEP). In each, the cone of tissue to be removed should be labeled in some way to allow proper orientation of the specimen during histologic evaluation. Reconstruction of the cervix may be carried out using sutures to reapproximate the edges of the cervical wound or the cervix may be left to heal spontaneously. With any of these techniques, significant distortion of the cervix can result. Following conization, cervical stenosis or incompetence are possible, but infrequent.

THERAPEUTIC/MANAGEMENT OPTIONS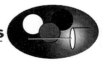

As with most aspects of medicine, the management of the abnormal Pap smear is neither universal nor immutable, but must be based on the abnormality reported and the individual patient's needs.

Studies looking at the relationship between the Pap smear abnormalities and the findings on repeated smears or cervical histology have found generally good, but not perfect, agreement. In one recent study, there was a 53% agreement between the initial and repeat Pap smears. When LSIL was diagnosed by Pap smear, there was an almost 90% agreement with the colposcopic impression. However, a colposcopic impression of high-grade squamous intraepithelial lesion (HSIL) was found in only one third of the women diagnosed with HSIL by smear. A comparison of the histology of the cervical biopsy and the electrosurgical loop specimen revealed 57% agreement. Therefore, patients with an initial Pap smear showing LSIL would benefit from a repeat Pap smear or colposcopically directed biopsies before proceeding with loop diathermy. More aggressive therapy appears warranted for those patients with HSIL findings.

Inadequate Specimen

The adequacy of the Pap smear specimen is now routinely assessed and reported. When the report is unsatisfactory, the smear must be repeated. Unsatisfactory smears may result from obscuring foreign material or from smears that are too thick or those with gross blood that prevents the squamous cells from being clearly seen. Smears reported to be" satisfactory but limited by the absence of endocervical cells" may be repeated; if the patient has had previously normal smears on a regular basis, routine follow-up may be acceptable.

Smears reported to be "satisfactory but limited by inflammation" are typical of patients with vaginal infections. The most common vaginal infection to disrupt the reading of the Pap smear is bacterial vaginitis. The strong inflammatory response found in true vaginitis, from whatever source, makes the reading of the smear difficult or impossible. When inflammation is less (or absent) the smear may be read and suspected infection reported in the form of "a shift in vaginal flora" or the presence of *Trichomonas* organisms. Both of these diagnoses are difficult to make on the basis of Pap smear changes. In the case of *Trichomonas* organisms, false-positive rates of up to 50% have frequently been reported. Therefore, therapy should be based on clinical suspicion or a reassessment.

Atypical Squamous Cells of Undetermined Significance (ASCUS)

One of the most perplexing aspects of management under the new reporting system is how to interpret smears reported as showing atypical squamous cells of undetermined significance (ASCUS). To understand current recommendations for the management of these patients it is important to note that this group is not equivalent to the previous "squamous atypias" or "class II" Pap smears of the past. These older designations accounted for almost 20% of all smears and were associated with cervical changes that ranged from benign inflammation to premalignant lesions. The ASCUS diagnosis has been developed to describe squamous cell changes that are more severe than reactive changes, but not as marked as those found in squamous intraepithelial lesions (SIL). Most feel that the ASCUS diagnosis should account for only about 5% of smears.

Management of patients with ASCUS is best determined by the presence and type of qualifications cytopathologists provide in their report. Patients with ASCUS for whom no qualification is offered or those reported to favor reactive change may be followed by repeated Pap smears every 2 to 6 months for 2 years or until three consecutive negative smears are obtained. Those with reactive or inflammatory aspects should be treated for specific infections present, followed by a repeat Pap smear in 2 to 3 months. Broad spectrum antibiotic therapy in the absence of documented infection is not warranted. ASCUS smears reported in postmenopausal patients not on hormonal replacement should be treated with topical estrogen (or systemic estrogen with topical boost) with the Pap smear repeated in 3 to 6 months. A familiarity with the style of the cytopathologist and open communications help establish the significance of the ASCUS report and the best management of these patients.

Colposcopy is generally not required to evaluate ASCUS smears except for those patients who have a second ASCUS smear within 2 years. Patients who have had previous

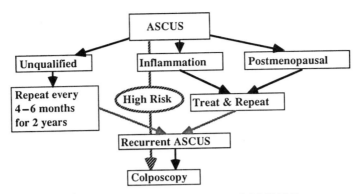

Figure 13.1. A schematic approach to the management of ASCUS Pap smears. Any patient at high risk for abnormality, poor compliance, or recurrent abnormality should proceed directly to colposcopic evaluation.

abnormal smears or those with poor compliance should also be considered for more aggressive management. A summary of management strategies for ASCUS smears is shown in Figure 13.1.

Early Changes, Intraepithelial Lesions, and Cervical Intraepithelial Neoplasia

Low-grade squamous intraepithelial lesions (LSIL) encompass changes associated with human papillomavirus (HPV), mild dysplasia, and cervical intraepithelial neoplasia (CIN I). These lesions have been grouped together because of their similarity in appearance, behavior, and treatment. As noted, 60% of patients with these findings will undergo spontaneous regression of the underlying process, resulting in a return to normal smears. Only 15% of patients with LSIL progress to HSIL. For this reason, compliant patients at low risk may be followed by serial Pap smears. As long as these remain satisfactory for evaluation and are negative, continued follow-up is all that may be required.

Those patients with inflammatory change, metaplasia, and HPV changes have been treated in the past with topical antibiotics, vaginal acidification, or electrodesiccation of the transformation zone or any nonstaining areas found on colposcopy. These therapies are currently not recommended.

For many patients with LSIL, colposcopy, colposcopically directed biopsy, and endocervical curettage are appropriate to establish the source of the cytologic abnormality. If colposcopy is adequate (the entire transformation zone and margins of any lesions present are seen) and the histologic abnormality found is mild, follow-up Pap smears at 4- to 6-month intervals is suitable. After 2 years or three normal smears, routine annual screening can be resumed. Continued therapy for these patients will be based on the histologic findings obtained by the conization, patient compliance with continuing surveillance, and the patient's wishes. Patients with adequate colposcopy and a well-circumscribed lesion may be treated by desiccation or ablation of the lesion. Ablation should not be performed without histologic confirmation of the diagnosis.

If colposcopy is inadequate to delineate any lesions present or the entire transformation zone cannot be seen, diagnostic conization is required.

Dysplasia (HSIL, CIN I, II, III)

High-grade squamous intraepithelial lesions (HSIL) include CIN II and III, as well as carcinoma in situ (CIS). These abnormalities, which are more likely to progress, warrant aggressive evaluation and treatment. The evaluation of HSIL is not dependent on the severity of the lesion. All patients with HSIL should be evaluated by colposcopy, colposcopically directed biopsy, and endocervical curettage. The results of this evaluation will determine therapy: cryotherapy, electrocautery, LEETZ or LEEP, laser ablation, or conization. Treatment must be based on an accurate diagnosis and the extent of the lesion involved. Ablative therapy must only be used when invasive cancer has been excluded and the cytologic, colposcopic, and histologic evaluation are all consistent. The conditions necessary for safe ablative therapy are summarized in Table 13.4. An overview of the management of LSIL and HSIL is shown in Figure 13.2.

Table 13.4. Conditions Necessary for Safe Cervical Ablative Therapy

Cytologic, colposcopic, and histologic examinations correlate
Entire lesion visible
Invasive cancer excluded
No endocervical involvement
No endocervical cellular abnormality on ECC

ECC = endocervical curettage.

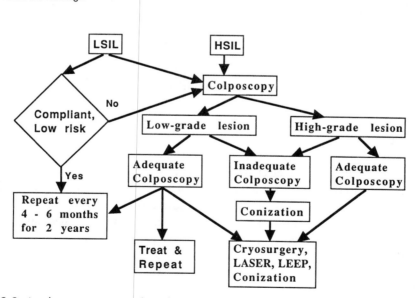

Figure 13.2. A schematic approach to the management of LSIL/HSIL Pap smears. Any patient at high risk for abnormality, poor compliance, or recurrent abnormality must be evaluated colposcopically. The management of low-grade cervical lesions must be based on patient history, type of lesion found, and preferences of both the patient and the provider.

Cryotherapy

Cryotherapy is most often used to treat cervical eversion, chronic infections, or mild dysplastic changes. The formation of ice crystals within the cells of the cervix leads to tissue destruction and slough. Most authors advocate a freeze-thaw-freeze technique with an ice ball that extends 4 mm to 5 mm beyond the edge of the probe. For this reason, cryotherapy tends to destroy moderately large areas of the cervix and thus is best for moderate sized, shallow lesions. (Because of the rich underlying blood supply that transfers heat removed by the cryosurgery probe, cryotherapy provides only relatively shallow destruction of the tissue.) Smaller lesions are often better managed with more precise tools.

Cryotherapy is associated with mild cramping during the procedure and a copious watery discharge that lasts for 4 to 5 weeks as tissue slough and healing occur. Cryotherapy should not be attempted in patients with a grossly distorted cervical os or in very obese patients, in whom avoidance of inadvertent vaginal wall injury may be more difficult.

Electrocautery

The term electrocautery is often indiscriminately applied to both electrosurgery (electrodesiccation) and actual cautery ("hot" cautery). Either technique may be used to destroy well-localized cervical lesions. Both provide more control over the area and depth of destruction than is available with cryotherapy, but they are otherwise similar. While there will be a watery discharge caused by cervical healing with electrocautery, it is generally less than that caused by cryotherapy.

Conization

Surgical conization remains the "gold standard" by which other methods are judged; it still plays a significant role in the evaluation and treatment of significant cervical lesions. Although surgical conization is generally done in a hospital or ambulatory surgery setting, it does provide for the greatest flexibility in biopsy size, shape, and depth. Surgical conization specimens can be more easily marked for correlation with lesions found during colposcopy and they lack the thermal artifact common to both electrosurgical loop excisions and laser techniques.

LEETZ/LEEP

Currently very popular are methods of excising a button of cervical tissue using an electrosurgical unit and thin wire loop electrode. Variously called LEETZ or LEEP, this procedure can be carried out in the office with a minimum of equipment, discomfort, complications, or time. Unfortunately, there is a tendency to remove too shallow or too narrow a portion of tissue, resulting in incomplete treatment of the cervical lesion or an inadequate specimen for histologic evaluation. In addition, thermal artifacts often cause problems with histologic interpretation, especially at the critically important edges of the specimen. In the right hands, this may be an excellent alternative to surgical conization, but excessive or indiscriminate use must still be avoided.

Laser Ablation and Laser Conization

Vaporization or excision of cervical lesions may also be accomplished by laser techniques. Energy, in the form of laser-generated light, is delivered to the tissue in a tightly focused beam that can cut through tissue or vaporize portions of tissue under fairly precise control. This technique most often uses infrared light generated by a CO_2 laser. Laser excision or conization is similar to that accomplished by knife or electrosurgical techniques, but generally demonstrates less thermal artifact in the histologic specimen. Vaporization of small lesions can be carried out with precise control of margins and depth, but results in no histologic specimen. Laser is best suited for lesions that extend into the endocervical canal or have deep glandular involvement.

Laser ablation of lesions produces only mild cramping and can be carried out under local infiltration of the cervix, a paracervical block, or without anesthesia. If more extensive evaluations or manipulations are required, general or regional anesthesia may be desirable. A vaginal discharge is generally present for 10 to 14 days.

The expense of the required equipment, the need for surgical time and privileges, a lack of proved superiority of the technique, and concerns about the possibility of viral spread via the smoke plume generated, have all blunted the initial enthusiasm for laser therapy.

Hysterectomy

For very selected patients, hysterectomy for HSIL lesions may be appropriate. This recommendation is generally be reserved for those with recurrent lesions or those whose lesions cannot be treated in a more conservative manner. In most cases, other gynecologic indications, in addition to the cervical abnormality, will suggest this approach.

AGCUS

The category of "atypical glandular cells of undetermined significance" (AGCUS) includes a range of findings from benign reactive changes in endocervical or endometrial cells to adenocarcinoma. If the cytology report indicates a probability of carcinoma, the endocervical canal and endometrial cavity should be evaluated. Cone biopsy and hysteroscopy may be required to adequately evaluate these patients. Referral is in order for the evaluation of these sometimes enigmatic findings.

Follow-Up

A vital part of the management of patients with abnormal Pap smears is continuing follow-up after the investigation and resolution of immediate abnormality. For even the most worrisome lesions, there are good data to support monitoring by cytology only. Frequent colposcopy in the absence of other indications of abnormality is not cost-effective.

All of the commonly employed surgical and ablative therapies used to treat cervical abnormalities carry a recurrence rate of approximately 10%, requiring frequent follow-up cytologic evaluations. For patients who have had preinvasive lesions, Pap smears should be repeated every 3 months for the first year. If these smears remain negative, a return to annual examinations can be recommended. For patients with invasive lesions, a somewhat more aggressive plan should be used. For these women, Pap smears should be repeated every 3 months for the first 2 years, then a 6-month schedule should be maintained for the next 2 to 3 years, after which annual examinations may be sufficient. Patients who have had a hysterectomy for a significant cervical abnormality (e.g., carcinoma in situ), should also be followed in this manner.

Recent studies indicate that compliance with follow-up recommendations can be greatly increased through the use of educational booklets. For this reason, serious consideration should be given to having educational brochures routinely accompany or immediately follow notification about abnormal Pap smears.

Any patient who undergoes conization must be monitored for the possibility of postoperative complications, most commonly excessive bleeding, which usually occurs 5 to 10 days after surgery. Some vaginal spotting or a slightly foul creamy-yellow discharge in the immediate postoperative period is normal.

HINTS AND COMMON QUESTIONS

For a follow-up Pap smear to be "negative," it must have normal or benign findings, but also be "satisfactory for interpretation."

One question that has yet to be resolved is the management and follow-up of immunosuppressed patients with abnormal Pap smears. There is evidence that cervical dysplasia and cancer behave in a more aggressive manner in these patients. A more determined effort at detection and follow-up is probably prudent for these women.

Endometrial cells may sometimes be found in the cervical cytology smears of postmenopausal women; however their presence carries a 10% chance that an endometrial cancer is present.

A small amount of water-soluble lubricant applied to the tip of the cryosurgery probe provides a better interface and more uniform freezing.

When LSIL or HSIL is found in pregnancy, some modification of the normal management is in order. In the absence of invasive carcinoma, conization is rarely needed and re-evaluation after delivery will suffice. These patients should be followed by frequent Pap smears. Colposcopically guided biopsy (but not ECC) may be carried out if needed, although most prefer to delay even biopsy if possible.

SUGGESTED READINGS

General References

Brinton LA, Hamman RF, Huggins GH, et al. Sexual and reproductive risk factors for invasive squamous cell cervical cancer. J Natl Cancer Inst 1987;79:23.

Carmichael JA, Maskens PD. Cervical intraepithelial neoplasia: examination, treatment and follow-up: review. Obstet Gynecol Surg 1985;40:545.

Christopherson WM, Lundin FE JR, Mendez WM, Parker JE. Cervical cancer control: a study of morbidity and mortality trends over a twenty-one-year peroid. Cancer 1976;38:1357.

Herbst AL. The Bethesda System for cervical/vaginal cytologic diagnoses. Clin Obstet Gynecol 1992;35:22.

Higgins RV, Hall JB, McGee JA, Laurent S, Alvarez RD, Partridge EE. Appraisal of the modalities used to evaluate an initial abnormal Papanicolaou smear. Obstet Gynecol 1994;84:174.

Kurman RJ, Henson DE, Herbst AL, Noller KL, Schiffman MH. Interim guidelines for management of abnormal cervical cytology. The 1992 National Cancer Institute Workshop. JAMA 1994;271:1866.

Kurman RJ, Malkasian GD JR, Sedlis A, Solomon D. From Papanicolaou to Bethesda: the rational for a new cervical cytologic classification. Obstet Gynecol 1991;77:779.

Montz FJ, Monk BJ, Fowler JM, Nguyen L. Natural history of the minimally abnormal Papanicolaou smear. Obstet Gynecol 1992;80:385.

Nasiell K, Roger V, Nasiell M. Behavior of mild cervical dysplasia during long-term follow-up. Obstet Gynecol 1986;67:665.

National Cancer Institute Workshop. The 1988 Bethesda system for reporting cervical/vaginal cytological diagnoses. JAMA 1989;262:931.

Richart RM. A modified terminology for cervical intraepithelial neoplasia. Obstet Gynecol 1990;75:131.

Specific References

August N. Cervicography for evaluating the atypical Papanicolaou smear. J Reprod Med 1991;36:89.

Bose J, Kannan V, Kline TS. Abnormal endocervical cells: Really abnormal? Really endocervical? Am J Clin Pathol 1994;101:708.

Carey P, Gjerdingen DK. Follow-up of abnormal Papanicolaou smears among women of different races. J Fam Pract 1993;37:583.

Cox JT, Schiffman MH, Winzelberg AJ, et al. An evaluation of human papillomavirus testing as part of referral to colposcopy clinics. Obstet Gynecol 1992;80:389.

Goff BA, Atanasoff P, Brown E, et al. Endocervical glandular atypia in Papanicolaou smears. Obstet Gynecol 1992;79:101.

Herbst AL. The Bethesda system for reporting cervical/vaginal cytological diagnoses: a note of caution. Obstet Gynecol 1990;76:449.

Kivlahan C, Ingram E. Papanicolaou smears without endocervical cells: are they inadequate? Acta Cytol 1986;30:258.

Kristenesen GB, Skyggebjerg K-D, Holund B, et al. Analysis of cervical smears obtained within three years of the diagnosis of invasive cervical cancer. Acta Cytol 1991;35:47.

Montz FJ, Bradley JM, Fowler JM, Nguyen L. Natural history of the minimally abnormal Papanicolaou smear. Obstet Gynecol 1992;80:385.

Nasiell K, Roger V, Nasiell M. Behavior of mild cervical dysplasia during long-term follow-up. Obstet Gynecol 1986;67:665.

Schiffman MH. Recent progress in defining the epidemiology of HPV infection in cervical neoplasia. J Natl Cancer Inst 1992;84:394.

Schiffman MH, Bauer HM, Hoover RN, et al. Epidemiologic evidence showing that human papillomavirus infection causes most cervical intraepithelial neoplasia. J Natl Cancer Inst 1993;85:958.

Sherlaw-Johnson C, Gallivan S, Jenkins D, Jones MH. Cytological screening and management of abnormalities in prevention of cervical cancer: an overview with stochastic modelling. J Clin Pathol 1994;47:430.

Stewart DE, Buchegger PM, Lickrish GM, Sierra S. The effect of educational brochures on follow-up compliance in women with abnormal Papanicolaou smears. Obstet Gynecol 1994;83:583.

Toon PG, Arrand JR, Wilson LP, Sharp DS. Human papillomavirus infection of the uterine cervix of women without cytological signs of neoplasia. BMJ 1986;293:1261.

14

Breast Disease

The significance of breast disease cannot be overemphasized. Society places a great deal of significance on the female breast and, for many women, it is a very visible affirmation, second only to pregnancy, of being female. Any process that alters the breast attacks a very basic part of a woman's self-image. Breast disease also poses a very real threat to a woman's health. Roughly one of four women will require medical attention for some form of breast problem. Breast cancer is the most common female cancer and the leading cause of death for women in their 40s. Women with breast symptoms often exhibit justifiable anxiety out of a fear of breast cancer, increasing the urgency and significance of timely evaluation and treatment. Failure to diagnose breast cancer is one of the leading causes for an allegation of malpractice in the United States.

Everyone who cares for women must be sensitive to the significance that breast disease carries. They must understand the basic approach to evaluating the common symptoms associated with the breast, which encompasses history, physical, and mammographic evaluations. This includes the management of women who present with a breast mass, tenderness, skin change, nipple discharge, or a complaint of breast pain. The clinician must be familiar with the presenting history and physical findings that suggest fibrocystic changes, fibroadenomas, intraductal papilloma, and carcinoma. Education regarding the importance of screening mammography and breast self-examination must also be a part of care.

BACKGROUND AND SCIENCE

The adult female breast weighs between 200 g and 300 g, made up primarily of fatty tissue and fibrous septa (80%), and the glandular structures themselves (20%), organized into 12 to

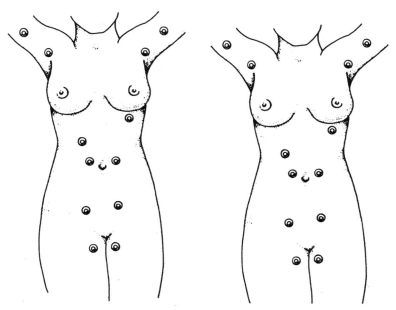

Figure 14.1. Location of milk lines and polythelia. (Adapted from: Mitchel GW, Bassett LW. The Female Breast and Its Disorders. Baltimore: Williams & Wilkins, 1990, p 10, 23.) (From Mitchell GW, Bassett LW. The female breast and its disorders. Baltimore: Williams & Wilkins, 1990:10,23.)

20 triangular shaped lobes. These lobes are constructed with a central duct, collecting ducts, and secretory cells arranged in alveoli, each of which drains at the nipple. Breast tissue may be located anywhere along the "milk lines" that run from the axilla to the groin (Fig. 14.1). Patients with one or more extra nipples (polythelia) are more common than those with true accessory breasts (polymastia). Breast asymmetry is not uncommon and is of only cosmetic significance. Significant asymmetry or hypertrophy may require surgical intervention.

Breast tissue is very sensitive to hormones, resulting in the development of the adult breast shape during puberty, cyclic variations that occur throughout the menstrual cycle, and changes associated with pregnancy and lactation. This sensitivity extends to pharmacologic manipulations such as oral contraception or estrogen replacement that sometimes cause undesirable side effects.

Each tissue type that makes up the breast may undergo pathologic change or be the source of clinical symptoms. The connective tissues of the breast give rise to fibrocystic changes and fibroadenomas. Fatty tissues may produce lipomas or necrose in response to trauma. The ductal system may become dilated (duct ectasia or galactocele), contain papillary neoplasms, or undergo malignant change. Although most common in nursing mothers, infections of the breast (mastitis) also occurs, potentially causing significant morbidity if not recognized and treated agresssively.

Fibrocystic Change

The term fibrocystic change encompasses a multitude of different processes or older terms, including "fibrocystic disease." It is the most common of all benign breast conditions, accounting for its linguistic demotion to "change" from the designation "disease." The prevalence of fibrocystic change is estimated to be from one third to three quarters of all women. Fibrocystic change produces symptoms for roughly half of these women. Although it is most common in women between age 30 and 50 years, 10% of those under the age of 21 will have some degree of change.

Fibrocystic changes appear in three steps. Initially there is a proliferation of stroma, especially in the upper outer quadrants of the breast, which produces the induration and tenderness experienced by these patients. In the next phase, marked proliferation of the ducts and alveolar cells occurs, adenosis ensues, and cysts are formed. During this phase cysts are small and range from microscopic to 1 cm in diameter. In the late stages of fibrocystic change, larger cysts are found and pain generally decreases. Proliferative changes may be extensive (though usually benign) in any of the involved tissues. When atypia is found in these hyperplastic ducts or in apocrine cells, there is a fivefold increase in the risk of developing carcinoma in the future. Diagnosis is based on symptoms and physical findings, rather than histology.

The cause(s), of fibrocystic change is unknown, but is postulated to arise from an exaggerated response to hormones. A role for progesterone has been suggested based on the common occurrence of premenstrual breast swelling and tenderness. Altered ratios of estrogen and progesterone or an increased rate of prolactin secretion are also proposed sources for fibrocystic changes, but neither has been conclusively established. There is no evidence that oral contraceptives increase the risk of these changes. Initial studies suggested a tie to methylxanthine intake, but more recent studies question this relationship. A family history of fibrocystic change is often present; however, because of the high prevalence of the condition, causality is difficult to establish.

Fibroadenoma and Cystosarcoma Phyllodes

Fibroadenomas are the second most common form of breast disease and the most common breast mass. These masses are firm, painless, mobile, and usually solitary. They are most common in teenagers and young women and may grow rapidly during adolescence or in high estrogen states (pregnancy, estrogen therapy). Rapid growth at other times suggest a re-evaluation of the diagnosis. Fibroadenomas are generally discovered incidentally or during breast self-examination and average 2 cm to 3 cm in diameter. Although generally solitary, multiple fibroadenomas develop in 15% to 20% of patients. They are bilateral in 10% to 20% of patients. Unlike fibrocystic change, these tumors do not change during the menstrual cycle and are generally slow growing.

Cystosarcoma phyllode is an infrequently encountered sarcoma thought to arise from fibroadenomas. These sarcomas account for only about 1% of breast cancers, although they are the most common type of sarcoma found in the breast. These tumors grow rapidly and are generally found in the fourth or fifth decade of life. Treated by wide local excision, only one in four are malignant and one in ten metastasizes.

Lipomas and Fat Necrosis

Fatty tissues of the breast may produce benign tumors that are difficult to distinguish from malignancy. Both lipomas and fat necrosis may present as ill-defined tumors. Lipomas are generally nontender, but their diffuse character may make them clinically suspicious for malignancy, although secondary signs suggestive of cancer (e.g., skin and nipple changes) are generally absent. The mammographic appearance of lipomas make them easy to distinguish from malignancy.

Fat necrosis is most often the result of trauma, although the causative event cannot be identified in roughly one half of cases. Fat necrosis is uncommon but gives rise to an irregular, tender mass that is easily confused with cancer. The patient usually presents with a solitary, tender, ill-defined mass. Skin retraction is sometimes present. Mammography often shows fine, stippled calcification and stellate or infiltrative fibrosis. Even with a history of trauma, the commonality of findings between fat necrosis and cancer found on physical examination, mammography, and ultrasonography, generally mandate further evaluation and biopsy.

Intraductal Papilloma

Intraductal papillomas are polypoid fibrovascular tumors, covered by benign ductal epithelium, that arise in the ducts of the breast. Although these tumors may range from 2 mm to 5 mm in diameter, they are typically not palpable. These lesions are most commonly discovered because of a spontaneous, intermittent, bloody, serous, or cloudy unilateral nipple discharge occurring in roughly 50% of cases. The amount of this discharge may vary from a few drops to a few milliliters of fluid. Intraductal papillomas are most often benign, but the similarity of symptoms to those of a carcinoma and a sometimes confusing histologic picture mandates excisional biopsy for most patients.

Mammary Duct Ectasia and Galactocele

Mammary duct ectasia arises from chronic intraductal and periductal inflammation, resulting in ductal dilatation and inspissation of normal secretions. Ductal ectasia is most common during the fifth decade of life, presenting with a thick gray to black nipple discharge, pain, and nipple tenderness. The characteristic discharge can be easily demonstrated during clinical examination. Thickening that may be difficult to distinguish from cancer is often present. Nipple retraction is common and ductal ectasia is the most common cause of an acquired nipple inversion. Biopsy will confirm the diagnosis and, once established, no further therapy is needed unless warranted by the patient's symptoms.

Ductal obstruction and inflammation during, or soon after, lactation may lead to cystic dilatation of a duct or ducts and the subsequent development of a galactocele. Galactoceles contain inspissated milk and desquamated epithelial cells that may become infected, resulting in acute mastitis or an abscess. When uncomplicated by infection, needle aspiration or drainage by gentle pressure is diagnostic and decompression is curative. Excision may be required for recurrences.

Mastitis

Mastitis is most common in nursing mothers 3 to 4 weeks after delivery. Infection comes from organisms carried in the nose and mouth of the nursing infant, most commonly *Staphylococcus aureus* and *Streptococcus* species. Pain, erythema, and fever mark the usual clinical presentation. Between 5% and 10% of patients will go on to abscess formation. Factors that increase the risk of puerperal mastitis include diabetes, steroid use, heavy cigarette smoking, and retracted (inverted) nipples. Some have suggested that the presence of breast implants (silicone or saline) may also increase the risk, but this has not been well established.

Nonpregnant and postmenopausal women may also suffer from mastitis, accompanied by squamous metaplasia. This condition usually presents as a palpable, recurrent mass, accompanied by a multicolored discharge from the nipple or an adjacent Montgomery's follicle. When well established, ductal thickening may lead to nipple retraction. It is unclear whether squamous metaplasia and swelling lead to obstruction and infection, or vice versa. Treatment consists of excisional biopsy.

Mondor Disease

Mondor disease, or superficial angiitis, is a superficial thrombophlebitis of the breast that may present as pain, with a dimpling of the skin or a distinct cord with erythematous margins. Although uncommon, it is most often linked to recent pregnancy, trauma, or operative procedures, but may occur spontaneously. Accentuation of dimpling, or the formation of a groove over the affected vein, often occurs when the ipsilateral arm is raised during physical examination. Mammography and, in some cases biopsy, may be required to establish the diagnosis. Analgesics and heat will improve symptoms. Mondor disease is self-limited, although full resolution may take 8 to 10 weeks.

Breast Cancer

Breast cancer is the most common malignancy found in women, accounting for almost one third of all their malignancies. Roughly one woman in ten will develop breast cancer in her lifetime. Breast cancer was the leading cause of cancer death for women until 1985, when it was replaced by lung cancer. With roughly 185,000 new cases annually and around 46,000 breast cancer deaths per year in the United States, breast cancer is still the most common cause of death in women in their 40s. Roughly one new case of breast cancer is diagnosed every 3 minutes and every 11 minutes there is a breast cancer death. Breast cancer accounts for approximately 18% of cancer deaths and results in about the same number of deaths per year as auto accidents. Although there has been little change in the overall mortality from breast cancer over the past 40 years, improved diagnostic techniques and increased awareness of breast problems by women and health care providers promise earlier diagnosis, resulting in more successful treatment.

A great deal has been written about risk factors for breast cancer (Table 14.1), but risk factors themselves are of limited clinical value. Only 21% of patients aged 30 to 54 years with breast cancer are identified by risk factors. Only the patient's gender and age are strongly correlated with the risk of developing breast cancer. However, risk factors may be useful in planning detection strategies. For example, 85% of all breast cancer occurs after the age of 40 and 75% after the age of 50. Because of this rising prevalence, current recommendations for mammographic screening are primarily dependent on the patient's age (Table 14.2).

Evolving research indicates that for a small number of women the presence of the BRCA-1 gene is a specific marker for a significantly increased risk of breast cancer. Those who carry this gene may have up to an 85% life-time risk of developing breast cancer. Currently this test is being applied only to those at increased risk owing to family history and

Table 14.1. Suggested Risk Factors for Breast Cancer

Factor	Relative risk
Gynecologic history	
Menarche < age 12	1.3
Greater than 40 menstrual years	1.5–2.0
Chronic annovulation	2–4
First delivery > age 35	2–3
Nulliparous	3
Oophorectomy < age 35	0.4
Family history	
First degree relative with breast cancer	1.2–3.0
Premenopausal, unilateral	3
Premenopausal, bilateral	9–10.5
Postmenopausal, bilateral	5
Neoplasms	
Contralateral breast cancer (approximately 1% per year since diagnosis)	5–10
Uterus or ovary	2
Major salivary gland	4
Other factors	
Age 60 vs. age 40	2
Atypical hyperplasia	4–6
High economic status	Suggested but unknown
Increased dietary fat	Suggested but unknown
Large bowel cancer	Suggested but unknown
Moderate alcohol use	1.5–2.0
North American (white or black)	5
Obesity	Suggested but unknown
Previous biopsy	1.9–2.1
Radiation exposure (>90 rads)	4
Urban dweller	Suggested but unknown

Table 14.2. American Cancer Society Guidelines for Mammographic Screening

- Baseline study between ages 35 and 40
- Mammography every 1 to 2 years from age 40 to 49
- Annual mammography from age 50 on

is not a screening tool for those at low risk. The absence of the BRCA-1 gene does not provide reassurance because those women who are candidates for screening generally carry other risk factors, possibly through other genes, that continue to place them at risk.

Often hotly debated, especially in the lay literature, is the relationship between oral contraceptive use, estrogen replacement, and breast cancer. It is generally agreed that below the age of menopause, there is no difference in the prevalence of breast cancer in women who have used oral contraceptives and those who have not. This is true even for prolonged contraceptive users if they began their use after the age of 25. A few studies suggest that if oral contraceptive use begins in a woman's teens or early 20s and is prolonged, there may be a slight increase in the risk of breast cancer during her 30s and 40s, although these same patients have a lower than average risk after this age. The largest American study to date has failed to support these findings, reporting no increased risk of cancer for young users, those with benign breast disease, or women with a family history of breast cancer. Similarly, meta-analysis of published papers dealing with estrogen replacement therapy and the risk of breast cancer have failed to show a relationship at commonly prescribed dosages. Evidence for a protective effect of progesterone as a part of estrogen replacement therapy is also lacking, resulting in the recommendation that patients without a uterus do not need routine progestin supplementation. (See also Chapter 12, Menopause.)

Many different cancer types can occur in the breast (Table 14.3), although most are related to ductal disease. Breast cancer survival depends less on cell type than it does on the size of the tumor and stage of disease. Breast tumors have a long latency from initial cellular aberration to clinically detectable lesions (Fig. 14.2). In the early stages of cancer growth, the tumor is usually painless, small, and may feel mobile, immitating benign fibrocystic changes. As the tumor enlarges, the borders become less distinct, with fixation to the supporting ligaments or underlying fascia common. Eighty percent of breast cancers present as a mass, with 75% of the masses found by the patients themselves. Nipple discharge (bloody or otherwise), skin changes ("peau d'orange" or orange peel skin), or ulceration are late occurrences and portend a bad prognosis.

Breast cancer disseminates by vascular and lymphatic routes, as well as by direct infiltration. There is also a growing trend to view breast cancer as a multifocal disease. The possibility of multiple sites of origin and early spread through multiple routes, means that breast can-

Table 14.3. Simplified Classification of Breast Cancer

Ductal cancers
    Infiltrating (80%)
        Papillary carcinoma
        Intraductal carcinoma
        Colloid carcinoma
        Medullary carcinoma
    Noninfiltrating (5%)
        Papillary carcinoma
        Intraductal carcinoma (comedocarcinoma)
        Intracystic carcinoma
Lobular cancers
    In situ and infiltrating (12%)
Sarcomas
    Cystosarcoma phyllodes
    Stromal sarcoma
    Liposarcoma
    Angiosarcoma
Lymphoma
Other (rare) cancers
    Sweat gland carcinoma
    Tubular carcinoma
    Adenoid cystic carcinoma
    Metaplastic lesions
    Inflammatory carcinoma (2%)
    Paget's disease (1%)
    Metastatic cancers

Work-up

The evaluation of a breast complaint is based on clinical suspicion derived from the history and physical examination, augmented by four modalities: imaging, aspiration, fine-needle biopsy, and open biopsy.

Imaging

Mammography is the best mode of screening for early lesions currently available. Mammography localizes, documents, objectifies, and identifies other occult pathology. Roughly 85% of breast cancers found by mammography are early stage lesions versus 54% to 70% found by physicians and 38% to 64% by the patient herself during breast self-examination. Wide-spread use of mammography has been credited with reducing the mortality rate from breast cancer by up to 30%. Unfortunately, not all women are appropriately screened on a regular basis. One study indicated that only 39% of women aged 50 to 59 and 36% of women aged 60 to 69 had had a mammogram in the preceding year. In another study, only 24% of women over the age of 65 followed the current recommendations for annual examinations. It has been estimated that breast cancer mortality could be reduced by as much as one half if all women over the age of 40 were screened annually. In one study, 6 cancers per 1000 screening mammograms were found, and 3 additional cancers were detected per 1000 annual repeat studies performed.

Roughly 35% of breast cancers are found by an abnormal mammogram, without a palpable mass present. Mammography can identify small lesions (1 mm to 2 mm), calcifications, or other changes suspicious for malignancy roughly 2 years before a lesion is clinically palpable; 10-year disease-free survival for these lesions is 90% to 95%. The average lesion found on breast self-examination is 2.5 cm, and half of these patients have nodal involvement. For these patients, 10-year survival falls to between 50% and 70%. Over one third of occult breast cancers have calcifications, making the otherwise undetected tumors visible on mammography. Clearly, mammography is an important screening tool if we are to reduce the impact of breast cancer.

Mammography is not without its drawbacks. Mammography in younger women is more difficult of interpret than in older women because of the greater tissue density present in the reproductive years. While the increasing ability to diagnose cancer in older women parallels their increasing risk, breast cancers in younger women are more easily missed. This diagnostic difficulty and the relatively higher rate of false-positive studies that necessitate further evaluation have raised questions about routine screening below the age of 50. Clusters of calcification that often are associated with cancer are nonspecific. Indeed, 75% of calcification clusters found on mammography are due to benign disease. Overall, mammography is approximately 85% accurate in diagnosing malignancy, with a 10% to 15% false-negative rate. For this reason, it provides an adjunct to clinical impressions and the definitive procedure of biopsy, but does not replace them. Roughly 10% of mammographic studies will require additional views. Between 1% and 2% of screening studies necessitate histologic evaluation to establish a diagnosis.

Patients sometimes express reservation about the radiation exposure involved with any radiographic procedure. Mammographic radiation exposure is minimal (less than 0.01 Gy). Based on this level of exposure, mammography might induce up to five new lifetime cancers for every one million women aged 40 to 44 screened, and fewer than one per 1 million for women aged 60 to 64. This is in contrast to a background risk of 115 and 292 for these age groups, respectively. In other words, the risk of death due to radiation exposure during mammography is roughly equivalent to the risk of death encountered by driving a car 220 miles, riding a bicycle for 10 miles, or smoking 1.5 cigarettes.

Other techniques for routine breast imaging have had little success. Ultrasonography is useful in differentiating solid and cystic breast masses, but it has limited spatial resolution and is unable to differentiate benign and malignant tissues. In one study of 64 women with breast cancer, ultrasonography was able to detect only 58% of lesions and only found 8% of tumors less than 1 cm in size. Ultrasonography does provide the possibility of repeated studies without radiation exposure. Beyond these distinctions, it provides little additional help in clinical management. Some authors suggest that for young women an ultrasound examination of a suspicious mass may be a more cost-effective tool than mammography and should be performed first, but this remains conjectural.

Other modalities, such as thermography and breast transillumination, have high false-positive and false-negative rates and have no proved value as either screening or diagnostic tools. Magnetic resonance imaging holds great promise because of its ability to provide detailed images of soft tissue. Expense and availability limit its applicability so that the exact role of magnetic resonance imaging is yet to be determined. In a similar way, digital radiography may improve the accuracy of mammography, but wide-spread evaluation and application appears to be far in the future.

Magnetic resonance imaging or computerized tomography of the pituitary gland should be considered in galactorrhea patients with elevated prolactin levels. These modalities are far more sensitive than the older "coned-down" or axial tomography techniques that they replace. Visual fields should also be evaluated in those patients suspected of having a pituitary adenoma.

Aspiration

If the patient has a cystic breast mass, needle aspiration with a 22- to 25-gauge needle may be both diagnostic and therapeutic (Fig. 14.4). If the cyst disappears completely and does not reform by a 1-month follow-up examination, no further therapy is required. Fluid aspirated from patients with fibrocystic changes customarily will be straw colored. Fluid that is dark brown or green occurs in cysts that have been present for a long time, but is equally innocuous. Bloody fluid requires further evaluation. Owing to high false-positive (up to 6%) and even higher false-negative rates (2% to 22%), cytologic evaluation of the fluid obtained is of little value. In women over the age of 35, mammography prior to aspiration should be considered because of the increased incidence of malignancy. Once aspiration has been attempted, mammography should be delayed several weeks owing to artifactual changes induced by the manipulation, which makes mammography difficult to interpret.

Fine-needle Biopsy

Fine-needle aspiration (FNA) of cells from a breast mass can provide histologic confirmation of malignancy and help direct definitive therapy. Although commercial devices are available, fine-needle aspiration may be performed using a 16- to 22-gauge needle mounted on a standard 10 cm^3 syringe (Fig. 14.5). The needle is inserted into the mass and negative pressure applied by the syringe. Multiple (15 or more) short passes through the tis-

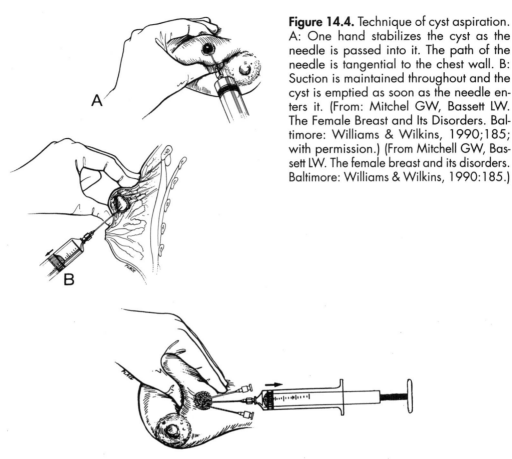

Figure 14.4. Technique of cyst aspiration. A: One hand stabilizes the cyst as the needle is passed into it. The path of the needle is tangential to the chest wall. B: Suction is maintained throughout and the cyst is emptied as soon as the needle enters it. (From: Mitchel GW, Bassett LW. The Female Breast and Its Disorders. Baltimore: Williams & Wilkins, 1990;185; with permission.) (From Mitchell GW, Bassett LW. The female breast and its disorders. Baltimore: Williams & Wilkins, 1990:185.)

Figure 14.5. Technique of fine-needle aspiration. Fine-needle aspiration (biopsy) using a standard 16- to 22-gauge needle and syringe. The needle is passed into the mass, suction is applied using the syringe, and multiple passes in various directions are made. Local anesthesia may be used at the discretion of the clinician. (Adapted from: Mitchell GW, Bassett LW. The Female Breast and Its Disorders. Baltimore: Williams & Wilkins, 1990, p 186.) (Modified from Mitchell GW, Bassett LW. The female breast and its disorders. Baltimore: Williams & Wilkins, 1990:186.)

sue are performed to obtain cells or tissue. The material obtained is expressed onto a glass slide, smeared, and fixed. This is then examined histologically or cytologically for evidence of malignancy. Fine-needle aspiration is 70% to 90% accurate, but carries a 20% false-negative rate. Hence, if the aspiration of a solid mass is negative, open biopsy is still required. Because of the possibility of hematoma formation or swelling after FNA, mammography if desired, should be performed prior to the procedure or delayed by 4 to 6 weeks.

Core biopsy or large-needle biopsy permits larger histologic specimens with better preservation of the architecture of the tissue sampled. Many feel, however, that if that degree of investigation is warranted, an excisional biopsy is more appropriate. Local custom and the preferences of the individual consultants are probably the best guide to the role of this modality in the absence of conclusive studies.

Open Biopsy

The definitive evaluation of any breast mass is open biopsy. This may be performed under local anesthesia through either radial or circumareolar incisions. Based on local custom, this biopsy may be performed by a general surgeon, plastic surgeon, gynecologist, or, in some cases, a family physician. Many feel that the biopsy is best performed by the person most likely to perform the ultimate surgical therapy, should such be required.

For small lesions or those difficult to localize, preoperative radiographically guided J-wire placement can provide operative guidance and ensure that the lesion is included in the histology specimen. Postoperative x-ray study of the pathology specimen may also confirm excision of the desired tissue.

Differential Diagnosis

The most common presenting breast complaints are pain and the presence of a mass. Both, which represent sources of great distress and a sense of emergency, deserve prompt, compasssionate evaluation.

Pain

Mastalgia is the nonspecific term used for breast pain of any etiology. Although patients are always concerned about the possibility of breast cancer, breast pain is a presenting complaint in less than 10% of patients with breast cancer. Mastalgia may be due to fibrocystic change, mastitis or breast abscess, trauma, or chest wall abnormalities. Fibrocystic changes most commonly present as cyclic, diffuse, bilateral pain and engorgement, with the worst symptoms occurring just prior to menses. The pain associated with fibrocystic change is diffuse, often with radiation to the shoulders or upper arms. On examination, scattered bilateral nodularity is typical. Well-localized breast pain may result from rapid expansion of a cyst, duct obstruction, trauma, or inflammation.

Mastalgia without an obvious pathology has been attributed to caffeine consumption and high-fat diets, although these connections are debated. Dorsal radiculitis or inflammatory changes in the costochondral junction (Tietze's syndrome) may also present as mastalgia. Noncyclic pain is also common in sclerosing adenosis, chest wall muscle spasms, costochondritis, neuritis, and referred pain.

Mass

Breast masses represent one of the most emotionally charged and difficult clinical problems the clinician will face. Firm, round and well-demarcated masses are most likely to be fibroadenomas. Smooth, round, mobile, tense masses are most often cystic; aspiration of these will be both confirmatory and therapeutic. Ropy thickening, especially in the upper outer quadrants of the breast, is common in fibrocystic disease, but more difficult to distinguish from more sinister changes. Less well-demarcated areas with a flattened, rubbery consistency are sugestive of malignancy, although fat necrosis may cause similar changes. With any mass, further evaluation (e.g., tissue confirmation by needle or open biopsy) is mandatory. Even in cases of obvious cancer, mammography is important to help detect multicentric disease and synchronous cancers, which are present in up to 5% of patients. One algorithm for evaluating a palpable breast mass is shown in Figure 14.6.

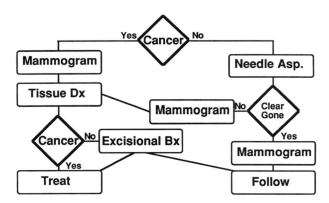

Figure 14.6. Management of breast masses. A clinical algorithm for the evaluation of a palpable breast mass. Mammography following an aspirated cyst that completely resolves is optional, athough recommended to diagnose and document other lesions elsewhere in the breast.

Discharge

Spontaneous discharge from the nipple is found in approximately 5% of nonlactating women, although up to 50% of menstrual age women may be able to express some secretions. Most physiologic discharge is white or green, or clear or yellow. Although bloody discharge from the nipple is the hallmark of intraductal papillomas, any unilateral spontaneous nipple discharge should cause suspicion. Serosanguineous or bloody nipple discharge is associated with malignancy in between 7% and 17% of cases, but the color or clarity of the fluid cannot diagnose or rule out carcinoma. Cytologic evaluation of the nipple discharge is associated with a false-negative rate of almost 20% and is, therefore, of little value. When the discharge comes from multiple ducts, carcinoma is more likely; mammography and biopsy are required to establish the diagnosis.

Bilateral, milky nipple discharge, especially when accompanied by amenorrhea, suggests the possibility of elevated prolactin levels. This may be due to continued lactation (after even a remote pregnancy), pituitary adenoma, medications, or other less common sources (Table 14.4). A simple fat stain of the discharge will confirm the physiologic character of the discharge in these cases. Laboratory study should include an evaluation of thyroid function in addition to serum prolactin levels. The possibility of an intercurrent pregnancy as a cause of galactorrhea should not be overlooked.

Nipple discharge associated with burning, itching, or local discomfort in older patients is suggestive of ductal ectasia. The discharge is usually thick or sticky, and gray to black in color. Excisional biopsy is often required to establish the final diagnosis.

Mastitis

Generalized pain, erythema over a portion of the breast (most often upper outer quadrant), and fever constitute the usual clinical presentation of mastitis. When these signs are present in a nursing mother 3 to 4 weeks after delivery, empiric therapy should be begun immediately. A mass present without signs of infection is suggestive of a galactocele, which is palpable in the central portion of the breast. Aspiration produces thick, creamy material. No specific therapy is required for a galactocele and the mass will subside in a few weeks.

Table 14.4. Differential Diagnosis of Galactorrhea

Failure of hypothalamic inhibition of prolactin release
    Central nervous system disease
    Drugs
        Alpha-methyldopa
        Butyrophenones
        Diazepams
        Isoniazid
        Metoclopramide
        Opioids
        Oral contraceptives
        Phenothiazines
        Reserpine
        Tricyclic antidepressants (e.g., Elavil, Tofranil)
        Verapamil
    Pituitary stalk section
Enhanced prolactin-releasing factor
    Hypothyroidism
Enhanced prolactin release (uncontrolled)
    Bronchogenic carcinoma
    Chorioepitheliomas
    Hydatidiform mole
    Hypernephroma
    Pituitary tumors (Forbes-Albright syndrome, Chromophobe adenoma)
Other (rare)
    Cervical spine lesions
    Cirrhosis
    Cushing's disease
    Hemodialysis
    Herpes zoster
    Persistent nipple stimulation
    Renal failure
    Sarcoid
    Stress/trauma
    Thoracotomy scarring

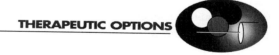

THERAPEUTIC OPTIONS

Selection of Therapy

Effective treatment of fibrocystic change is difficult and based mainly on the character and severity of symptoms experienced by the individual patient. Initial therapy consists of mechanical support (a well-fitting brassiere worn day and night), analgesics, and reassurance. An acute exacerbation may be helped with cold compresses or ice. Diuretics (such as spironolactone or hydrochlorothiazide given prior to periods); premenstrual restriction of salt or fluids; and reduction of caffeine, tobacco, oral contraceptives, or supplemental progestin, all of which are advocated, are successful for 50% to 70% of patients. For patients with severe symptoms, danazol, bromocriptine, tamoxifen, or gonadotropin-releasing hormone (GnRH) agonists may be needed; however, as with simpler modalities, success is not guaranteed and side effects with these agents are more significant. Rarely, patients with intractable pain refractory to medical management require subcutaneous mastectomy.

Many lay publications advocate vitamins B_6 or E, iodine (kelp tablets), evening primrose oil, or diuretic teas for mastalgia or fibrocystic change. Most of these lack rigorous trials and in some cases, such as diuretic teas, many contain caffeine or other agents that may actually worsen symptoms.

Fibroadenomas generally do not disappear, but rather tend to enlarge gradually. They are usually treated by simple local excision, often under local anesthesia, although up to 20% of women will have recurrences. Similarly, lipomas may be followed or excised, based on the size, location, and wishes of the patient.

Patients with puerperal mastitis require aggressive antibiotic therapy with agents such as penicillin G or erythromycin (250–500 mg orally four times a day; erythromycin ethylsuccinate [EES] 400, orally four times a day) for 10 days. First-generation oral cephalosporins (cephalexin 500 mg twice daily, cefaclor 250 mg three times daily) or amoxicillin/clavulanate (Augmentin, 250 mg, three times daily) may also be used. Dicloxacillin may be required for penicillin-resistant strains or sever infections. Nursing or breast pumping should continue during therapy. If tenderness or fever do not respond promptly, abscess formation must be suspected. Breast abscesses require prompt surgical drainage, usually under general anesthesia.

Patients with galactorrhea (with or without amenorrhea) should be treated based on the underlying cause and the patient's wishes for fertility. Patients with elevated prolactin levels not due to a pituitary tumor, may be treated medically with bromocriptine (Parlodel) in escalating doses beginning with 2.5 mg daily, advancing to three times a day. Good resolution of symptoms and return of fertility are generally reported with this therapy. Continuing follow-up of prolactin levels, pituitary imaging, and visual fields may be required based on the patient's clinical course and diagnosis.

Breast cancer treatment is directed toward three goals: local control of disease, treatment of distant disease, and improved quality of life. Early stage breast cancer is treated by breast-sparing surgical excision. (Radical mastectomy, once the standard surgical approach, is giving way to wide local excision or lumpectomy with axillary node dissection.) Surgery is generally followed by adjunctive therapy such as radiation therapy, chemotherapy, hormonal manipulations, or a combination of these three. In general, premenopausal women tend to respond better to cytotoxic chemotherapy, whereas older women have a better response to hormonal treatment. In later stage disease (stage III or IV) multiple therapy is the rule, often involving a multidisciplinary team. In these patients, attention to symptom relief and palliation may take precedence.

Therapy Follow-up

Patients with mastalgia but no dominant mass may be safely rechecked at a different stage of the next menstrual cycle. Following aspiration of a cyst (yielding clear fluid and complete loss of the mass), the patient should be rechecked in 2 to 4 weeks. Recurrence of the cyst or the presence of a palpable mass should prompt additional evaluation, such as fine-needle aspiration or open biopsy. Patients with a history of multiple cysts, diffuse fibrocystic change, or a strong family history of breast disease should be considered for a follow-up mammogram to delve for other occult lesions. Breast self-examination should be encouraged and screening mammography performed based on current guidelines.

Even though breast cancer patients will receive the majority of their follow-up care outside the primary care setting, support and general health issues will continue to be important parts of their care. These patients are at higher risk for developing a new cancer on the opposite side and two thirds of these patients may eventually develop distant metastasis. Primary care providers must keep this in mind as they follow the patient for routine care. These patients must be closely followed with physical examination and mammography (when appropriate). No biologic markers yet exist to allow for either serum-based detection or monitoring of those with breast cancer.

HINTS AND COMMON QUESTIONS

Breast self-examination is best done at the end of the menstrual flow. Hormones are at their lowest at this point, resulting in fewer physiologic "lumps" and less tenderness, making the examination easier. Therefore, when the patient finishes a monthly period or starts a new package of birth control pills, she should plan to perform a breast examination. For patients who have had a hysterectomy and do not have identifiable cyclic changes, or those who have undergone oophorectomy, the examination should be tied to something that happens in a monthly manner to provide a reminder. This may be the first or last day of the month, the patient's birth date, when the rent is due, or when the telephone bill comes. Anything that will act as a reminder will do. Patients with a uterus who are on cyclic hormonal replacement should perform their examination at the end of withdrawal bleeding, just as they would with a natural period.

When an indistinct lesion is found in young women, a repeat examination immediately following the next menstruation will reduce the effect of naturally occurring, hormonally dependent variations in the breast tissue.

Using a small amount of talcum powder or a soap solution (such as pHisoHex) to make the skin slippery greatly facilitates the discovery and characterization of small breast masses and changes in tissue texture.

When a patient reports finding a mass, but no mass is felt by the examiner, re-examination at a different phase of the menstrual cycle, evaluation by another clinician, or mammographic evaluation should be considered.

Obese patients and those with large breasts should be considered for mammography even before they would normally be screened based on their age. Despite careful clinical examinations, only the grossest of lesions is likely to be found without the help of imaging.

When evaluating patients with nipple discharge, two additional causes should be considered: jogging and aerobic exercise. Patients who jog several miles a day, especially without adequate breast support, may develop a spontaneous nipple discharge. Aerobic conditioning, especially when combined with weightlifting, may provide sufficient pectoral muscle stimulation to induce a discharge as well.

Many patients ask about cyclic increases in breast size or fullness occurring just prior to menstruation. For some patients this may lead to discomfort. These changes are normal. The average woman will have an increase in breast volume of roughly 10% (25–30 mL) owing to hormonally dependent increased blood flow, vascular engorgement, and fluid storage.

Breast cancer occurs infrequently during pregnancy, accounting for only 2% to 3% of all cancers. While pregnancy often causes a delay in diagnosis, there is little evidence that these tumors behave any differently, stage for stage, than those diagnosed outside of pregnancy.

At one time lactation was recommended as conferring some protection against breast cancer. A number of studies have now shown that this is not the case. Lactation does not have any independent protective effect on the likelihood of developing breast cancer.

For the purposes of counseling, it is important to remember that although a patient's lifetime risk of cancer is roughly 1 in 10, her risk by decade of life is much less. For patients between the ages of 30 and 40 years there is a risk of approximately 1 in 1000 of developing breast cancer. This doubles to 2 in 1000 between the ages 40 and 50, and becomes 3 in 1000 for women 50 to 60 years of age. Thus, when a 35-year-old patient is told that having a first-degree relative with breast cancer increases her risk threefold, this only brings her risk to 3 in 1000.

SUGGESTED READINGS

General References

American Cancer Society. Cancer facts and figures—1994. Atlanta: ACS, 1994.

American College of Obstetricians and Gynecologists. Carcinoma of the Breast. ACOG Technical Bulletin 158. Washington, DC: ACOG, 1991.

Fletcher SW, Black W, Harris R, Rimer BK, Shapiro S. Report of the International Workshop on screening for breast cancer. Bethesda, MD: National Cancer Institute, 1993.

Goodson WH III. Annual breast evaluation. In Glass RH (ed). Office Gynecology, 4th ed. Baltimore: Williams & Wilkins, 1992, p 121.

Marchant DJ, Sutton SM. Use of mammography—United States 1990. MMWR 1990;39:621.

Medical News and Perspectives: Breast cancer screening guidelines agreed on by AMA, and other medically related organizations. JAMA 1989;262:1155.

Mitchel GW, Bassett LW. The Female Breast and Its Disorders. Baltimore: Williams & Wilkins, 1990.

Seltzer V, ed. The role of the obstetrician-gynecologist in diagnosing and treating breast disease. Clin Obstet Gynecol 1994;37:877.

Specific References

Bailar JC. Mammography: a contrary view. Ann Intern Med 1976;84:77.

Bergkvist L, Adami HO, Persson I, Hoover R, Schairer C. The risk of breast cancer after estrogen and estrogen-progestin replacement. N Engl J Med 1989;321:293.

Boyle CA, Berkowitz GS, LiVolsi VA, et al. Caffeine consumption and fibrocystic breast disease: a case control epidemiologic study. J Natl Cancer Inst 1984;72:1015.

Butler JA, Vargas HI, Worthen N, Wilson SE. Accuracy of combined clinical-mammographic-cytologic diagnosis of dominant breast masses: a prospecitve study. Arch Surg 1990;125:893.

Colditz GA, Egan KM, Stampfer MJ. Hormone replacement therapy and risk of breast cancer: results from epidemiologic studies. Am J Obstet Gynecol 1993;168:1473.

Colditz GA, Hankinson SE, Hunter DJ, et al. The use of estrogens and progestins and the risk of breast cancer in postmenopausal women. N Engl J Med 1995;332:1589.

Colditz GA, Stampfer MJ, Willet WC, et al. Prospective study of estrogen replacement therapy and risk of breast cancer in post-menopausal women. JAMA 1990;264:2648.

Committee on Gynecologic Practice. Estrogen replacement in women with previously treated breast cancer. Washington, DC: American College of Obstetricians and Gynecologists Committee Opinion No. 135, April 1994.

Donegan WL. Evaluation of a palpable breast mass. N Engl J Med 1992;327:937.

Dupont WD, Page DL. Menopausal estrogen replacement therapy and breast cancer. Arch Intern Med 1991;151:67.

Eddy DM, Hasselblad V, McGivney W, et al. The value of mammography screening in woman under age 50 years. JAMA 1988;259:1512.

Ferguson CM, Powel RW. Breast masses in young women. Arch Surg 1989;124:1338.

Foster RS, Costanza MC. Breast self-examination practices and breast cancer survival. Cancer 1984;53:999.

Freig SA. Decreased breast cancer mortality through mammography screening: results of clinical trials. Radiology 1988;167:659.

Greenwald P, Nasca PC, Lawrence CE, et al. Estimated effect of breast self-examination and routine physician examinations on breast-cancer mortality. N Engl J Med 1978;299:271.

Isaacs JH. Other nipple discharge. Clin Obstet Gynecol 1994;37:898.

Miller BA, Ries LA, Hankey BF, Kosary CL, Edwards BK, eds. Cancer Statistics Review: 1973–1989. Washington, DC: US Department of Health and Human Services, National Cancer Institute. HIH Publication No. 92–2789, 1992.

Minton JP, Foecking MK, Webster DJT, et al. Caffeine, cyclic nucleotides and breast disease. Surgery 1979;86:105.

Moskowitz M. Predictive value, sensitivity, and specificity in breast cancer screening. Radiology 1988;167:576.

Recht A, Come SE, Gelman RS, et al. Integration of conservative surgery, radiotherapy, and chemotherapy for the treatment of early-stage node-positive breast cancer: sequencing, timing, and outcome. J Clin Oncol 1991;9:1662.

Schlesselman JJ. Cancer of the breast and reproductive tract in relation to use of oral contraceptives. Contraception 1989;40:1.

Smart CR. The role of mammography in the prevention of mortality from breast cancer. Cancer Prevention 1990;June:1.

Steinberg KK, Thacker SB, Smith SJ, et al. A meta-analysis of the effect of estrogen replacement on the risk of breast cancer. JAMA 1991;265:1985.

15

Infertility

The inability to conceive and bear children affects between 8% and 18% of the American population. At one time, there was little that could be done to help these couples. With improved understanding of the physiology of conception and a wide range of technologies that may be brought to bear to assist with procreation, 85% of "infertile" couples can be helped. Much of the evaluation and initial treatment of these couples can be carried out in the outpatient primary care setting. Interest and facility with the emotional and interpersonal impacts of the inability to conceive is clearly the strength of the primary care provider.

BACKGROUND AND SCIENCE

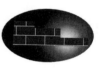

"Infertility"

Under ordinary circumstances, 80% to 90% of normal couples will conceive during a year of attempting pregnancy (Fig. 15.1). Although public awareness of infertility and media interest in assisted reproduction technologies have increased, rates of infertility have remained relatively stable over the 30 years for which data have been available. The prevalence of infertility does, however, increase with the age of the woman (Fig. 15.2). Delayed childbearing by women who have deferred families to complete an education or further a career together with a greater awareness of, and wider access to, infertility services have contributed to the perception of increased fertility problems.

Infertility is generally defined as failure to conceive after 1 year of regular, unprotected intercourse. Infertility can be further subdivided into primary and secondary types based on the patient's reproductive history; nulligravida infertility patients are classified as primary; those who have achieved a pregnancy more than a year previously, regardless of the

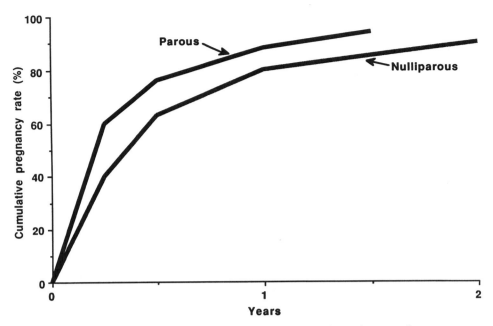

Figure 15.1. Cumulative conception rates for normal couples. The cumulative conception rates for normal parous and nulliparous women is shown. Conception rates are often even higher for patients in their teens and early 20s. (Data from: Lenton ES, Eston GA, Cooke ID. Long-term follow-up of the apparently normal couple with a complaint of infertility. Fertil Steril 1977;28:913.)

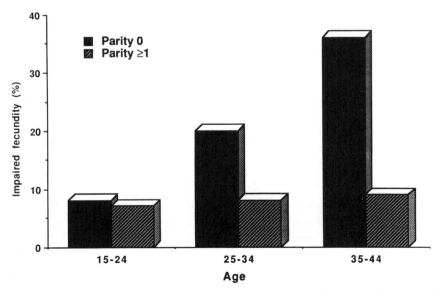

Figure 15.2. Impaired fecundity by age and parity status in currently married women. As age increases, fecundity impairment rate increases for those who have never born children, while it remains relatively stable for those who have had previous pregnancies. Infertility over the age of 45 approaches 70% in some studies. (Data from: Mosher WD, Pratt WF. Fecundity and infertility in the United States, 1965–1988. Advance Data 1990;192:1.)

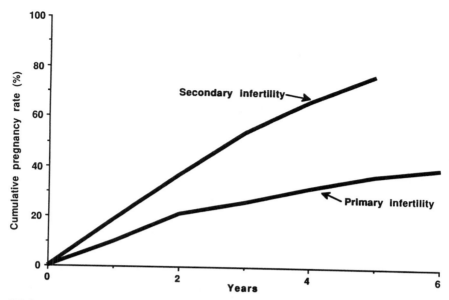

Figure 15.3. Cumulative conception rates for infertile couples. The cumulative conception rates for infertile couples are shown. (Data from: Lenton ES, Weston GA, Cooke ID. Long-term follow-up of the apparently normal couple with a complaint of infertility. Fertil Steril 1977;28:913.)

outcome of that pregnancy, are grouped as secondary infertility. Slightly more than half of infertility patients fall into the primary group. Some authors base the primary versus secondary designation on the male partner's reproductive history as well, labeling as secondary infertility a couple made up of a woman has never conceived and a man who has fathered at least one child. For the purposes of this chapter, we will use the more prevalent convention of basing the classification of infertility on the reproductive history of the woman. Although the distinction between primary and secondary infertility is somewhat artificial, the outlook for successful achievement of pregnancy varies significantly between the two groups (Fig. 15.3).

The medical definition of infertility differs from that of fecundity, which refers to the physical ability of a woman to have children. Women with impaired fecundity include those who find it physically difficult or medically inadvisable to conceive, and those who fail to conceive after 36 months of regular, unprotected intercourse. In short, fecundity deals with childbearing ability, whereas fertility deals with childbearing performance.

Some authors include as a form of infertility recurrent or habitual abortion. Although this does result in an inability to have children, it reflects a different set of pathophysiologies and therapeutic problems than does the inability to conceive. This aspect of impaired childbearing is discussed in Chapter 5, Complications of Early Pregnancy.

Physiology of Conception

To achieve pregnancy, three critical elements must be in place: 1) a sperm must be available, 2) an egg must be available, and 3) the sperm and egg must meet at a time and place

Table 15.1. Characteristics of a Normal Ejaculate

Volume	2–15 mL
	(Average 2.5 mL)
Viscosity	Full liquefaction within 1 h
pH	7.2–7.8
Count (per mL)	>20 million
Motility	>60% after 4 h
	(>50% with forward progression immediately, or >25% with forward progression after 1 h)
Abnormal sperm morphology	<25%
White blood cells (WBC)	<1 million/mL
	(2–5 WBC/high power field)

conducive to fertilization. It is the investigation of these three elements that constitutes the evaluation of the infertile couple.

The male partner brings to the union sperm-laden semen, deposited in the vagina during intercourse. The average ejaculate has a volume of between 1 and 15 mL, and contains over 20 million spermatozoa (Table 15.1). The survival of sperm in the female genital tract is thought to be at least 96 hours, and it may be as long as 8 days. However, it is probable that sperm are capable of fertilizing an egg for only the first 24 to 48 hours after ejaculation. This would indicate that the deposition of normal amounts of semen into the genital tract every 2 to 3 days is probably sufficient for fertilization to occur.

The woman's gametic contribution—the oocyte—is released from the ovary during the midcycle process of ovulation. In normal ovulatory cycles, this takes place 14 days before the onset of menstruation, regardless of the total cycle length. Therefore, in the hypothetically normal cycle of 28 days, ovulation takes place on day 14; but when the cycle is longer or shorter, the time of ovulation varies, maintaining the 14-day luteal phase. Once ovulation takes place, progesterone is produced by the luteinized follicle. This increased progesterone produces a characteristic rise of between 0.5°F and 1°F in basal body temperature. Elevated progesterone levels associated with ovulatory cycles may also produce the characteristic preperiod symptoms of abdominal bloating, increased heaviness, fullness and tenderness of the breasts, decreased vaginal secretions, mild peripheral edema, and mood changes. This collections of symptoms is referred to as preperiod molimina, which can be used clinically as presumptive evidence of ovulation.

It is estimated that the oocyte may be fertilized only during the first 24 hours after ovulation. Fertilization generally takes place in the distal portion of the fallopian tube. For this to happen, sperm must be deposited in the upper vagina, traverse the cervical mucus, become capacitated, pass through the endometrial cavity and proximal tubes, and reach the distal tube. The oocyte must have been picked up by the fimbria and delivered to the distal fallopian tube; both egg and sperm must be present within the appropriate time frame.

Even if fertilization does occur, pregnancy will not result unless the zygote passes into the uterine cavity at the correct time (approximately 3 to 5 days after fertilization), encounters a receptive endometrium, and can successfully implant and grow. Obstruction in the fallopian tubes, inappropriate transport time, distortion of the uterine cavity, or a hostile endometrium may all result in loss of the zygote.

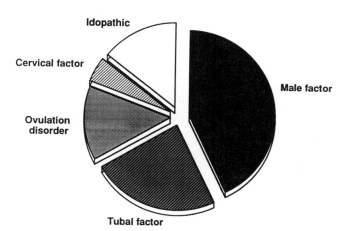

ESTABLISHING THE DIAGNOSIS

When dealing with the question of infertility, establishing the diagnosis is not the problem; rather it is identifying the underlying pathophysiology. Unlike most areas of medicine, except obstetrics, the provider must deal with two patients at the same time, for it is the couple that is infertile, not the man or woman. When the relative frequency of causes is considered (Fig. 15.4), it is apparent that male and female factors are present in roughly equal proportion, with only a small number of the remaining being idiopathic. This is important to keep in mind when counseling. The distribution of causes is also helpful in designing a logical and efficient strategy for the evaluation of the infertile couple (Fig. 15.5).

Before embarking on testing, it is important that the couple understand the nature, duration, limitations, and expense of an infertility evaluation. Reticence or ambivalence on the part of one or both partners may signal problems with motivation or interest or the presence of hidden agendas. The couple's interest in an infertility evaluation may be prompted by pressure from relatives or be an outgrowth of marital discord. The evaluation will not solve these problems, and a tenuous marriage is only weakened by a pregnancy. These couples deserve a different form of diagnosis and support.

History and Physical Examination

As with most conditions, the evaluation of the complaint of infertility should begin with a history, obtained from both partners. The gynecologic portion addresses the age of the patient, her gravidity and parity, and menstrual, contraceptive, medical, and surgical histo-

Figure 15.4. Approximate distribution of infertility causes. Approximately 35% to 50% of infertility is due to a male factor, such as azoospermia. Female factors, such as tubal disease (20% to 30%), ovulation disorders (10% to 15%), and cervical factors (5%), contribute to the roughly 50% to 60% of female causes. The remaining 10% to 20% of couples have no identifiable cause for their infertility (idiopathic).

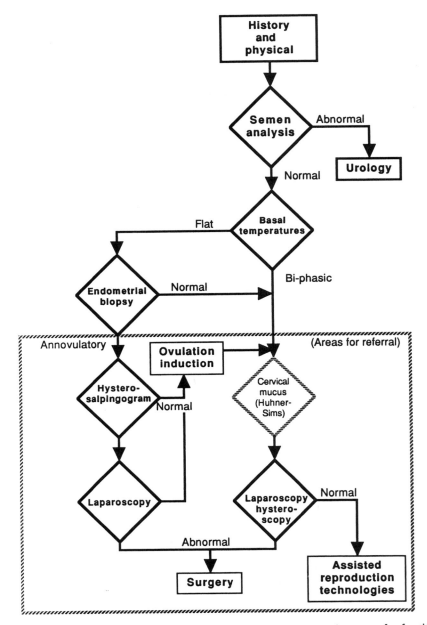

Figure 15.5. Algorithm for the evaluation of infertility. While the evaluation of infertility proceeds, couples should be instructed to continue attempting pregnancy through intercourse timed to the most fertile days of the cycle. Between one third and one half of all infertility problems may be diagnosed in the first phase of evaluation. This portion of the evaluation is well within the purview of the primary care team. For those who wish to perform more extensive evaluations of the male factor, the flow chart shown in Figure 15.6 expands on this phase of testing. When anovulation or oligo-ovulation is suspected, it may be evaluated as shown in Figure 19.4.

ries, including sexually transmitted diseases and pelvic infections. Her partner's age, medical, and surgical history must also be reviewed. The duration of the current partnership, duration of the infertility, previous marital history, and the results of any previous evaluations should be obtained. Medication use and exposure to toxins or illicit drugs, for either partner, should be established. The frequency of intercourse, its distribution throughout the week or month, and the use of adjuncts, such as lubricants, must be noted. Postcoital practices, including douching, must be explored. Everything from hot tubs to the type of underwear worn must be explored. Even the obvious, such as extravaginal intercourse must be considered. Some authors suggest that more candid answers may be forthcoming if the partners are interviewed separately.

Physical examination of both partners is directed toward the detection of illness or physical conditions that might impair fertility, as well as a general assessment of health. For the male partner this must include testicular size, the presence of a varicocele (present in 25% of infertile men), genitourinary infection, and hypospadias. For the woman, a general examination is performed, including the breast and pelvic areas. At the time of the pelvic examination cervical cultures may be taken and the cervical mucus assessed. Some authors suggest that a maturation index be obtained at the same time, although without reason to suspect significant estrogen deficit this is unlikely to be of significant value.

Male Factors

The first investigation performed for any infertile couple should be a semen analysis. This is the least invasive of all infertility tests and it has the greatest potential to find a cause of any single test. If the semen analysis is normal, roughly one half of all identifiable causes of infertility will have been ruled out. Even when a coexistent female factor is found, no pregnancy will result from treatment of the female partner if the male cannot supply the needed sperm.

Classification of male fertility is based on two to three semen analyses. Semen analysis is carried out after a minimum of 48 hours of abstinence. Ejaculate is obtained by masturbation in the office or laboratory, so that immediate assessment of the sample may be carried out. A prewarmed, clean, wide-mouthed jar or sample container is adequate. For those men who find masturbation unacceptable for religious or other reasons, samples obtained during intercourse, followed by withdrawal, or a special silastic sheath can be used. These samples or those obtained by masturbation at home must be kept at body temperature and transported to the laboratory within 2 hours of collection. A condom should not be used for sample collection because of spermicidal effects that even unmedicated condoms may have.

Anticipated normal values for a semen analysis are shown in Table 15.1. A normal semen analysis excludes a male factor in more than 90% of couples. Men with sperm counts of between 5 and 20 million are classed as subfertile, although as many as 20% of couples with sperm counts between 10 and 20 million will conceive without further assistance. Counts below 5 million carry a poor prognosis for fertility. Significant abnormalities of volume, pH, morphology, or motility are similarly associated with impaired fertility. A partial list of causes of male infertility is shown in Table 15.2. Some authors advocate a sperm penetration assay when inconclusive semen analysis or persistent infertility without other identifiable cause is encountered (Fig. 15.6). The role of this test and the full range of other evaluations performed for the subfertile or infertile male, beyond the obvious, is outside the scope of this book.

Table 15.2. Possible Causes of Male Infertility

Pretesticular and hormonal causes
    Central gonadotropin deficiency
        Hypothalamic (congenital GnRH deficiency, tumor, trauma, infection)
        Pituitary (congenital FSH/LH deficiency, tumor, trauma, infection, infarction)
        Metabolic (sarcoidosis, hemachromatosis)
    Endocrin excess
        Androgen (congenital adrenal hyperplasia, androgen-producing tumors)
        Estrogen (adrenal tumors, cirrhosis)
        Glucocorticoid (Cushing's syndrome, exogenous steroids)
    Other
        Hypothyroidism
        Diabetes mellitus
Testicular causes
    Anatomic abnormality (varicocele)
    Androgen insensitivity syndrome
    Chemotherapy
    Chromosomal abnormalities (Klinefelter's syndrome, 47, XXY)
    Cryptorchidism (unilateral or bilateral)
    Idiopathic maturation arrest
    Radiation
    Sertoli-cell-only syndrome
    Thermal stress
    Torsion
    Toxin exposure (smoking, marijuana)
    Trauma
    Viral orchitis (mumps)
Posttesticular and extratesticular causes
    Acquired ductal obstruction (infection, surgical)
    Antisperm antibodies
    Congenital ductal obstruction (vas deferens, epididymis)
    Hypospadias
    Impaired motility syndromes
    Medication (phenothiazines, adrenergic inhibitors, nitrofurantoin, sulfasalazine, colchicine, cimetidine, spironolactone)
    Retrograde ejaculation

GnRH = gonadotropin-releasing hormone; FSH = follicle-stimulating hormone; LH = luteinizing hormone.

Female Factors

Ovulatory Disorders

Disorders of ovulation are found in up to 30% of infertile couples. Documenting the presence and timing of ovulation is, therefore, an important early part of any infertility evaluation. Although there are a number of ways to establish conclusive or presumptive evidence of ovulation (Table 15.3), one of the easiest methods is the basal body temperature chart. This simple test can provide presumptive evidence of ovulation, assess the adequacy of the luteal phase, provide a glimpse of coital frequency and timing, and assist in the scheduling of other infertility studies. The clinical utility of the basal body temperature (BBT) graph is limited by the manner in which the patient obtains and records the data. For this reason, a few moments of careful instruction will prevent the loss of days or months worth of in-

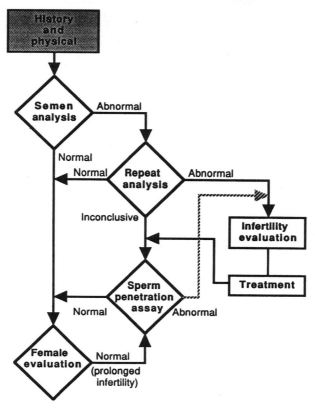

Figure 15.6. Algorithm for the evaluation of infertility. When an abnormal semen analysis is obtained, a second or third assay should be performed before proceeding with further testing. The sperm penetration assay is best used to evaluate men with inconsistent or inconclusive semen analysis, those undergoing treatment for infertility (prior to expensive or invasive tests or therapies), or for couples with prolonged unexplained infertility.

vestigation and may prevent unnecessary, costly, or potentially dangerous further evaluations.

Patients who have been asked to record their BBT should be instructed to obtain their temperature in a uniform manner. They should take their temperature at the same time, on awakening, and before arising from the bed even to visit the bathroom. The thermometer must be correctly placed and left in place for 5 minutes, timed by the clock. The temperature reading thus obtained is then plotted on the graph. Coital activity for the preceding 24 hours and the presence of bleeding or other symptoms should be recorded as well. Some authors advocate recording additional information, such as the presence and character of cervical secretions, breast tenderness, or mood, although many feel that this provides little additional information and only increases the already heavy burden of tasks asked of the infertile couple.

More than 90% of ovulatory women will have the characteristic biphasic temperature graph shown in Figure 15.7. It must be kept in mind that the temperature rise actually occurs after ovulation when progesterone produced by the corpus luteum influences tempera-

Table 15.3. Diagnostic Tests for Ovulation

Presumptive
 Biphasic basal temperature graph
 Cervical mucus change
 Cul-de-sac fluid documented by ultrasound
 Endometrial biopsy
 Follicle collapse documented by ultrasound
 LH surge (serum or urinary)
 Plasma 17 α-hydroxyprogesterone
 Plasma estradiol
 Plasma or salivary progesterone
 Premenstrual molimina
 Regularity of menstrual cycles
 Urinary pregnanediol
 Vaginal cytology
 Vaginal pH change
 Visualization of corpus luteum (laparoscopy or ultrasound)
Conclusive
 Observation of ovulation (laparoscopy)
 Pregnancy
 Recovery of oocyte (tubal or uterine flushing)

LH = luteinizing hormone.

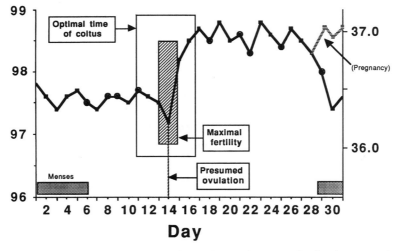

Figure 15.7. Basal body temperature graphs in the evaluation of infertility. Graphs of basal body temperature, which are taken on awakening before any physical activity has taken place, may be useful in evaluating ovulatory function and in timing of intercourse. Here the temperature graph suggests an ovulatory pattern with reasonable coital frequency (circles), but unfortunate timing. Had a pregnancy occurred, the temperature would have remained elevated (dotted line).

ture control mechanisms. For this reason, BBT graphs are good for supporting the presumption of ovulation during the preceding month, but are poor predictors of when to have intercourse during the cycle at hand. Evaluation of cervical mucus character and ferning (Fig. 15.8) can be used in a similar way to infer ovulation. Endometrial biopsy can provide a more direct picture of hormonal effects, but at a high price and risk of morbidity.

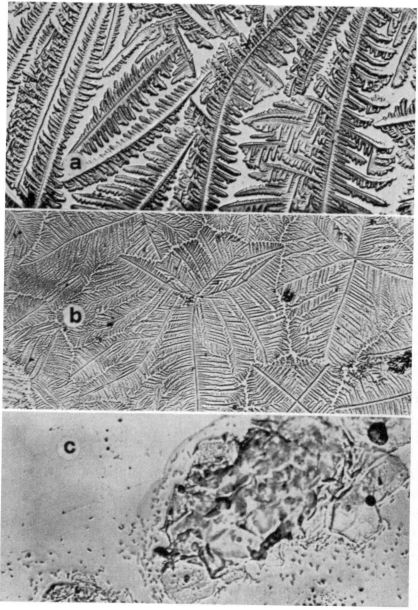

Figure 15.8. Presumptive ovulation determined by cervical mucus changes. Ovulation occurs at the time when fern formation is strongly positive (**a** and **b**); when progesterone is present the mucus shows a negative reaction or only a slight fern pattern (**c**). (From Jones HW, Wentz AC, Burnett LS. Novak's textbook of gynecology. 11th ed. Baltimore: Williams & Wilkins, 1988:269.)

Tubal Factors

Although tubal factors are a more common cause of infertility than are ovulation disorders, tubal patency evaluation is much more invasive and, therefore, delayed until after the semen analysis and assessment of ovulation has taken place. Tubal infection and pelvic adhesive disease are the most common causes of tubal obstruction and dysfunction. Endometriosis, scarring and adhesion formation following pelvic surgery, and anatomic distortion from tumors or congenital malformations may all contribute to tubal factor infertility. Previously, the most common tool for assessing tubal patency was the hysterosalpingogram. Although this test still plays an important role in the evaluation of infertility, for some patients it may be more cost-effective to proceed directly to laparoscopy, with simultaneous hysteroscopy.

Hysterosalpingography (HSG) provides information about the inside contour of the uterine cavity and presumptive evidence of tubal patency (Fig. 15.9). It does not provide information about the outside contour of the uterus or the presence of periovarian and paratubal adhesions that can interfere with ovum transport. Even when signs of tubal obstruction are detected by HSG, they are not always borne out by other studies. For example, spasm of the proximal fallopian tubes may provide a false impression of obstruction during hystesosalpingography. As a result, the diagnostic accuracy of the HSG is estimated to be

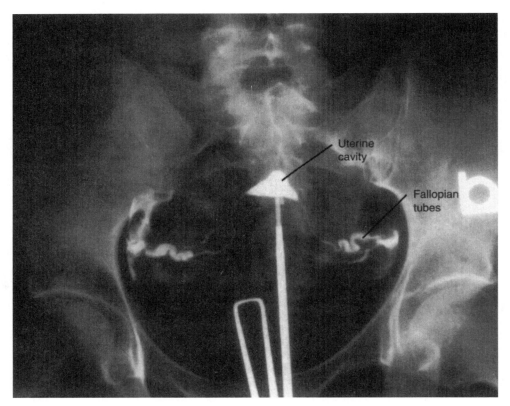

Figure 15.9. Hysterosalpingogram showing normal genital tract anatomy and architecture. (From Beckmann RB, Ling FW, Barzansky BM, et al. Obstetrics and gynecology. 2nd ed. Baltimore: Williams & Wilkins, 1995:396.)

only 70%. The combination of laparoscopy, chromotubation (the injection of colored fluid into the uterine cavity during laparoscopy to detect tubal spill), and hysteroscopy provides more direct information. Approximately 50% of women undergoing endoscopy will have one or more abnormalities detected, usually pelvic adhesions or endometriosis. These procedures also offer the possibility of direct therapeutic intervention if an abnormality is found, potentially offsetting the increased cost and morbidity of these more invasive techniques.

Although most primary care providers choose to refer patients for hysterosalpingography, a passing familiarity with the technique facilitates counseling and patient selection. Hysterosalpingography is generally performed between the seventh and thirteenth day of the menstrual cycle to avoid iatrogenic retrograde menstruation or interference with ovum transport and implantation after ovulation. Mild to moderate cramping and some vaginal bleeding may be encountered during or after the procedure. Although HSG is associated with improved subsequent fertility, presumably through mechanical lysis of small adhesions and distension of the tubal lumen, it is also associated with an increased risk of upper genital tract infection. Any complaint of fever, chills, or abdominal pain that persists or occurs soon after the procedure should be promptly investigated.

Cervical and Other Factors

A frequently employed test to evaluate cervical mucus and sperm deposition, density, and motility is the postcoital test (Sims-Huhner test). This test is best performed just before anticipated ovulation when cervical mucus is abundant and facilitates sperm transport and survival. The couple is asked to have normal intercourse 2 to 8 hours before the scheduled test. The cervix is visualized using a speculum and a small sample of cervical mucus is aspirated and placed on a microscope slide. In a normal test, eight to ten motile sperm will be found per high power field of view. Clumping of the sperm or excessive numbers of white

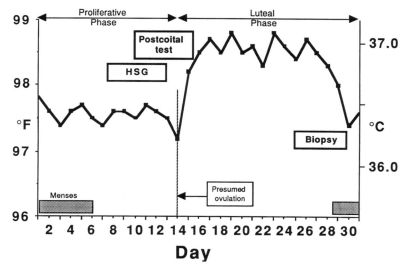

Figure 15.10. Timing of a specialized infertility test throughout the menstrual cycle. Infertility tests should be timed to specific phases of the menstrual cycle. The hysterosalpingogram should be performed in the proliferative phase, whereas endometrial biopsy is carried out just before menstruation. Postcoital testing should be done just before or at the time of ovulation.

blood cells are abnormal and suggest antisperm antibodies or inflammation, respectively. When normal, the postcoital test provides information about the adequacy of intercourse, sperm deposition, sperm pickup, and motility. The postcoital test does not substitute for a semen analysis, nor does it provide a good appraisal of ovulatory function.

The relative timing of the postcoital test, hysterosalpingography, and endometrial biopsy are shown in Figure 15.10.

Immunologic testing to detect the presence of antisperm antibodies in either partner, specialized andrology studies, evaluation of luteal phase defects, biochemical studies, and other testing is the province of specialists and will not be covered here. Referral to these specialists is even required of most general gynecologists.

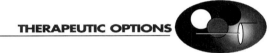

THERAPEUTIC OPTIONS

The treatment of an infertile couple is based on identifying the impediment to fertility and overcoming or bypassing it to achieve pregnancy. A number of techniques are available to accomplish this end. Most are less exotic than their acronyms would suggest (Table 15.4). Among infertile couples seeking treatment, 85% to 90% can be treated with conventional medical and surgical procedures and will not require assisted reproductive technologies such as in vitro fertilization.

Treatment success depends to a great extent on the identified cause of infertility (Fig. 15.11), as some problems are more easily overcome than others. It must be recognized that success is also a function of the age of the woman (Fig. 15.12). It is also true that the rate of spontaneous pregnancy loss also increases rapidly after the age of 35. This poses a

Table 15.4. Commonly Encountered Abbreviations Associated with Assisted Reproduction

Abbreviation	Technique
AID	Artificial insemination, donor (using donor sperm, occasionally referred to as TDI or therapeutic donor insemination)
AIH	Artificial insemination, homologous (using the partner's sperm)
BBT	Basal body temperature
GIFT	Gamete intra-fallopian transfer (gametes are placed in the fallopian tube for fertilization)
HSG	Hysterosalpingogram, or uterine cavity x-ray
IUI	Intrauterine insemination; placement of either donor or husband sperm directly into the uterine cavity
IVF/ET	In vitro fertilization with embryo transfer
PCT	Post-coital test or Huhner-Sims test
SPA	Sperm penetration assay (also known as a hamster egg test, or zona-free egg penetration test)
ZIFT	Zygote intra-fallopian transfer (fertilization takes place in vitro and the zygote is transferred to the fallopian tube to be transported into the uterine cavity)

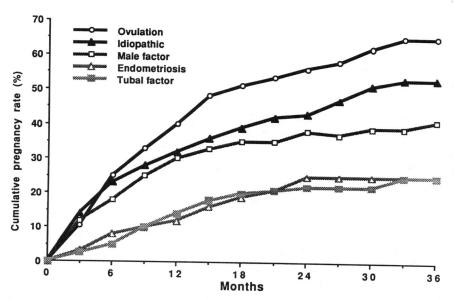

Figure 15.11. Cumulative pregnancy rates by type of underlying disorder. Cumulative pregnancy rates and success of therapy varies by the nature of the underlying cause. Success is greatest when a problem with ovulation exists and poorest when the infertility is based on a tubal factor. Data shown is based on 1297 couples reported by: Collins JA, So Y, Wilson EH, Wrixon W, Casper RF. Clinical factors affecting pregnancy rates among infertile couples. Can Med Assoc J 1984;130:269.

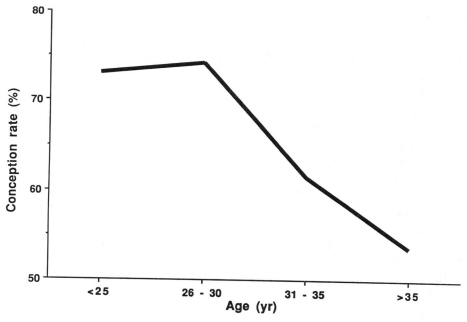

Figure 15.12. Success of artificial insemination by age of the woman. The success of infertility treatment is influenced by the age of the woman treated. There is a significant decline in success as age increases, as demonstrated in this data taken from experience with donor insemination programs. (Data from: Federation CECOS, Schwartz D, Mayaux MJ. Female fecundity as a function of age: Results of artificial insemination in 2193 nulliparous women with azoospermic husbands. N Engl J Med 1982;306:404.)

dilemma: How aggressive should the evaluation and treatment of infertility be for women after the age of 40? Although pregnancy does occur after this age, indeed even after the age of 50, aggressive intervention risks exploitation of couples who may be unrealistic and vulnerable. Ultimately, the final decision must rest with the patient, her partner, and the health care team, but realistic counseling about the chance of success is mandatory in this age group. The couple may be better served by realistic advice about alternatives, such as adoption, than by attempts to bend the rules of biology.

Often a good starting point in the treatment of infertility is a frank and open discussion about sexuality and the physiology of conception. Many couples do not understand the process, inadvertently compromising their chances through myth and misunderstanding. Assisting couples to understand the relationship between coital frequency, timing of intercourse, and the chance of fertilization, may significantly increase their probability of conception. When couples have intercourse four or more times per week, over 80% will achieve pregnancy in the first 6 months of trying. By contrast, only about 15% of couples conceive when intercourse happens less than once a week.

Because the timing of ovulation can never be known with any precision, asking the couple to abstain from intercourse for 5 to 7 days prior to presumed ovulation to save sperm, may result in missing the most fertile time. A more realistic suggestion is that intercourse be maintained on an every other day cycle from 3 to 4 days prior to and 2 to 3 days after the time of the presumed ovulation.

Male Factors

When low sperm counts are present, greater effectiveness may be made of those available through the use of the first portion of the ejaculate, coupled with artificial insemination. In this technique the most concentrated semen is placed in proximity to the cervix through the use of a cervical cap or placed into the uterine cavity using a cannula and syringe. The cervical cap technique may even be used by the couple at home, with some authors reporting over 50% pregnancy rates using this approach. This technique is most successful in cases involving problems with the deposition of semen, such as paraplegia, retrograde ejaculation, impotence, or vaginismus.

A slight improvement in success rates for subfertile men may be obtained by the use of washed and centrifuged samples that are then placed directly into the uterine cavity. More technically complex and prone to complications such as vasovagal syncope, these techniques are best left to those with specialized experience.

More successful is insemination with donor sperm. This provides normal sperm numbers, often from donors with proved fertility. The loss of direct biologic descendants, cost, and a small risk of disease transmission, make this option unacceptable for some couples. It is also not a guarantee of success. A 1987 study by the U.S. Office of Technology Assessment found that almost 175,000 women underwent artificial insemination, resulting in approximately 65,000 births, representing a success rate of 38%. Donor insemination programs and the use of frozen semen samples carry a number of technical, ethical, and legal controls that are best left to those who do them on a regular basis.

When a varicocele is present, surgical treatment is associated with a fertility rate of approximately 30% to 50%.

Ovulation Disorders

When ovulation disorders are encountered, ovulation induction or control may be used to enhance the likelihood of pregnancy. Clomiphene citrate may be used to induce ovulation. Ovulation is successfully achieved in 70% of patients, but is associated with only a 40% pregnancy rate. Furthermore, the incidence of twin gestations is increased to 5% to 10%. The use of human menopausal gonadotropins (HMG) may also be used to control ovulation, but this is generally reserved for in vitro fertilization programs where superovulation and exact timing are required. The use of these techniques falls to the specialist, necessitating referral.

Tubal Factors

Tubal factor infertility may be addressed by either surgical repair of the damage or by bypassing the tubes completely through in vitro fertilization and embryo transfer (IVF/ET). Success rates for surgical repair, including the reversal of previous sterilization procedure, are highly variable. Success is based on the degree of damage, the extent of the surgery required, the length and patency of the remaining tube, the age of the patient, the skill of the surgeon, and other factors. Success rates of 25% to 40% are typical. Success rates of in vitro fertilization programs also vary, but are generally in the range of 10% to 30%. Possible indications for IVF/ET are shown in Table 15.5.

HINTS AND COMMON QUESTIONS

Infertility patients are extremely motivated, following to the letter any suggestion made by the health care team. For this reason, care must be taken that in the process of evaluating and treating infertility, we do not destroy the couple's relationship. In the end, there is no guarantee that our efforts will result in a conception, so we must not damage what is present in the quest of something that may not be. Couples should be reminded that: "If you miss having intercourse at the 'right time' on a given month, remember that ovulations are like commuter trains—there is probably another one on its way." If the couple is in the mood for making love, in any of its myriad forms, they should not worry about what the temperature chart is doing. To do otherwise is the fodder of cinematic comedy and divorce lawyers.

Because infertility threatens neither life nor health, many insurance providers will not cover the cost of its evaluation or treatment. A frank and open discussion about the time

Table 15.5. Clinical Indications for In Vitro Fertilization and Embryo Transfer (IVF/ET)

Abnormal cervical factor
Fallopian tube obstruction
Immunologic infertility
Oligospermia
Significant fimbrial disease
Unexplained infertility

and expense involved in an infertility evaluation allows the couple to make informed choices and avoids unnecessary financial or emotional hardship in the future.

Some of the tests and procedures required during an infertility evaluation may violate some couple's religious prohibitions. For example, the collection of a semen sample by masturbation poses a problem for some Catholic men and having intercourse within 7 days of menstrual bleeding is prohibited by Orthodox Jewish law. Inquiry about the religious beliefs of a couple early in the evaluation process will save embarrassment later and will allow specific accommodations to be made.

It is not enough to determine that a couple has intercourse three times a week. In this era of dual or even triple incomes, partners may pass each other on the way to work. The only time they may be at home together may be the weekend. The result is multiple episodes of coitus concentrated into a short period, which is no more likely to result in a pregnancy than a single exposure during the same time interval. Intercourse that occurs over 3 separate days is more likely to result in pregnancy than are three episodes on the same day. While both may be sexually satisfying, they are not the same for the purposes of conception.

When it comes to the frequency of intercourse, too much can be as bad as too little. Frequent ejaculation may result in a loss of seminal volume and sperm numbers, potentially dropping below the threshold need for fertilization. Couples attempting pregnancy will occasionally increase their coital frequency to several times a day in an attempt to overcome their lack of success, further decreasing their chances. The best sperm counts and motility are obtained with coital intervals of about 36 hours.

Sperm generation time is approximately 72 to 84 days. As a result, events that took place more than 2 months prior are reflected in the semen analysis. Conversely, any attempt at therapeutic intervention to facilitate sperm production will take a comparable amount of time to have an effect.

Sperm production is very temperature-sensitive. A rise in testicular temperature of only 1°F to 2°F is sufficient to impair sperm production. Hot baths, hot tubs, wearing tight brief-style underwear, or occupations that required prolonged sitting may all decrease fertility. Cooling the scrotum has been advocated, but this has not been thoroughly evaluated.

Women who experience absent or irregular menses; or who have signs of hirsutism, severe acne, or galactorrhea; or abnormally scant vaginal secretions may be presumed to be anovulatory, and, therefore, need not record basal body temperatures. The evaluation of these women should proceed in the same manner as for secondary amenorrhea (Chapter 19, No Periods [Amenorrhea]).

Home test kits to detect the luteinizing hormone (LH) surge are available. These may be used to help detect the preovulatory surge of LH, but they are expensive, must still be used in conjunction with a calendar or temperature graph to conserve tests, and do not confirm the actual ovulation. These kits should not be used routinely, but may be helpful for the timing of artificial insemination.

Half of all women found to have tubal factor infertility have no history of antecedent infections or surgery, supporting the need to evaluate tubal patency in patients regardless of their past history.

Premedication with a nonsteroidal anti-inflammatory drug will significantly reduce the discomfort of hysterosalpingography or endometrial biopsy. The dosage and agents used are those used to treat primary dysmenorrhea. Over-the-counter equivalents may also be used.

SUGGESTED READINGS

General References

American College of Obstetricians and Gynecologists. Infertility. ACOG Technical Bulletin 125. Washington, DC: ACOG, 1989.

American College of Obstetricians and Gynecologists. New reproductive technologies. ACOG Technical Bulletin 140. Washington, DC: ACOG, 1990.

American College of Obstetricians and Gynecologists. Male infertility. ACOG Technical Bulletin 142. Washington, DC: ACOG, 1990.

Bresnick E, Taymor ML. The role of counseling in infertility. Fertil Steril 1979;32:154.

Davajan V. The postcoital tests. J Reprod Med 1977;18:132.

Mosher WD. Reproductive impairments in the United States 1965–1982. Demography 1985;22:415.

Office of Technology Assessment. Infertility: medical and social choices. Washington, DC: Congress of the United States, 1988, p 25.

Olive DL, Schwartz LB. Endometriosis. N Engl J Med 1993;328:1759.

Pratt WF, Mosher WD, Bachrach CA, Horn MC. Understanding U. S. fertility: Findings from the National Survey of Family Growth, Cycle III. Population Bulletin 1984;39:27.

Speroff L, Glass RH, Kase NG. Clinical Gynecologic Endocrinology and Infertility, 5th ed. Baltimore: Williams & Wilkins, 1994.

Wentz AC. Infertility. In Jones HW III, Wentz AC, Burnett LS (eds). Novak's Textbook of Gynecology, 11th ed. Baltimore: Williams & Wilkins, 1988, p 263.

Wilcox LS, Mosher WD. Characteristics associated with impaired fecundity in the United States. Fam Plann Perspect 1994;26:218.

Specific References

Allen NC, Herbert CM, Maxson WS, Rogers BJ, Diamond MP, Wentz AC. Intrauterine insemination: a critical review. Fertil Steril 1985;44:569.

Asch RH, Smith CG. Effects of marijuana on reproduction. Contemporary Ob/Gyn 1983;22:217.

Bateman BG, Kolp LA, Mills S. Endocscopic versus laparotomy management of endometriomas. Fertil Steril 1994;62:690.

Beck WW JR. A critical look at the legal, ethical, and technical aspects of artificial insemination. Fertil Steril 1976;27:1.

Bergquist CA, Rock JA, Miller J, Guzick DS, Wentz AC, Jones GS. Artificial insemination with fresh donor semen using the cervical cap technique: a review of 278 cases. Obstet Gynecol 1982;60:195.

Bronson R, Cooper G, Rosenfeld D. Sperm antibodies: their role in infertility. Fertil Steril 1984;42:171.

Buxton CL, Olson LE. Endometrial biopsy inadvertently taken during conception cycle. Am J Obstet Gynecol 1969;105:702.

Carter JE, Trotter JP. GnRH analogs in the treatment of endometriosis. Female Patient 1995;20:13.

Chung PH, Verkauf BS, Eichberg RD, Casady L, Sanford EJ, Maroulis GB. Electroejaculation and assisted reproductive techniques for anejaculatory infertility. Obstet Gynecol 1996;87:22.

Collins JA, So Y, Wilson EH, Wrixon W, Casper RF. Clinical factors affecting pregnancy rates among infertile couples. Can Med Assoc J 1984;130:269.

Collins JA, So Y, Wilson EH, Wrixon W, Casper RF. The postcoital test as a predictor of pregnancy among 355 infertile couples. Fertil Steril 1984;41:703.

Diamond MP, Christianson C, Daniell JF, Wentz AC. Pregnancy following use of the cervical cap for home artificial insemination utilizing homologous semen. Fertil Steril 1983;39:480.

Federation CECOS, Schwartz D, Mayaux MJ. Female fecundity as a function of age: results of artificial insemination in 2193 nulliparous women with azoospermic husbands. N Engl J Med 1982;306:404

Goldfarb JM, Austin C, Lisbona H, Peskin B, Clapp M. Cost-effectiveness of in vitro fertilization. Obstet Gynecol 1996;87:18.

In vitro fertilization-embryo transfer (IVF-ET) in the United States: 1989 results from the IVF-ET Registry. Fertil Steril 1991;55:14.

Kulikauskas V, Blaustein D, Ablin RJ. Cigarette smoking and its possible effects on sperm. Fertil Steril 1985;44:526.

Lenton ES, Weston GA, Cooke ID. Long-term follow-up of the apparently normal couple with a complaint of infertility. Fertil Steril 1977;28:913.

Miller PB, Soules MR. The usefulness of a urinary LH kit for ovulation prediction during menstrual cycles of normal women. Obstet Gynecol 1996;87:13.

Moghissi KS, Sacco AG, Borin K. Immunologic infertility. I. Cervical mucus antibodies and postcoital test. Am J Obstet Gynecol 1980;136:941.

Mosher WD, Pratt WF. Fecundity and infertility in the United States, 1965–1988. Advance Data 1990;192:1.

Office of Technology Assessment. Artificial insemination practices in the United States: summary of a 1987 survey. Washington, DC: Congress of the United States, 1988.

Perez-Pelaez M, Cohen MR. The split ejaculation in homologous insemination. Int J Fertil 1965;10:25.

Rasmussen F, Lindequist S, Larsen C, Justesen P. Therapeutic effect of hysterosalpingography: Oil versus water soluble contrast media—A randomized prospective study. Radiology 1991;179:75.

Rogers BJ. The sperm penetration assay: its usefulness reevaluated. Fertil Steril 1985;43:821.

Schiller P, Blake RE, Nolan GH. Sexual behavior and infertility. Infertility 1985;8:293.

Smith KD, Rodriguez-Rigau LJ, Steinberger E. Relationship between indicies of semen analysis and pregnancy rate in infertile couples. Fertil Steril 1977;28:1314.

Soules MR, Spadoni LR. Oil versus aqueous media for hysterosalpingography: a continuing debate based on many opinions and few facts. Fertil Steril 1982;38:1.

Sutton CJG, Ewen SP, Whitelaw N, Hanes P. Prospective, randomized, double-blind, controlled trial of laser laparoscopy in the treatment of pelvic pain associated with minimal, mild, and moderate endometriosis. Fertil Steril 1994;62:696.

The American Fertility Societiy: New guidelines for the use of semen donor insemination: 1990. Fertil Steril 1990;53(suppl 1):1s.

Thomas AJ JR. Ejaculatory dysfunction. Fertil Steril 1983;39:445.

Vermeulen A, Vandeweghe M. Improved fertility after vericocele correction: Fact or fiction. Fertil Steril 1984;42:249.

Zavos PM. Seminal parameters of ejaculates collected from oligospermic and normospermic patients via masturbation and at intercourse with the use of a silastic seminal fluid collection device. Fertil Steril 1985;44:517.

Zorgniotti AW, Sealfon AI, Toth A. Chronic scrotal hypothermia as a treatment for poor semen quality. Lancet 1980;1:904.

Zukerman Z, Rodriguez-Rigau LJ, Smith KD, Steinberger E. Frequency distribution of sperm counts in fertile and infertile males. Fertil Steril 1977;28:1310.

16

Heavy Periods and Toxic Shock Syndrome

Between 10% and 15% of women experience excessive menstrual flow. This represents a significant medical and social problem. Multiple causative pathologies, combined with a past lack of effective treatments, has made the diagnosis and treatment of menorrhagia a frustrating clinical task. Although establishing the existence of heavy menses would appear to be simple, it has proven to be an arduous task. A better understanding of prostaglandin pathophysiology, improved clinical tools, such as ultrasonography and office endometrial biopsy, and new therapies have changed this picture. Now most cases of heavy menstruation can be diagnosed and managed successfully in the primary care setting.

BACKGROUND AND SCIENCE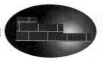

As noted in Chapter 2, Physiology of Menstruation, the average blood loss during a normal menstrual period is between 30 and 50 mL. Menstrual periods generally last 4 to 7 days, with 80% of menstrual blood loss occurring during the first 48 hours. Menstrual loss of greater than 80 mL constitutes menorrhagia and may result in anemia. This level has been operationally defined based on both the statistical average of menstrual loss and the likelihood of developing anemia. While it is possible to have menstrual losses in excess of

80 mL and not be anemic, anemia in the absence of any other cause is almost always associated with menstrual bleeding greater than this level.

Some authors include menstrual flow that last more than 7 days under the classification of menorrhagia. This is more closely tied to dysfunctional bleeding patterns than to the pathophysiologies that are responsible for heavy blood loss, and will be considered along with other forms of dysfunctional uterine bleeding in the next chapter.

As with menstrual pain, menorrhagia is categorized by the presence or absence of a clinically identifiable cause. Where such a process can be identified, the bleeding is classed as secondary menorrhagia; when no cause is evident, primary menorrhagia is presumed. The latter has also been referred to as "essential" menorrhagia. Because therapy is chosen on the basis of the underlying pathophysiology, this distinction is not trivial. Care in establishing the diagnosis greatly improves the likelihood of successful treatment.

Secondary menorrhagia can originate from a number of potential pathologies. These may be further classified as those processes that arise within the uterus and those that are external to the uterus (Table 16.1). Some of these processes have a high degree of association with heavy periods, some do not. For example, roughly one third of women with uterine leiomyoma complain of menorrhagia, whereas endocervical polyps are much more likely to be asymptomatic or cause mild, intermenstrual spotting. In some cases, there is an association only by extension through another process. For instance, endometriosis is associated with menorrhagia, but most likely it is due to the coexistence of adenomyosis in 20% of these patients. Adenomyosis, in turn, is associated with menorrhagia in 40% to 50% of patients. Most of the conditions responsible for secondary menorrhagia may be either suspected or diagnosed in the office setting or by a few simple tests. In some cases the mechanisms involved in producing heavier menses are well understood; in others they are not.

The prevalence of secondary menorrhagia parallels that of the underlying pathology. During adolescence, anovulation and blood dyscrasia are most common, whereas climacteric changes, fibroids, and neoplasia predominate in older patients. Although not a cause

Table 16.1. Possible Causes of Secondary Menorrhagia or Acute Bleeding

Uterine causes	Extrauterine causes
Abortion (threatened, incomplete, retained products of conception)	Chronic anovulation
Adenomyosis	Endometriosis (vaginal, vulvar)
Cervical lesions (including cancer)	Nongynecologic causes (blood dyscrasia or coagulopathy, hypothyroidism, leukemia, liver
Endometrial cancer	disease, systemic lupus erythematosus, thyroid
Endometrial hyperplasia	disease)
Infection (cervicitis, chronic endometritis)	Tumors
Intrauterine contraceptive devices (IUCDs)	Benign or malignant tumors of ovary
Myomas (generally intracavitary or intramural)	
Polyps (endometrial or cervical)	

of a recurrent, cyclic heavy vaginal bleeding, a pregnancy-related process is a possibility that must always be considered. This is especially true for any sudden onset bleeding or the abrupt emergence of heavy bleeding at the time of expected menstruation for a patient who has not previously experienced menorrhagia.

Patients at either end of their reproductive years are more likely to experience prolonged intervals of anovulation. This chronic, unopposed estrogen stimulation results in an endometrium that proliferates to a critical height beyond which it becomes unstable, resulting in irregular, sometimes heavy, bleeding. When unopposed estrogen stimulation persists, hyperplasia or neoplasia may result, both of which may be associated with heavy bleeding episodes. Roughly 75% of adolescent menorrhagia is due to coagulation disorders.

Current evidence supports an overproduction or an imbalance in the relative ratios of uterine prostaglandins as the cause of primary menorrhagia. The dominant prostaglandin (PG) in menorrhagia appears to be PGE_2. This prostaglandin, along with prostacyclin (PGI_2), act as vasodilators and smooth muscle relaxants; they may also act to disperse platelets, counteracting the actions of thromboxane A_2. It is probable that PGE_2 may also mediate the excessive bleeding found in some forms of secondary menorrhagia as well. Some evidence suggests that patients with primary menorrhagia may also have increased fibrinolysis, further enhancing a tendency to bleed.

Women who experience prolonged or heavy periods are more likely to wear tampons for more days or for longer periods at a time. This places them at risk for an uncommon, but potentially fatal complication: toxic shock syndrome. Toxic shock syndrome (TSS) is caused by toxins produced by an often asymptomatic infection with *Staphylococcus aureus*. For toxic shock to develop, three conditions must be met: There must be colonization by the bacteria, it must produce toxin, and there must be a portal of entry for the toxin. While most commonly associated with prolonged tampon use, about 10% of TSS cases are associated with other conditions (Table 16.2). The presence of foreign bodies, such as a tampon, is thought to reduce magnesium levels which promote the formation of toxin by the bacteria.

Table 16.2 Conditions Associated with Toxic Shock Syndrome

Surgical wounds (including dilatation and curettage)
Nonsurgical focal infections
    Cellulitis
    Subcutaneous abscesses
    Mastitis
    Infected insect bites
Postpartum (including transmission to the neonate)
Nonmenstrual vaginal conditions
    Vaginal infection
    Contraception with diaphragm or sponge (now removed from market)
    Pelvic inflammatory disease
    Steroid cream use

It is difficult to assess the amount of menstrual flow a woman experiences. This has led to both the over- and under diagnosis of menorrhagia and rare cases of factitious complaints. It is appropriate to ask about the use of tampons or pads, the number used per period, the frequency with which they must be changed, or the presence of clots. These give a broad indication of the amount of flow, although objective studies have shown a poor correlation with the actual measured blood loss. In classic studies carried out in the 1980s, it was demonstrated that one third of women who described light menstrual flow actually had losses of greater than 80 mL. By contrast, one half of patients who described their menses as heavy had losses of less than the 80 mL traditionally used to define menorrhagia. Studies by other investigators have demonstrated that a woman's perception of heavy bleeding has a positive predictive value of only 55% for the presence of menorrhagia. Several recent studies have attempted to use semiobjective methods of estimating loss based on the degree of sanitary napkin or tampon soiling or through the use of menstrual cups. From a practical standpoint, these are not useful in the clinical setting. As a result, any patient who presents with the complaint of heavy bleeding deserves at least a cursory evaluation. In addition, any patient who has unexplained anemia must be presumed to have menorrhagia, regardless of the perceived amount of menstrual loss.

Historical review for the patient with presumed menorrhagia must contain the standard elements of a gynecologic history (menarche, normal menstrual pattern, obstetric history, and contraception), but must also include inquiries that will suggest processes associated with menorrhagia or factors that might increase the risk of such processes. The latter might include a history of diabetes, obesity, or chronic anovulation, which would place the patient at higher risk for endometrial hyperplasia or malignancy. Screening should also include those signs and symptoms that suggest systemic disease, metabolic disturbances, or anemia. For patients with abrupt bleeding, the possibility of a pregnancy must be explored.

A careful pelvic examination is critical to establishing the presence of processes responsible for secondary menorrhagia. In addition to routine measures, such as Pap smears, special attention should be directed toward the detection of pelvic masses, anatomic or other distortions of the uterus, and changes in the position or character or the uterus itself. Irregular enlargement of the uterus suggests leiomyomas, whereas a "boggy" or "woody" enlargement of the uterus suggests adenomyosis. Uterine leiomyomas are the single most common cause of secondary menorrhagia and are generally easy to palpate in cooperative patients. Although more often associated with dysfunctional bleeding, signs of cervical change (including infection, eversion, or polyps) should be noted.

The role of ultrasonography in the diagnosis of menorrhagia is limited to the detection of secondary sources that may be difficult to document by history or clinical examination alone. For most patients, such studies are unnecessary. Imaging should be considered for the evaluation of patients who do not respond to medical therapy or for whom an adequate pelvic examination could not be performed. One New Zealand study of treatment failures found that almost two thirds of these women had pathologic processes identified. Identification of these secondary causes helps refine the therapeutic options offered the patient and thus improve success.

Patients who are at risk for endometrial hyperplasia, neoplasia, or those who do not respond to initial therapy may require endometrial biopsy, hysteroscopy, or diagnostic curettage. The wide acceptance of office endometrial sampling has made this easier to accomplish with reasonable reliability. Studies indicate that office sampling has a diagnostic sensitivity of greater than 95%. Inadequate samples or continued bleeding should prompt referral for hysteroscopy or curettage. Laparoscopy is almost never indicated for the evaluation of menorrhagia alone.

Aside from documenting anemia, there are no routine laboratory tests that can establish the presence or cause of menorrhagia. Liver function tests, a sensitive thyroid stimulating hormone (sTSH) assay, or measures of coagulation and bleeding time should be ordered when appropriate. A pregnancy test should be considered for patients who exhibit acute bleeding.

Table 16.3. Presenting Symptoms of Toxic Shock Syndrome

Most common
    Fever >38.9° C (102° F)
    Diffuse rash
    Hypotension
Other typical findings
    Agitation
    Arthralgias
    Confusion
    Diarrhea
    Erythema of pharynx, vulva or vagina, conjunctiva
    Headache
    Myalgias
    Nausea
    Vomiting

Table 16.4. Characteristics that Define Toxic Shock Syndrome

Fever >38.9° C (102° F)
Diffuse macular, erythematous rash
Desquamation of palms and soles 1 to 2 weeks after onset
Hypotension (<90 mm Hg systolic, or orthostatic change)
Negative blood, pharyngeal, and cerebrospinal fluid culture
Negative serologic tests for measles, leptospirosis, Rocky Mountain Spotted Fever
Three or more of the following organ systems
    Cardiopulmonary (respiratory distress, pulmonary edema, heart block, myocarditis)
    Central nervous system (disorientation or altered sensorium)
    Gastrointestinal (vomiting, diarrhea)
    Hematologic (thrombocytopenia of ≤100,000/mm³)
    Hepatic (>2 fold elevation of total bilirubin or liver enzymes, serum albumin <2 gm/dL)
    Mucous membrane inflammation (vaginal, oropharyngeal, conjunctival)
    Musculoskeletal (myalgia, >2 elevation of creatine phosphokinase)
    Renal (pyuria, >2 fold elevation of blood urea nitrogen (BUN) or creatinine)

Table 16.5. Differential Diagnosis of Toxic Shock Syndrome

Other exanthems
    Acute rheumatic fever
    Bullous impetigo
    Drug reaction
    Erythema multiforme
    Kawasakis disease
    Leptospirosis
    Meningococcemia
    Rocky Mountain Spotted fever
    Rubella
    Rubeola
    Scarlet fever
    Viral disease
Gastrointestinal illness
    Appendicitis
    Dysentery
    Gastroenteritis
    Pancreatitis
    Staphylococcal food poisoning
Other disorders
    Acute pyelonephritis
    Hemolytic uremic syndrome
    Legionnaires' disease
    Pelvic inflammatory disease
    Reye's syndrome
    Rhabdomyolysis
    Septic shock
    Stevens-Johnson syndrome
    Systemic lupus erythematosus
    Tick typhus
    Tularemia

Patients with toxic shock syndrome are generally unaware of a staphylococcal infection or the production of toxin until they experience the abrupt onset of high fever, myalgia, nausea, vomiting, diarrhea, and a diffuse, sunburnlike rash (Table 16.3). Hypotension may quickly ensue, with frank shock common by the time the patient first presents for care. Criteria that make up the strict description of TSS are shown in Table 16.4. Other conditions that must be distinguished from TSS are listed in Table 16.5.

THERAPEUTIC OPTIONS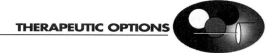

The specific therapy for menorrhagia is based on a number of factors: acuity of symptoms, patient age, and desire for contraception. The primary goals of therapy are to control excess bleeding, correct anemia, and detect occult pathology. Some authors have suggested that the patient's hemoglobin may be used as a guide to the selection of possible interventions (Fig. 16.1). This, however, lacks flexibility and ignores the possibility of menorrhagia that does not result in anemia. For this reason a more general approach seems appropriate (Fig. 16.2). It should be unnecessary to point out that secondary menorrhagia is best managed by treating the underlying process; therefore, most of the discussion on therapeutic options is directed toward the treatment of primary menorrhagia.

Acute Bleeding

Although patients with acute uterine bleeding are uncommon, they do require rapid evaluation and intervention. When the patient is hemodynamically unstable, fluid and blood resuscitation should be instituted immediately. This type of potentially life-threatening bleeding is most often pregnancy related, and may require immediate curettage once the patient has been stabilized. Curettage is generally successful in arresting the bleeding and provides tissue for evaluation. Neoplasia or blood dyscrasia must also be considered in these patients. Any patient who has evidence of significant acute blood loss or a hemoglobin of less than 8 g, should be considered for hospitalization while stabilization and evaluation are performed.

Less voluminous acute bleeding can occur with primary menorrhagia. Therapies with intravenous conjugated estrogen (20–25 mg) or intramuscular progestins have been widely advocated. As an alternative, oral estrogen (conjugated estrogen: 2.5 mg; micronized estradiol: 3 to 6 mg) may be given every 2 hours until the bleeding lessens. Estrogen therapy is then maintained for 20 to 25 additional days, with a progestin added for the last 10 days of

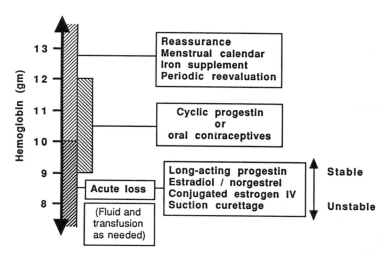

Figure 16.1. Menorrhagia therapy based on hemoglobin and acuity of blood loss. For patients with little or no reduction in hemoglobin, reassurance and monitoring are appropriate. When acute blood loss occurs, the first line of management must be stabilization and determination of pregnancy status. Unstable patients must be stabilized and considered for curettage. Less-threatening blood loss can be treated with long-acting progestins, intravenous (IV) conjugated estrogen (25 mg every 4 h up to a maximum of six doses), or oral contraceptive agents (see text).

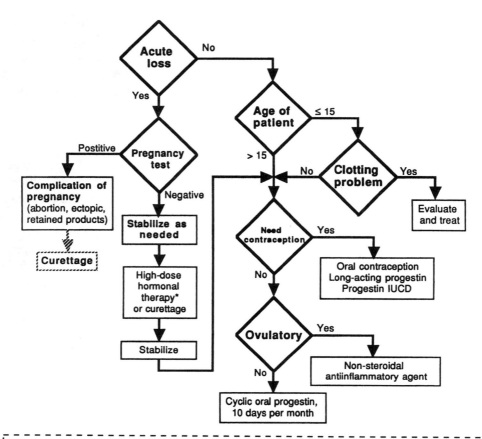

Figure 16.2. Algorithm for the treatment of primary menorrhagia. IUCD = intrauterine contraceptive device; IM = intramuscular; IV = intravenous.

treatment. The exact mechanism by which these agents accomplish the short-term control of bleeding is uncertain, but clinical experience has found them to be effective for many patients. High-dose combination oral contraceptives containing estradiol and norgestrel, such as Ovral, have also been used to provide acute control of idiopathic menorrhagia. Oral contraceptives used in this manner are usually given as four tablets a day for 3 to 5 days or until bleeding stops, followed by one a day for the duration of the 21-day pack. An alternative dosage regimen is four tablets the first day of therapy, followed by three per day for 1 day, two the next day, and then one daily for the remainder of the package. This 4-3-2-1 patterns is generally well tolerated and may be a good choice when bleeding is not aggressive.

When the endometrium is reasonably intact, high-dose progestin may be used to stop acute uterine bleeding. This may take the form of oral medroxyprogesterone acetate (MPA [10 mg, three times daily]) or intramuscular depot medroxyprogesterone acetate (DMPA [150 to 300 mg]). These agents will not provide satisfactory hemostasis if there has been prolonged bleeding resulting in a denuded or atrophic endometrium. Such patients will require estrogen therapy. For most patients, estrogen therapy provides a more rapid response.

Once acute control has been gained, cyclic estrogen plus progestin therapy should be continued for an additional 3 months. During this interval, additional diagnostic studies may be considered and plans laid for long-term management, should it be necessary.

Any patient who has bled to anemia, either acutely or chronically, will benefit from iron supplementation, using either ferrous sulfate or gluconate (300 mg) given two or three times daily.

Continuing Symptoms

The desire for contraception helps determine the optimal treatment of menorrhagia. If contraception is desired, oral combination contraceptives or continuously dosed progestogens (orally, by injection, or as a medicated intrauterine device) are reasonable for patients with primary menorrhagia and for some patients with secondary menorrhagia. Oral contraceptives, either monophasic or polyphasic, generally provide lighter, shorter, less crampy periods because of the thinner, more atrophic endometrium they engender. In the absence of this contraceptive need, oral contraceptives require 21 days of therapy for 2 to 5 days of benefit, reducing their cost-effectiveness. Although studies are lacking, many clinicians prefer monophasic preparations when they are used for this purpose.

Long-acting progestins, such as depot medroxyprogesterone acetate, are associated with amenorrhea in 50% to 60% of long-term users. Levonorgestrel-releasing intrauterine contraceptive devices (IUCDs) produce a thin, atrophic endometrium, resulting in lighter menstrual flow, but must be replaced annually. These progesterone-based therapies provide contraception and avoid the problem of short-term compliance. A significant incidence of random bleeding early in therapy and the continuing need for quarterly follow-up visits in the case of DMPA, combined with the established noncontraceptive benefits of oral contraceptives, all suggest an oral contraceptive may be a better choice for many patients.

In intractable cases of menorrhagia or in patients being prepared for extirpative surgery or endometrial ablation, therapy with gonadotropin-releasing hormone (GnRH) agonists may be considered. These agents, however, can be used only for a maximum of 6 months. This therapeutic approach is further limited by cost and the common occurrence of side effects.

If contraception is not an issue, the first choice of treatment generally is among drugs that are administered only during menstruation, such as prostaglandin synthesis inhibitors or antifibrinolytics. Of these, antifibrinolytics reduce menstrual blood loss to the greatest extent, whereas prostaglandin synthesis inhibitors have the lowest incidence of side effects.

Multiple studies have shown both objective and subjective improvement with nonsteroidal anti-inflammatory agents (NSAIDs) such as meclofenamate sodium, mefenamic acid, or flurbiprofen. These agents cause a reduction in myometrial blood flow and may help to correct either excess prostaglandin production or a disruption of the relative concentration of counterbalancing eicosanoids. Some agents, such as meclofenamate and mefenamic acid have the ability to block the actions of prostaglandins in addition to suppressing their formation, further enhancing their efficacy. Therapy with these agents is restricted to the time of menstrual flow; many patients require fewer than 10 doses over the duration of flow. Patients with primary menorrhagia experience 30% to 50% reductions in blood loss while taking these agents. Interestingly, the greatest decreases in volume of menstruation are found in those patients with the greatest pretreatment loss. Nonsteroidal therapy addresses the specific cause of these patients' symptoms, provides excellent symptom relief, and requires a small number of doses of relatively inexpensive medication. Prostaglandin synthesis inhibitors also have the extra advantage of diminishing dysmenorrhea, a common complaint for those with menorrhagia. There is no place for ergometrine in the treatment of menorrhagia. Nonsteroidal therapy will not work as well with secondary-type bleeding; however, it is often an excellent choice for initial therapy.

Antifibrionlytics, such as ethamsylate or tranexamic acid (1 g four times daily for the first 4 days of flow), have been studied, but have not enjoyed wide clinical acceptance. Published studies have found reductions in blood loss of up to 50% with these agents, making them a reasonable alternative for patients who cannot use estrogen or NSAIDs. In comparative trials, mefenamic acid caused more rapid changes in menstrual blood loss than ethamsylate, but ethamsylate provided better long-term efficacy with less rebound after treatment cessation. Antifibrinolytic therapy carries a greater risk of serious complications, such as stroke.

Danazol sodium (200 mg daily) has also been used in some studies to treat menorrhagia. Side effects, cost, and poor response has limited the enthusiasm for this approach. Head-to-head studies have not found statistical differences between hormonal, NSAID, and danazol treatments. Typical responses, taken from two recent comparative studies, are shown in Figure 16.3.

Cyclic treatment with progestins is effective for menstrual irregularity and may improve symptoms in climacteric patients or in adolescents who have heavy anovulatory bleeding patterns. A commonly employed regimen is medroxyprogesterone acetate, given at a dose of 10 mg a day for 10 days, taken from cycle day 14 onward. For patients who are ovulatory, progestin therapy may cause even greater endometrial growth and heavier menstrual flow. Estrogen should be added to progesterone anytime the endometrium is likely to be denuded or atrophic (Table 16.6).

Surgical therapy for menorrhagia has undergone a number of changes. Where once a significant number of hysterectomies were done for the complaint of menorrhagia, improved medical therapy and less extensive surgical procedures have diminished the role that hysterectomy should play. The greatest change in surgical therapy has been the introduction of hysterscopic evaluation and operative intervention. Endometrial ablation, polypectomy, or the resection of submucous myomata has become an option. Although these procedures are performed in the outpatient setting, they are not uniformly successful. They carry all the risks that are associated with any surgery and have a not inconsiderable learning curve associated with their application. In some series, failure rates approach 50%. Most authors advocate placing patients on GnRH agonist therapy for awhile before endometrial therapy is attempted. This significantly increases the cost of therapy and, by itself, may be effective. The exact role of surgical therapy is still being defined. The final choice of therapy for a given patient should be based on the patient's pathology, significance of symptoms, available treatment options, and her reproductive desires.

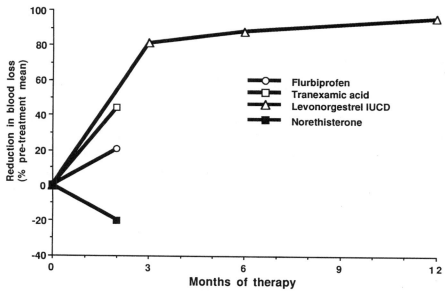

Figure 16.3. Comparative effectiveness of flurbiprofen, tranexamic acid, norethisterone, and a levonorgestrel-releasing intrauterine contraceptive device. Reductions in menstrual loss may be obtained by the use of nonsteroidal anti-inflammatory agents, antifibrinolytic therapy, or progesterone, given orally or by way of a medicated intrauterine contraceptive device (IUCD). The greatest response was found with the progesterone-medicated IUCD, but in one study oral progestin actually worsened blood loss. Other studies of nonsteroidal anti-inflammatory agents find reductions of 30% to 50%, which is comparable to the 45% response documented for antifibrinolytic agents in this data from two separate studies. (Data from: Milsom I, Andersson K, Andersch B, Rybo G. A comparison of flurbiprofen, tranexamic acid, and a levonorgestrel-releasing intrauterine contraceptive device in the treatment of idiopathic menorrhagia. Am J Obstet Gynecol 1991;164:879; and Preston JT, Cameron IT, Adams EJ, Smith SK. Comparative study of tranexamic acid and norethisterone in the treatment of ovulatory menorrhagia. Br J Obstet Gynaecol 1995;102:401.)

Table 16.6. Reasons to Add Estrogen to Progestin Therapy for Menorrhagia

Following prolonged, heavy bleeding when the endometrium is likely to be denuded.
Following prolonged progestin therapy.
When endometrial biopsy shows minimal benign tissue or only proliferative changes.
Uncertain history or likelihood of follow-up.

Toxic Shock Syndrome

Although the prognosis for patients with toxic shock syndrome is generally good, mortality rates of 5% to 10% are common. The treatment of TSS is both supportive and specific. Aggressive support and treatment of the attendant shock is paramount. The site of infection must be identified and drained, most commonly by removing the contaminated tampon. Antibiotic therapy with a beta-lactamase–resistant antistaphylococcal agent should be started, but it does not alter the initial course of the illness. Adult respiratory distress syndrome is a common sequelae of TSS and patients must be monitored for the development of this complication. Although the risk of recurrence is unknown, patients who have had TSS should refrain from the use of tampons in the future.

HINTS AND COMMON QUESTIONS

From time to time menstrual cups or tassettes are touted as either methods of measuring menstrual blood loss or as an alternative for menstrual hygiene. Most studies have found that 40% or more of women with normal menstrual flow, and virtually 100% of women with heavy flow, have found these devices unacceptable.

Because adolescents are often reluctant to discuss contraception, the complaint of heavy or crampy periods may provide an excuse to seek care. This "hidden agenda" should be explored in a confidential manner.

Patients often blame menstrual changes on sterilization. Objective studies have failed to show any consistent difference in menstrual blood loss after sterilization or with various sterilization methods.

If ultrasonographic imaging is chosen to assist in the diagnosis of patients with menorrhagia, the most reliable information about the endometrium and myometrium will be gained by transvaginal techniques.

The value of endometrial thickness measured by vaginal ultrasonography is still being evaluated. Although endometrial thickening would suggest hyperplasia or neoplasia, the test has neither sufficient positive nor negative predictive values to allow clinical application at this time.

Because of the possibility of a coexistent neoplasm, endometrial biopsy should be considered for most patients over the age of 40 who experience heavy bleeding, even when uterine fibroids are present.

The rare patient with a coagulopathy as the source of menorrhagia is at high risk for bleeding complications if endometrial biopsy or curettage is carried out. For this reason, any patient suspected of having blood dyscrasia or young patients with menorrhagia who may have an undiagnosed bleeding tendency, should be evaluated with a bleeding time before any procedure is contemplated.

Not all nonsteroidal anti-inflammatory agents are alike in their ability to reduce menstrual blood loss. For example, even high doses of aspirin have been shown to be ineffective in the treatment of menorrhagia. As a result, the choice of agent should be restricted to those drugs that have been tested and found to be efficacious (Table 16.7).

It was once thought that to be effective for the control of heavy bleeding, NSAIDs had to be given 1 day before the onset of menses. This is both difficult to accomplish and unnecessary. All of the agents studied to date will work if started at the onset of menstrual flow.

If an endometrial biopsy is considered, it is best performed before hormonal therapy is instituted, which confounds the histologic interpretation.

If endometrial biopsy shows simple or cystic hyperplasia, cyclic progestin therapy for a minimum of 3 months is generally curative, but does require follow-up biopsy as a test of cure. Atypical adenomatous hyperplasia is believed to be a premalignant condition, carrying a 20% to 30% chance of progression, necessitating referral for evaluation and therapy.

Table 16.7. Nonsteroidal Anti-inflammatory Agents for Menorrhagia*

Drug	Initial dose (mg)	Subsequent dose
Flurbiprofen	100	50 tid or 100 bid
Ibuprofen	400–600	400–600 q4h
Ketoprofen	75	75 tid
Meclofenamate	100	50–100 q4–6 h
Mefenamic acid	500	250 q4–6 h
Naproxen	500	250 q4–6 h
Naproxen sodium	550	275 q6–8 h

*Consult full prescribing information before using any of these drugs.
All agents should be used for the full duration of menstrual flow. bid = twice daily; tid = three times daily; q = every.

Occasionally patients receiving depot medroxyprogesterone acetate experience depression, headaches, or nausea. Changing to norethindrone (0.35 to 0.7 mg daily) may relieve some of these symptoms.

It is exceedingly rare for patients with non–pregnancy-related bleeding to require a hysterectomy under emergency conditions. Patients may, therefore, be reassured that the bleeding found in most cases of menorrhagia is neither life-threatening nor is it likely to result in emergency surgery.

Even when uterine bleeding is heavy, vaginal packing should never be used. Such packing will not affect the rate of bleeding and only render it occult, making continuing assessment difficult.

The rash of toxic shock syndrome is commonly absent in places where clothing presses tightly against the skin.

SUGGESTED READINGS

General References

Adelantado JM, Rees MCP, Bernal AL, Turnbull AC. Increased uterine prostaglandin E receptors in menorrhagic women. Br J Obstet Gynaecol 1988;95:162.

Cameron I. Management of menorrhagia. Practitioner 1992;236:650.

Claessens EA, Cowell CA. Acute adolescent menorrhagia. Am J Obstet Gynecol 1981;139:377.

Cohen BJB, Gibor J. Anemia and menstrual blood loss. Obstet Gynecol Surv 1980;35:597.

Duncan KM, Hart LL. Nonsteroidal antiinflammatory drugs in menorrhagia. Ann Pharmacother 1993;27:1353.

Hallberg I, Hogdahl AM, Nilsson L, Rybo G. Menstrual blood loss—A population study. Acta Obstet Gynaecol Scand 1966;45:320.

Higham JM. The medical management of menorrhagia. Br J Hosp Med 1991;45:19.

Higham J, Reid P. A preliminary investigation of what happens to women complaining of menorrhagia but whose complaint is not substantiated. J Psychosom Obstet Gynecol 1995;16:211.

Liddell H. Menorrhagia. Aust N Z J Med 1993;106:255.

Long CA, Gast MJ. Menorrhagia. Obstet Gynecol Clin N Am 1990;17:343.

Nelson L, Rybo G. Treatment of menorrhagia. Am J Obstet Gynecol 1971;110:713.

Neinstein LS. Menstrual problems in adolescents. Med Clin N Am 1990;74:1181.

Rees MCP. Human menstruation and eicosanoids. Reprod Fertil Dev 1990;2:467.

Rees MCP. Menorrhagia. BMJ 1987;294:759.

Shaw RW. Treating the patient with menorrhagia. Br J Obstet Gynaecol 1994;101 (suppl 11):1.

van Eijkeren MA, Christiaens GC, Scholten PC, Sixma JJ. Menorrhagia. Current drug treatment concepts. Drugs 1992;43:201.

Wood C. Treatment of menorrhagia. Aust Fam Physician 1995;24:825.

Ylikorkala O. Prostaglandin synthesis inhibitors in menorrhagia, intrauterine contraceptive device-induced side effects and endometriosis. Pharmacol Toxicol 1994;75 (suppl 2):86.

Specific References

Physiology

Adelantado JM, Rees MC, Lopez-Bernal A, Turnbull AC. Increase uterine prostaglandin E receptors in menorrhagic women. Br J Obstet Gynaecol 1988;95:162.

Blessin NE, Hambley H. Early hypothyroidism in patients with menorrhagia. Am J Obstet Gynecol 1990;163:697.

Christiaens GCML, Sizma JJ, Haspels AA. Haemostasis in menstrual endometrium in the presence of an intrauterine device. Br J Obstet Gynaecol 1981;88:825.

Fraser IS, McCarron G, Markham R, Resta T. Blood and total fluid content of menstrual discharge. Obstet Gynecol 1985;65:194.

Fraser IS, McCarron G, Markham R, Resta T, Watts A. Measured menstrual blood loss in women with menorrhagia associated with pelvic disease or coagualtion disorder. Obstet Gynecol 1986;68:630.

Greer IA, Lowe GD, Walker JJ, Forbes CD. Haemorrhagic problems in obstetrics and gynaecology in patients with congenital coagulopathies. Br J Obstet Gynaecol 1991;98:909.

Hourihan HM, Sheppard BL, Bonnar J. The morphologic characteristics of menstrual hemostasis in patients with unexplained menorrhagia. Int J Gynecol Pathol 1989;8:221.

Makarainen L, Ylikorkala O. Primary and myoma-associated menorrhagia: role of prostaglandins and the effect of ibuprofen. Br J Obstet Gynaecol 1986;93:974.

Raju GC, Naraynsingh V, Woo J, Jankey N. Adenomyosis uteri: a study of 416 cases. Aust N Z J Obstet Gynaecol 1988;28:72.

Rees MC, Anderson ABM, Demers LM, Turnbull AC. Endometrial and myometrial prostaglandin release during the menstrual cycle in relation to menstrual blood loss. J Clin Endocrinol Metab 1984;58:813.

Rybo G. Menstrual blood loss in relation to parity and menstrual pattern. Acta Obstet Gynecol Scand 1966;45:119.

Smith SK, Abel MH, Kelly RW, Baird DT. A role of prostacyclin (PGI$_2$) in excessive menstrual bleeding. Lancet 1981;1:522.

Taw RL. Review of menstrual disorders in which a secretory endometrium was found. Am J Obstet Gynecol 1975;122:490.

van Eijkeren MA, Christiaens GC, Geuze HJ, Haspels AA, Sixma JJ. Morphology of menstrual hemostasis in essential menorrhagia. Lab Invest 1991;64:284.

van Eijkeren MA, Christiaens GC, Haspels AA, Sixma JJ. Measured menstrual blood loss in women with a bleeding disorder or using oral anticoagulatnt therapy. Am J Obstet Gynecol 1990;162:1261.

Wilansky DL, Greisman B. Early hypothyroidism in patients with menorrhagia. Am J Obstet Gynecol 1989; 160:673.

Diagnosis

Bakri YN, Jabbar JA. Munchausen syndrome presenting as uncontrolled menorrhagia. Int J Gynaecol Obstet 1992;39:338.

Broome CV. Epidemiology of toxic shock syndrome in the United States. Rev Infect Dis 1989;11:S14.

Cheng M, Kung R, Hannah M, Wilansky D, Shime J. Menses cup evaluation study. Fertil Steril 1995;64:661.

Chimbira TH, Anderson ABM, Turnbull AC. Relation between menstrual blood loss and patient's subjective assessment of loss, duration of bleeding, number of sanitary towels used, uterine weight and endometrial surface area. Br J Obstet Gynaecol 1980;87:603.

Eddows HA, Read MD, Codling BW. Pipelle: a more acceptable technique for outpatient endometrial biopsy. Br J Obstet Gynaecol 1990;97:961.

Fedele L, Bianchi S, Dorta M, Arcaini L, Zanotti F, Carinelli S. Transvaginal ultrasonography in the diagnosis of diffuse adenomyosis. Fertil Steril 1992;58:94.

Fothergill DJ, Brown VA, Hill AS. Histological sampling of the endometrium— A comparison between formal curettage and the Pipelle sampler. Br J Obstet Gynaecol 1992;99:779.

Fraser IS, McCarron G, Markham R. A preliminary study of factors influencing perception of menstrual blood loss volume. Am J Obstet Gynecol 1984;149:788.

Fraser IS. Hysteroscopy and laparoscopy in women with menorrhagia. Am J Obstet Gynecol 1990;165:1264.

Gimpleson RJ, Rappold HD. A comparative study between panoramic hysteroscopy with directed biopsies and dilatation and curettage. Am J Obstet Gynecol 1988;158:489.

Gleeson N, Devitt M, Buggy F, Bonnar J. Menstrual blood loss measurement with gynaeseal. Aust N Z J Obstet Gynaecol 1993;33:79.

Hallberg L, Nilsson L. Determination of menstrual blood loss. Scand J Clin Lab Invest 1964;16:244.

Haynes PJ, Hodgson H, Anderson ABM, Turnbull AC. Measurement of menstrual blood loss in patients complaining of menorrhagia. Br J Obstet Gynaecol 1977;84:763.

Higham J, O'Brien PM, Shaw RW. Assessment of menstrual blood loss using a pictorial chart. Br J Obstet Gynaecol 1990;97:734.

Janssen CA, Scholten PC, Heintz AP. A simple visual assessment technique to discriminate between menorrhagia and normal menstrual blood loss. Obstet Gynecol 1995;5:977.

Loffer FD. Hysteroscopy with selective endometrial sampling compared with D&C for abnormal uterine bleeding: the value of negative hysteroscopic view. Obstet Gynecol 1989;73:16.

Nolan TE, Smith RP, Smith MT, Gallup DC. A prospective evaluation of an endometrial suction curette. Obstet Gynecol Surv 1993;48:471–473.

Rees MCP, Chimbira TH, Anderson ABM, Turnbull AC. menstrual blood loss: measurement and clinical correlates. Research Clinical Forums 1982;4:69.

Rees MCP. Role of menstrual blood loss measurements in management of complaints of excessive menstrual bleeding. Br J Obstet Gynaecol 1991;98:327.

Reingold AL, Shards KN, Dan BB, Broome CV. Toxic-shock not associated with menstruation. A review of 54 cases. Lancet 1982;1:1.

Rome ES, Emans SJ. Hypermenorrhea and anovulatory cycles in the adolescent. Current Therapy in Endocrinology and Metabolism 1994;5:210-.

Silver MM, Miles P, Rosa C. Comparison of Novak and Pipelle endometrial biopsy instruments. Obstet Gynecol 1991;78:828.

van Eijkeren MA, Scholten PC, Christiaens GCML, Alsbach GPJ, Haspels AA. The alkaline hematin method for measuring blood loss: a modification and its clinical use in menorrhgia. Eur J Obstet Gynecol Reprod Biol 1986;22:345.

Wood C, Hurley VA, Leoni M. The value of vaginal ultrasound in the management of menorrhagia. Aust N Z J Obstet Gynaecol 1993;33:198.

Treatment

Achirron A, Gornish M, Melamed E. Cerebral sinus thrombosis as potential hazard in antifibrinolytic treatment of menorrhagia. Stroke 1990;21:817.

Andersch B, Milsom I, Rybo G. An objective evaluation of flurbiprofen and tranexamic acid in the treatment of idiopathic menorrhagia. Acta Obstet Gynaecol Scand 1988;67:645.

Anderson ABM, Haynes PJ, Guillebaud J, Turnbull AC. Reduction of menstrual blood loss by prostaglandin-synthetase inhibitiors. Lancet 1976;1:774.

Anderson JK, Rybo G. Levonorgestrel-releasing intrauterine device in the treatment of menorrhagia. Br J Obstet Gynaecol 1990;97:690.

Bergqvist A, Rybo G. Treatement of menorrhagia with intrauterine release of progesterone. Br J Obstet Gynaecol 1983;90:255.

Bonduelle M, Walker JJ, Calder AA. A comparative study of danazol and norethisterone in dysfunctional uterine bleeding presenting as menorrhagia. Postgrad Med J 1991;67:833.

Cameron IT, Haining R, Lumsden MA, Thomas VR, Smith SK. The effects of mefenamic acid and norethisterone on measured menstrual blood loss. Obstet Gynecol 1990;76:85.

Chamberlain G, Freeman R, Price F, Kennedy A, Green D, Eve L. A comparative study of ethamsylate and mefenamic acid in dysfunctional uterine bleeding. Br J Obstet Gynaecol 1991;98:707.

Coulter A, Peto V, Doll H. Patients' preferences and general practitioners' decisions in the treatment of menstrual disorders. Fam Pract 1994;11:67.

DeCherney AH, Diamond MP, Lavy G, Polan ML. Endometrial ablation for intractable uterine bleeding: hysteroscopic resection. Obstet Gynecol 1987;70:668.

DeCherney AH, Polan ML. Hysteroscopic management of intrauterine lesions and intractable uterine bleeding. Obstet Gynecol 1983;61:392.

DeVore GR, Owens O, Kase N. Use of intravenous premarin in the treatment of dysfunctional uterine bleeding—A double-blind randomized control study. Obstet Gynecol 1982;59:285.

Dwyer N, Hutton J, Stirrat GM. Randomized controlled trial comparing endometrial resection with abdominal hysterectomy for the surgical treatment of menorrhagia. Br J Obstet Gynaecol 1993;100:237.

Fraiser IS. Treatment of ovulatory and anovulatory dysfunctional uterine bleeding with oral progestogens. Aust N Z J Obstet Gynaecol 1990;30:353.

Fraiser IS, Angsuwathana S, Mahmoud F, Yezerski S. Short and medium term outcomes after rollerball endometrium ablation for menorrhagia. Med J Aust 1993;158:454.

Fraiser IS, McCarron G. Randomized trial of 2 hormonal and 2 prostaglandin-inhibiting agents in women with a complaint of menorrhagia. Aust N Z J Obst Gynaecol 1991;31:66.

Fraiser IS, McCarron G, Markham R, et al. Long-term treatment of menorrhagia with mefenamic acid. Obstet Gynecol 1983;61:109.

Fraiser IS, Pearce C, Sherman RP, Elliott PM, McIlveen J, Markham R. Efficacy of mefenamic acid in patients with a complaint of hemorrhagia. Obstet Gynecol 1981;58:543.

Garry R, Erian J, Grochmal SA. A multi-centre collaborative study into the treatment of menorrhagia by Nd-YAG laser ablation of the endometrium. Br J Obstet Gynaecol 1991;98:357.

Goldfarb HA. A review of 35 endometrial ablations using the Nd-YAG laser for recurrent menometrorrhagia. Obstet Gynecol 1990;76:833.

Goldrath MH, Fuller TA, Segal S. Laser photovaporization of endometrium for the treatment of menorrhagia. Am J Obstet Gynecol 1981;140:14.

Hall P, Maclachlan N, Thorn N, Nudd MWE, Taylor CG, Garrioch DB. Control of menorrhagia by the cyclo-oxygenase inhibitors naproxen sodium and mefenamic acid. Br J Obstet Gynaecol 1987;94:554.

Higham JM, Shaw RW. A comparative study of danazol, a regimen of decreasing doses of danazol, and norethindrone in the treatment of objectively proven unexplained menorrhagia. Am J Obstet Gynecol 1993;169:1134.

Indman PD. Hysteroscopic treatment of menorrhagia associated with uterine leiomyomas. Obstet Gynecol 1993; 81:716.

Jakubowicz DL, Wood C. The use of the prostaglandin synthetase inhibitor mefenamic acid in the treatment of menorrhagia. Aust N Z J Obstet Gynaecol 1978;18:135.

Kasonde JM, Bonnar J. Aminocaproic acid and menstrual loss in women using intrauterine devices. BMJ 1975;4:17.

Lamb MP. Danazol in menorrhagia: a double blind placebo controlled trial. J Obstet Gynecol 1987;7:212.

Milsom I, Andersson K, Andersch B, Rybo G. a comparison of flurbiprofen, tranexamic acid, and a levonorgestrel-releasing intrauterine contraceptive device in the treatment of idiopathic menorrhagia. Am J Obstet Gynecol 1991;164:879.

Need JA, Forbes KL, Milazzo L, McKenzie E. Danazol in the treatment of menorrhagia: the effect of a 1 month induction does (200 mg) and 2 month's maintenace therapy (200 mg, 100 mg, 50 mg or placebo). Aust N Z J Obstet Gynaecol 1992;32:346.

Osei E, Tharmaratnam S, Opemuyi I, Cochrane G. Laser endometrial ablation with the neodynium:yttrium-aluminium garnet (Nd-YAG) laser: a review of ninety consecutive patients. Acta Obstet Gynecol Scand 1995;74:619.

Pedron N, Lozano M, Gallegos AJ. The effect of acetylsalicylic acid on menstrual blood loss in women with IUDs. Contraception 1987;36:295.

Preston JT, Cameron IT, Adams EJ, Smith SK. Comparative study of tranexamic acid and norethisterone in the treatment of ovulatory menorrhagia. Br J Obstet Gynaecol 1995;102:401

Sculpher MJ, Bryan S, Dwyer N, Hutton J, Stirrat GM. An economic evaluation of transvaginal endometrial resection versus abdominal hysterectomy for the treatment of menorrhagia. Br J Obstet Gynaecol 1993;100:244.

Shaw RW. Assessment of medical treatments for menorrhagia. Br. J Obstet Gynaecol 1994;101 (suppl 11):15.

Shaw RW, Fraser HM. Use of a superactive luteinizing hormone releasing hormone (LHRH) agonist in the treatment of menorrhagia. Br J Obstet Gynaecol 1984;91:913.

Tauber PF, Wold AS, Herting W, Zaneveld LJD. Hemorrhage induced by intrauterine devices: control by local proteinase inhibition. Fertil Steril 1977;28:1375.

Thomas EJ, Okuda KJ, Thomas NM. The combination of a depot gonadotrophin releasing hormone agonist and cyclical hormone replacement therapy for dysfunctional uterine bleeding. Br J Obstet Gynaecol 1991;98:1155.

Toppazada M. Treatment of increased menstrual blood loss in IUD users. Contraception 1987;36:145.

Townsend DE, Richart RM, Paskowitz RA, Woolfork RE. Rollerball coagulation of the endometrium. Obstet Gynecol 1990;76:310.

Turnbull AC, Rees MCP. Gestrione in the treatment of menorrhagia. Br J Obstet Gynaecol 1990;97:713.

van Eijkeren MA, Christiaens GC, Geuze HJ, Haspels AA, Sixma JJ. Effects of mefenamic acid on menstrual hemostasis in essential menorrhagia. Am J Obstet Gynecol 1992;166:1419.

Vargas JM, Campeau JD, Mishell DR JR. Treatment of menorrhagia with meclofenamate sodium. Am J Obstet Gynecol 1987;157:944.

Vercellini P, Trespidi L, Bramante T, Panazza S, Mauro F, Crosignani PG. Gonadotropin releasing hormone agonist treatment before hysteroscopic endometrial resection. Int J Gynaecol Obstet 1994;45:235.

Ylikorkala O, Pekonen F. Naproxen reduces idiopathic but not fibromyoma-induced menorrhagia. Obstet Gynecol 1986;68:10.

17

Irregular Periods and Dysfunctional Bleeding

Abnormal vaginal bleeding can be disruptive: It makes work and social planning difficult, its messiness and inconvenience are troublesome, and it may portend the presence of significant pathology. The frequent occurrence of abnormal bleeding makes this a common clinical problem accounting for 10% to 15% of all gynecologic visits. Fortunately, most of the processes responsible for these maladies can be discovered and treated in the primary care setting.

BACKGROUND AND SCIENCE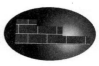

Abnormal uterine bleeding (AUB) encompasses a wide range of menstrual disturbances and clinical complaints, including irregular menses, prolonged or abnormal amounts of menstrual flow, and intermenstrual bleeding. There is often confusion over the nomenclature applied to these conditions (Table 17.1) and to the broad nonspecific term, "dysfunctional uterine bleeding." The latter is generally reserved for those patients in whom no clinically identifiable underlying cause is found. Some authors further restrict this term to those patients who are anovulatory and they have proposed that the term "anovulatory uterine bleeding" would be more accurate. Because the ovulatory status of the patient is not always obvious, the more liberal definition is probably more useful. Under either definition, the diagnosis of dysfunctional uterine bleeding (DUB) is one of exclusion.

Table 17.1. Terms Commonly Applied to Abnormal Bleeding Patterns

Term	Cycle	Timing of bleeding	Character
Hypomenorrhea	Regular	Menstrual	Decreased or scant amount
Intermenstrual bleeding	Regular	Between periods	Light bleeding between otherwise regular menses
Menometrorrhagia	Irregular	Menstrual	Excessive, prolonged bleeding
Menorrhagia (hypermenorrhea)	Regular	Menstrual	Excessive amount and duration
Metrorrhagia	Irregular	Menstrual	Normal character
Oligomenorrhea	Irregular	Menstrual	Usually at intervals >40 d
Polymenorrhea	Regular, frequent	Menstrual	Generally with intervals <21 d

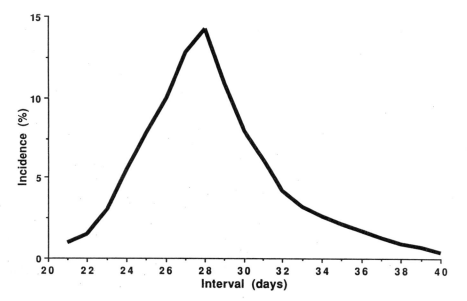

Figure 17.1. Normal variation in menstrual cycle length. Menstrual cycle interval is generally regarded as being 28 days, yet less than 15% of women have this interval. (After: Dysfunctional uterine bleeding. In Speroff L, Glass RH, Kase NG (eds). Clinical Gynecologic Endocrinology and Infertility, 5th ed. Baltimore: Williams & Wilkins, 1994;183–230.)

To understand abnormal uterine bleeding, it must be appreciated that there is a wide variation in what is considered normal (Fig. 17.1). Most patients have only their own experience as a standard for comparison. As a result, some clinical concerns actually represent normal variants, requiring only reassurance. For the remainder of patients, there are many possible causes for AUB. As with menorrhagia and dysmenorrhea, the processes responsible for menstrual disturbances vary with the age of the patient (Fig. 17.2). Abnormal uterine bleeding is most often encountered in adolescents and climacteric patients. These two groups are most likely to experience irregular or absent ovulation as the source of their complaints.

The rather long list of possible causes for AUB can be made more manageable by dividing it into those processes related to anovulation and those in which ovulation is un-

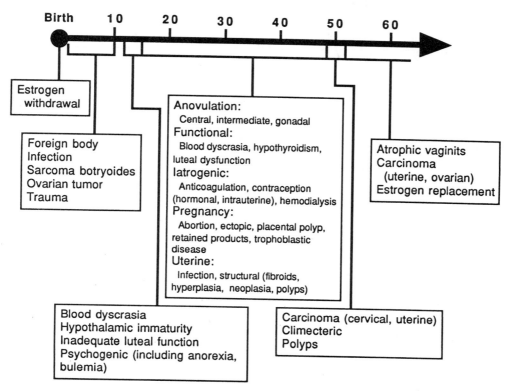

Figure 17.2. Causes of abnormal bleeding throughout life. Possible causes of abnormal bleeding vary over the life of a woman.

changed or occurs, but in an altered rhythm (Table 17.2). Anovulation is generally associated with bleeding that is less regular and of longer interval than usual. When anovulation occurs, for whatever reason, the lining of the uterus may experience unbalanced estrogen and progesterone exposure or unopposed estrogen stimulation. As a result of unopposed stimulation, proliferation of the endometrial tissues continues, albeit at a slower rate, until they becomes unstable. Once instability is reached, the lining may slough all at once, resulting in menorrhagia or in irregular fragments that are lost over a period of time. The latter pattern is typical of dysfunctional uterine bleeding. A similar growth and instability does not occur with exposure to progestin alone. As a result, progesterone withdrawal bleeding only occurs if the endometrium has had sufficient estrogen priming. The cause of anovulation is seldom directly responsible for abnormal bleeding, it is only the resulting noncyclic hormonal pattern that is responsible. Conditions that may account for amenorrhea are summarized in Tables 19.1 and 19.2 (Chapter 19, No Periods [Amenorrhea]).

In cases of iatrogenic anovulation (hormonal contraception) and climacteric and postmenopausal bleeding, the physiology is slightly different. In these patients the endometrium is often thin and atrophic. This endometrium is also prone to irregular sough, resulting in erratic, although generally light, bleeding. Because the endometrial tissue is so denuded, it does not respond well to progestational agents. Estrogen, alone initially or in combination

Table 17.2. Differential Diagnosis of Dysfunctional Uterine Bleeding

Anovulatory patients
    Chemotherapy
    Chronic illness
    Climacteric changes
    Endometrial carcinoma
    Endometrial hyperplasia
    Hormonal contraception (oral, injectable, intrauterine)
    Iatrogenic (anticoagulation, hormone replacement)
    Idiopathic
    Medications (anticholinergic agents, monoamine oxidase inhibitors, morphine, phenothiazines, reserpine)
    Nutritional disruption (anorexia, bulimia, excess physical activity)
    Obesity
    Pituitary-hypothalamic-ovarian axis immaturity
    Pituitary tumor
    Polycystic ovary syndrome
    Stress
    Systemic disease (hepatic, renal, thyroid)
Ovulatory patients
    Anatomic lesions (adenomyosis, cervical neoplasia, cervical polyps, endometrial carcinoma, endometrial polyps, leiomyomata, sarcoma)
    Bleeding at ovulation
    Coagulopathies (natural or iatrogenic)
    Endometritis
    Fallopian tube disease (infection, tumor)
    Foreign body (intrauterine contraceptive device, pessary, tampon)
    Idiopathic
    Injested substances (estrogens, ginseng)
    Leukemia
    Luteal phase dysfunction
    Pelvic inflammatory disease (including tuberculosis)
    Pregnancy-related (abortion, ectopic, hydatidiform mole, retained products of conception)
    Repeated trauma
    Systemic disease (hepatic, renal, thyroid)

with progestin therapy, is required to induce initial growth and development of progestin receptors, which affects endometrial stabilization.

Nonphysiologic levels of estrogen and progestin can be found in anovulatory patients. Excess estrogen may be present in obese patients, those with polycystic ovary disease, or those exposed to exogenous estrogen sources. Low-dose oral contraceptives, hypogonadism, or pre- and postmenopausal changes may result in insufficient estrogen, resulting in an unstable atrophic endometrium. Excess progestin may occur through the use of progestin-based contraception (depot medroxyprogesterone acetate, levonorgestrel implants) or when a persistent corpus luteum is present. Without adequate estrogen, this may also yield an atrophic endometrium. In each of these cases, the altered ratio or timing of hormonal exposure may result in desynchronous endometrial growth or maturation, leading to irregular bleeding.

Because some of the biologic processes that result in anovulation represent a threat to the overall health of the patient, aggressive evaluation and treatment is appropriate (Chapter 19, No periods). It should also be kept in mind that chronic unopposed estrogen stimulation of the endometrium may predispose to the development of endometrial cancer. Endometrial carcinoma is the most frequent malignancy of the female reproductive tract and irregular vaginal bleeding is the most common presenting symptom. Endometrial carcinoma is found most commonly among postmenopausal women, although 5% of endometrial cancers occur to women between the ages of 30 and 40 years. Endometrial cancer is often associated with obesity, nulliparity, and anovulation. It must always be borne in mind that anovulatory patients may still have an anatomic process that accounts for their bleeding, as well as any contribution made by their anovulatory status.

Patients who are, or might reasonably be expected to be, ovulatory represent a smaller group with abnormal uterine bleeding. The bleeding these women experience may be related to the processes of ovulation and cycling or may be independent of them. Examples of the latter are anatomic processes that give rise to bleeding. Most of these pathologies (e.g., adenomyosis, cervical neoplasia, cervical polyps, endometrial carcinoma, endometrial polyps, leiomyomata, and sarcoma) will be readily identified as long as clinical suspicion is maintained. These antecedents are most likely to present with bleeding that is independent of the background menstrual rhythm. Indeed, the relationship between the perceived menstrual rhythm and the bleeding experienced can be used to assist in the differential diagnosis of abnormal bleeding (Fig. 17.3). Additional causative processes that are independent of ovula-

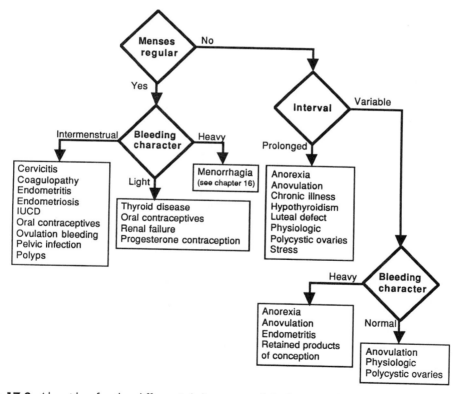

Figure 17.3. Algorithm for the differential diagnosis of dysfunctional uterine bleeding. IUCD = intrauterine contraceptive device.

tion include coagulopathies, endometriosis, endometritis and pelvic infection, foreign bodies (including pessaries, tampons, and intrauterine contraceptive devices), trauma, and complications of pregnancy. Although many of these will not cause recurrent bleeding abnormalities, they must be considered in the differential diagnosis of abnormal vaginal bleeding.

The character and timing of ovulatory-driven menstrual periods can be influenced by a number of factors. Ovulation can be delayed by a number of processes, such as psychosocial conditions (anorexia, bulimia, stress), chronic illness, renal or hepatic failure, and thyroid disease. Ovarian changes that lead to polycystic ovaries, luteal phase defects, or, rarely, tumors, can also delay the ovulation process. The ingestion of estrogenlike substances (most notably ginseng) or unregulated estrogen production, as seen in obesity, may produce irregular menstrual cycles and should be considered in the differential diagnosis.

ESTABLISHING THE DIAGNOSIS

One of the first tasks to be accomplished in the evaluation of patients with the complaint of abnormal menses is to be sure that the patient and provider are discussing the same thing. Because patterns of bleeding can help to separate possible causes, it is vital that the exact pattern involved is known and understood. Often, critical aspects of the bleeding (e.g., timing, duration, character, and associated symptoms) may be hazy or unavailable. An extremely useful tool to assist in this assessment is the menstrual calendar (Fig. 17.4). This simple tool can rapidly distinguish abnormalities in the rhythm or duration of menses and document the presence and timing of intermenstrual bleeding. Because some types of abnormal bleeding will self-correct over one to two menstrual cycles, the maintenance of a menstrual calendar provides both information and opportunity for spontaneous resolution without intervention.

The history and physical examination of the patient with abnormal bleeding patterns is focused on the detection of possible accountable pathologies. The duration and evolution of the patient's symptoms should be evaluated. New onset symptoms suggest a different set of pathologies than do periods that have been heavy or irregular since their inception (e.g., complication of pregnancy vs. a coagulopathy). In addition to characterizing the patient's complaint, the history should seek to elicit symptoms suggestive of somatic disease, such as thyroid dysfunction, galactorrhea, hepatic or renal disease, or coagulopathy. Coincident symptoms, including pain or dyspareunia, should be noted. The use of medications, both prescription and over-the-counter, and current contraception method, if any, should be ascertained. Any previous medical or surgical treatments should be explored, especially if they had been directed toward similar symptoms. Symptoms suggestive of ovulation, such as breast tenderness, bloating, or mood change, may help narrow the list of possible diagnoses. Presumptive and diagnostic tests for the presence of ovulation are shown in Table 15.3 (Chapter 15, Infertility).

In a similar manner, the physical examination should be wide-ranging to detect evidence of processes capable of influencing uterine function. Hirsutism, acne, galactorrhea, striae, or thyroid enlargement support an endocrine cause. Pale sclera or multiple bruises

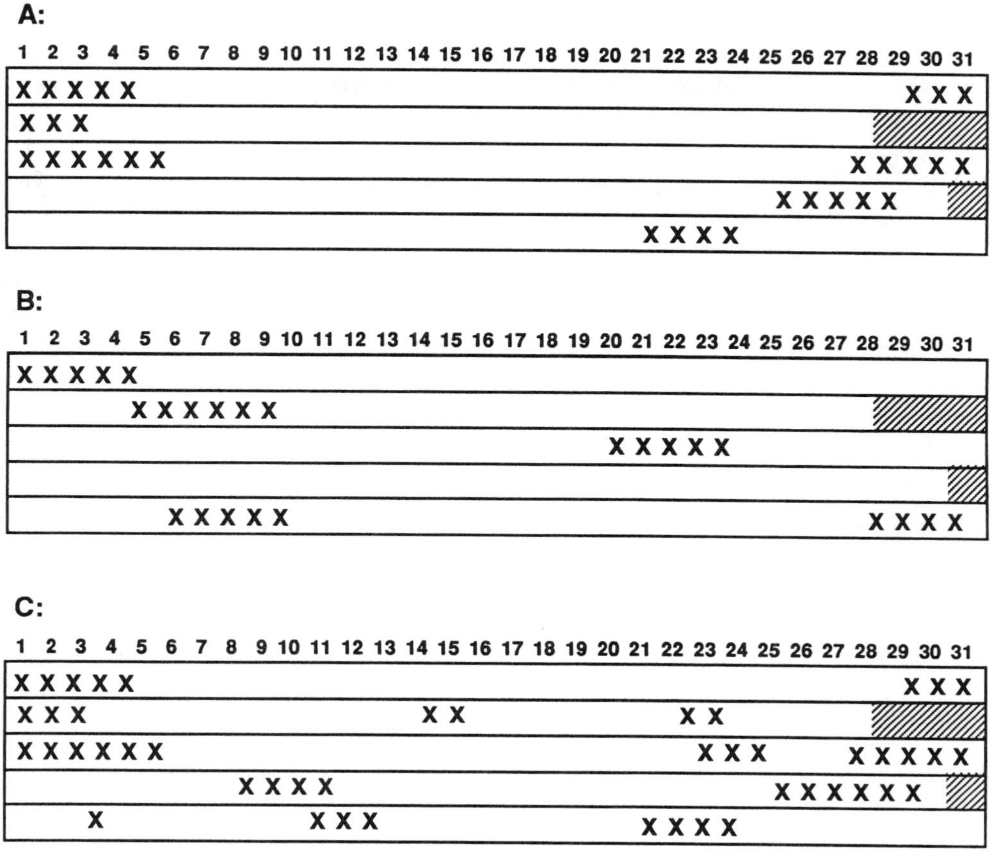

A:

| 1 | 2 | 3 | 4 | 5 | 6 | 7 | 8 | 9 | 10 | 11 | 12 | 13 | 14 | 15 | 16 | 17 | 18 | 19 | 20 | 21 | 22 | 23 | 24 | 25 | 26 | 27 | 28 | 29 | 30 | 31 |

```
X X X X X                                               X X X
X X X                                                   /////
X X X X X X                                     X X X X X
                                    X X X X X        /////
                        X X X X
```

B:

| 1 | 2 | 3 | 4 | 5 | 6 | 7 | 8 | 9 | 10 | 11 | 12 | 13 | 14 | 15 | 16 | 17 | 18 | 19 | 20 | 21 | 22 | 23 | 24 | 25 | 26 | 27 | 28 | 29 | 30 | 31 |

```
X X X X X
    X X X X X X                                          /////
                            X X X X X
                                                        /////
        X X X X X                               X X X X
```

C:

| 1 | 2 | 3 | 4 | 5 | 6 | 7 | 8 | 9 | 10 | 11 | 12 | 13 | 14 | 15 | 16 | 17 | 18 | 19 | 20 | 21 | 22 | 23 | 24 | 25 | 26 | 27 | 28 | 29 | 30 | 31 |

```
X X X X X                                               X X X
X X X                      X X                  X X      /////
X X X X X X                                 X X X   X X X X X
                X X X X                          X X X X X X /////
        X                X X X                X X X X
```

Figure 17.4. Examples of menstrual calendars used in the evaluation of abnormal uterine bleeding. A menstrual calendar can greatly facilitate the evaluation of abnormal uterine bleeding. **A.** A patient who complains of "two periods a month" may demonstrate regular, 28–29 day interval periods, allowing reassurance. **B.** Patients who are infrequently ovulatory or anovulatory tend to have cycles that have variable interval and duration. **C.** Patients with anatomic causes for abnormal bleeding may have intermenstrual bleeding to the extent that detecting the background menstrual cycle may be difficult. Basal body temperature information may be combined with or substituted for the menstrual calendar to provide information about the presence and timing of ovulation (Figure 2.7).

Table 17.3. Possible Indications for Hysteroscopic Evaluation

Amenorrhea
Complications of intrauterine contraceptive device use
Infertility
Menometrorrhagia
Menorrhagia unresponsive to therapy
Metrorrhagia
Postmenopausal bleeding
Recurrent pregnancy loss
Suspected uterine anomaly

propound anemia or a coagulopathy, respectively. Pelvic examination may detect the uterine enlargement typical of fibroids, identify a cervical polyp, or discover the string of a forgotten intrauterine contraceptive device.

There are no laboratory tests specific for the diagnosis of abnormal uterine bleeding. Testing should be chosen on the basis of the differential diagnoses under deliberation. Tests that evaluate liver or renal function or that assess coagulation and bleeding time should be ordered when appropriate. Because thyroid abnormalities may be found in up to 20% of clinically euthyroid patients with abnormal uterine bleeding, a sensitive thyroid stimulating hormone (sTSH) test should be considered. Patients thought to be climacteric or to have polycystic ovary disease may benefit from a measurement of serum follicle-stimulating hormone (FSH) and luteinizing hormone (LH). Cervical cultures may be helpful when cervicitis or endometritis is considered possible, but a negative culture does not rule out the diagnosis. A pregnancy test should be considered for patients who complain of amenorrhea or acute bleeding.

Imaging modalities may assist in detecting pathology in some patients in whom it may be difficult to document by clinical examination alone. Ultrasonography, computed axial tomography, or magnetic resonance imaging may be useful for selected patients. For most patients, however, such studies are unnecessary. Transvaginal ultrasonography may be of help in identifying endometrial polyps or documenting endometrial cavity distortion by leiomyomata, but these will generally be suspected based on physical findings or the lack of

Table 17.4. Potential Sources of Nonuterine Bleeding

Cervical sources
    Carcinoma
    Cervical eversion
    Cervicitis
    Condyloma
    Polyps
Vaginal sources
    Adenosis
    Atrophic change
    Carcinoma
    Foreign bodies (condom, pessary, tampon)
    Infection
    Lacerations (abortion attempts, coital injury, trauma)
Vulvar and extragenital sources
    Atrophy
    Condyloma
    Cystitis/urethritis
    Gastrointestinal (cancer, diverticulitis, inflammatory bowel disease)
    Hematuria
    Hemorrhoids
    Infection
    Labial varices
    Neoplasm
    Trauma
    Urethral caruncle
    Urethral diverticula
    Urethral prolapse/eversion

response to hormonal therapy. Diagnostic hysteroscopy, with or without direct operative therapy, is gradually replacing ultrasonography and blind curettage for this purpose.

For some patients, sampling of the endometrium may be appropriate to aid in the diagnosis of DUB. This may be done by way of office endometrial biopsy or by curettage. Hysteroscopy has replaced blind curettage in many centers, owing in part to studies indicating that lesions can be missed in 10% to 35% of blind procedures. This technique provides a direct view of the endometrial cavity; it may help direct biopsy sites and may be used as a route for therapies such as polypectomy, adhesiolysis, myomectomy, or endometrial ablation. Commonly used indications for diagnostic hysteroscopy are shown in Table 17.3.

Care must be taken to differentiate uterine bleeding from other sources of genital blood loss (Table 17.4). This can be both obvious and challenging. When a determination cannot be made during physical examination, placement of a tampon for a period of time with subsequent inspection (of the tampon) may point toward an approximate location.

THERAPEUTIC OPTIONS

Abnormal uterine bleeding is only a symptom. As such, care must be taken to rule out serious causes of the bleeding prior to instituting therapy. As with menorrhagia, the goals of management for abnormal uterine bleeding are simple: control acute bleeding, restore normal menses, and detect potentially dangerous conditions. Traditional treatment methods have had their shortcomings (Table 17.5), due, in part, to their indiscriminate application without attention to attendant pathology or physiology. Ultimately, the most successful therapy is one directed toward the specific causative condition responsibe for the patient's symptoms.

When definitive therapy is not an option (e.g., a hysterectomy for adenomyosis in a patient who wishes to preserve fertility), symptomatic treatment must be offered based to an extent on the presence or absence of ovulation.

Patients who are anovulatory and experiencing moderate bleeding may be managed as shown in Figure 17.5. This protocol addresses the immediate need to control distressing symptoms and provides long-term management based on the fertility plans of the patient. Patients who do not wish either pregnancy or contraception should be managed with cyclic progestin therapy such as medroxyprogesterone acetate, 5 to 10 mg per day for 10 days each month. This provides good control of bleeding, supplies predictable withdrawal bleeding, and prevents the sequella of unopposed estrogen stimulation. It does not, however, provide contraception should it be a necessity, currently or at a later date.

Patients who experience lighter bleeding and who have been ovulatory in the recent

Table 17.5. Failings of Management Strategies for Dysfunctional Bleeding

Dilatation and curettage: no evidence for long-term effect
Hormonal: anovulatory bleeding only
Sclerosis (medical or irradiation): significant side effects
Hysterectomy: overused
Intrauterine surgery: evolving

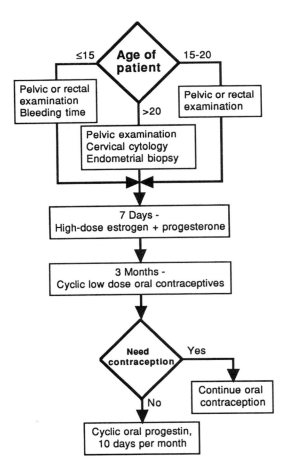

Figure 17.5. Suggested management of anovulatory (dysfunctional) bleeding. Once the possibility of an anatomic cause (or blood dyscrasia for adolescent patients) has been evaluated and a pregnancy ruled out, acute management consists of high-dose combined estrogen and progestin such as multiple tablets of combination contraceptives or a mixture of estrogen and progestin prescribed separately. Treatment with combination contraceptive for 3 months is then followed by therapy dictated by the patient's desire for contraception. Patients wishing pregnancy should be managed as outlined in Chapter 15, Infertility.

past may be reassured and observed or be treated with a single cycle of progestin therapy. In roughly 85% of cases, this single cycle provides adequate response. It has been postulated that ovulation is restored through progestin therapy, but the mechanism is unknown and it is unlikely that it will result in the face of chronic ovulation disorders. When used in this manner, progestin is given beginning on day 14 of the cycle and continued for 10 days. Patients should be warned that while they are taking their medication there may be no change in symptoms; the efficacy of the treatment will be determined by the behavior of subsequent menses. Patients should also be warned that the withdrawal bleeding that follows such therapy may be heavy, crampy, or prolonged as a result of the medication. While the period is often atypical, it need not be so for the treatment to be effective. Cyclic progestin therapy as discussed or combination estrogen-progestin therapy, should be considered for those patients who experience recurrence of symptoms after a single month of treatment. Estrogen therapy alone is not usually appropriate in the management of dysfunctional bleeding without the addition of progestin in some form.

For many patients, regardless of ovulation status, combination oral contraceptive agents provide good cycle control, contraception, and noncontraceptive benefits. Low-dose agents may even be considered in older women who have no other contraindications. Good cycle control is offered by most of the products currently available. Should midcycle break-through bleeding occur on phasic agents, switching to a monophasic product will generally relieve the problem.

Patients who are ovulatory, have no clinically identifiable pathologic process, and who have experienced only one or two abnormal cycles, may be reassured and followed. Many of the pa-tients will experience spontaneous resolution of their symptoms and will require no additional therapy. This is especially true of processes such as a persistent corpus luteum. When interven-tion is initiated, it will generally be successful after only one or two cycles and then may be dis-continued. If symptoms reoccur, an intensified search for underlying processes must be made.

As an alternative to estrogen or progestin therapy, some have advocated the used of dana-zol or gonadotropin-releasing hormone (GnRH) agonists. Although both can be used with good effect, their higher cost and side effect profiles have blunted enthusiasm for them. Non-steroidal anti-inflammatory agents, so effective in the treatment of menorrhagia, provide only limited effectiveness for dysfunctional bleeding. The greatest response gained from these drugs tends to be in women who are ovulatory and experience either heavy or painful flow.

If an endometrial biopsy has been performed, the results can help guide effective ther-apy. If the biopsy shows proliferative endometrium, benign hyperplasia, or disordered mat-uration, progestin therapy will generally be successful in restoring cycle control. If the biopsy shows secretory endometrium or atrophy, estrogen with progestin should be the therapy of choice. This may be given as combination oral contraceptives or customized us-ing individual prescriptions for both agents. If endometrial biopsy indicates the presence of endometritis, it may be treated with doxycycline (100 mg twice daily for 10 days).

In rare instances, hormonal manipulation does not give satisfactory control of the pa-tient's symptoms. Reconsideration of the original diagnosis is in order, with special atten-tion directed toward the possibility of intrauterine lesions. In these cases, dilatation and curettage, endometrial ablation, or hysterectomy may be necessary. These should never be considered as first line therapy. A trial of GnRH agonist therapy may be appropriate prior to surgical intervention, but this is a only a temporizing method in these cases. Consulta-tion is warranted when hormonal management fails.

HINTS AND COMMON QUESTIONS

Only one sixth of menstrual cycles are 28 days long.

The color and character of menstrual fluid has no prognostic significance. In general, the darker the flow the longer the hemoglobin component has been out of the systemic circulation. The patient may be reassured that such variations of character are normal and it is the pattern of bleeding that is most important.

Between 20% and 25% of adolescents with dysfunctional bleeding will be found to have a coagulation defect.

During the first 2 years of a woman's menstrual cycles, 50% to 80% of cycles are anovu-latory, making these women at risk for dysfunctional bleeding patterns.

Postcoital bleeding suggests cervicitis, a cervical polyp, or cervical carcinoma, all of which may be easily diagnosed by pelvic examination.

Anytime a delay or absence of menstruation is being evaluated, the possibility of a pregnancy must be considered.

An abrupt change in menstrual timing or character associated with abdominal pain (especially unilateral) should raise the possibility of an ectopic pregnancy. A pregnancy test is almost never inappropriate.

Midcycle spotting is not uncommon for women with endometriosis. Although the mechanism by which this occurs is unknown, it is a common clinical finding. When midcycle spotting is accompanied by cyclic pain, dyspareunia, or infertility, endometriosis should be considered.

Laborlike cramps at times other than menses should suggest the possibility of an endometrial polyp or pedunculated intracavitary myoma.

Endometrial biopsy is seldom necessary in teenagers with dysfunctional bleeding.

Postmenopausal bleeding should be presumed to indicate the presence of a malignancy, until proved otherwise. The only exception to this is the withdrawal bleeding that occurs as a part of cyclic estrogen-progesterone hormone replacement therapy.

There is no consistent evidence that sterilization alters the occurrance rate of abnormal uterine bleeding. Because fertility is no longer an issue for these patients, the treatments offered are more likely to be surgical, although studies indicate that this decision is often affected by other nonmedical factors.

In general, oral contraceptives result in a lighter, better tolerated menstrual period than does sequential estrogen-progestin therapy.

The discomfort of an office endometrial biopsy may be greatly reduced by premedication with a nonsteroidal anti-inflammatory agent, given 30 to 60 minutes before the procedure.

Cervical polyps can be easily removed in the office without the use of anesthesia. A cervical biopsy forceps may be used to remove the polyp, or it can be twisted from its base using a hemostat or packing forceps. The base of the polyp must be excised or it may be cauterized with silver nitrate. Although rarely malignant, any tissue removed should be sent for histologic evaluation. By contrast, endometrial polyps carry a 1% risk of malignancy.

SUGGESTED READINGS

General References

Aksel S, Jones GS. Etiology and treatment of dysfunctional uterine bleeding. Obstet Gynecol 1974;44:1.

American College of Obstetricians and Gynecologists. Dysfunctional uterine bleeding. ACOG Technical Bulletin 134. Washington, DC: ACOG, 1989.

Baker ER. Menstrual dysfunction and hormonal status in athletic women. Fertil Steril 1981;36:691.

Bayer RL, DeCherney AH. Clinical manifestations and treatment of dysfunctional uterine bleeding. JAMA 1993;269:1823.

Emans SJ, Grace E, Goldstein DP. Oligomenorrhea in adolescent girls. J Pediatr 1980;97:815.

Neese RE. Managing abnormal vaginal bleeding. Postgrad Med 1991;89:205.

Neinstein LS. Menstrual problems in adolescents. Med Clin N Am 1990;74:1181.

Rees MCP. Human menstruation and eicosanoids. Reprod Fertil Dev 1990;2:467.

Shangold M, Rebar RW, Wentz AC, Schiff I. Evaluation and management of menstrual dysfunction in athletes. JAMA 1990;263:165.

Speroff L, Glass RH, Kase NG. Clinical Gynecologic Endocrinology and Infertility, 5th ed. Baltimore: Williams & Wilkins, 1994, pp 183–230.

Specific References

Physiology

Baird DT, Glasier AF. Menstrual bleeding patterns and contraception. International Planned Parenthood Foundation Medical Bulletin 1991;254:1.

Bierman M, Nolan GH. Menstrual function and renal transplantation. Obstet Gynecol 1977;49:186.

Deligish L, Loewenthal M. Endometrial changes associated with myomata of the uterus. J Clin Pathol 1970;23:676.

DeStafano F, Perlman J, Peterson HB, Diamond E. Long-term risk of menstrual disturbances after tubal sterilization. Am J Obstet Gynecol 1985;152:835.

Duckman S, Sese L, Suarez J, Tantakesem P. Myoma uteri and abnormal uterine bleeding. South Med J 1972;65:1356.

Emans SJ, Grace E, Goldstein DP. Oligomenorrhea in adolescent girls. J Pediatr 1980;97:815.

Farhi B, Nosanchuk J, Silverberg S. Endometrial adenocarcinoma in women under 25 years of age. Obstet Gynecol 1986;68:741.

Field CS. Dysfunctional uterine bleeding. Prim Care 1988;15:561.

Fraser IS, Michie EA, Wide L, Baird DT. Pituitary gonadotropins and ovarian function in adolescent dysfunctional uterine bleeding. J Clin Endocrinol Metab 1973;37:407.

Higgins GR. IUD use and unexplained vaginal bleeding. Obstet Gynecol 1981;58:409.

Kjer J, Knudsen L. Hysterectomy subsequent to laparoscopic sterilization. Eur J Obstet Gynecol 1990;35:63.

Murphy NJ, Wallace DL, Behrend AE. Menometrorrhagia in an oral contraceptive user. J Fam Pract 1993;36:229.

Nedoss BR. Dysfunctional uterine bleeding: relation of endometrial histology to outcome. Am J Obstet Gynecol 1971;109:103.

Rulin MC, Davidson AR, Philliber SG, Graves WL, Cushman LF. Changes in menstrual symptoms among sterilized and comparison women: a prospective study. Obstet Gynecol 1989;79:749.

Rulin MC, Davidson AR, Philliber SG, Graves WL, Cushman LF. Long-term effect of tubal sterilization on menstrual indices and pelvic pain. Obstet Gynecol 1993;82:118.

Rulin MC, Turner JH, Dunworth R, Thompson D. Post tubal sterilization syndrome: a misnomer. Am J Obstet Gynecol 1985;151:13.

Sehgal N, Haskins AL. The mechanism of uterine bleeding in the presence of fibromyomas. Am Surg 1960;26:21.

Shy KK, Stergachis A, Grothaus, Wagner EH, Hecth J, Anderson G. Tubal sterilization and risk of subsequent hospital admission for menstrual disorders. Am J Obstet Gynecol 1992;166:1698.

Siegberg R, Nilsson CG, Stenman UK, Widholm O. Sex hormone profiles in oligomenorrheic adolescent girls and the effect of oral contraceptives. Fertil Steril 1984;41:888.

Smith SK, Abel MH, Kelly RW, Baird DT. Prostaglandin synthesis in the endometrium of women with ovular dysfunctional uterine bleeding. Br J Obstet Gynaecol 1981;88:434.

Taw RL. Review of menstrual disorders in which a secretory endometrium was found. Am J Obstet Gynecol 1975;122:490.

Venturoli S, Porcu E, Fabbri R, Paradisi R, Orsini LF, Flamigni C. Ovaries and menstrual cycles in adolescence. Gynecol Obstet Invest 1984;17:219.

Wilcox LS, Martinez-Schnell B, Peterson HB, Ware JH, Hughes JM. Menstrual function after tubal sterilization. Am J Epidemiol 1992;135:1368.

Diagnosis

Bayer SR, DeCherney AH. Clinical manifestations and treatment of dysfunctional uterine bleeding. JAMA 1993;269:1823.

Brooks PG, Serden SP. Hysteroscopic findings after unsuccessful dilatation and curettage for abnormal uterine bleeding. Am J Obstet Gynecol 1988;158:1354.

Eddows HA, Read MD, Codling BW. Pipelle: a more acceptable technique for outpatient endometrial biopsy. Br J Obstet Gynaecol 1990;97:961.

Fedele L, Bianchi S, Dorta M, Brioschi D, Zanotti F, Vercellini P. Transvaginal ultrasonography versus hysteroscopy in the diagnosis of uterine submucous myomas. Obstet Gynecol 1991;77:745.

Fothergill DJ, Brown VA, Hill AS. Histological sampling of the endometrium—A comparison between formal curettage and the Pipelle sampler. Br J Obstet Gynaecol 1992;99:779.

Gimpleson RJ. Panoramic hysteroscopy with directed biopsies versus dilatation and curettage for accurate diagnosis. J Reprod Med 1984;29:575.

Gimpleson RJ, Rappold HD. A comparative study between panoramic hysteroscopy with directed biopsies and dilatation and curettage. Am J Obstet Gynecol 1988;158:489.

Indman PD. Abnormal uterine bleeding: accuracy of vaginal probe ultrasound in predicting abnormal hysteroscopic findings. J Reprod Med 1995;40:545.

Loffer FD. Hysteroscopy with selective endometrial sampling compared with D&C for abnormal uterine bleeding: the value of negative hysteroscopic view. Obstet Gynecol 1989;73:16.

Mahmood TA, Templeton AA, Thomson L, Fraser C. Menstrual symptoms in women with pelvic endometriosis. Br J Obstet Gynaecol 1991;98:558.

Silver MM, Miles P, Rosa C. Comparison of Novak and Pipelle endometrial biopsy instruments. Obstet Gynecol 1991;78:828.

Valle RF. Hysteroscope evaluation of patients with abnormal uterine bleeding. Surg Gynecol Obstet 1981;153:521.

Management

Brooks PG, Clouse J, Morris LS. Hysterectomy vs resectoscopic endometrial ablation for the control of abnormal uterine bleeding: a cost-comparative study. J Reprod Med 1994;39:755.

Brooks PG, Loffer FD, Serden SP. Resectoscopic removal of symptomatic lesions. J Reprod Med 1989;34:435.

Brooks PG, Serden SP. Hysteroscopic findings after unsuccessful dilatation and curettage for abnormal uterine bleeding. Am J Obstet Gynecol 1988;158:1354.

Cooperman AB, DeCherney AH. Endometrial cancer following endometrial ablation. Obstet Gynecol 1993; 82:640.

Corson Sl, Brooks PG. Resectoscopic myomectomy. Fertil Steril 1991;55:1041.

Cowan BD, Morriaon JC. Management of abnormal genital bleeding in girls and women. N Engl J Med 1991;324:1710.

DeCherney AH, Diamond MP, Lavy G, Polan ML. Endometrial ablation for intractable uterine bleeding: hysteroscopic resection. Obstet Gynecol 1987;70:668.

DeVore GR, Owens O, Kase N. Use of intravenous Premarin in the treatment of dysfunctional uterine bleeding— a double-blind randomized control study. Obstet Gynecol 1982;59:285.

Diaz S, Croxatto HB, Pavez M, Belhadj H, Stern J, Sivin I. Clinical assessment of treatments for prolonged bleeding in users of Norplant implants. Contraception 1990;42:97.

Fortney JA. Oral contraceptives for older women. International Planned Parenthood Foundation Medical Bulletin 1990;243:3.

Fraiser IS. Treatment of ovulatory and anovulatory dysfunctional uterine bleeding with oral progestogens. Aust N Z J Obstet Gynaecol 1990;30:353.

Goldfarb HA. A review of 35 endometrial ablations using the Nd-YAG laser for recurrent menometrorrhagia. Obstet Gynecol 1990;76:833.

Hamilton JV, Knab DR. Suction curettage: therapeutic effectiveness in dysfunctional uterine bleeding. Obstet Gynecol 1975;45:47.

Livio M, Mannucci PM, Vigano G, et al. Conjugated estrogens for the management of bleeding associated with renal failure. N Engl J Med 1986;315:731.

Petrucco OM, Fraser IS. The potential for the use of GnRH agonists for treatment of dysfunctional uterine bleeding. Br J Obstet Gynaecol 1992;99(suppl 7):34.

Pinion SB, Parking DE, Abramovich DR, et al. Randomized trial of hysterectomy, endometrial laser ablation, and transcervical endometrial resection for dysfunctional uterine bleeding. BMJ 1994;309:979.

Serden SP, Brooks PG. Treatment of abnormal uterine bleeding with the gynecologic resectoscope. J Reprod Med 1991;36:697.

Thomas EJ, Okuda KJ, Thomas NM. The combination of a depot gonadotrophin releasing hormone agonist and cyclical hormone replacement therapy for dysfunctional uterine bleeding. Br J Obstet Gynaecol 1991;98:1155.

Townsend DE, Richart RM, Paskowitz RA, Woolfork RE. "Rollerball" coagulation of the endometrium. Obstet Gynecol 1990;76:310.

Valle RF. Endometrial ablation for dysfunctional uterine bleeding: role of GNRH agonists. Int J Gynaecol Obstet 1993;41:3.

Valle RF. Hysterscopic removal of submucous leiomyomas. J Gynecol Surg 1990;6:89.

Vancaillie TG. Electrocoagulation of the endometrium with the ball-end resectoscope ("rollerball"). Obstet Gynecol 1989;74:425.

18

Menstrual Pain

The high prevalence, repetitive nature, and potentially debilitating severity of dysmenorrhea obligates those who care for women to have a thorough knowledge of this problem. Dysmenorrhea represents the single greatest source of lost productivity. Its incidence is as high as 70% for women during their late teens and early 20s, with one half of these women experiencing a least some loss of function: time out of school, home, or work. Of all menstrual-age women, 10% to 15% suffer significant disability with every period, losing from 1 to 3 days each month. It has been estimated that dysmenorrhea accounts for over 600 million lost working hours annually in the United States.

Despite a predilection for young women, dysmenorrhea can affect any woman no matter what her age, race, or parity. One indication of the pervasiveness of this affliction is the observation that few, if any, colloquial terms for menstruation are better than neutral in connotation. Most are decidedly negative, derogatory, or sinister.

BACKGROUND AND SCIENCE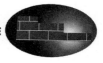

"Dysmenorrhea," which is derived from Greek, means difficult monthly flow. Despite this venerable root, the term did not make its appearance in the English language until about 1810. Clinically, dysmenorrhea is divided into two broad classifications: primary and secondary. Unlike diagnoses where "primary" and "secondary" have a temporal meaning (e.g., primary infertility or secondary amenorrhea), in dysmenorrhea these terms relate to causality. In secondary dysmenorrhea there is a clinically identifiable cause. History and physical examination are usually sufficient to establish the diagnosis and rarely will diagnostic procedures be required. In primary dysmenorrhea the cause is biochemical, with the diagnosis suggested by history and supported by the absence of physical abnormalities.

Because the common causes of secondary dysmenorrhea (e.g., fibroids, pelvic adhesions, adenomyosis, and so forth) are more frequent in older patients, secondary dysmenorrhea is more common in this age group as well. The incidence of primary dysmenorrhea is greatest in adolescents and women in their 20s.

The symptoms of both primary and secondary dysmenorrhea may be similar, making diagnosis based solely on history unreliable. The distinction between the two is important because successful therapy must target the underlying cause.

Secondary Dysmenorrhea

In secondary dysmenorrhea, identifiable pathologic or iatrogenic conditions act on the uterus, tubes, ovaries, or pelvic peritoneum causing pain. The perception of pain generally results when these processes alter pressure in or around the pelvic structures, release chemical messengers or irritants, change or restrict blood flow, or cause irritation of peritoneal surfaces. These pathologies may act in combination with normal physiologic changes to create discomfort or they may act independently with their symptoms becoming noticeable during menstruation.

The possible causes of secondary dysmenorrhea can be broadly classified as being intrauterine and extrauterine (Table 18.1). Diffuse lower abdominal cramping, back or thigh pain, nausea, diarrhea, and headache may occur with either intrauterine or extrauterine sources of secondary dysmenorrhea. Extrauterine sources most likely provide hints of their presence through additional nonmenstrual symptoms. Musculoskeletal, gastrointestinal, or urinary pathologies may cause symptoms at the time of menstruation, but their effects are rarely restricted to the time of flow. For example, irritable bowel syndrome often significantly worsens around the time of menstruation, but a careful history usually reveals postprandial cramping, food intolerance, or episodic diarrhea or constipation. Pelvic scarring (from surgery or inflammatory processes such as infection) or endometriosis may cause overlooked symptoms of pain with intercourse, bowel movements, or physical activity. Intermenstrual spotting is sometimes found in patients with endometriosis. Somatization may focus symptoms on the pelvis that can worsen with the stress of menstruation, but it is rare for these patients not to exhibit symptoms at other times of the month or not to have signs of stress, anxiety, depression, or personality disorders.

Table 18.1. Possible Causes of Secondary Dysmenorrhea

Uterine causes	Extrauterine causes
Adenomyosis	Endometriosis
Cervical stenosis and cervical lesions	Inflammation and scarring (adhesions)
Congenital abnormalities (outflow obstructions, uterine anomalies)	Nongynecologic causes Musculoskeletal, gastrointestinal, urinary
Infection (chronic endometritis)	"Pelvic congestive syndrome" (debated)
Intrauterine contraceptive devices (IUCDs)	Psychogenic (rare)
Myomas (generally intracavitary or intramural)	Tumors Myomas, benign or malignant tumors of
Polyps	ovary, bowel, or bladder

Intrauterine sources of dysmenorrhea are thought to cause menstrual pain by disrupting the normal contractile activities of the uterus, through the liberation of compounds such as prostaglandins, or both contractions and prostaglandins. Mechanical disruption of normal uterine function occurs when the uterine wall (as in the case of myomas, adenomyosis, congenital anomalies) or the cavity itself is distorted (as in intracavitary polyps or intrauterine contraceptive devices). The uterus normally has low amplitude contractions that occur every few minutes throughout the menstrual cycle. These contractions, which increase near ovulation and during menstruation, are thought to assist in expelling menstrual fluid. Mechanical disruption of the uterine wall muscle bundles is postulated to cause local spasms, ischemia, or abnormal stretch, all of which could result in pain. Large intrauterine polyps or pedunculated myomas may stimulate excess uterine activity as the uterus undergoes laborlike contractions to expel them. Cervical lesions, stenosis, or congenital malformations that restrict uterine outflow may result in elevated intrauterine pressures and the sensation of cramps, although this is an uncommon cause of dysmenorrhea.

Much has been made over the years about the role of psychogenic factors in the development of menstrual pain. Some studies have indicated that "high-strung" or "supersensitive" women, those with unstable personalities, or those unable to accept their role as women were prone to develop dysmenorrhea. Although it may be true that women with neuroses, paranoia, emotional instability, or immaturity may have dysmenorrhea, there is no evidence that this is any more common than other somatic complaints in these same patients. Much of the writing implicating psychosocial factors in dysmenorrhea was published before the pathophysiology of dysmenorrhea was understood. As is often the case, it is sometimes easier to blame something than it is to admit ignorance. Psychosocial factors may be involved in the complaint of dysmenorrhea, but rarely are they the only cause.

Primary Dysmenorrhea

Although dysmenorrhea is uncommon during the first 6 months of menstruation, roughly 38% of women experience it in their first year and 80% of those with pain develop it within 3 years (Fig. 18.1). Unfortunately, primary dysmenorrhea often creates more severe

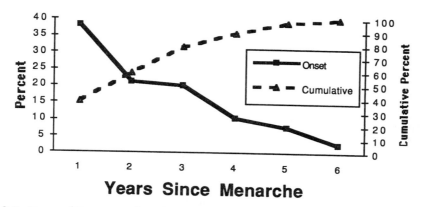

Figure 18.1. Onset of Dysmenorrhea. Years since menarche. Data from: Andersch B, Milson I. An epidemiologic study of young women with dysmenorrhea. Am J Obstet Gynecol 1982;144:655.

symptoms than those experienced by patients with secondary dysmenorrhea. These women experience sharp, spasmodic, laborlike midline pain that comes and goes in waves. The pain may radiate to the back or legs and may be accompanied by nausea, vomiting, hypotension, and collapse. The onset and severity of primary dysmenorrhea mimics the menstrual flow itself, beginning within a few hours of the onset of flow and reaching maximal severity during the heaviest portion of the period. Physical examination will not demonstrate any mechanical abnormality, which led many of these patients to be classed as malingerers or worse. Until the responsible pathophysiology was established, little could be done to ameliorate the symptoms these patients experienced short of narcotics or inhibition of menstruation.

Traditionally, menstrual pain has been attributed to absolute intrauterine pressure, the rate of intrauterine pressure change, and the quality of rest between contractions. These characteristics appear broadly related to the pain of dysmenorrhea, although even today the exact relationship remains unclear. Two lines of research have come together to provide an understanding of the cause of primary dysmenorrhea: electromechanical activity of the uterus and the pathophysiology of uterine prostaglandins.

Uterine Activity Studies

The first successful attempts to measure uterine contractile activity predate the development of the sphygmomanometer and efforts to record intrauterine pressure from the nonpregnant uterus date from 1889. Increased uterine electrical and mechanical activity were proposed as causes of dysmenorrhea and by the late 1930s objective findings began to support the concepts. Dysmenorrhea was still viewed as a woman's weakness, rather than a physiologic disturbance, but by the late 1940s this was beginning to change. There was growing acceptance that women with dysmenorrhea had fundamental differences in uterine activity.

The most detailed and influential studies of dysmenorrhea and uterine activity came in the late 1940s and early 1950s. These studies found a direct correlation between intrauterine pressure and pain. It was found that patients with dysmenorrhea have stronger more frequent contractions, poorly coordinated contractile patterns, along with poorer relaxation and higher pressures between contraction waves (Fig. 18.2). Thus, by the middle of this century three main mechanisms seemed established for the creation of pain in dysmenorrhea: 1) High intrauterine pressures (sometimes in excess of 400 mm Hg); 2) "poor rest" between contractions because of elevated "tone," decreased time between contraction waves, or both; and 3) altered contraction patterns, including irregular "notched" waves, uncoordinated or asynchronous contractions.

Despite these observations, there was no ready explanation for why the increased uterine activity occurred until biochemical studies entered the picture.

Uterine Prostaglandins

In parallel with uterine activity studies were investigations that attempted to find a biochemical disturbance. In 1957, Pickles reported that acetone and ether extracts of menstrual fluid contained a powerful "plain muscle stimulant." These studies were expanded and the source localized to the sloughing endometrium. By the early 1960s, these stimulants had been identified as prostaglandins.

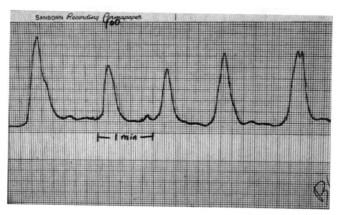

Figure 18.2. Intrauterine pressures in primary dysmenorrhea. Intrauterine pressure recordings made during menses in dysmenorrheic women demonstrate high pressures, prolonged contractions, and poor rest between contraction waves. (Full scale pressure in the tracing shown is 400 mm Hg.)

The stage was set for the connection between prostaglandins and uterine activity to be drawn. It came in 1965, when Pickles reported elevated levels of prostaglandin $F_{2\alpha}$ in the menstrual fluid of dysmenorrheic women. A causative role for prostaglandin $F_{2\alpha}$ in dysmenorrhea was supported with additional studies and the connections seemed complete between excess uterine prostaglandin $F_{2\alpha}$, increased uterine activity, and the pain of dysmenorrhea.

Current evidence indicates that women with primary dysmenorrhea produce between two and seven times the normal amount of prostaglandin $F_{2\alpha}$. This results in the strong, poorly coordinated uterine activity found and helps explain the great success that has been obtained through the use of prostaglandin inhibitor therapy. Excess prostaglandins may also be responsible for the smooth muscle activity noted in the gastrointestinal tract of these women. Hypermobility of the gut may be responsible for the frequent coexistence of nausea, vomiting, and diarrhea in these patients. Prostaglandins may also act as initiators or potentiators of nociceptive pain signals, further contributing to the symptoms experienced.

Endometrial prostaglandin production is tied to endometrial changes throughout the menstrual cycle. Prostaglandin is stored in the endometrium as it thickens in preparation for implantation or menstruation. With the onset of menstruation, preformed prostaglandins are liberated and large amounts of arachidonic acid is released from the cell walls of sloughed endometrial cells. Arachidonic acid is the prime substrate for prostaglandin production. This large increase in substrate results in a tremendous increase in prostaglandin production, which augments the supplies liberated from the sloughed endometrial cells. Anything that results in a thin, atrophic endometrium, such as that found in anovulatory cycles or while taking oral contraceptives, reduces prostaglandin production, resulting in a less painful period.

Why these women make excess prostaglandin is unknown, but there is good evidence that primary dysmenorrhea runs in families. How much of this observation is due to genetic predisposition to excess prostaglandin production and how much to anticipation and expectations ingrained by rearing, is also unknown.

Just as mysterious, is the spontaneous improvement over time that women with primary dysmenorrhea experience. Some have postulated that aging and childbirth may reduce the number of α-adrenergic receptors found in the uterine wall. These receptors, which help mediate uterine contractility, are affected by hormonal changes and even by psychogenic factors. Destruction of some of these receptors may take place due to stretch of the uterine wall during pregnancy. Despite this hypothesis, up to one third of women with primary dysmenorrhea reported in some series, have been parous.

Although our understanding of dysmenorrhea has advanced greatly over the past years, there is still much left to be discovered.

ESTABLISHING THE DIAGNOSIS

Almost any other process that can affect the pelvic viscera or cause acute pain can be a source for cyclic pain and dysmenorrhea (Table 22.1, Chapter 22, Pelvic Pain). For this reason, care must be taken when obtaining the history to separate pain that occurs only during menses from that which changes or that worsens, but is present at other times of the cycle as well. The history should include the age of onset, the character, location, radiation, and associated factors that make the symptoms better, worse, or different. The exact relation to the onset of menstrual flow must be determined. For example, pain that begins 1 to 2 days before the onset of flow and improves once flow is established, is more apt to be due to endometriosis than it is to be an example of primary dysmenorrhea.

When developing a differential diagnosis, it is easy to be lulled into a narrow field of possible causes. The association of cyclic pain and the menstrual cycle implies a causal relationship to the genital tract or ovaries that may not be present. Care must be taken to consider other sources of pain as well. Any cyclic pelvic pain, including dysmenorrhea, may be caused by gynecologic, urologic, gastrointestinal, musculoskeletal, and other processes. It is important to separate menstrual pain (dysmenorrhea) from pelvic pain occurring in a cyclic manner. The distinction between cyclic pain, which is more closely associated with chronic pain syndromes (see Chapter 22, Pelvic Pain), and true dysmenorrhea, is vital to establishing a correct diagnosis and subsequently achieving successful therapy. Anything that increases the likelihood of finding the underlying process, increases the probability of a successful therapy. This necessitates a wide-ranging approach to the diagnosis. Therefore, when the symptoms are suprapubic, the temptation to jump automatically to gynecologic or urologic sources risks missing the patient with referred musculoskeletal pain or somatization. Irritable bowel syndrome will be missed as a cause for crampy left lower abdominal pain that worsens during the time of menstrual flow unless it is included in the differential diagnosis. Careful attention to the patient's history, and a well-thought-out approach to physical, laboratory, and other evaluations, will result in a correct diagnosis and facilitate successful treatment.

Secondary Dysmenorrhea

The signs and symptoms of secondary dysmenorrhea are often nonspecific and are more referable to the underlying pathophysiology. The symptoms may be slightly milder, and more general in nature, than those of primary dysmenorrhea. The specific ailment an individual experiences is more likely to be determined by the underlying pathology. Frequently, a careful history will suggest the ongoing causative process and direct further evaluations. For example, a complaint of heavy menstrual flow accompanying dysmenorrhea suggests adenomyosis, myomas, or polyps. The coexisting complaint of infertility may suggest endometriosis. Pelvic heaviness, pressure, or a change in abdominal contour, should raise the possibility of intra-abdominal neoplasia or fibroids. Gastrointestinal symptoms, urinary difficulties, back complaints, or the like should alert the physician to the possibility of nongynecologic or even extra-pelvic processes. If the patient noted that her symptoms started only after placement of an intrauterine contraceptive device (IUCD), it is appropriate to think of the IUCD as a probable cause. Therefore, the most sensitive diagnostic studies for secondary dysmenorrhea are a careful history and a thoughtful physical examination.

Observation of the patient's movement, careful examination of the upper and lower abdomen, as well as the pelvic examination, are all required if a correct diagnosis is to be established. Even the pelvic examination must be modified in patients with dysmenorrhea. Careful examination of the urethra, adenexa, uterosacral ligaments, posterior cul-de-sac, and other areas often examined in only a cursory way, must be singled out for special attention in these patients. Asymmetric enlargement of the uterus suggests myomas or other tumors. Symmetric enlargement of the uterus is often present in adenomyosis and also occasionally when intrauterine polyps are present. Painful nodules in the posterior cul-de-sac with restricted motion of the uterus is suggestive of endometriosis. Restricted motion of the uterus may also be present with pelvic scarring from adhesions or inflammation. This specifically should be suspected when there is thickening of adnexal structures.

Ultrasonography, computed tomography (CT) scanning, and magnetic resonance imaging (MRI) are seldom of assistance except in the face of a grossly inadequate clinical examination. One exception to this rule may be those patients in whom it is difficult or impossible to distinguish uterine enlargement from an adnexal mass. Here ultrasonography or CT scanning may resolve the issue, resulting in a change in diagnosis or therapy. Diagnostic laparoscopy may be required to establish a diagnosis, but it should be reserved until other diagnostic measures and clinical trials of therapy have been exhausted. Although roughly one third of diagnostic laparoscopies find no pathology, there is often a discordance between the pelvic examination and the findings at laparoscopy, which underscores the value of this procedure for selected patients.

The role of laboratory evaluation for patients with secondary dysmenorrhea or cyclic pelvic pain is limited and nonspecific. Blood counts may help to evaluate ongoing or excessive blood loss that occurs in patients with fibroids or adenomyosis. Sedimentation rates may help to identify the presence of a chronic inflammatory process, but, of necessity, are imprecise in providing a diagnosis.

Primary Dysmenorrhea

Young women with primary dysmenorrhea generally have typical sharp lower abdominal pain which takes place during the first 1 to 3 days of menstruation. The suprapubic location with radiation to the back, sacrum, or the inner thighs, accompanied by moderate to severe nausea, vomiting, and diarrhea should suggest the diagnosis. Patients often double up into a fetal position to gain relief. They frequently report using a heating pad or hot water bottle to decrease their discomfort. Dyspareunia (even during menstruation) is not a feature of primary dysmenorrhea and should suggest the presence of secondary causes. Although the diagnosis of primary dysmenorrhea may be suspected by history alone, it is fundamentally a diagnosis of exclusion.

Because the very definition of primary dysmenorrhea is one in which there is no clinically identifiable cause, the physical examination of a patient with primary dysmenorrhea should be normal. There should be no palpable abnormalities of the uterus or adnexa. If the patient is examined during menstruation she often appears pale and "shocky," but her abdomen will be soft and nontender. As in patients suspected of having secondary dysmenorrhea, imaging, laboratory studies, and invasive measures such as laparoscopy should be carefully reserved. Often, a therapeutic trial may be more appropriate as a diagnostic measure.

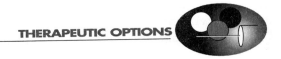

THERAPEUTIC OPTIONS

Over the years, many interventions have been used to relieve the discomfort of menstruation. These have varied from the admonition to have "right thoughts," eat a balanced diet, and exercise regularly to patent medicines that contain more alcohol than any other ingredient. Time, and a greater understanding of the pathophysiology of dysmenorrhea, has led to a wide range of therapies that can be used (Table 18.2). The most effective of these approaches is tailored to the needs of the individual patient and the processes thought to be at work.

Secondary Dysmenorrhea

The best therapy for secondary dysmenorrhea is one directed toward the underlying source. Although analgesics, antispasmodics, and oral contraceptives may provide some symptomatic relief, only therapy aimed at correcting the cause is ultimately successful. This may range from removing an IUCD to gonadtropin-releasing hormone (GnRH) therapy for endometriosis, to removing an endometrial polyp, to hysterectomy for fibroids. In each in-

Table 18.2. General Therapeutic Options for Dysmenorrhea

Type of approach	Example
General measures	Heat, exercise, diet, mild diuretics (caffeine)
Analgesics	Nonprescription medications, nonnarcotics
Pain prevention	Nonsteroidal anti-inflammatory drugs
Modification of periods	Oral contraceptives, GnRH agonists
Nonpharamacologic analgesia	Transcutaneous electrical nerve stimulation (TENS), biofeedback
Tocolysis	Alcohol, calcium channel blockers (limited by side effects)
Surgery	Presacral neurectomy, polypectomy, myomectomy, hysterectomy

GnRH = gonatropin-releasing hormone.

stance, a specific, effective therapy aimed at the root of the symptoms, not the symptoms themselves, is best. Care must be taken that the therapies suggested are those appropriate for the proposed pathology, and are not colored by compassion for the degree of disability reported by the patient. That is, surgical therapy should be reserved for those patients in whom a specific, surgically correctable diagnosis is established, and for whom other forms of therapy have either failed or are deemed inappropriate. Many studies have shown that hysterectomy performed without a specific preoperative diagnosis other than dysmenorrhea or chronic pelvic pain, is unlikely to resolve the patient's complaints. Further investigation in the form of imaging, diagnostic laparoscopy, or medical hysterectomy (through the use of GnRH agonists) may be a more appropriate step. Short-term use of GnRH agonists may be useful both as therapy and to confirm a cycle-based disturbance. Clearly, if these agents do not provide relief of the menstrual pain, surgical removal of the uterus or ovaries will not be of benefit and is contraindicated.

Presacral neurectomy or laser ablation of the uterosacral ligaments has been advocated for patients where no specific diagnosis has been established and intractable, debilitating midline pain is present. Here, too, these interventions should be reserved for those patients in whom no other therapy has been successful, and who recognize that their symptoms may be unchanged or even worsened by the intervention. Although some reports claim good relief from pain, these procedures are far from innocuous and their use should be limited.

For patients where specific therapy is not available and for those who are not surgical candidates, other, less invasive, modalities (e.g., analgesics, cycle modification, biofeedback, or transcutaneous electrical nerve stimulation [TENS]) may be equally or more effective. Analgesics are probably the first treatment that patients, if not physicians, turn to for menstrual pain. For most women, over-the-counter analgesic and menstrual pain products will be inadequate for relief beyond the mildest symptoms. Significant dysmenorrhea often requires moderate strength analgesics, sometimes including narcotics. Extreme care must be taken in the use of potent analgesics. Not only may we be substituting one disability for another, due to sedation or side effects, we may also potentiate or sustain drug-seeking behavior in those few patients with somatization, personality disorders, or depression as a source for their pain. (For a more complete discussion of this problem and the analgesics available for treating moderate to severe pain see Chapter 22, Pelvic Pain.)

Dysmenorrhea may be improved with the use of low-dose oral contraceptives in those patients who desire contraception and have no contraindications to their use. Low-dose oral contraceptives, either monophasic or triphasic, provide lighter, shorter, and less painful cycles, resulting in improvement of symptoms for roughly 80% of patients. In addition, the predictable timing of menstrual flow may facilitate the use of analgesics to anticipate, rather than react to, pain.

TENS therapy is often overlooked because it is not familiar to many outside the fields of sports medicine and physical therapy. This modality provides excellent relief for many patients with dysmenorrhea (including those with primary dysmenorrhea) without the systemic side effects associated with analgesic and other therapies. The battery-operated, small signal generators used may be easily carried or worn by the patient as she goes about her usual activities. Electrodes can be placed in a triangular pattern of two periumbilical and one lower quadrant sites (Fig. 18.3), or may be applied on either side of the low back, based on the patient's symptoms and empiric trials of efficacy.

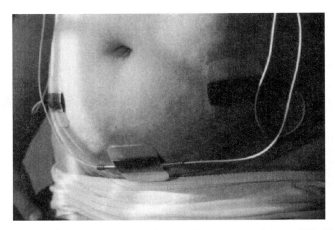

Figure 18.3. Placement of transcutaneous electrical nerve stimulation (TENS) electrodes.

Primary Dysmenorrhea

The same philosophy of treatment that was applied to secondary dysmenorrhea pertains to primary dysmenorrhea as well: treat the ultimate cause, not just the symptoms. Hence, therapy for primary dysmenorrhea is directed toward reducing the production or action of the causative prostaglandins. Indeed, in this way it is possible to refer to pain prevention, rather than to pain relief (analgesia).

Patients with primary dysmenorrhea generally experience exceptional pain relief through the use of nonsteroidal anti-inflammatory drugs (NSAIDs). A number of NSAIDs are available and may be used for the treatment of primary dysmenorrhea (Table 18.3). These may be broadly grouped into families as shown in Table 18.4. The importance of these families is that similarities between drugs in a single family are far greater than their differences. As a result, if an agent is ineffective when given in the proper way, other members of the same family are also unlikely to be successful. However, patients who receive only partial relief from one drug may benefit from a trial of a compound from another family. Tissue specificity as well as subtle differences in the site or mechanism of action of these drugs accounts for this phenomenon. Response rates for all of these agents exceed 75% to 80% and are often much better. No clear advantage of one drug over another has yet been demonstrated.

Nonsteriodal Anti-inflammatory Drug Families

Some drugs that inhibit prostaglandin synthesis are not effective treatments for dysmenorrhea. Some have only weak antiprostaglandin activity; some require metabolic transformation to become active or have side effects limiting their usefulness. These drugs (e.g., aspirin, phenacetin, phenylbutazone, paracetamol, or indomethacin) can be used to treat dysmenorrhea, but have generally been replaced by more effective compounds.

There are two major classifications of NSAID (carboxylic acids, enolic acids), each with subgroups, as shown in Table 18.3. Carboxylates are the most familiar. These drugs have the most utility for dysmenorrhea. Within this major group there are four subgroups of compounds that have individual characteristics.

Table 18.3. Nonsteroidal Anti-inflammatory Drugs for Dysmenorrhea*

Drug	Initial dose (mg)	Subsequent dose (mg)
Diclofenac (potassium)	50–100	50 bid
Diclofenac (sodium)	75–150	75 bid
Diflunisal	1000	500 q12 h
Etodolac	400	400 q4–6 h
Fenoprofen calcium	200	200 q4–6 h
Flurbiprofen	50	50 tid
Ibuprofen[†]	600	600 q4 h
Indomethacin	25	25 tid
Ketoprofen	75	75 tid
Ketorolac	10	10 q4–6 h
Meclofenamate[†]	100	50–100 q4–6 h
Mefenamic acid[†]	500	250 q4–6 h
Naproxen[†]	500	250 q4–6 h
Naproxen sodium[†]	550	275 q6–8 h
Sulindac	200	200 bid
Suprofen	200	200 q4 h
Tolmetin	400	400 tid

*Consult full prescribing information before using any of these drugs.
†FDA approved for primary dsymenorrhea.
bid = twice a day; tid = three times daily; q = every.

Table 18.4. Families of Nonsteroidal Anti-inflammatory Drugs

Drug	Trade Name
CARBOXYLATES	
Salicylic acids	
Aspirin	(various)
Diflunisal	Dolobid
Salicylate	Disalcid, Mono-Gesic, Salflex, Salsalate, Salsitab
Indoleacetic acids	
Diclofenac potassium	Cataflam
Diclofenac sodium	Voltaren
Etodolac	Lodine
Indomethacin	Indocin
Ketorolac tromethamine	Acular, Toradol
Sulindac	Clinoril, Sulindac
Tolmetin	Tolectin, Tolmetin
Propionic acids	
Fenoprofen calcium	Nalfon, Fenoprofen
Flurbiprofen	Ansaid
Ibuprofen*	Motrin, IBU, Rufen
Ketoprofen	Orudis, Oruvail, Ketoprofen
Naproxen sodium*	Aflaxen, Anaprox
Naproxen*	Naprosyn
Fenimates	
Meclofenamate*	Mecolmen
Mefenamic acid*	Ponstel
ENOLIC ACIDS	
Pyrazolones	
Oxyphenbutazone	
Phenylbutazone	Azolid, Butazolidin
Oxicams	
Piroxicam	Feldene, Piroxicam

*FDA approved for primary dysmenorrhea.

The first group is the salicylic acid group. Aspirin has a very low potency for reducing prostaglandin synthesis in the uterus; therefore, aspirin has had little clinical utility in preventing moderate or severe dysmenorrhea. Diflunisal (Dolobid) has a long half-life allowing twice a day dosage, but its slow onset of action limits use for most patients.

Increased potency against dysmenorrhea is found in the acetic acid group. Most of the drugs in this group are directly effective and do not undergo metabolism into an active form. Indomethacin (Indocin) has been used to treat dysmenorrhea, but a moderate incidence of side-effects limits the use of this and most other drugs in this group.

The most commonly used drugs for dysmenorrhea come from the two remaining carboxylate groups: arylalkanoic acids (propionic acid derivatives) and anthranilic acids (fenamates).

Of the propionic acid derivatives currently available, ibuprofen (Motrin, Rufen) and naproxen (Naprosyn, Anaprox) are commonly used for dysmenorrhea. Other drugs of this class have been used for pain relief or arthritis therapy, but are not currently approved for dysmenorrhea.

The fenamates are potent prostaglandin synthetase inhibitors, which have been shown to antagonize the actions of preformed prostaglandins. Subjective and objective studies have consistently shown these agents to be very effective. In this country, mefenamic acid (Ponstel) is approved for dysmenorrhea and clinical studies supporting the use of meclofenamate (Meclomen) have shown it to be very effective. The dual action of synthesis inhibition and direct antagonism should give these agents an edge in efficacy, although clinical advantages have not been proved.

The most commonly used treatments include mefenamic acid (Ponstel) 500 mg followed by 250 mg every 4 to 6 hours; Ibuprofen 1200 to 1600 mg followed by 600 to 800 mg three times a day; or diclofenac sodium (Voltaren) 150 mg followed by 75 mg three times a day. Over-the-counter dosages of ibuprofen or other NSAIDs can be used in many patients with mild to moderate symptoms.

Choice of Agents

How should an appropriate therapy for the patient with primary dysmenorrhea be chosen? The evidence seems to slightly favor the fenamates over the propionic acid agents, but both groups are sufficiently effective that the differences may be moot. Once an agent has been selected, it should be tried over two to four menstrual cycles before success or failure is determined. If therapy is unsuccessful, some patients may still have favorable response to another NSAID chosen from a different family.

One must always be aware of the potential for side effects with these medications. Although side effects are infrequent and generally mild, serious side effects are possible. The short duration of use in dysmenorrhea therapy limits these risks. Patients with aspirin-sensitive asthma, ulcers, or inflammatory bowel disease should not use these drugs.

Other Treatments

In addition to NSAIDs, oral contraceptives are appropriate if contraception is desired. As with secondary dysmenorrhea, the thinner, more atrophic endometrium that results with these drugs will give a lighter, shorter and more tolerable period. Some patients may consider the use of both oral contraceptives and NSAIDs to give even greater relief.

Strong analgesics, TENS, and other therapies are seldom needed to treat primary dysmenorrhea. When these are considered, the probability that a secondary cause is involved must also be heavily weighed.

HINTS AND COMMON QUESTIONS

If a patient complains of painful menstruation, but has not had dysmenorrhea in the past, careful consideration must be given to complications of pregnancy as a cause. Ectopic pregnancy, threatened, or incomplete abortion may all be confused with dysmenorrhea.

Dysmenorrhea that occurs with a girl's first one or two menses suggests the possibility of a congenital obstruction to flow.

Dysmenorrhea that begins after the age of 25 is most often secondary, not primary.

Patients with primary dysmenorrhea often describe their pain using the example of a fist opening and closing, which is similar to the contractions found in the uterus.

The value of oral contraceptives for patients who do not need contraception must be weighed carefully: costs and possibility of side effects from 21 days of medication versus 2 to 3 days of symptom relief. For these patients, a trial of nonsteroidal anti-inflammatory agents may be a better first therapy.

Nonsteroidal anti-inflammatory drug therapy for primary dysmenorrhea is so effective that at least moderate response should be anticipated. Any patient who does not show this expected improvement should have the diagnosis reconsidered and be re-evaluated for signs of secondary dysmenorrhea.

One exception to the rule of switching drug families when treatment fails is the use of ibuprofen. Many patients will tell you that this drug does not work for their menstrual pain. It is wise to inquire about the actual dose used that accounted for this failure. Most patients know that the over-the-counter ibuprofen drugs are "just the same as the prescription brand," but do not realize that the nonprescription type is only 200 mg, or about a quarter the dose required for patients with severe pain. Drugs in the propionic acid family may still be a good choice for trial, even though you may not want to use ibuprofen by name.

If pain relief is not complete using NSAID therapy, patients should be warned not to add additional analgesics, especially other NSAIDs, because of possible potentiation of gastrointestinal and other side effects. Adding a second NSAID doubles the risk of side effects with doubling the therapeutic benefits.

Patients, and frequently physicians, believe that menstrual pain will improve after delivering a child. Unfortunately, the incidence of primary dysmenorrhea is not directly affected by childbearing. Growing older by a year, combined with a year of amenorrhea during which the pain of dysmenorrhea may be forgotten, likely causes any apparent changes that occur. Objective studies do not support a causal relationship between pain improvement and pregnancy.

Little or no data are available regarding the duration or character of labor for women who have had primary dysmenorrhea. Many patients report that their labors were not as uncomfortable as menstrual periods, but the subjective aspects of pain and the very nature of the birth process make these observations anecdotal, at best.

Does the 15% to 20% response rate to placebo medication indicate a psychological component to dysmenorrhea? Although there may be some psychological component to any recurring ailment, these figures are equally consistent with the observation that pain is extraordinarily difficult to measure. As a result of this difficulty, any study wherein pain relief is an outcome measure will have a high degree of variability and placebo response due to the vagaries of estimation alone.

Many patients have been told that menstrual pain is "all in the head" and that little can be done to treat it. It is important to reassure the patient (and sometimes her family) that dysmenorrhea is real and that, with therapy, a return to full and normal activities can be expected.

SUGGESTED READINGS

General References

Though somewhat older, excellent reviews of the pathophysiology of dysmenorrhea may be found in:
Akerlund-M. Pathophysiology of dysmenorrhea. Acta Obstet Gynecol Scand 1979;87(suppl):27.
Coupey SM, Ahlstrom P. Common menstrual disorders. Pediatr Clin North Am 1989;36:551.
Dawood MY. Dysmenorrhea. J Reprod Med 1985;30:154.
Dawood MY. Dysmenorrhea. Clin Obstet Gynecol 1990;33:168.
Dawood MY. Current concepts in the etiology and treatment of primary dysmenorrhea. Acta Obstet Gynecol Scand 1986;113:63–67.
Rosenwaks Z, Seegar-Jones G. Menstrual pain: Its origin and pathogenesis. J Reprod Med 1980;25:207.
Ylikorkala O, Dawood M Y. New concepts in dysmenorrhea. Am J Obstet Gynecol 1978;30:833.
An excellent compilation of articles on primary dysmenorrhea can be found in Dawood MY, McGuire JL, Demers LM, eds. Premenstrual Syndrome and Dysmenorrhea. Baltimore: Urban & Schwarzenberg, 1985.

Specific References

Åkerlund M. Pathophysiology of dysmenorrhea. Acta Obstet Gynecol Scand 1979;87(suppl):27.
Åkerlund M, Andersson K-E. Effects of terbutaline on human myometrial activity and endometrial blood flow. Obstet Gynecol 1976;47:529.
Andersch B, Milson I. An epidemiologic study of young women with dysmenorrhea. Am J Obstet Gynecol 1982;144:655.
Anderson ABM, Hanes PJ, Fraser IS, Turnbull AC. Trial of prostaglandin-synthesis inhibitors in primary dysmenorrhoea. Lancet 1978;1:345.
Andersson K-E, Ulmsten U. Effects of nifedipine on myometrial activity and lower abdominal pain in women with primary dysmenorrhea. Br J Obstet Gynaecol 1978;85:142.
Asch RH, Greenblatt RB. Primary and membranous dysmenorrhea. South Med J 1978;71:1247.
Benedetto C. Eicosanoids in primary dysmenorrhea, endometriosis and menstrual migraine. Gynecol Endocrinol 1989;3:71.
Bickers W. Uterine contractions in dysmenorrhea. Am J Obstet Gynecol 1941;42:1023.
Boehm FH, Sarratt H. Indomethacin for the treatment of dysmenorrhea: a preliminary report. J Reprod Med 1975;15:84.
Brotanek V, Hendricks CH, Yoshida T. Changes in uterine blood flow during uterine contractions. Am J Obstet Gynecol 1969;103:1108.
Chambers PL. Further studies on the plain muscle stimulant present in human endometrium. J Endocrinol 1960;20:6.
Chambers PL, Pickles VR. Plain-muscle stimulants in extracts of menstrual fluid and of endometrial curettings. J Physiol 1958;144:68.
Chan WY, Dawood MY. Prostaglandin levels in menstrual fluid of nondysmenorrheic and dysmenorrheic subjects with and without oral contraceptive or ibuprofen therapy. Adv Prostaglandin Thromboxane Leukot Res 1980;8:1445.

Chan WY, Dawood MY, Fuchs F. Prostaglandins in primary dysmenorrhea: comparison of prophylactic and non-prophylactic treatment with ibuprofen and use of oral contraceptives. Am J Med 1981;70:535.

Chan WY, Hill JC. Menstrual prostaglandin levels in non-dysmenorrheic and dysmenorrheic subjects. Prostaglandins 1978;15:365.

Corson SL, Bolognese RJ. Ibuprofen therapy for dysmenorrhea. J Reprod Med 1978;20:246.

Csapo AI. The diagnostic significance of the intrauterine pressure. I. General considerations and techniques. Obstet Gynecol Surv 1970;25:403.

Csapo AI. The diagnostic significance of the intrauterine pressure. II. Clinical considerations and trials. Obstet Gynecol Surv 1970;25:515.

Csapor AI. A rationale for the treatment of dysmenorrhea. J Reprod Med 1980;25(suppl):198.

Csapo AI, Pulkkinen MO, Henzl MR. The effect of Naproxen-sodium on the intrauterine pressure and menstrual pain of dysmenorrheic patients. Prostaglandins 1977;13:193.

Dawood MY. Overall approach to dysmenorrhea. In Dawood MY, McGuire JL, Demers LM (eds). Premenstrual Syndrome and Dysmenorrhea. Baltimore: Urban & Schwarzenberg, 1985, p 177.

Dingfelder JR. Primary dysmenorrhea treatment with prostaglandin inhibitors: a review. Am J Obstet Gynecol 1981;140:874.

Ekström P, Juchnicka E, Laudanski T, Åkerlund M. Effect of an oral contraceptive in primary dysmenorrhea—Changes in uterine activity and reactivity to agonists. Contraception 1989;40:39.

Filler WW, Hall WC: Dysmenorrhea and its therapy: a uterine contractility study. Am J Obstet Gynecol 1970;106:104.

Forman A, Ulmsten U, Andersson K-E. Aspects of inhibition of myometrial hyperactivity in primary dysmenorrhea. Acta Obstet Gyencol Scand 1983;113(suppl):71.

Halbert DR, Demers LM. A clinical trial of indomethacin and ibuprofen in dysmenorrhea. J Reprod Med 1978;21:219.

Hayashi RH. Clinical management of dysmenorrhea and labor. In Garfield RE (ed). Uterine Contractility: Mechanisms of Control. Norwell, MA: Serono Symposia, 1990;309.

Heltzel JA, Senta TA, Weeks ME. Effective control of primary dysmenorrhea pain using transcutaneous electrical nerve stimulation (TENS). Pain 1987;29(suppl):S370.

Hendricks CH. Inherent motility patterns and response characteristics in the nonpregnant human uterus. Am J Obstet Gynecol 1966;96:824.

Henzl MR, Ortega-Herrera E, Rodriguez C, Izu A. Anaprox in dysmenorrhea: reduction of pain and intrauterine pressure. Am J Obstet Gynecol 1979;134:455.

Henzl MR, Izu A. Naproxen and naproxen sodium in dysmenorrhea: development from in vitro inhibition of prostaglandin synthesis to suppression of uterine contractions in women and demonstration of clinical efficacy. Acta Obstet Gynecol Scand 1979;87(suppl):105.

Irwin J, Morse E, Riddick D. Dysmenorrhea induced by autologous transfusion. Obstet Gynecol 1981;58:286.

Lumsden MA, Baird DT. Intra-uterine pressure in dysmenorrhea. Acta Obstet Gynecol Scand 1985;64:183.

Lundeberg T, Bondesson L, Lunström V. Relief of primary dysmenorrhea by transcutaneous electrical nerve stimulation. Acta Obstet Gynecol Scand 1985;64:491.

Lundström V, Gréen K, Svanborg K. Endogenous prostaglandins in dysmenorrhea and the effects of prostaglandin synthetase inhibitors (PGSI) on uterine contractility. Acta Obstet Gynecol Scand 1979;87 (suppl):51.

Lundström V, Gréen K, Wiqvist N. Prostaglandin, indomethacin and dysmenorrhea. Prostaglandins 1976;11:893.

Lundström V. Treatment of primary dysmenorrhea with prostaglandin synthetase inhibitors—A promising therapeutic alternative. Acta Obstet Gynecol Scand 1978;57:421.

McRae MA, Kin MH. Dysmenorrhea in uterus unicornis with rudimentary uterine cavity. Obstet Gynecol 1979;53:134.

Metheny WP, Smith RP. The relationship among exercise, stress, and primary dysmenorrhea. J Behav Med 1989;12:569.

Milsom I, Hedner N, Mannheimer C. A comparative study of the effect of high-intensity transcutaneous nerve stimulation and oral naproxen on intrauterine pressure and menstrual pain in patients with primary dysmenorrhea. Am J Obstet Gynecol 1994;170:123.

Morrison JC, Ling FW, Forman EK, et al. Analgesic efficacy of ibuprofen for treatment of primary dysmenorrhea. South Med J 1980;73:999.

Novac E, Reynolds SRM. The cause of primary dysmenorrhea. JAMA 1932;99:1466.

Osler M. Standard treatment of dysmenorrhea with special reference to treatment with spasmolytics and hormones. Acta Obstet Gynecol Scand 1979;87(suppl):69.

Owen PR. Prostaglandin synthetase inhibitors in the treatment of primary dysmenorrhea. Am J Obstet Gynecol 1984;148:96.

Pickles VR. A plain muscle stimulant in the menstrual fluid. Nature (London) 1957;180:1198.

Pickles VR. Some evidence that the endometrium produces a hormone that stimulates plain muscle. J Endocrinol 1959;18:1.

Pickles VR. Myometrial responce to the plain-muscle stimulant. J Endocrinol 1959;19:150.

Pickles VR. Prostaglandins and dysmenorrhea. Acta Obstet Gynecol Scand 1979;87(suppl):7.

Pickles VR, Hall WJ, Best FA, Smith GN. Prostaglandins in endometrium and menstrual fluid from normal and dysmenorrheic subjects. Br J Obstet Gynaecol 1965;72:185.

Pulkkinen MO. Suppression of uterine activity by prostaglandin synthestase inhibitors. Acta Obstet Gynecol Scand 1979;87(suppl):39.

Pickles VR, Hall WJ, Best FA, Smith GN. Prostaglandins in endometrium and menstrual fluid from normal and dysmenorrheic subjects. Br J Obstet Gynaecol 1965;72:185.

Pulkkinen MO. Relief of menstrual discomfort and dysmenorrhea and simultaneous suppression of uterine activity by isoxepac. Acta Obstet Gynecol Scand 1980;59:367.

Pulkkinen MO. Prostaglandins and the non-pregnant uterus. The pathophysiology of primary dysmenorrhea. Acta Obstet Gynecol Scand 1983;113(suppl):63.

Pulkkinen MO, Csapo AI. The effect of ibuprofen on the intrauterine pressure and menstrual pain of dysmenorrheic patients. Prostaglandins 1978;15:1055.

Pulkkinen MO, Kaihola H-L. Mefenamic acid in dysmenorrhea. Acta Obstet Gynecol Scand 1977;56:75.

Rucker MP. Contractions of a non-pregnant multiparous human uterus. Am J Obstet Gynecol 1925;9:255.

Smith RP. A brief history of intrauterine pressure measurement. Acta Obstet Gynecol Scand 1984;129 (suppl):1.

Smith RP. Intrauterine pressure analysis in nonpregnant dysmenorrheic women. Medical Instrumentation 1984;185:137.

Smith RP. Objective changes in intrauterine pressure during placebo treatment of dysmenorrhea. Pain 1987;29:59.

Smith RP. The dynamics of nonsteroidal anti-inflammatory therapy for primary dysmenorrhea. Obstet Gynecol 1987;70:785.

Smith RP, Heltzel JA. Interrelation of analgesia and uterine activity in women with primary dysmenorrhea. J Reprod Med 1991;36:260.

Smith RP, Powell JR. Intrauterine pressure changes during mefenamic acid treatment of primary spasmodic dysmenorrhea. Am J Obstet Gynecol 1982;143:286.

Smith RP, Powell JR. The objective evaluation of dysmenorrhea therapy. Am J Obstet Gynecol 1980;137:314.

Smith RP, Powell JR. Simultaneous objective and subjective evaluation of meclofenamate sodium in the treatment of primary dysmenorrhea. Am J Obstet Gynecol 1987;157:611.

Walker JB, Katz RL. Peripheral nerve stimulation in the management of dysmenorrhea. Pain 1981;11:355.

Widholm O. Dysmenorrhea during adolescence. Acta Obstet Gynecol Scand 1979;87(suppl):61.

Willman EA, Collins WP, Clayton SG. Studies in the involvement of prostaglandins in uterus symptomatology an pathology. Br J Obstet Gynaecol 1976;83:337.

Wilson L, Kurzrok R. Studies on the motility of the human uterus in vivo. Endocrinology 1983;23:79.

Wilson L, Kurzrok R. Uterine contractility in functional dysmenorrhea. Endocrinology 1940;27:23.

Woodbury RA, Torpin R, Child GP, Watson H, Jarboe M. Myometrial physiology and its relation to pelvic pain. JAMA 1947;134:1081.

19

No Periods
(Amenorrhea)

For good or ill, the monthly return of menstruation signals reproductive health. When menstruation fails to develop or is absent, it can represent both a physiologic warning and a source of psychological stress. The causes of absent menstruation range from the physiologic to major disruptions of enzyme systems or the body's genome. Efficient evaluation and appropriate intervention are necessary for the continuing health and peace of mind of the patient.

Despite what may appear to be a daunting array of possible causes, most patients with amenorrhea have relatively simple problems that are easily within the purview of the primary care setting. Managing patients with amenorrhea can be effectively accomplished by using simple schemes for diagnosis and treatment that can be applied by all primary care providers.

BACKGROUND AND SCIENCE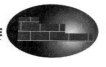

Amenorrhea occurs anytime there is a disruption in the delicate coordination of the hypothalamic-pituitary-ovarian system or when some process alters the ability of the uterus or the genital outflow tract to manifest cyclic hormonal function. Ultimately, amenorrhea is a symptom that may result from a number of reasons and is not a disease unto itself.

Amenorrhea is clinically divided into two broad classifications based on timing: 1) primary amenorrhea, in which the patient has failed to begin menstruation despite appropriate age and development and 2) secondary amenorrhea, in which a patient suffers the loss of previously established periods. A third type, physiologic amenorrhea, is most common, and by definition not abnormal. The designations of primary and secondary amenorrhea by themselves do not reflect either the severity of the underlying pathophysiology or the prospects for restoring normal cycling. The separation into primary and secondary types does facilitate the clinical evaluation. This is because the relative frequency of pathophysiologic processes varies within the two groups, even though the majority of causes are not unique to either type.

A number of classification schemes can be used to help organize the multiple possible sources of absent menstruation. Based on the normal physiology of menstruation, it is logical to classify the causes of amenorrhea into four groups: physiologic, hypothalamic and pituitary dysfunction, ovarian dysfunction, and alterations to the genital outflow tract. This general classification scheme works well for the clinical evaluation of either primary or secondary amenorrhea.

Often, the level of gonadotrophin is used to distinguish possible causes of amenorrhea. When used, this segregates patients into three groups: those with high gonadotrophin levels, such as menopausal patients; those with normal levels, such as those with endometrial or outflow problems; and those with abnormally low values, such as found in prepubertal women and those with pituitary or hypothalamic dysfunction. This meshes well with the above classification scheme and differentiates between the second and third types listed (hypothalamic and pituitary dysfunction vs. ovarian dysfunction). Although this works well in providing tables of pathologic processes, the clinical evaluation is often more pragmatic, searching for causes based on frequency or ease of testing.

Nonphysiologic amenorrhea occurs to less than 5% of women during their reproductive lives. This value varies widely based on the population studied. Patient groups such as athletes, prisoners, psychiatric patients, and others have rates that range to 100%.

Two forms of secondary amenorrhea that deserves special attention are those in which galactorrhea or virilization are present. Galactorrhea, the presence of spontaneous milky breast discharge, may result from a number of causes, but when paired with amneorrhea warrants a slighly modified diagnostic approach. Virilization results in more sweeping changes than just the loss of menstruation, changes that can profoundly affect a woman's self-image and function in society. True virilization is usually the harbinger of significant pathologic processes that may jeopardize the patient's overall health. Even with normal menstrual function, patients often express concern about the presence of excess body hair, worried that it portends virilization. The evaluation of hirsutism and virilization, therefore, carry both medical and social import, warranting their separate discussion.

Physiologic Amenorrhea

Physiologic amenorrhea is the expected absence of menstruation before the age of menarche, after the age of menopause, and during pregnancy or lactation. Iatrogenic amenorrhea due to hysterectomy is generally ignored as a trivial classification. In each instance of physiologic amenorrhea, the absence of menstrual bleeding is normal, expected, and reflects well-elucidated physiologic processes. Although these forms of menstrual absence are generally inconsequential in clinical practice, the possibility of their existence must always be kept in mind. To overlook them risks missing an early pregnancy or premature menopause.

Lactating women have highly variable patterns of amenorrhea. It is unknown if this variation arises from differences in suckling stimulus, variable sensitivity of the pituitary-hypothalamic system, or a combination of factors. It has been well established that lactating women will resume normal ovulation while breast-feeding, resulting in a pregnancy risk before the first period heralds the return of fertility.

Menopause occurs when there is a depletion of oocytes capable of responding to gonadotropins. The median age of menopause in the United States is 51.5 years, with 95% of women experiencing this event between the ages of 44 and 55. Less than 1% of women undergo a spontaneous menopause younger than the age of 40, although premature ovarian failure does account for 10% of nonphysiologic secondary amenorrhea. Although menopause is a physiologic process, strong evidence of a detrimental sequella of estrogen withdrawal has led to the view that menopause is an endocrinopathy that requires treatment. (See Chapter 12, Menopause.)

Primary Amenorrhea

Most of the pathophysiologic processes that cause secondary amenorrhea may be responsible for primary amenorrhea as well. Primary amenorrhea, however, can also result from a number of causes unique to delayed or absent menarche, markedly expanding the list of possible diagnoses.

Potential causes for primary amenorrhea may be classified as gonadal or extragonadal (Table 19.1). The most common cause of failure to begin menstruation is gonadal dysgenesis. In about 60% of women with primary amenorrhea, an abnormality of gonadal differentiation or function has occurred during the fetal or neonatal period. When this occurs, it may be accompanied by incomplete or inappropriate development of the external genitalia.

Table 19.1. Etiologic Classification of Primary Amenorrhea

Gonadal abnormalities (60% of cases)
    Autoimmune ovarian failure (Blizzard syndrome)
    Gonadal dysgenesis
        Pure gonadal dysgenesis
        45, XO (Turner's syndrome)
        46, XY gonadal dysgenesis (Swyer's syndrome)
        46, XX q5 X chromosome long-arm deletion
        Mixed or mosaic
    Follicular depletion
        Autoimmune disease
        Infection (e.g., mumps)
        Infiltrative disease processes (e.g., tuberculosis, galactosemia)
    Iatrogenic ovarian failure (e.g., alkylating chemotherapy, irradiation)
    Ovarian insensitivity syndrome (Savage's syndrome)
    17 α-hydroxylase deficiency
    Chronic anovulation of pubertal onset
Extragonadal anomalies (40% of cases)
    Congenital absence of uterus and vagina (müllerian agenesis)
    Imperforate hymen
    Male pseudohermaphroditism (testicular feminization syndrome)
    Pituitary-hypothalamic dysfunction
    Transverse vaginal septum

Puberty is often delayed, with primary amenorrhea bringing the patient to medical attention. Much of gonadal dysgenesis is due to a lack of part or all of an X chromosome. Based on the amount of missing genetic material, the clinical impact varies from simple failure of sexual maturation to the full stigmata of Turner's syndrome (45, XO). Patients with Turner's syndrome suffer a number of abnormalities that include short stature (< 150 cm), minimal or absent secondary sexual changes, webbing of the neck, low neck hairline, multiple nevi, a high arched palate, an increased carrying angle of the arms (cubitus valgus), and coarctation of the aorta. It is estimated that Turner's syndrome occurs in about 1 of every 2700 female births.

The terms "pure gonadal dysgenesis" and "mixed gonadal dysgenesis" are used to distinguish patients who do not carry the stigmata of Turner's syndrome but still suffer absent menarche due to chromosomal abnormalities. These patients are generally tall (> 150 cm) with normal appearance. They are a more chromosomally heterogeneous group, with individuals who are 46,XX, 46,XY, or have mosaic X/XY karyotypes. Gonad development may be absent or grossly abnormal.

Some patients with primary menstrual failure will be phenotypically female but genetically male (male pseudohermaphroditism or testicular feminization). These patients have a normal male karyotype but a genetic alteration that results in somatic cells that cannot recognize or respond to testosterone. Testosterone and gonadotropin levels are essentially normal (there may be a slight increase in luteinizing hormone), but the testosterone is biologically ineffective because of the body's inability to utilize it. As a result, masculinization does not take place, and the normal production of müllerian-inhibiting factor results in regression of the upper genital tract and a blind vaginal pouch. These patients undergo normal female breast development, although immature nipples and hypopigmented areolae are common. The patients have scant or no pubic or axillary hair and are often above average in height. Gonads may be palpable in the inguinal canal or labioscrotal folds. When testicular feminization is found or there is a mosaicism involving a Y chromosome, surgical extirpation of the gonads must be performed because of a 25% to 30% risk of malignant gonadal tumor formation.

Enzymatic defects, such as 17 α-hydroxylase deficiency, may result in sexual infantilism and absent menarche. These patients often have hypertension and hypokalemic alkalosis in addition to elevated levels of progesterone and corticosterone. Other enzyme defects may result in virilization or hirsutism and are discussed in that context.

Obstruction or agenesis of the genital outflow tract, due to congenital abnormalities in the development or canalization of the müllerian ducts, results in absent or covert menstrual bleeding. Uterine and vaginal agenesis, or an imperforate hymen are the most commonly encountered abnormalities of this type, but transverse vaginal septi or cervical agenesis can occur. When present and if neglected, there is a high prevalence of upper tract damage, resulting in a very poor reproductive prognosis. This is true for even the easily correctable imperforate hymen, which is associated with a high prevalence of endometriosis, vaginal adenosis, and other anomalies that result in long-term reproductive problems.

Complete lack of müllerian development (Mayer-Rokitansky-Küster-Hauser syndrome), which is the most frequently encountered anatomic cause of primary amenorrhea, is found in about 1 of 4000 female births. These otherwise normal women lack a vagina. A partial endometrial cavity may exist in 10% of patients, resulting in cyclic abdominal pain and the development of a pelvic mass before the diagnosis is made. A high prevalence of co-existing renal (30% to 50%) and skeletal abnormalities (10% to 15%) require additional evaluation. The high degree of similarity between this syndrome and male pseudohermaphroditism (testicular feminization), supports the value of a karyotype.

As indicated in Table 19.1 and in Chapter 7, Pediatric and Adolescent Care, there are an additional number of highly unusual causes of absent menarche, including enzyme defects, autoimmune syndromes, and other chromosomal abnormalities not discussed here. These conditions involve highly specialized evaluations and expertise. The initiation of the clinical investigation is appropriate in the primary care setting, but early referral of patients with primary amenorrhea should be seriously entertained.

Secondary Amenorrhea

The most common cause of secondary amenorrhea, other than pregnancy, is anovulation. This may come about because of problems at the level of the hypothalamus or the ovary itself. The distinction between these two sites is often the basis by which diagnoses are classified or evaluated. The ovary may fail to respond to gonadotropins for a number of reasons, including the depletion of functional oocytes, which results in menopause, or a large number of processes may be responsible for pituitary-hypothalamic dysfunction (Table 19.2). Many, if not most, of these may be suspected clinically.

Anovulation does not invariably lead to amenorrhea. It is estimated that between 50% and 60% of patients with anovulation are amenorrheic with the remainder having bleeding patterns that vary between regular, unpredictable and light, to frank dysfunctional bleeding.

Anovulation is associated with hypothalamic or pituitary dysfunction in roughly one half of cases. Of these patients, the hypothalamus is the source of dysfunction in two thirds of cases, whereas pituitary problems make up the rest. Even factors outside of these structures may act through them, resulting in menstrual disruption. For example, constitutional factors, such as weight loss, exercise, or stress, which influence hypothalamic function, may be responsible for the disruption in menstrual function. Even when constitutional factors are obviously present, a careful evaluation for other sources is fitting.

Outflow tract abnormalities are an infrequent (< 10%) cause of secondary amenorrhea. Scarring or occlusion of the uterine cavity (Asherman's syndrome) can occur following curettage, especially when performed after septic abortion or in the immediate postpartum period. Any instrumentation of the uterine cavity that is complicated by infection may cause sufficient endometrial damage to result in hypomenorrhea or frank amenorrhea. Endometrial damage by infection unrelated to instrumentation, such as tuberculosis or schistosomiasis, and cervical stenosis occurring after conization may also result in secondary loss of menstrual bleeding.

Anovulation and secondary amenorrhea are common in elite athletes, patients who diet excessively or have major nutritional deficiencies, and those with significant eating disorders such as anorexia nervosa. The impact of significant emotional stress may be manifest in menstrual irregularity or hypothalamic amenorrhea. Some studies have reported that 5% to 20% of recreational runners experience amenorrhea and up to two thirds of competitive runners experience luteal phase disruptions. These patients may have delays in menarche by up to 3

Table 19.2. Causes of Pituitary-Hypothalamic Amenorrhea

Functional
    Exercise (excessive)
    Malnutrition
    Obesity
    Weight loss
Drug induced
    Hormonal contraception
    Marijuana
    Tranquilizers
Neoplasia
    Craniopharyngioma
    Hypothalamic hamartoma
    Pituitary adenoma (prolactin secreting)
    Small cell carcinoma of lung
Psychogenic
    Anorexia nervosa
    Anxiety
    Pseudocyesis
    Stress
Other
    Adrenal androgenization
    Central nervous system trauma
    Chronic medical illness
    Hemochromatosis
    Hystiocytosis X
    Internal carotid artery aneurysms
    Irradiation
    Juvenile diabetes mellitus
    Polycystic ovary syndrome
    Sheehan's syndrome (postpartum ischemic necrosis)
    Syphilitic gummas
    Tuberculosis
    Uremia

years when training is begun before puberty. The exact mechanism for these delays is not known, but evidence suggests that it is related to body fat levels (Fig. 19.1).

Galactorrhea

Milky nipple discharge is not always galactorrhea. It is not uncommon for women, especially those who have been pregnant, to be able to express a milky discharge from one or both breasts. Galactorrhea is characterized by spontaneous, bilateral nipple leakage, which may be due to disruptions in thyroid or prolactin (PRL) hormone levels. Hypothyroidism, as manifested by elevated thyroid-stimulating hormone (TSH), is readily corrected, although often overlooked as a cause of galactorrhea.

Prolactin is responsible for preparing the breast for nursing in the later stages of pregnancy and the early postpartum period. When prolactin levels are elevated, breast stimulation, milk formation and discharge, and suppression of the normal control of menstrual cycling may all result. The most common cause of elevated serum prolactin is a pituitary

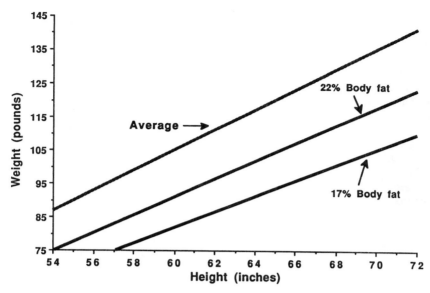

Figure 19.1. Body fat thresholds for menstruation. It has been estimated that menarche will not occur until body fat exceeds 17% and regular menstruation will be lost if body fat drops below 22%. These levels are not absolute, but provide guidelines for assessment and counseling.

adenoma. These can vary in size, occasionally growing out of the bounds of the sella turcica. When this occurs, impingement on the optic nerve or adjacent structures may be clinically apparent. There is a poor correlation between serum PRL levels and the size or detectability of a pituitary lesion. Only about a third of women with elevated prolactin levels experience loss of menstrual function, although elevated levels are detected in between 10% and 20% of patients with amenorrhea. Elevated PRL levels are not universally associated with galactorrhea, which may be absent in 25% or more of patients. Conversely, roughly one-half of women with galactorrhea will have a normal PRL. There are a number of potential causes for elevated prolactin, the most common of which are shown in Table 19.3.

Virilization and Hirsutism

Virilization and hirsutism are often found in the absence of amenorrhea, but because they represent a special subset of amenorrheas, they are reasonably discussed under this wider umbrella. Virilization refers to the loss of female sexual characteristics, such as body contour, and the acquisition of masculine qualities, such as increased muscle mass, temporal balding, deepening of the voice, and clitoromegaly. In contrast, hirsutism refers only to increased or excessive hair growth, which may be idiopathic (hypertrichosis) or due to androgen-stimulated excessive growth. Hypertrichosis, which involves increased hair on the extremities, tends to be ethnic, racial, or familial in origin.

Excessive hair growth is based on a number of factors including the rate and amount of androgen secretion present, the concentration of sex hormone-binding globulin (SHBG), the rate of peripheral conversion of weak androgens to potent androgens, and the sensitivity of the pilosebaceous unit to the androgens present. A change in one or more of these factors can result in an increase in hair growth or a change in hair distribution. Both

Table 19.3. Sources of Elevated Prolactin Levels

Pharmacologic (examples)	Pathophysiologic causes
Anesthetics	Central nervous system
CNS-dopamine depleting agents	Cavernous sinus thrombosis
α-Methyldopa	Infection
Monoamine oxidase inhibitors	Neurofibromas
Reserpine	Temporal arteritis
Dopamine receptor blocking agents	Tumors and cysts (all types)
Domperidone	Hypothalamic
Haloperidol	Craniopharyngioma
Metoclopramide	Glioma
Phenothiazines	Granulomas
Pimozide	Histocytosis disease
Sulpiride	Sarcoid
Dopamine re-uptake blockers	Tuberculosis
Nomifensine	Irradiation damage
Histamine H_2-receptor antagonists	Pituitary stalk transection
Cimetidine	Surgical
Hormones	Traumatic
Estrogens	Pseudocyesis (functional)
Oral contraceptives	Pituitary lesions
TRH	Acromegaly
Opiates	Mixed growth hormone or
Serotoninergic system stimulators	ACTH-PRL secreting adenoma
Amphetamines	Prolactinoma
Hallucinogens	Somatic sources
	Breast augmentation or reduction
	Bronchogenic carcinoma
	Chest wall trauma
	Chronic nipple stimulation
	Cushing's syndrome
	Herpes zoster
	Hypernephroma
	Hypothyroidism
	Pregnancy
	Renal failure
	Upper abdominal surgery

CNS = central nervous system; TRH = thyrotropin-releasing hormone; ACTH-PRL = adrenocorticotropin hormone-prolactin.

may be distressing to a woman and both deserve at least a cursory evaluation. When accompanied by amenorrhea, signs of defeminization, or frank virilization, aggressive and thorough evaluation is required, with referral to a specialist advisable.

Hyperandrogenism may be caused by four main mechanisms (Table 19.4). Increased androgen production by the adrenal gland may signal the presence of a metabolic or enzyme derangement, such as congenital adrenal hyperplasia. Congenital enzyme defects are present in 10% to 15% of hirsute women. These generally follow an autosomal recessive inheritance pattern with a carrier rate of 2% to 6%. For most of these patients, hirsutism dates from puberty and true virilization is rare. With most enzyme defects, menstrual ir-

Table 19.4. Cause of Hyperandrogenism

Altered androgen metabolism (in skin)
    Idiopathic (most common)
Increased androgen production
        Hypersecretion of precursors
        Direct secretion of testosterone
        Conversion of dihydrotestosterone
    Adrenal sources
      Virilizing congenital adrenal hyperplasia
        21-hydroxylase deficiency
        3 β-hydroxysteroid dehydrogenase deficiency
        11 β-hydroxylase deficiency (partial)
      Cushing's syndrome
      Virilizing adrenal tumors (90% benign)
      Hyperprolactinemia
    Ovarian sources
      Polycystic ovary syndrome
      Hyperthecosis
      Virilizing tumors
Decreased sex hormone-binding globulin
Exogenous androgen intake

regularity may or may not be present. These patients are difficult to distinguish clinically from those with polycystic ovary disease (PCOD).

Hirsutism is present in approximately 60% of women with Cushing's disease, whereas amenorrhea occurs in 50% and acne is found in 40% of these patients. The classic findings of truncal obesity, facial rounding, cervicodorsal fat deposition (buffalo hump), and red or purple striae are often not fully developed by the time the patient notes a change in her menstrual pattern. Roughly 60% of these patients have increased secretion of adrenocorticotropin hormone (ACTH) by a pituitary adenoma. The remaining patients have increased ACTH due to ectopic production, such as with oat cell carcinoma of the lung, or an ACTH-independent process, such as an adrenal adenoma.

Patients with ovarian sources of increased androgen will have an ovarian enlargement palpable during pelvic examination between 50% and 90% of the time. Despite the ability of transvaginal ultrasonography and computerized tomography to detect 90% of virilizing tumors, 5% to 10% of tumors may not be detected, necessitating surgical exploration.

The most commonly encountered ovarian abnormality associated with hirsutism is polycystic ovary syndrome. Polycystic ovary syndrome is estimated to account for up to 30% of secondary amenorrhea. Excessive hair growth, primarily along the angle of the jaw, upper lip, and chin, is found in 70% of PCOD patients. Roughly half of these patients are obese and 75% to 80% will be anovulatory. The ovaries of these women are enlarged with a thickened white capsule. The ovaries contain multiple follicles in varying stages of development. The exact pathophysiology of PCOD is not well established, but abnormal secretion of follicle-stimulating hormone (FSH) and luteininzing hormone (LH) during puberty is thought to result in androgen excess. Elevated levels of LH persist and may be used to help establish the diagnosis.

ESTABLISHING THE DIAGNOSIS

The evaluation of both primary and secondary amenorrhea is very similar. This similarity is sufficiently strong that some authors suggest that the distinction is both artificial and archaic. The differences in diagnostic methods usually applied to these two groups is based on the prevalence of possible diagnoses, with the strategies honed to provide the most expeditious evaluation possible. For this reason, there is still merit in discussing the sequence of evaluation in this clinical context.

The evaluation of patients with amenorrhea begins with a history, which will reveal the diagnosis in 85% of patients. The history must explore events and processes present over the months preceding and not just the time of the first missed period. Special attention should be directed toward the patient's family history, her developmental history, the use of drugs, and exposure to chemicals or irradiation. Menstrual abnormalities experienced by other members of the family and the chronology of the individual patient's sexual development milestones are of particular interest. The development of sexual hair or breasts provides an outward sign of androgen and estrogen production, respectively. Information about dietary and exercise habits may impart insight into acquired amenorrhea. Sources of work or family stress should also be sought.

The physical evaluation of amenorrheic patients is directed toward assessing structural normality and detecting the stigmata of endocrine disease. Subtle findings during the physical evaluation can indicate nutritional status, skin pigmentation change, nipple discharge, and altered hair patterns or suggest underlying processes that may be responsible for the patient's absence of menstruation. Even the patient's estrogen status may be grossly estimated by the appearance of the vagina, cervix, and cervical mucous. Care in the evaluation of historical and physical findings often obviates the need for extensive or expensive additional testing.

The diagnosis of physiologic amenorrhea is suggested by history and confirmed by simple investigations, such as pregnancy tests or the measurement of gonadotropins. The latter is especially useful in identifying menopause and prepubertal hypogonadotropic states.

Table 19.5. Anticipated Serum Levels of Gonadotropins in Selected Conditions

	FSH (mlU/mL)	LH (mlU/mL)
Normal adult	5–30	5–20
Ovulatory peak	2 fold increase	3 fold increase
Exogenous estrogen	<10	5–20
Hypogonadotropic	<5	<5
Prepubertal, hypothalamic, and pituitary dysfunction		
Hypergonadotropic		
Postmenopausal, gonadal failure, castrate	>40	>25
Impending menopause	>40	5–20
Pregnancy, trophoblastic disease	5–20	>40
Polycystic ovary syndrome	5–30	>25

FSH = follicle-stimulating hormone; LH = luteinizing hormone.

Measurements of FSH and LH are important in the evaluation of both primary and secondary amenorrhea (Table 19.5).

Primary Amenorrhea

Primary amenorrhea is far less common than are the physiologic and secondary types. The less frequently encountered conditions and syndromes, the possibility of enzyme or chromosomal defects, and the need for more involved testing make the assessment of primary amenorrhea daunting at best. For this reason alone, many primary care providers choose to refer these patients for specialized care. Some preliminary evaluations are within the scope of the primary care setting, especially when collaborative consultation is available.

An overall algorithm for the evaluation of primary amenorrhea is presented in Figure 19.2. This algorithm begins with the assessment of the breasts and whether vaginal and uterine development is normal. Breast development acts as a surrogate indicator of estrogen secretion, whereas uterine development provides a quick way of assessing müllerian anomalies. Based on the results of these evaluations, karyotyping or measuring serum testosterone, prolactin, or FSH may be indicated.

Because roughly one third of patients with primary amenorrhea have a chromosomal abnormality, some authors suggest a different algorithm based on an initial assessment of chromatin (Fig. 19.3). A buccal smear will be positive in genotypic female patients, but negative in those with only one X chromosome or in genotypic males. Results may be mixed when mosaicism is present. Because only about a third of patients with a mosaicism involving a Y chromosome show signs of virilization, a chromosomal analysis should be considered even when the patient is phenotypically normal.

When suspecting a patient of a global delay in puberty, begin the evaluation with a general history, including general health, weight, and height records, and a family history, including the pubertal experience of others in the family. As noted in Chapter 7, Pediatric and Adolescent Care, the physical examination should evaluate the type and degree of sexual development present. Breast development provides an indication of estrogen production, whereas the growth of pubic or axillary hair indicates the presence of androgens. These are useful markers to help direct further evaluations.

Laboratory evaluation of patients with disordered puberty should include serum FSH, LH, and prolactin measurements, skull x-ray study, thyroid function studies, bone age, and chromosomal or cytologic studies. Pelvic ultrasonography or other imaging studies may also be indicated. Because of the significance of disordered puberty, referral for specialized evaluation is required.

Secondary Amenorrhea

As with primary amenorrhea, evaluating secondary amenorrhea can be expedited by using a simple algorithm that may be easily implemented in the primary care setting. Such an algorithm is shown in Figure 19.4. Even when psychosocial or behavior factors are suggestive of the cause, all patients deserve at least a sufficient evaluation to rule out serious disease and confirm hypothalamic-based anovulation.

Because the most common cause of secondary loss of cyclic menstruation is pregnancy, the first step in any evaluation must be to exclude it. Even in patients using reliable contra-

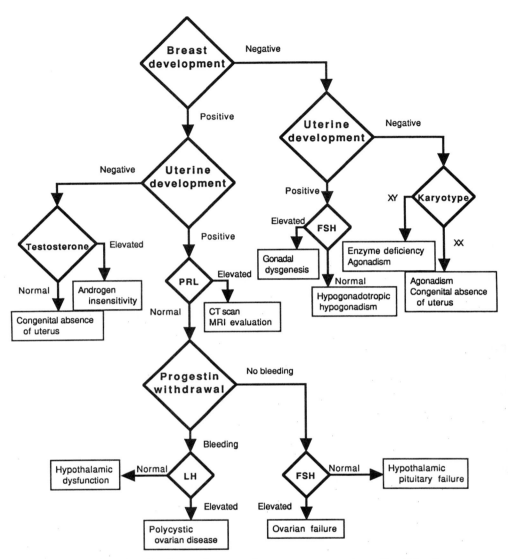

Figure 19.2. An algorithm for the evaluation of primary amenorrhea. Possible diagnoses are shown. Enzyme deficiencies that must be considered include 17 α-hydroxylase, and 17, 20-desmolase. FSH = follicle-stimulating hormone; LH = luteinizing hormone; PRL = prolactin.

ception, including sterilization, this possibility must be considered. Although the diagnosis may be suggested by secondary symptoms of breast fullness, weight gain, nausea, or fatigue, a urine or serum pregnancy test should be performed. Not only will this eliminate a large proportion of patients with physiologic amenorrhea and allay the patient's concerns, it also avoids unnecessary testing and exposure of the conceptus to hormonal manipulations or imaging.

Once the possibility of an ongoing pregnancy has been eliminated, a progesterone challenge may be used to assess the level of endogenous estrogen and the competence of the genital tract. This is carried out by prescribing a pure progesterone, such as medroxyproges-

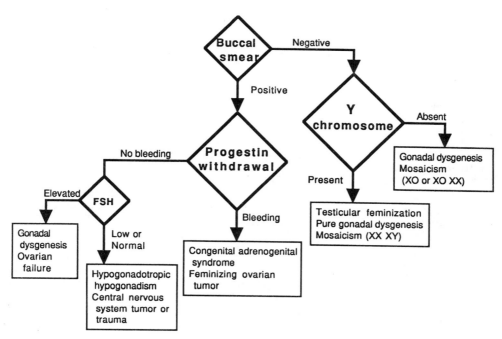

Figure 19.3. Evaluation of primary amenorrhea based on chromosome analysis. A buccal smear or chromatin analysis may be used initially to separate causes of primary amenorrhea. If this is negative, the presence of a Y chromosome must be sought by quinacrine mustard staining, immunologic detection of the H-Y antigen, or other method. It should be noted that in pure gonadal dysgenesis and XX/YY mosaicism, a uterus is present. FSH = follicle-stimulating hormone.

terone acetate (10 mg, orally) for 5 days. Within 2 to 7 days after the last dose, bleeding should take place. Any bleeding beyond a few spots supports a diagnosis of anovulation. This bleeding also demonstrates estrogen priming of an intact and responsive endometrium and a normal outflow tract. Because estrogen levels may be inferred to be normal, by extension, this bleeding also indicates that the ovaries, pituitary, and central nervous systems are at least minimally functional. In the absence of reasons to believe thyroid function or prolactin levels are abnormal, no further evaluation is required and the issue of management may be addressed. An exception to this general rule is the patient with anovulation associated with hirsutism or virilization who must be evaluated for the possibility of a hyperandrogenic state.

If the patient fails to have withdrawal bleeding after a progesterone challenge, the possibility of damage to the uterine lining must be considered. This may take the form of intrauterine synechia (Asherman's syndrome), infection (e.g., tuberculosis or schistosomiasis), or irradiation. The diagnosis of intrauterine synechia is made based on the history of an immediately preceding intrauterine procedure, usually a dilatation and curettage, and confirmed by hysteroscopy or hysterosalpingography. Patients with endometrial damage will fail to have withdrawal bleeding with either progesterone or estrogen plus progesterone hormonal challenges. Combined estrogen and progesterone withdrawal testing is done by prescribing estrogen, at a dose comparable to 1.25 mg of conjugated estrogen or 0.1 μg of transdermal estrogen, given for 21 to 30 days, with medroxyprogesterone acetate (10 mg/d)

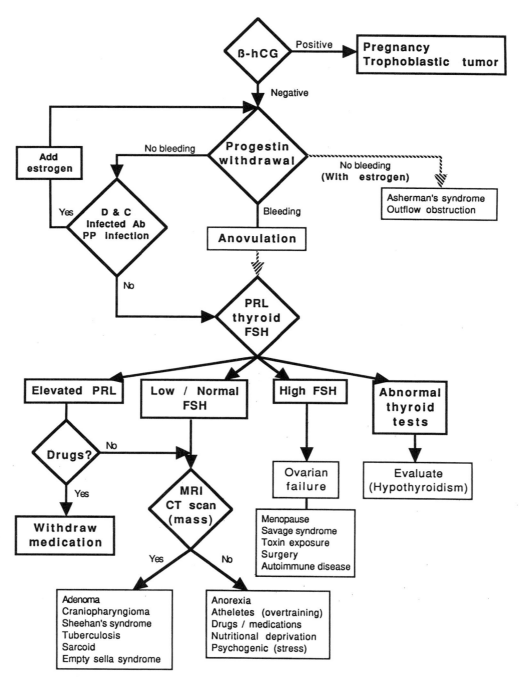

Figure 19.4. An algorithm for the evaluation of secondary amenorrhea. Pathways shown in dashed arrows are conditional or optional; interventions are in bold boxes. In some centers, MRI has replaced CT as the procedure of choice for detecting pituitary and hypothalamic lesions.β-HCG = human chorionic gonadotrophin; CT = computed tomography; FSH = follicle-stimulating hormone; LH = luteinizing hormone; PRL = prolactin; PP = postpartum; CNS = central nervous system; D & C = dilatation and curretage.

added for the last 5 to 10 days of treatment. If withdrawal bleeding is not forthcoming, a second 1-month trial of the same therapy is justified before drawing any conclusions.

For most patients, the combined estrogen-progestin challenge will be unnecessary. When the patient's physical examination is normal and there is no history of trauma or instrumentation, abnormalities of the endometrium and outflow tract are unlikely.

Galactorrhea

The evaluation of patients with galactorrhea is independent of menstrual history (Fig. 19.5). Although less than 5% of patients with galactorrhea, with or without amenorrhea,

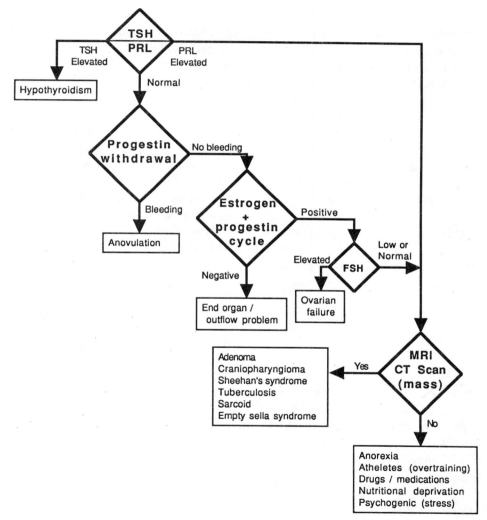

Figure 19.5. An algorithm for the evaluation of galactorrhea with amenorrhea. Patients with amenorrhea and galactorrhea are evaluated with a slightly different approach than that used for patients with secondary amenorrhea and no breast symptoms. FSH = follicle-stimulating hormone; TSH = thyroid-stimulating hormone; PRL = prolactin; CT = computed tomography; MRI = magnetic resonance imaging.

have hypothyroidism that is not clinically apparent, TSH measurement is reasonable. Because of the ease of testing, the significance of hypothyroidism, and the ready reversal of the symptoms, TSH testing is warranted in the early phases of the clinical evaluation.

When significant elevations in prolactin levels are found, radiologic evaluation of the pituitary is necessary to search for prolactin-secreting tumors. In the past this was accomplished by coned down lateral views of the sella turcica. While still valuable, this has been replaced in many centers by computed tomography or magnetic resonance imaging. When a pituitary lesion is suspected, consultation with imaging specialists is recommended to determine the best evaluation modality.

Virilization and Hirsutism

Whenever there is a question of excessive hair growth, loss of femininity, or frank virilization, care must be taken to seek subtle signs of adrenal or other endocrine abnormalities. A careful family history and chronology of the current concern are important in assessing familial hypertrichosis. A rapid onset of symptoms suggests diseases such as ectopic production of ACTH, whereas a slow or stable process may be due to familial, racial, or ethnic propensities. The presence of galactorrhea, amenorrhea, or the recent onset of symptoms suggestive of diabetes or thyroid failure should also be sought. Check for signs of virilization, the stigmata of Cushing's syndrome, or a pelvic mass in the physical examination.

A good indication of virilization is the clitoral index. This is defined as the vertical dimension times the horizontal dimension, in millimeters. The normal range is from 9 to 35 mm, with borderline values in the range of 36 to 99 mm. Values above 100 mm indicate severe hyperandrogenicity and should prompt aggressive evaluation and referral.

Patients suspected of having adrenal sources of hyperandrogenicity can be screened by measuring 24-hour urinary-free cortisol or by ACTH stimulation tests or an overnight dexamethasone suppression test. Measurement of other hormone levels may be advisable, based on consultation with specialists.

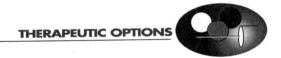

THERAPEUTIC OPTIONS

Treatment of amenorrhea is predicated on first establishing a cause, then determining the patient's need for therapy. It should be kept in mind that amenorrhea, in and of itself, is not an indication for therapy. Once the cause is determined, specific therapies are often highly successful in restoring menstruation, if not fertility, although this is dependent on the source; hypothalamic and pituitary dysfunction may be successfully treated whereas ovarian failure is usually irreversible.

Primary Amenorrhea

Of patients with primary amenorrhea, only about 20% have treatable conditions. Although this number is small, the benefits of early diagnosis and therapy are great.

Patients with hypogonadotropic hypogonadism causing their amenorrhea can be successfully treated with hormonal therapy. For patients with pubertal delay, this will initiate and sustain the development of normal secondary sex characteristics, allow for normal height, and encourage bone mass deposition. Adolescents are much more sensitive to the effects of estrogen than are postmenopausal women, allowing doses in the range of 0.3 mg of conjugated estrogen, 0.5 mg estradiol, or their equivalent, daily. After 6 to 12 months of therapy at this level, the dose should be doubled and a progestin (e.g., medroxyprogesterone acetate, 10 mg for the first 12 days of the month) added. This generally results in regular menstruation and normal pubertal development proceeds on its own when the patient reaches a bone age of 13. Because ovulation may occur during these therapies, contraception must be discussed and provided as appropriate.

The timing of gonadal removal in patients with a Y chromosome is controversial. Some authors advocate removal as soon as the diagnosis is made, whereas others suggest delaying removal until pubertal changes are complete. Surgical management should be individualized and carried out in conjunction with consultants. Progestin replacement is not required for these patients.

Secondary Amenorrhea

Patients who experience physiologic amenorrhea generally require no intervention except reassurance and whatever normal management is appropriate to the process, such as prenatal care or consideration of postmenopausal hormonal replacement. When the loss of menstruation falls outside the normal parameters of physiologic loss (e.g., premature menopause), it should be investigated and treated in the same way as any other case of secondary amenorrhea.

The management of anovulatory patients is based on their reproductive desires. Those who are ready to pursue a pregnancy will require ovulation induction, usually with clomiphene citrate administered by a specialist. Those who do not wish pregnancy, should receive periodic progestin therapy, such as medroxyprogesterone acetate (10 mg/d for 10 to 12 days) each month. This is aimed at providing progestin withdrawal and endometrial slough, to protect from endometrial hyperplasia induced by unopposed estrogen. This periodic progestin challenge also allows recurring assessment of the original diagnosis. If the patient fails to have withdrawal bleeding, a re-evaluation, done in the same manner as the initial scheme, must be implemented. There is limited research that suggests that this periodic exposure to progestin may also provide some decrease in the overall risk of breast cancer, when compared with women who have prolonged unopposed estrogen. Some authors suggest that this periodic estrogen/progestin therapy may be given every 2 to 3 months, rather than monthly. This may be more acceptable to some patients, but has been less well studied.

Patients with behaviorally-based hypothalamic amenorrhea, such as competitive runners or anorectics, almost always respond by reversing the patterns responsible. Until cyclic ovarian function is restored, periodic estrogen and progestin therapy may be necessary, as well as calcium supplementation to provide additional prophylaxis for osteoporosis. If avoidance of withdrawal bleeding is a significant goal, these patients can be placed on continuous estrogen and progestin therapy, such as 0.625 mg conjugated estrogen or its equivalent, and 2.5 mg medroxyprogesterone acetate.

Patients with intrauterine scarring require surgical therapy. The endometrial cavity must be opened, usually through dilatation and curettage or hysteroscopy, and the endometrial lining regenerated. Estrogen therapy is given to promote endometrial regrowth and an intrauterine contraceptive devise or Foley catheter is generally inserted to help hold the uterine walls apart while this regrowth takes place. This is type of intervention is not suitable for the primary care office setting and referral is required. A 90% success rate for hysteroscopic adhesiolysis is reported, including a 35% fertility rate, with 80% of these women carrying the pregnancy to term.

Galactorrhea

When prolactin levels are low and the coned-down view of the sella turcica is normal, observation alone may be sufficient; if so, periodic re-evaluation is required to check for the emergence of slow-growing tumors. When prolactin levels are elevated, but not excessive (PRL < 100 ng/mL), medical therapy with bromocriptine and periodic reassessment may be appropriate. Treatment with bromocriptine is recommended for patients who desire pregnancy, those with distressing degrees of galactorrhea, or to suppress intermediate sized pituitary tumors. Bromocriptine will reduce PRL levels and restore menstruation in 80% to 90% of patients. There is no evidence that long-term bromocriptine therapy permanently suppresses elevations of PRL or eliminates small tumors. Rapidly growing tumors, tumors that are large at the time of discovery, or those that do not respond to bromocriptine therapy may have to be treated surgically. When imaging shows a pituitary abnormality or prolactin level is greater than 100 ng/mL, referral to an endocrine specialist is recommended.

Virilization and Hirsutism

Patients with adrenal hyperandrogenicity will respond well to cortisol administration, which reduces the production of androgenic precursors. The treatment of Cushing's disease depends on the form of the disorder and is beyond the scope of this discussion.

Patients with polycystic ovary disease often do well on oral contraceptive suppression of ovarian function or use of spironolactone (100 to 200 mg/d). Because spironolactone is teratogenic, patients who use it and are at risk for pregnancy must use reliable contraception. Weight loss is often associated with an improvement in symptoms and a return of menstrual function in patients with polycystic ovary disease. Other therapies, including gonadtropin-releasing hormone (GnRH) analogs and clomiphene citrate can be used, but cost and other considerations suggest that these are best reserved for a limited number of patients who fall outside the primary care setting.

Suppressive therapies will reduce the growth of new hair, but once a hair follicle is induced, or turned on, it will continue to grow. For this reason, shaving, depilatories, or electrolysis may be required. These will only be satisfactory if combined with other therapies to reduce growth.

HINTS AND COMMON QUESTIONS

Amenorrhea should not be confused with oligomenorrhea (menses occurring with an interval of between 40 and 180 days) and hypomenorrhea (defined as a reduction in the number of days of flow, regardless of menstrual interval).

During the first several years after menarche, it is not uncommon for a girl to skip menstrual periods. This is found in up to 20% of girls and may last for 2 to 12 months without adverse consequences.

Because of a high prevalence of chromosomal abnormalities, patients with primary amenorrhea and short stature should have a karyotype performed early in their evaluation.

When prescribing progestins to induce withdrawal bleeding, an agent with purely progestational effects should be used. Agents used in oral contraception, including oral contraceptive formulations themselves, should not be used because of their potentially confounding estrogen effects that could lead to incorrect clinical impressions.

If the patient fails to have withdrawal bleeding after a progesterone challenge, in addition to problems with the outflow system, consider the possibility of noncompliance or inadequate therapy based on body habitus (obesity).

It is important to recognize that cyclic progesterone therapy is insufficient to provide contraception and adequate protection from pregnancy must be addressed.

If hyperandrogenism is detected in the process of evaluating amenorrhea, adrenal function should be carefully checked.

Because menopause is unusual prior to age 30, any patient below this age who has high gonadotropin levels should be evaluated for the possibility of a chromosomal mosaicism.

When premature ovarian failure occurs, the possibility of an autoimmune disease must be considered. Between 30% and 50% of these patient will have circulating antibodies present. This autoimmunity is most commonly manifested by abnormal thyroid function, which is easily detected by thyroid testing. These patients also require annual surveillance for the possible emergence of a generalized autoimmune reaction. Assessment of TSH, morning cortisol, serum calcium, phosphorous, and glucose should be considered.

FSH is a more sensitive marker than LH for impending or current ovarian failure. Both FSH and LH will be elevated if, by chance, the sample is drawn during the midcycle surge. If this is the case, menstruation or pregnancy should be detected within 3 weeks of the time the sample was drawn.

Only about a third of patients with elevated prolactin levels are amenorrheic. This may be owing to the hypoestrogenic state that often is found when prolactin is elevated or to other factors.

Patients suspected of having Kallmann's syndrome (hypogonadotropic hypogonadism associated with anosmia) can be identified by their inability to recognize common odors. Clinically, the most readily available odors used to challenge olfactory function include alcohol skin preparation pads, coffee, or breath mints. These karyotypic females are distinctive for their primary amenorrhea, infantile sexual development, low gonadotropins, and anosmia.

If gonadotropins are to be assayed as a part of the evaluation of a patient with amenorrhea, at least 2 weeks must elapse following any steroid given for diagnosis or therapy.

The measurement of blood or urinary estrogen has little clinical value in quantifying endogenous estrogen production. Similarly, a single measurement of a specific estrogen does not provide clinically useful information.

Amenorrhea that follows the use of hormonal contraception, the so-called "postpill amenorrhea," is not causally related to the use of these agents. Studies indicated that the relationship is temporal and coincidental, not causal. As a result, patients who experience this type of amenorrhea must be evaluated in the same manner as any amenorrhea patient.

The possibility of iatrogenic hirsutism should not be overlooked. Patients may use steroids for a number of reasons, legal and otherwise, and may not recognize the possibility of virilizing side effects. The use of danazol sodium, as in endometriosis therapy, may be associated with increased hair growth as well.

There is no evidence that cyclic administration of progestins, the use of oral contraceptive agents to regulate periods, or ovulation induction results in the long-term return of normal ovulatory function if it is currently absent. Prolonged use of these modalities may exacerbate suppression of the hypothalamic-pituitary-ovarian axis, further aggravating the problem.

Anovulation and amenorrhea are not contraindications to the use of low-dose oral contraceptives, either for contraception or for the protection of the endometrium through a return of regular menstruation.

The only reason to attempt ovulation induction in anovulatory patients is to achieve pregnancy. Unless the patient is actively pursuing a pregnancy, it should not be undertaken.

SUGGESTED READINGS

General References

Bachmann GA, Kemmann E. Prevalence of oligomenorrhea and amenorrhea in a college population. Am J Obstet Gynecol 1982;144:98.

Brenner S, Lessing J, Quagliarello J, et al. Hyperprolactinemia and assoicated piruitary prolactinomas. Obstet Gynecol 1985;65:661.

Buttram VC JR, Bibbons WE. Mülllerian anomialies: a proposed classification (an analysis of 144 cases). Fertil Steril 1979;32:40.

Drew FL. The epidemiology of secondary amenorrhea. Journal of Chronic Disease 1961;14:396.

Jaffe SB, Loucopoulos A, Jewelewicz R. Cytogenetics of müllerian agenesis. J Reprod Med 1992;13:242.

L'hermite M, Caufriez A, Vekemans M, et al. Pharmacological and pathological aspects of human prolactin secretion. Progress in Reproductive Biology 1977;2:244.

Liu JH. Hypothalamic amenorrhea: clinical perspectives, pathophysiology, and management. Am J Obstet Gynecol 1990;163:1732.

Maxson WS, Wentz AC. The gonadotropin resistant ovary syndrome. Semin Reprod Endocrinol 1983;1:2.

McDonough PG, Byrd JR. Gonadal dysgenesis. Clin Obstet Gynecol 1977;20:565.

Pettersson F, Fries H, Nillius SJ. Epidemiology of secondary amenorrhea. I. Incidence and prevalence rates. Am J Obstet Gynecol 1973;117:80.

Reindollar RH, Novak M, Thomas SPT, McDonough PG. Adult-onset amenorrhea: a study of 262 patients. Am J Obstet Gynecol 1986;155:531.

Singh KB. Menstrual disorders in college students. Am J Obstet Gynecol 1981;140:299.

Soules MR. Adolescent amenorrhea. Pediatr Clin North Am 1987;34:1083.

Speroff L. Amenorrhea. In Glass RH (ed)., Office Gynecology, 4th ed. Baltimore: Williams & Wilkins, 1992, p 263.

Yen SSC. Prolactin in human reporduction. In Yen SSC, Jaffe RB (eds). Reproductive Endocrinology, 3rd ed. Philadelphia: WB Saunders 1991, p 357.

Specific References

Effects of Exercise

Baker ER. Menstrual dysfunction and hormonal status in athletic women. Fertil Steril 1981;36:691.

Bullen B, Skrinar G, Beitins I, et al. Induction of menstrual disorders by strenuous exercise in untrained women. N Engl J Med 1985;312:1349.

Cumming D, Vickovic M, Wall S, et al. Defects in pulsatile LH release in normally menstruating runners. J Clin Endocrinol Metab 1985;60:810.

DeSouza MJ, Metzger DA. Reproductive dysfunction in amenorrheic athletes and anorexic patients: a review. Med Sci Sports Exerc 1991;23:995.

Drinkwater BL, Nilson K, Ott S, Chestnut CH. Bone mineral density after resumption of menses in amenorrheic athletes. JAMA 1986;256:380.

Frisch RE. Body fat, menarche, and reproductive ability. Semin Reprod Endocrinol 1985;3:45.

Hale RW. Exercise, sports, and menstrual dysfunciton. Clin Obstet Gynecol 1983;26:728.

Henley K, Vaitukaitis JL. Exercise-induced menstrual dysfunction. Ann Rev Med 1988;39:443.

Loucks AB, Vaitukaitis J, Cameron JL, et al. The reproductuive system and exercise in women. Med Sci Sports Exerc 1992;24:S288.

Marcus R, Cann C, Madvig P, et al. Menstrual function and bone mass in elite women distance runners: endocrine and metabolic features. Ann Intern Med 1985;102:158.

Prior JC. Luteal phase defects and anovulation: adaptive alterations occurring with conditioning exercise. Semin Reprod Endocrinol 1985;3:27.

Rivier C, Revier J, Vale W. Stress-induced inhibition of reproductive functions: role of endogenous corticotropin-releasing factor. Science 1986;231:607.

Russel JV, Mitchell D, Musey PI, Collins DC. The relationship of exercise to anovulatory cycles in female athletes: hormonal and physical characteristics. Obstet Gynecol 1984;63:452.

Samuels MH, Sanborn CF, Hofeldt R, et al. The role of endogenous opiates in athletic amenorrhea. Fertil Steril 1991;55:507.

Sanborn CF, Albrecht BH, Wagner WW JR. Athletic amenorrhea: Lack of association with body fat. Med Sci Sports Exerc 1987;19:207.

Sforzo GA. Opioids and exercise: an update. Sports Med 1988;7:109.

Shangold M. Exercise and amenorrhea. Semin Reprod Endocrinol 1985;3:35.

Shangold M, Rebar RW, Wentz AC, Schiff I. Evaluation and management of menstrual dysfunction in athletes. JAMA 1990;263:165.

Skonich AA. Medical news and perspective: the female athlete triad, risk for women. JAMA 1993;270:8.

Warren WP. The effect of exercise on pubertal progression and reproductive function in girls. J Clin Endocrinol Metab 1980;51:1150.

Wentz AC. Body weight and amenorrhea. Obstet Gynecol 1980;56:482.

Galactorrhea

Chang RJ, Keye WR, Young JR, et al. Detection, evaluation, and treatment of pituitary microadnomas in patients with galactorrhea and amenorrhea. Am J Obstet Gynecol 1977;128:356.

Reinche M, Allolio B, Saeger W, Menzel J, Winkelmann W. The "incidentaloma" of the pituitary gland. JAMA 1990;263:2772.

Schlechte J, Dolan K, Sherman B, Chapler F, Luciano A. The natural history of untreated hyperprolactinemia: a prospective analysis. J Clin Endocrinol Metab 1989;68:412.

Stein Al, Levenick MN, Kletzky OA. Computed tomography versus magnetic resonance imaging for the evaluation of suspected pituitary adenomas. Obstet Gynecol 1989;73:996.

Teasdale E, Teasdale G, Mohsen F, MacPherson P. High-resolution computed tomography in pituitary microadenoma: Is seeing believing? Clin Radiol 1986;37:227.

Virilization and Hirsutism

Carr BR, Breslau NA, Givens C, Byrd W, Barnett-Hamm C, Marshburn PB. Oral contraceptive pills, gonadotropin-releasing hormone agonist, or use in combinations for treatment of hirsutism: a clinical research center study. J Clin Endocrinol Metab 1995;80:1169.

Fruzzetti F, De Lorenzo D, Parrini D, Ricci C. Effects of Finasteride, a 5 α-reductase inhibitor, on circulating androgens and gonadotropin secretion in hirsuite women. J Clin Endocrinol Metab 1994;79:831.

Hall JE. Polycustic ovarian disease as a neuroendocrine disorder of the female reproductive axis. Endocrinol Metab Clin North Am 1993;22:75.

Rittmaster RS, Loriaux DL. Hirsuitism. Ann Int Med 1987;106:95.

Tagitz GE, Kopher RA, Nagel TC, Okagaki T. The clitoral index: a bioassay of androgenic stimulation. Obstet Gyencol 1979;54:562.

Other

Akinkuge A. Vaginal atresia and cryptomenorrhea. Obstet Gynecol 1975;46:317.

Alpert MM, Garner PR. Premature ovarian failure: Its relationship to autoimmune disease. Obstet Gynecol 1985;66:27.

Cann CE, Martin MC, Genant HK, Jaffe RB. Decreased spinal mineral content in amenorrheic women. JAMA 1984;251:626.

Coulam CB, Adamson SC, Annegers JF. Incidence of premature ovarian failure. Obstet Gynecol 1986;67:604.

Coulam CB, Annegers JF, Kraz JS. Chronic anovulation syndrome and associated neoplasia. Obstet Gynecol 1983; 61:403.

Diaz S, Cardenas H, Brardeis A. Early difference in the endocrine profile of long and short lactational amenorrhea. J Clin Endocrinol Metab 1989;72:196.

Fedele L, Ferrazzi E, Dorta M, Vercillini P, Candiani GB. Ulatrasonography in the differential diagnosis of "double" uteri. Fertil Steril 1988;50:361.

Fedele L, Dorta M, Brioschi D, Giudici MN, Candiani GB. Magnetic resonance imaging in Mayer-Rokitansky-Hauser Syndrome. Obstet Gynecol 1990;76:593.

Fore SR, Hammond CB, Parker RT, et al. Urologic and genital anomalies in patients with congenital absence of vagina. Obstet Gynecol 1975;46:410.

Griffin JE, Edwards C, Maddden JD, et al. Congenital absence of the vagina: Mayer-Rokitansky-Kuster-Hauser syndrome. Ann Intern Med 1976;85:224.

Jacobs H, Knuth U, Hull M, et al. Post-"pill" amenorrhea: cause or coincidence? BMJ 1977;2:940.

Johnston CC, Miller JZ, Slemenda CW, et al. Calcium supplementation and increases in bone mineral density in children. N Engl J Med 1992;327:82.

March CM, Israel R, March AD. Hysteroscopic management of intrauterine adhesions. Am J Obstet Gynecol 1978;130:653.

Morris JM. The syndrome of testicular feminization in male pseudohermaphrodites. Am J Obstet Gynecol 1953;65:1192.

Niver DH, Barrette G, Jewelewicz R. Congenital atresia of the uterine cervix and vagina: three cases. Fertil Steril 1980;33:25.

Rebar RW, Connolly HV. Clinical features of young women with hypergonadotropic amenorrhea. Fertil Steril 1990;53:804.

Short RV, Lewis PR, Renfree MB, et al. Contraceptive effects of extended lactational amenorrhoea: beyond the Bellagio Consensus. Lancet 1991;337:715.

Warren MP, Vande Wiele RL. Clinical and metabolic features of anorexia nervosa. Am J Obstet Gynecol 1973; 117:435.

White CM, Hergenroeder AC, Klish WJ. Bone mineral density in eumenorrheic and amenorrheic, 15–21 year old females. Am J Dis Child 1992;146:31.

20

Premenstrual Syndrome

Although interest in perimenstrual syndromes seems recent, descriptions of these sufferings date back further than many would imagine. In 1835, Prichard wrote: "Some females, at the period of catamenia, undergo a considerable degree of nervous excitement: morbid dispositions of mind are displayed by them at these times, a wayward and capricious temper, excitability in the feelings, moroseness in disposition, a proneness to quarrel with their dearest relatives, and sometimes a dejection of mind approaching to melancholia." The essential character of the syndrome was published in 1931, by Frank, who described it as a severe syndrome of "indescribable tension and irritability from ten to seven days preceding menstruation which, in most instances, continues until the time that the menstrual flow occurs." The term "premenstrual tension," encompassing the triad of depression, irritability, and lethargy, was changed to "premenstrual syndrome" in 1953, by Green and Dalton.

Despite the universality of experience, significance of the distress, number of years being the focus of medical interest, and vast literature, premenstrual syndromes remain poorly understood, plagued by skepticism and controversy. In the absence of a solid physiologic understanding, cynicism about the existence of the condition, evangelism over causes and cures, exploitation of frustrated patients, and anger over the lack of significant progress in diagnosis and treatment have all flourished. Answers are emerging, however, that allow the primary care team to establish the diagnosis and institute effective therapy with a reasonable certainty of success.

BACKGROUND AND SCIENCE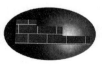

The classification of menstrually related phenomena may be conceptionalized as shown in Figure 20.1. Although all menstrually related occurrences can be broadly classified as being

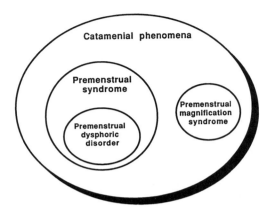

Figure 20.1. Summary of menstrually related diagnoses. All menstrually related diagnoses fall into the broad classification of "catamenial" phenomena. Within this grouping are the premenstrual syndromes (PMS, PMDD, and PMM). (Areas shown do not reflect the relative frequency of occurrence.)

"catamenial," this term is generally reserved for specific, single entity pathologies such as recurrent headaches (catamenial migraine) or menstrually related recurrent pneumothorax. Women who experience mild cyclic physical or emotional symptoms also fall into this group, although the label is seldom applied to these patients. Under the umbrella of catamenial processes are the premenstrual syndromes and premenstrual magnification.

Premenstrual syndromes encompass both the physiologic and emotional complaints known by the familiar "PMS," and the predominantly psychological symptoms of premenstrual dysphoric disorders (PMDD) as defined by the American Psychiatry Association. Patients in these two groups experience absence of symptoms during the follicular phase of the menstrual cycle. Patients with premenstrual magnification (PMM) experience variable symptoms that persist throughout the cycle, but undergo significant worsening just prior to menses. Even these distinctions are somewhat artificial; all of these conditions can occur in women who have undergone hysterectomy without oophorectomy, making the term "premenstrual" meaningless.

The prevalence and impact of premenstrual syndromes varies widely with age and other factors, making generalizations difficult. Although premenstrual distress can occur during any part of a woman's reproductive life, it appears most commonly to women in their 30s and 40s. It is estimated that between 25% and 85% of reproductive age women experience some reproducible changes tied to the premenstrual or menstrual phase of their cycles. Approximations of the proportion of women who experience significant work or lifestyle disruption are harder to establish with certainty, but range from 2% to 15% (Fig. 20.2). Most authors currently agree that only 2% to 5% of reproductive age women meet the strict criteria for the diagnosis of PMS or PMDD. When mood symptoms predominate, 60% of patients have a PMM pattern rather than PMDD.

The physiologic basis of PMS, PMDD, and PMM have yet to be established. Many different causes for these disorders have been proposed, often with evangelistic zeal, but objective studies have failed to show evidence for any consistent causation or differences between those with the condition and those without (Table 20.1). Even the existence of a physiologic cause has been called into question. Research in which the investigators convinced study subjects that they were in the premenstrual phase of their menstrual cycle found a worsening of symptoms, even when the patients were actually in the follicular phase. Studies of this type suggest that an element of anticipation, social conditioning, or expectation may also be present.

The linkage between the patient's symptoms and the regular occurrence of menstruation immediately suggests a causal relationship with ovarian steroid production (Table 20.2). Widely suggested is the possibility of over or under production of one or more ovarian hormones, although no change has even been documented and therapies based on these assumed abnormalities have generally not withstood scientific evaluation. Indeed, in studies where men-

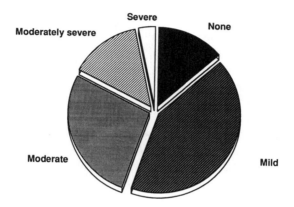

Figure 20.2. Relative severity of premenstrual symptoms. In a study of a nonclinic population, over 15% of women had moderately severe or severe premenstrual symptoms. (After: Johnson SR, McChesney C, Bean J. Epidemiology of premenstrual symptoms in a nonclinical sample. J Reprod Med 1984;33:340.)

Table 20.1. Biologic Theories (not proved) of Premenstrual Syndrome

Altered aldosterone
Altered mineral levels (magnesium, zinc)
Altered testosterone
Central changes in catecholamines
Changes in estrogen:progesterone ratios
Elevated monoamine oxidase (MAO)
Endogenous endorphin withdrawal
Endometrial infection
Excess prolactin secretion
Falling estrogen levels
High estrogen levels
Increased adrenal activity
Increased aldosterone activity
Increased renin-angiotensin activity
Low progesterone levels
Response to prostaglandins
Steroid allergy
Subclinical hypoglycemia
Vitamin deficiencies (A, B_6, E, thiamin)

Table 20.2. Evidence Linking Premenstrual Syndrome and Cyclic Ovarian Function

- Premenstrual syndrome is not present in prepubertal, postmenopausal (surgical, medical, or natural), anovulatory, ovulation suppressed, or pregnant women
- Premenstrual syndrome does not occur in women with hypothalamic hypogonadism
- Cyclic estrogen-progestin replacement therapy can cause symptoms that mimic premenstrual syndrome
- Cyclic oral contraceptives are more likely to cause premenstrual syndrome than are monophasic products
- Some animals (Rhesus monkey) demonstrate similar cyclic changes linked to ovarian cycles

strual bleeding was induced at various points during the ovarian cycle, no effect on the timing or severity of PMS symptoms could be identified, further confounding perception of the underlying pathophysiology. It is clear, however, that steroid hormones can have both direct and indirect impact on central nervous system functions, including behavior, mood, and cognitive function. It is still probable that normal physiologic variations in hormone levels over the menstrual cycle set the stage for other, yet undefined, mechanisms to be set in motion.

The most promising research into a cause of PMS has been in the areas of β-endorphins and serotonin. Studies of β-endorphins suggest that women with PMS have a decrease in peripheral levels during the luteal phase compared with controls. This difference is not found in studies of cerebrospinal fluid, however. Serotonin plays a key role in integrative functions, behavior, appetite, temperature control, and hormone release. Some studies have suggested lower serum levels and an abnormal uptake of serotonin during the luteal phase in women with PMS. This evidence, along with the therapeutic success of serotoninergic agents, suggests a major role for serotonin in PMS. The high degree of symptom variability and the contradictory findings of those who have attempted to find a hormonal cause, present the possibility of a mixed etiology: Those with somatic symptoms may have hormonally mediated mechanisms, whereas those with emotional symptoms may experience more involvement of neurotransmitters. Both mechanisms may have some role for most patients.

In the absence of physiologic markers and with almost 200 symptoms associated with these complaints, all premenstrually related syndromes must be defined in an operative manner. The broadest definition thus becomes: The periodic recurrence in the luteal phase of the ovarian cycle of a combination of distressing physical, psychological, and behavioral changes of sufficient severity to result in interference in normal daily activities or relationships. In 1987, the American Psychiatric Association (APA) attempted to formalize the diagnosis of premenstrual syndromes by its incorporation into the Diagnostic and Statistical Manual-III. Because of the way this was listed in that manual, many presumed that it implied a psychogenic cause or "mental disorder." Special interest groups objected and the term was modified to "Late Luteal Phase Dysphoric Disorder (LLPDD)," and relegated to an appendix. In the fourth edition, this has been further modified to become "Premenstrual Dysphoric Disorder (PMDD)" and is listed with mood disorders under the category of "depression, not otherwise specified." The criteria for establishing the diagnosis of PMDD are shown in Table 20.3. The National Institute of Mental Health has added their own operational definition, which requires a 30% increase in the severity of symptoms during the 5 days prior to menses compared with the 5 days following menstruation. This standard has been most useful in defining premenstrual magnification syndromes.

Table 20.3. Diagnostic Criteria for Premenstrual Dysphoric Disorder

All of the following
    Symptoms NOT an exacerbation of another underlying psychiatric disorder
    Symptoms clustered in luteal phase; absent within first few days of the follicular phase
    Symptoms cause significant disability
Plus, five or more of the following
    At least one
      Marked affective lability
      Marked anxiety, tension, feelings of being "keyed up" or "on edge"
      Markedly depressed mood, feelings of hopelessness, or self-deprecating thoughts
      Persistent and marked anger or irritability
    One or more of the following:
      Avoidance of social activities
      Decreased interest in usual activities
      Decreased productivity and efficiency
      Increased sensitivity to rejection
      Interpersonal conflicts
      Lethargy, easy fatigability, lack of energy
      Marked change in appetite, cravings
      Physical symptoms (reproducible pattern of complaints)
      Sleep disturbances (hypersomnia, insomnia)
      Subjective sense of being "out of control"
      Subjective sense of being overwhelmed
      Subjective sense of difficulty in concentration

Modified from: Reid RL, Yen SSC. Premenstrual syndrome. Am J Obstet Gynecol 1981;139:85.

It should be apparent from these definitions that the character of the patient's symptoms is less important than is the temporal relationship to cyclic ovarian function. It is this pattern of premenstrual worsening, with absence or improvment in postmenstrual phase, that is required to establish the diagnosis (Fig. 20.3).

ESTABLISHING THE DIAGNOSIS

Cultural expectations, memory inaccuracies, and a desire to substantiate the patient's own perception of her condition, all result in inaccurate and frequently misleading, retrospective reporting of symptoms. Research has shown that up to 80% of patients who present with self-diagnosed PMS fail to meet strict criteria for this diagnosis. Most will be determined to have other conditions that range from mood disorders to physical conditions, such as irritable bowel disease or endometriosis. This observation makes it imperative that no therapy be instituted until the diagnosis can be firmly established.

Although the diagnosis of PMS should be seen as one of exclusion, there are several steps that can establish the diagnosis in a positive manner. The diagnosis and treatment of any menstrually related complaint must begin with a general history and physical examination (Fig. 20.4). These are directed toward the detection of conditions that may have a cyclic character and thus mimic premenstrual syndromes. These range from endometriosis

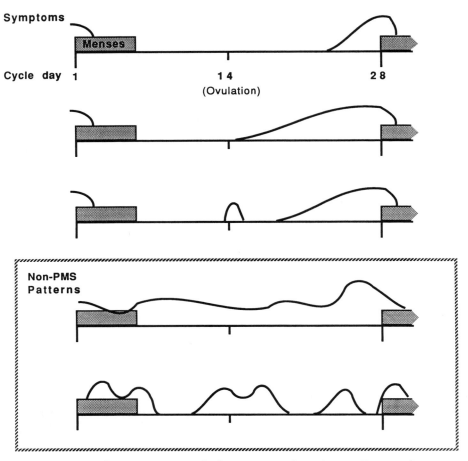

Figure 20.3. Patterns of symptoms typical of premenstrual syndrome. To meet the criteria of PMS, symptoms must be present only in the luteal phase and disappear completely during the follicular portion of the menstrual cycle. The character of the symptoms is not important; only the timing of their appearance. Symptoms that are present at all times but worsen prior to menses or those that appear at irregular intervals do not meet the criteria for PMS.

and irritable bowel syndrome to hypothyroidism and climacteric hormonal changes (Table 20.4). Psychosocial and family stresses, depression, mood and personality disorders must also be evaluated. As noted, a high percentage of patients with self-diagnosed PMS will prove to have one or more identifiable physical or emotional conditions that may be addressed specifically, and do not constitute a premenstrual-type disorder.

Many authors suggest augmenting the usual office-style history with structured questionnaires or tests. A number of such tools have been published, the most popular of which are Moos' Menstrual Distress Questionnaire (MMDQ), Patient Report of Increased Symptoms with Menses (PRISM), Endicott Symptom Checklist, Minnesota Multiphasic Personality Inventory (MMPI), and Beck's Depression Inventory (BDI). Many specialists find the PRISM and the BDI to be the most useful, although many providers prefer to rely on a personalized self-reporting scale. If static scales such as the MMPI or the BDI are used,

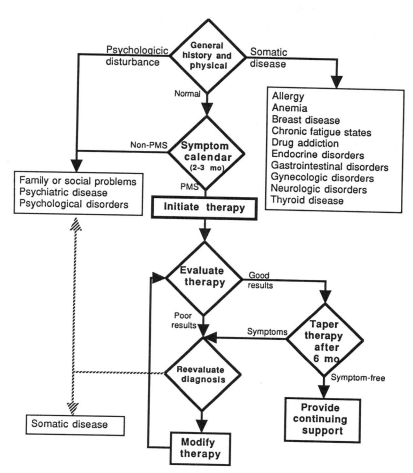

Figure 20.4. Algorithm for the management of premenstrual syndrome. The diagnosis of PMS is predicted on the elimination of other physical and psychologic conditions mimicking PMS, and the use of a 2- to 3-month prospective calendar of symptoms. Once the diagnosis of PMS is established, pharmacologic and supportive (nonpharmacologic) therapy is begun. If successful, the pharmacologic therapy is withdrawn after 6 months and careful, supportive follow-up continued. Failure of any therapy suggests the need for a critical re-evaluation of the diagnosis. If this reassessment continues to support the diagnosis of PMS, the therapy is modified and the process of monitoring begins anew.

they should be administered during both the follicular and luteal phases of the cycle, and the results compared.

There are no laboratory or imaging studies that are useful in diagnosing premenstrual syndromes. Laboratory studies may be helpful when conditions mimicking PMS are under consideration (Table 20.5). The most likely condition to be detected by laboratory screening is hypothyroidism, which is often overlooked and underdiagnosed in these patients.

Once other physical and emotional processes have been eliminated from consideration, the diagnosis of a premenstrual syndrome should be positively established. This is accomplished by using a prospectively maintained symptom diary, covering a minimum of two

Table 20.4. Differential Diagnosis of Premenstrual Syndrome

Allergy
Breast disorders (fibrocystic change)
Chronic fatigue states
    Anemia
    Chronic cytomegalovirus infection
    Lyme disease
Connective tissue disease (lupus erythematosus)
Drug and substance abuse
Endocrinologic disorders
    Adrenal disorders (Cushing's syndrome, hypoadrenalism)
    Adrenocorticotropic hormone-mediated disorders
    Hyperandrogenism
    Hyperprolactinemia
    Panhypopituitarism
    Pheochromocytoma
    Thyroid disorders (hypothyroidism, hyperthyroidism)
Family, marital, and social stress (physical or sexual abuse)
Gastrointestinal conditions
    Inflammatory bowel disease (Crohn's disease, ulcerative colitis)
    Irritable bowel syndrome
Gynecologic disorders
    Dysmenorrhea
    Endometriosis
    Pelvic inflammatory disease
    Perimenopause
    Uterine leiomyomata
Idiopathic edema
Neurologic disorders
    Migraine
    Seizure disorders
Psychiatric and psychologic disorders
    Anxiety neurosis
    Bulimia
    Personality disorders
    Psychosis
    Somatoform disorders
    Unipolar and bipolar affective disorders

menstrual cycles. A number of such diaries have been published, but the most useful approach appears to be any open-ended system that allows the patient to record those symptoms that are most distressing, rather than those provided by a pre-printed form. Diary assessments should be performed and recorded at the same time each day to ensure consistency. For ease of interpretation, a graphic method of plotting this information is preferred, but not required. Examples of this type of graph are shown in Figure 20.5. It is common for there to be a discordance between the pattern of complaints offered during the initial description of symptoms and the pattern found in the prospective diary.

Once a premenstrual syndrome has been documented, the predominant type of menstrually related process should be established. Some authors do not distinguish between

Table 20.5. Useful Laboratory Studies to Consider in the Evaluation of Premenstrual Complaints

General studies
    Complete blood count (CBC)
    Liver enzyme studies
Cultures
    Chlamydia cultures and antibody testing
Endocrin studies
    Androgens
    Follicle-stimulating hormone/luteinizing hormone (FSH/LH)
    Glucose tolerance test
    Prolactin
    Thyroid function studies
        Highly sensitive thyroid-stimulating hormone (TSH)
        Thyronine (T_4)
        Thyrotropin-releasing hormone (TRH) stimulation

PMS, PMDD, and PMM; however, it is useful to group those patients with significant emotional symptoms separately from those with more somatic complaints. Although these distinctions may seem artificial, experience has shown that these patients respond to different management approaches based on these groupings.

PMS

Patients classified as having true PMS are very heterogeneous in the symptoms they experience. Most troubling are physical complaints such as breast tenderness, bloating, and weight gain. Generalized aches and pains, peripheral and facial edema, and headache are also common. While many patients with PMS also have anxiety, irritability, or depression, these symptoms do not predominate.

PMDD

Patients with PMDD may have physical complaints, but these are secondary to the mood and behavioral disturbances these patients experience. By definition, these patients most closely fit the APA description of symptom patterns (see Table 20.3). Just as in PMS, care must be taken to establish the diagnosis in a prospective manner.

PMM

The diagnosis of premenstrual magnification syndrome is established in much the same manner as other menstrually related processes: through the use of a prospective evaluation of symptoms. To be classed as PMM, the symptoms reported by the patient must be present at a low level throughout the month, with an increase of more than 30% during the premenstrual phase of the cycle. As with other premenstrual syndromes, the exact nature of the symptoms reported is not important, just the timing. Patients who experience random swings in symptom severity throughout the month do not have PMM syndrome and other conditions must be sought.

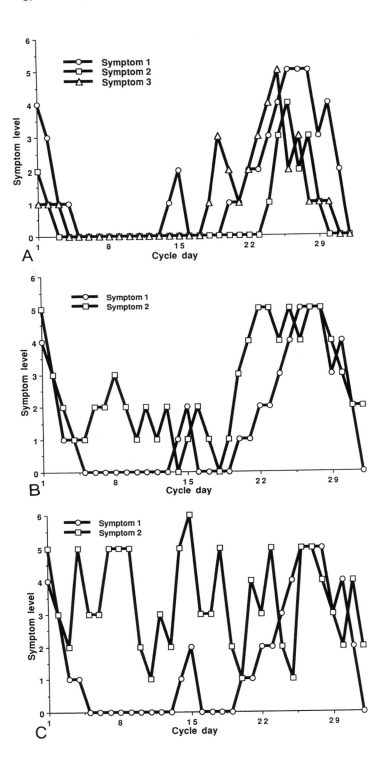

By the very nature of this syndrome, patients with PMM are likely to have an underlying physical or emotional process that may be directly identified and treated, independent of the menstrual cycle. Even while these patients are undergoing general treatment, a continuing effort should be made to identify a specific causative process. Finding such a process will result in more specific and successful treatment.

THERAPEUTIC OPTIONS

Effective therapies are now available for PMS, PMDD, and PMM. As a result, a favorable response should be expected for 80% of PMS patients and 50% of those with PMM. Therapy must be individualized to the needs of the patient, but will generally consist of education, counseling regarding lifestyle interventions, pharmacologic intervention for specific symptoms, and referral for significant or unresponsive psychological or psychosexual problems.

It is not uncommon for some women to report an improvement in their symptoms during the initial evaluation phase of treatment. The process of symptom charting often gives insight and credence to the patient's symptoms. Strategies for managing symptoms often emerge by virtue of a better understanding of their timing. In a manner similar to biofeedback, these patients gain some level of control, often reporting that their symptoms no longer intrude to the extent they did before they sought help. It should also be recognized that in some studies, over 50% of patients have a positive response to placebo therapy. Whatever their origin, these improvements are just as real as those produced by pharmacologic interventions.

Once the diagnosis of PMS, PMDD, or PMM is established, therapeutic intervention may begin (see Figure 20.4). The first step in this process must be one of education. The patient must be reassured of the veracity of her complaints, the commitment of the health care team to help her, and her ability to help herself manage the changes she experiences. Awareness of the pattern involved may help her plan activities to minimize stress, social or physical demands, and work obligations to allow for the smoothest transition through the luteal phase. Lifestyle patterns that may be contributing to the severity of symptoms can be recognized and discussed. Simple lifestyle changes may be suggested (Table 20.6). Although many of these are of unproved value, few are dangerous, most promote healthy behaviors,

Figure 20.5. Examples of graphic symptom recording. Graphic records for the symptoms experienced by the patient make establishing the diagnosis of menstrually related syndromes simpler. The number and type of symptoms tracked should be individualized to the needs of the patient. The severity scale is arbitrary, but should be consistent from month to month. The typical pattern of symptoms present in PMS is seen in panel **A**. These may be contrasted with PMM which is shown in **B**. Panel **C** illustrates patterns typical of nonmenstrually related symptoms, which do not fall within the definition of PMS, PMM, or PMDD. Symptoms may worsen or be less tolerable near the time of menstruation, but they are clearly not as directly related as they are in the other two patterns. This pattern may be found in up to 75% of patients who complete charts.

Table 20.6. Lifestyle and Dietary Interventions for Women with Premenstrual Syndromes

Lifestyle changes
    Aerobic exercise (20 to 45 min, 3 times weekly)
    Smoking cessation
    Stress reduction
Dietary changes and supplementation
    Diet
        Adequate protein and complex carbohydrates
        Avoidance of alcohol, caffeine, and simple sugars
        Frequent small meals
        Fresh fruits and vegetables
        Reduce dietary fat to <15%
        Salt restriction
        Increased dietary or supplemental fiber
    Supplementation
        Calcium 1000 mg/d
        Magnesium 200 mg/d during luteal phase
        Vitamin B_6 50–200 mg/d
        Vitamin E 150–300 IU/d

Table 20.7. Pharmacologic Therapy for Specific Symptoms of Premenstrual Syndrome

Symptom	Possible therapies
Cravings	High-protein, low fat and low-sugar diet*
	Pyridoxine 50 mg/d*
Fluid retention	Spironolactone 50–100 mg/d, luteal phase*
	Hydrochlorothiazide 25–50 mg/d, luteal phase
Irritability (agitation and anxiety)	Alprazolam 0.25 mg three to four times daily
	Atenolol 25 mg two to three times daily
Mastalgia/mastodynia	Bromocriptine 2.5–5 mg/d, luteal phase
	Danazol sodium 200 mg/d, luteal phase or continuous
Migrane	Atenolol 25 mg two to three times daily
Mood swings	Buspirone 5 mg three times daily
	Fluoxetine 20 mg/d (in the morning)
Pelvic or joint pain, headache, dysmenorrhea	Nonsteroidal anti-inflammatory agents
	Meclofenamate sodium 50–100 mg three times daily as needed for pain
	Naproxen 250 mg every 6 to 8 h as needed for pain
	Ibuprofen 600–800 mg every 4 h as needed for pain

*Unproven in blinded studies.

and all give some element of control back to the patient. In addition to the above measures, support groups or individual counseling may be of value, based on the availability of resources and the needs of the patient.

The symptoms that the patient finds most distressing should be identified so that they are specifically addressed by any treatment plan. When these are somatic, therapy specific to the complaint may be successful (Table 20.7). No one therapy is successful for all patients. Frequently, a sequence of therapies must be tried to find the one most effective for the individual patient.

More global complaints and those within the realm of PMDD require a more generalized approach. Either hormonal or central nervous system modifications have been advocated, several of which have been shown to be effective in controlled trials (Table 20.8). Past experience with oral contraceptives suggests that only about one quarter of patients experience improvement on these agents, whereas an equal number have a worsening of their symptoms. Contraceptives using the newer progesterones, such as desogestrel, appear to do better than older formulations, but long-term experience is lacking. If the patient requires contraception, a trial of these agents may be reasonable. Progesterone, natural or synthetic, in any of its forms and routes, has not been shown to be effective and, in some cases, may cause a worsening of symptoms. Therefore, its use is not endorsed. Similarly, estrogen-testosterone combinations should not be used to treat these women.

Danazol sodium has proved to be effective for many patients. It may be given at the onset of symptoms or on a continuous basis. Danazol is most effective when mastalgia is a predominant complaint. The presence of distressing side effects, such as hirsutism, increased appetite, and hepatic dysfunction, are unusual with the usual dose for PMS. Danazol is a teratogen, making concomitant nonhormonal contraception necessary.

Medical oophorectomy with gonadtropin-releasing hormone (GnRH) agonists has proved very effective in treating PMS and PMDD. The effectiveness of this therapy is such that if symptoms persist after the first month of therapy, serious reconsideration of the diagnosis must be entertained. Cost and concerns about bone loss during prolonged therapy limit wide application of this approach. Many reserve this therapy for patients with the most severe problems or those for whom the diagnosis is in doubt.

Excellent results have been reported for the serotonergic agents such as buspirone and fluoxetine. These agents are well tolerated and often have half-life profiles that allow intermittent dosing. These agents have proved themselves in randomized trials. Although other serotonergic drugs are now available, they should not be substituted for these agents until clinical studies support their effectiveness. Alprazolam is the benzodiazepine of choice when agitation or anxiety are dominant symptoms. The possibility of dependency may be minimized by restricting the use of this agent to the luteal phase. Tranquilizers such as Val-

Table 20.8. Pharmacologic Therapy for Generalized Symptoms of Premenstrual Syndrome and Premenstrual Dysphoric Disorder

Therapeutic class	Typical agents
Central nervous system modifiers	Alprazolam 0.25 mg three to four times daily Buspirone 5 mg three times daily Fluoxetine 20 mg/d, luteal phase or continuous (taken in the morning)

Hormonal	Third-generation oral contraceptives (e.g., desogestrel-containing)
	Danazol sodium 200 mg/d, luteal phase or continuous
	GnRH agonists
	    Depot-luprolide 3.75 mg intramuscularly monthly for a maximum of 6 months,
	    Nafarelin acetate nasal spray, 200 µg twice daily for a maximum of 6 months

GnRH = gonatropin-releasing hormone.

ium and meprobamate should not be used because of their addictive potential and depressive side effects.

All hormonal and central nervous system agents should be gradually withdrawn after 6 months of therapy. For most patients, symptoms will not recur or will return in a sufficiently mild form that minimal disruption occurs. When intervention is necessary, a different therapeutic modality is often chosen and the cycle of therapy, assessment, and eventual withdrawal is begun again. Surgical extirpation of the ovaries is only indicated for those rare patients with significant disability who respond only to GnRH agonist therapy. Even for these patients, a trial of GnRH agonist with hormone replacement should be undertaken to assess the possibility of recurrence with postoperative replacement hormone treatment.

HINTS AND COMMON QUESTIONS

Patients who present for the evaluation of PMS have had their symptoms for an average of 5 years before they seek help. As a result, many arrive with unrealistic expectations and a string of failed self-medication attempts that must be recognized and addressed.

Because there is no evidence of corpus luteum dysfunction or hormonal abnormality associated with premenstrual syndromes, patients can be reassured that the presence of these symptoms does not reflect on their ability to have children.

There is no evidence that childbearing has any effect on the development or evolution of premenstrual syndromes, even though they are commonly improved or absent during the course of the pregnancy itself.

Common historical findings in women with PMS include poor exercise, young age, high parity, and other women in the family with depression or PMS. A history of postpartum depression, affective disorders, migraine headaches, or high intakes of alcohol, caffeine, or chocolate are also common. These histories are not diagnostic, however, and diagnosis must be established for each patient as noted above.

When reviewing the patient's history, specific questions about the use of medications and diet supplements must be posed. These most commonly contain ineffective or minimally effective combinations of mild diuretics, vitamins, and sedatives. Many of the over-the-counter treatments for PMS contain caffeine and other agents that may actually worsen symptoms. These agents also encourage self-medication for a condition that affects less than 50% of those who believe they are sufferers.

Symptoms, including difficulty thinking or concentrating, indecision, memory loss, obsessional thinking, depersonalization, and poor judgment are common in women with PMS, but they are also common presenting complaints for patients with depression. This must always be a part of the differential diagnosis for these patients.

It is unusual for patients to object to the need for a prospective diary. Those who get angry because they "already know" they have PMS are the most likely to have a personality disorder and not true PMS. These women are often reacting to past experience, stress, or abuse. They should be reassured that they are being taken seriously and that care in establishing the exact nature of their condition makes effective therapy possible.

As in other conditions lacking physical findings (e.g., chronic pain states), the possibility of substance or alcohol abuse and physical or sexual abuse must be considered in all patients with the complaints of PMS. Ill-defined symptoms may be a cry for help.

Despite the common perception, women with PMS do not have any documentable change in cognitive function during the luteal phase of their menstrual cycle. When such a change is suspected or documented, other sources must be sought.

The high prevalence of placebo response found in premenstrual disorders is not evidence that they do not exist. The placebo response is a powerful reality that may be exploited to the benefit of the patient. It really does not matter who or what gets the credit if the condition improves.

Significant lifestyle changes are often difficult to achieve. For this reason, it is sometimes advisable to institute major changes (e.g., exercise, smoking cessation, or diet) one at a time. Although this approach is slower, it may be more realistic.

Some nonprescription PMS remedies contain toxic (> 200 mg) levels of vitamin B_6. Doses at or above this level have been associated with the development of peripheral neuropathies. This level of use should be checked for in any patient who uses self-medication and the patient advised accordingly.

Oral contraceptives are least effective in treating patients with premenstrual magnification disorders.

If a GnRH agonist is used to treat PMS or PMDD, less initial worsening of symptoms will occur if the first dose is given during the midluteal phase rather than the usual early follicular start. As with any hormonal manipulation, the possibility of a pregnancy must be evaluated prior to initiation of therapy or when a period does not occur as expected.

It is estimated that up to 10% of women may develop anxiety and restlessness if alprazolam is abruptly discontinued. Progressive reduction from three times daily to twice daily for 2 days, followed by once a day for 2 days prior to complete withdrawal, will avoid this complication.

SUGGESTED READINGS

General References

American College of Obstetricians and Gynecologists. Premenstrual syndrome. ACOG Committee Opinion 155. Washington, DC: ACOG, 1995.

American Psychiatric Association. Diagnostic and Statistical Manual of Mental Disorders, 4th ed. Washington, DC: American Psychiatric Association, 1994.

Dawood MY, McGuire JL, Demers LM. Premenstrual Syndrome and Dysmenorrhea. Baltimore: Urban & Schwarzenberg, 1985.

d'Orban RT. Medicolegal aspects of the premenstrual syndrome. Br J Hosp Med 1983; December.

Endicott J, Nee J, Cohen J, et al. Premenstrual changes: Patterns and correlates of daily ratings. J Affect Disord 1986;10:127.

Freeman E, Rickels K, Sondheimer S, Scharlop B. Diagnostic classifications from daily symptom ratings of women who seek treatment for premenstrual symptoms. American Journal of Gynecologic Health 1987;1:17.

Freeman E, Sondheimer S, Weinbaum PJ, Rickels K. Evaluating premenstrual syndrome in medical practice. Obstet Gynecol 1985;65:500.

Garris PD, Sokol MS, Kelly K, Witman GF, Plouffe L Jr. Leuprolide acetate treatment of catamenial pneumothorax. Fertil Steril 1994;61:173.

Gise LH, Lebovits AH, Paddison PL, Strain JJ. Issues in the identification of premenstrual syndrome. J Nerv Ment Dis 1990;178:228.

Greene R, Dalton K. The premenstrual syndrome. BMJ 1953;1:1007.

Halbreich U, Endicott J. Methodological issues in studies of premenstrual changes. Psychoneuroendocrinology 1985;10:15.

Keye WR JR. The Premenstrual Syndrome. Philadelphia: WB Saunders, 1988.

Moline ML. Pharmacologic strategies for managing premenstrual syndrome. Clin Pharm 1993;12:181.

Moos RH. The development of a menstrual distress questionnaire. Psychosom Med 1968;30:85.

Moos RH. Typology of menstrual cycle symptoms. Gynecology 1968;103:390.

Newmark ME, Penry JK. Catamenial epilepsy: a review. Epilepsia 1980;21:281.

Plouffe L Jr, Khreim IM, Rausch JL, Stewart K. Premenstrual syndrome: update on diagnosis and management. Female Patient 1994;19:53.

Plouffe L JR, Trott EA. Premenstrual syndrome: new concepts and recent therapeutic breakthroughs. Postgraduate Obstetrics and Gynecology 1995;15:1.

Rapkin AJ, ed. Premenstrual syndrome. Clin Obstet Gynecol 1992;35:585.

Rausch JL, Parry BL. Treatment of premenstrual mood symptoms. Psychiatr Clin North Am 1993;16:829.

Reid RL, Yen SSC. Premenstrual syndrome. Am J Obstet Gynecol 1981;139:85.

Rubinow DR. The premenstrual syndrome: new views. JAMA 1992;268:1908.

Severino SK. Premenstrual dysphoric disorder. Primary Care Update Ob/Gyn 1995;2:12.

Smith S, Schiff I. The premenstrual syndrome: diagnosis and management. Fertil Steril 1989;52:527.

Steiner M, Haskett RF, Carrol BJ. Premenstrual tension syndrome: the development of research diagnostic criteria and new rating scales. Acta Psychiatr Scand 1980;62:177.

Stenchever MA. Dysmenorrhea and premenstrual syndrome. In Herbst AL, Mishell DR, Stenchever MA, Droegemueller WR (eds). Comprehensive Gynecology, 2nd ed. St Louis: CV Mosby, 1992, p 1074.

Specific References

Frequency and Impact

Andersh B, Wendetam C, Hahn L, Ohman R. Premenstrual complaints. I. Prevalence of premenstrual syndrome in a Swedish urban population. Journal of Psychosomatic Obstetrics and Gynecology 1986;5:39.

Chaturvedi SK, Chandre PS, Issac MK, et al. Premenstrual experiences: the four profiles and factorial patterns. Journal of Psychosomatic Obstetrics and Gynecology 1993;14:223.

Ekholm U-B, Hammarback S, Backstrom T. Premenstrual tension syndrome: a study comparing symptom ratings during two consecutive menstrual cycles. Journal of Psychosomatic Obstetrics and Gynecology 1991;12:291.

Ekholm U-B, Hammarback S, Backstrom T. Premenstrual syndrome: changes in symptom pattern between two menstrual cycles. Journal of Psychosomatic Obstetrics and Gynecology 1992;13:107.

Freeman EW, Rickles K, Sondheimer SJ. Premenstrual symptoms and dysmenorrhea in relation to emotional distress factors in adolescents. Journal of Psychosomatic Obstetrics and Gynecology 1993;14:41.

Johnsom SR, McChesney C, Bean J. Epidemiology of premenstrual symptoms in a nonclinical sample. J Reprod Med 1984:33:340.

Logue CM, Moos RH. Perimenstrual symptoms: prevalence and risk factors. Psychosom Med 1986;48:388.

Ramcharan S, Love EJ, Fick GH, Goldfine A. The epidemiology of premenstrual symptoms in a population-based sample of 2650 urban women: Attributable risk and risk factors. J Clin Epidemiol 1992;45:377.

Walsh RM, Budtz-Olsen I, Leader C, Cummins RA. The menstrual cycle, personality, and academic performance. Arch Gen Psychiatry 1981;38:219.

Woods NF, Most A, Dery GK. Prevalence of perimenstrual symptoms. Am J Public Health 1982;72:1257.

Physiology and Causation

AuBuchon PG, Calhoun KS. Menstrual cycle symptomatology: the role of social expectancy and experimental demand characteristics. Psychosom Med 1985;47:35.

Chuong CJ, Coulam CB, Bergstralh EJ, O'Fallon WM, Steinmetz GI. Clinical trial of naltrexone in premenstrual syndrome. Obstet Gynecol 1988;72:332.

Chuong CJ, Coulam CB, Kao PC, Bergstralh EJ, Go VLW. Neuropeptide levels in premenstrual syndrome. Fertil Steril 1985;44:760.

Dennerstein L, Brown JB, Gotts G, Morse CA, Farley TMM, Pinol A. Menstrual cycle profiles of women with and without premenstrual syndrome. Journal of Psychosomatic Obstetrics and Gynecology 1993;14:259.

Endicott J, Halbreich U. Retrospective report of premenstrual depressive changes: factors affecting confirmation by daily ratings. Psychopharmacol Bull 1983;18:109.

Facchinetti F, Martignoni E, Petraglia F, Sances MG, Mappi G, Genazzanit AR. Premenstrual fall of plasma β-endorphin in patients with premenstrual syndrome. Fertil Steril 1987;47:570.

Frank RT. The hormonal causes of premenstrual tension. Arch Neurol Psychiatry 1931;26:1053.

Gannon FL. Evidence for a psychological etiology of menstrual disorders: a critical review. Psychol Rep 1981;48: 287.

Hammarbäch S, Damber JE, Backstrom T, et al. Relationship between symptom severity and hormone changes in women with premenstrual syndrome. J Clin Endocrinol Metab 1989;68:125.

Israel SL. Premenstrual tension. JAMA 1934;110:1721.

Kimmel S, Gonsalves L, Youngs D, Gidwani G. Fluctuating levels of antidepressants premenstrually. Journal of Psychosomatic Obstetrics and Gynecology 1992;13:277.

Mira M, Stewart PM, Abraham SF. Vitamin and trace element status in premenstrual syndrome. Am J Clin Nutr 1988;47:636.

Olasov B, Jackson J. Effects of expectancies on women's reports of moods during the menstrual cycle. Psychosom Med 1987;49:65.

Parry BL, Gerner RH, Wilkins JN, et al. CSF and neuroendocrine studies of premenstrual syndrome. Neuropsychopharmacology 1991;5:127.

Prichard JC. A Treatise on Insanity. London: Sherwood, Gilbert, and Piper, 1835.

Rapkin AJ, Edelmuth E, Chang LE, et al. Whole-blood serotonin in premenstrual syndrome. Obstet Gynecol 1987;70:533.

Reid RL, Yen SSC. Premenstrual syndrome. Am J Obstet Gynecol 1981;139:85.

Rubinow DR, Hoban G, Grover GN, et al. Changes in plasma hormones across the menstrual cycle in patients with menstrually related mood disorders and in control subjects. Am J Obstet Gynecol 1988;158:5.

Rubinow DR, Roy-Byrne P. Premenstrual syndromes: overview from a methodologic perspective. Am J Psychiatry 1984;141:163.

Rubinow DR, Schmidt PJ. Premenstrual syndrome: a review of endocrine studies. Endocrinologist 1992;2:47.

Ruble CN. Premenstrual symptoms: A reinterpretation. Science 1977;197:219.

Schagen van Leeuwen JH, te Velde ER, Kop WJ, vander Ploeg HM, Haspels AA. a simple strategy to detect significant premenstrual changes. Journal of Psychosomatic Obstetrics and Gynecology 1993;14:211.

Schagen van Leeuwen JH, te Velde ER, Koppeschaar HPF, et al. Is premenstrual syndrome an endocrine disorder? Journal of Psychosomatic Obstetrics and Gynecology 1993;14:91.

Schmidt PJ, Grover GN, Roy-Byrne PP, Rubinow DR. Thyroid function in women with premenstrual syndrome. J Clin Endocrinol Metab 1993;76:671.

Schmidt PJ, Nieman LK, Grover GN, Muller KL, Merriam GR, Rubinow DR. Lack of effect of induced menses on symptoms in women with premenstrual syndrome. N Engl J Med 1991;324:1174.

Sommer B. The effect of menstruation on cognitive and preceptual-motor behavior: a review. Psychosom Med 1973;35:515.

Steege JF, Stout AL, Knight DL, et al. Reduced paltelet tritium-labeled imipramine binding sites in women with premenstrual syndrome. Am J Obstet Gynecol 1992;167:168.

Tulenheimo A, Laatikainen T, Salminen K. Plasma β-endorphin immunoreactivity in premenstrual tension. Br J Obstet Gynaecol 1987;94:26.

Watts JFF, Butt WR, Edwards LR, et al. Hormonal studies in women with premenstrual syndrome. Br J Obstet Gynaecol 1985;92:247.

Therapy and Counseling

Backstrom T, Hansson-Malmstrom Y, Lindhe BA, Cavalli-Bjorkman B, Nordenstrom S. Oral contraceptives in premenstrual syndrome: a randomized comparison of triphasic and monophasic preparations. Contraception 1992;46:253.

Berger CP, Presser B. Alprazolam in the treatment of two subsamples of patients with late luteal phase dysphoric disorder: a double-blind, placebo-controlled crossover study. Obstet Gynecol 1994;84:379.

Pearlstein TB, Stone AB. Long-term fluoxetine treatment of late luteal phase dysphoric disorder. J Clin Psychiatry 1994;55:332.

Burnet RB, Radden HS, Easterbrook EG, McKinnon RA. Premenstrual syndrome and spironolactone. Aust N Z J Obstet Gynaecol 1991;31:366.

Cason P, Hahn PM, Van Vugt DA, Reid RL. Lasting response to ovariectomy in severe intractable predmenstrual syndrome. Am J Obstet Gynecol 1990;162:99.

Casper RF, Hearn MT. The effect of hysterectomy and bilateral oophorectomy in women with severe premenstrual syndrome. Am J Obstet Gynecol 1990;162:105.

Collins A, Cerin A, Coleman G, Landgren B-M. Essential fatty acids in the treatment of premenstrual syndrome. Obstet Gynecol 1993;81:93.

Corney RH, Stanton R, Newell R, Clare AW. Comparison of progesterone, placebo and behavioral psychotherapy in the treatment of premenstrual syndrome. Journal of Psychosomatic Obstetrics and Gynecology 1990;11:211.

Elks ML. Open trial of fluoxetine therapy for premenstrual syndrome. South Med J 1993;86:503.

Facchinetti F, Borella P, Kangasniemi P, et al. The efficacy and safety of subcutaneous sumatriptan in the acute treatment of menstrual migraine. Obstet Gyencol 1995;86:911.

Facchinetti F, Borella P, Sances G, Fioroni L, Nappi RE, Genazzani AR. Oral magnesium successfully relieves premenstrual mood changes. Obstet Gynecol 1991;78:177.

Freeman EW, Rickels K, Sondheimer SJ, Polansky M. A double-blind trial of oral progesterone, alprazolam, and placebo in treatment of severe premenstrual syndrome. JAMA 1995;274:51.

Freeman EW, Rickels K, Sondheimer SJ, Polansky M. Ineffectiveness of progesterone suppository treatment of premenstrual syndrome. JAMA 1990;264:349.

Graham CA, Sherwin BS. A prospective treatment study of premenstrual symptoms using a triphasic oral contraceptive. J Psychosom Res 1992;36:257.

Hagen I, Nesheim BI, Tuntland T. No effect of vitamin B-6 against premenstrual tension. Acta Obstet Gynecol Scand 1985;64:667.

Harrison WM, Endicott J, Nee J. Treatment of premenstrual dysphoria with alprazolam. Arch Gen Psychiatry 1990;47:270.

Hellberg D, Claesson B, Nilsson B. Premenstrual tension: a placebo-controlled efficacy study with spironolactone and medroxyprogesterone acetate. Int J Gynecol Obstet 1991;34:243.

Hussain SY, Massil JH, Matta WH, Shaw RW, O'Brien PMS. Buserelin in premenstrual syndrome. Gynecol Endocrinol 1992;6:57.

Khoo SK, Munro C, Battistutta D. Evening primrose oil and treatment of premenstrual syndrome. Med J Aust 1990;153:189.

Lichten EM, Bennett RS, Whitty AJ, Daoud Y. Effecacy of danazol in control of hormonal migraine. J Reprod Med 1991;36:419.

Maddocks S, Hahn P, Moller F, Reid RL. A double-blind placebo-controlled trial of progesterone vaginal suppositories in the treatment of premenstrual syndrome. Am J Obstet Gynecol 1986;154:573.

Menkes DB, Taghavi E, Mason PA, Howard RC. Fluoxetine's spectrum of action in premenstrual syndrome. Int Clin Psychopharmacol 1993;8:95.

Metclaf MG, Livesey JH, Wells JE. Mood and physical symptom cyclicity in women with the premenstrual syndrome: unexpected response to placebo treatment. J Psychosom Obstet Gynaecol 1991;12:273.

Mezrow G, Shoupe D, Spicer D, Lobo R, Leung B, Pike M. Depot leuprolide acetate with estrogen and progestin add-back for long-term treatment of premenstrual syndrome. Fertil Steril 1994;62:932.

Mira M, McNeil D, Fraser IS, Vizzard J, Abraham S. Mefanamic acid in the treatment of premenstrual sydnrome. Obstet Gynecol 1986;68:395.

Mortola JF, Girton L, Fischer U. Successful treatment of severe premenstrual syndrome by combined use of gonadotropin-releasing hormone agonist and estrogen/progestin. J Clin Endocrinol Metab 1991;72:250.

Mortola JF. A risk-benefit appraisal of drugs used in the management of premenstrual syndrome. Drug Safety 1994;10:160.

Mortola JF. Applications of gonadotropin-releasing hormone analogues in the treatment of premenstrual syndrome. Clin Obstet Gynecol 1993;36:753.

Muse K, Cetel NS, Futterman LA, Yen SSC. The premenstrual syndrome: effects of "medical oophorectomy." N Engl J Med 1984;311:1345.

Muse K. Hormonal manipulation in the treatment of premenstrual syndrome. Clin Obstet Gynecol 1992;35:658.

Plouffe L JR, Stewart K, Craft KS, et al. Diagnostic and treatment results from a southeastern academic center-based premenstrual syndrome clinic: the first year. Am J Obstet Gynecol 1993;169:295.

Prior JC, Vigna Y, Sciarretta D, Alojado N, Schulzer M. Conditioning exercise decreases premenstrual symptoms—A prospective, controlled 6-month trial. Fertil Steril 1987;47:402.

Rausch JL, Weston S, Plouffe L. Role of psychotropic medication in the treatment of affective symptoms in premenstrual syndrome. Clin Obstet Gynecol 1992;35:667.

Rickels K, Freeman E, Sondheimer S. Buspirone in treatment of premenstrual syndrome. Lancet 1989;1:777.

Sarno AP, Miller EJ, Lundblad EG. Premenstrual syndrome: beneficial effects of periodic, low-dose danazol. Obstet Gynecol 1987;20:33.

Schaumburg H, Kaplan J, Windebank A, et al. Sensory neuropahty from pyridoxine abuse: A new megavitamin syndrome. N Engl J Med 1983;309:445.

Schmidt PJ, Grover GN, Rubinow DR. Alprazolam in the treatment of premenstrual syndrome. A double-blind, placebo-controlled trial. Arch Gen Psychiatry 1993;50:467.

Smith S, Rinehart JS, Ruddock VE, Schiff I. Treatment of premenstrual syndrome with alprazolam: results of a double-blind, placebo-controlled, randomized cross-over clinical trial. Obstet Gynecol 1987;70:37.

Steiner M, Steinberg S, Stewart D, et al. Fluoxetine in the treatment of premenstrual dysphoria. Canadian Fluoxetine/Premenstrual Dysphoria Collaborative Study Group. N Engl J Med 1995;332:1529.

Stone AB, Pearlstein TB Brown WA. Fluoxetine in the treatment of late luteal phase dysphoric disorder. J Clin Psychiatry 1991;52:290.

Tobin MB, Schmidt PJ, Rubinow DR. Reported alcohol use in women with premenstrual syndrome. Am J Psychiatry 1994;151:1503.

Toth A, Lesser ML, Nus G, et al. Effect of doxycycline on premenstrual syndrome: A double-blind randomized clinical trial. J Int Med Res 1988;16:270.

Vellacott ID, Shroff NE, Pearce MY, Stratford ME, Akbar FA. A double-blind, placebo-controlled evaluation of spironolactone in the premenstrual syndrome. Curr Med Res Opin 1987;10:450.

Williams MJ, Harris RA, Dean BC. Controlled trial of pyridoxine in the premenstrual syndrome. J Int Med Res 1985;13:174.

Wood SH, Mortola JF, Chan YF, Moossazadeh F, Yen SS. Treatment of premenstrual syndrome with fluoxetine: a double-blind placebo-controlled, crossover study. Obstet Gynecol 1992;80:339.

21

Pelvic Masses

Despite the fact that most pelvic masses found in asymptomatic women are benign, the discovery of a pelvic mass is of concern to all. Conservative therapy for asymptomatic or nonacute patients is often appropriate, but the management of pelvic masses is neither uniform nor inflexible. Management is based on how the mass was found and its characteristics as well as the age, menstrual, and medical status of the patient. Evaluation and management that might be reasonable for one patient may be inappropriate for another. An asymptomatic mass found during an annual evaluation requires a different course of evaluation and treatment than the mass found in a patient experiencing shock and abdominal pain.

Because of the nature of mass lesions and the frequent necessity for surgical evaluation or therapy, consultation is most often required. It is highly likely, however, that a non-emergent patient may receive most of her initial evaluation in the primary care setting. When referral is required, a familiarity with the management and expected outcomes associated with these pathologies greatly enhances the primary care provider's ability to counsel and provide continuing care.

BACKGROUND AND SCIENCE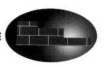

Almost any structure in or abutting the pelvis may be the source of enlargement, distention, or neoplasia, resulting in the formation of a mass. For convenience, pelvic masses may be classified anatomically by their origin. The location and character of the mass can be used to develop a manageable differential diagnosis and plan of therapy.

Uterine Masses

The most common pelvic masses found in women during their reproductive years are related to the uterus: pregnancy and leiomyomata (fibroids). The possibility of a pregnancy, intrauterine or otherwise, must always be considered when a pelvic mass is found. This is especially true when the mass is midline and there is a history of a menstrual disturbance.

Fibroids represent the most common pelvic tumor in nonpregnant women. Indeed, up to 30% of hysterectomies performed in the United States, and almost half of those performed on women between the ages of 35 and 50 years, are for "fibroids." Clinically identifiable fibroids occur in one fourth of white and one half of black women, reaching their peak incidence in the fifth decade of life when they are found in about 40% of all patients. Fibroids are more common in nulliparous women and those with early menarche. They vary in size from microscopic to more than 100 lbs. Up to one half of women with fibroids will have symptoms, most commonly pelvic pain and abnormal bleeding, which occurs in about 30% of cases.

A number of complications, which may necessitate intervention or induce significant morbidity, can occur with fibroids. Fibroids may undergo torsion, infarction, degeneration, or become infected. Submucous fibroids may prolapse through the cervical canal (a rare cause for uterine inversion) or fibroids may cause the uterus to become incarcerated in the pelvic cavity. More commonly, fibroids cause pressure on adjacent structures, infrequently causing urinary retention or hydroureter to develop.

In pregnancy, fibroids may grow rapidly or undergo hemorrhage or necrosis, and may occasionally even be a cause for disseminated intervascular coagulopathy. Large fibroids may obstruct delivery or cause obstacles to the progress of labor. It is thought that between 2% and 3% of unexplained infertility is caused by the presence of fibroids.

Uterine leiomyomata represent a clone of cells arising from a single smooth muscle cell. It is unknown whether these arise from embryonic cells within the myometrium or from smooth muscle cells in the vascular wall. The cause of this proliferation is unknown, although it is known that these cells have more estrogen than progesterone receptors on their surface, accounting for their sensitivity to estrogen levels and their growth during periods of increased estrogen, such as with pregnancy or estrogen therapy. There is some evidence that fibroids may be sensitive to epidermal growth factor as well, although the exact role that this plays in their cause or growth is not well outlined. During conditions of rapid growth, fibroids may undergo degeneration or infarction. The most common forms of degeneration include hyalin, myxomatous, and calcific changes.

Seventy to 80% of uterine fibroids are found within the wall of the uterus, with 5% to 10% lying below the endometrium and fewer than 5% arising in or near the cervix. Multiple fibroids are found in up to 85% of cases; most individual fibroids span more than one location. Occasionally, fibroids may develop long pedicles, which places them at risk for torsion or prolapse through the cervix when in an intracavitary location. The location, size, and number of fibroids often determines the type and severity of symptoms encountered by the patient: Those with fibroids on the outer surface of the uterus have the fewest symptoms; those with fibroids that impinge on the uterine cavity develop the most complaints.

Other, less common processes may also lead to uterine enlargement. These are summarized in Table 21.1. Endometrial cancer rarely causes significant uterine enlargement; it

Table 21.1. Sources of Uterine Enlargement Presenting as a Pelvic Mass

Adenomyosis
Hematometra (congenital, acquired)
Leiomyoma(s)
Malignant tumor (endometrial, cervical, metastatic)
Pregnancy (intrauterine, cornual)
Pyometra

Table 21.2. Adnexal Masses

Ovarian masses
    Benign
        Corpus luteum cysts
        Cystadenoma
        Cystic teratoma (dermoid)
        Endometrioma
        Fibroma
        Follicular cysts
    Malignant
        Epithelial tumors
        Germ cell tumors
        Metastatic tumors
        Stromal tumors
Nonovarian
    Actinomycosis
    Ectopic pregnancy (tubal or abdominal)
    Endometriosis
    Fallopian tube malignancy
    Hydrosalpinx
    Leiomyoma (broad ligament or pedunculated)
    Paraovarian cysts
    Tubo-ovarian abscess

is generally suspected on the basis of bleeding abnormalities and diagnosed by tissue obtained at endometrial biopsy or curettage.

Adnexal Masses

Adnexal masses constitute the fourth most common reason for hospital admission for women in the United States. Unfortunately, almost two thirds of women under the age of 40 who undergo surgery for ovarian enlargement, are found to have only functional ovarian changes, such as corpus luteum or follicular cysts. Differentiating these functional changes from the more deleterious changes of benign neoplasm or ovarian cancer is sometimes difficult. Much of the evaluation necessary, however, can be done in the primary care setting, allowing for conservative management or timely referral, as appropriate.

The significance, and often the management, of pelvic masses depends on their origin. Those that arise from the ovary are most common, but tubal and paraovarian pathology may also present as a mass lesion (Table 21.2). Distinguishing these different pathologies is often not possible short of surgical exploration, although imaging studies sometimes provide clues.

Ovarian Masses

Ovarian cystic masses come and go as a normal part of the monthly process of ovulation. As a result, a functional cyst is the most common cause of ovarian enlargement and the most common finding at the time of surgery. Such cysts arise during the process of follicle maturation prior to ovulation or from the corpus luteum after the ovum has been released. The dominant follicle often becomes greater than 2 cm in diameter prior to ovulation, making it readily palpable in thin, cooperative patients.

True ovarian tumors may be either solid or cystic and arise from any of the histologic elements of the ovary (Table 21.3). Most common of these are the benign serous and mucinous cystadenomas of epithelial origin. Approximately two thirds of ovarian tumors are derived from coelomic epithelium. About 20% of ovarian masses arise from germ cells, 10% from the ovarian stroma, and the remainder are metastatic to the ovary from other sites.

BENIGN TUMORS. Approximately 90% of ovarian tumors encountered in younger women are benign and metabolically inactive. Benign ovarian tumors are most often diagnosed at the time of routine examination and are asymptomatic. When symptoms do occur, they are generally either catastrophic, as when bleeding, rupture, or torsion occurs, or they are indolent and nonspecific, such as a vague sense of pressure or fullness.

Over three quarters of the benign adnexal masses encountered in clinical practice are functional. Functional cysts are not true neoplasms, but rather anatomic variants resulting from the normal function of the ovary. Follicular cysts occur when ovulation fails to take place, with the developing follicle continuing to grow beyond its normal time. These unilateral cysts may grow to over 5 cm in diameter and may cause abdominal pain and a delay in menses. Follicular cysts are filled with estrogen-rich fluid, which may contribute to endometrial growth and irregular shedding. Rupture of these cyst may engender pain or their unruptured bulk may set the stage for torsion. Only in the latter case is therapeutic intervention needed. In a similar manner, the corpus luteum may persist or, through internal bleeding, enlarge and become symptomatic. The triad of unilateral pelvic pain, delayed menses with irregular spotting, and adnexal fullness (Halban's syndrome) is identical to that of an ectopic pregnancy. The diagnosis of corpus luteum cyst is, therefore, difficult to make clinically and often is not confirmed until the patient's pregnancy status has been ascertained. If the diagnosis can be established, symptomatic support is adequate except in the rare instance of a frankly surgical abdomen.

About 25% of ovarian enlargements in reproductive age women represent true neoplasia, with only about 10% being malignant. As noted in Table 21.3, the largest group of benign ovarian tumors are those that arise from the epithelium of the ovary and its capsule. Despite the diversity of tumors with epithelial beginnings, the most common ovarian tumor in young reproductive age women is the cystic teratoma, or dermoid, which originates in a germ cell. These tumors are derived from primary germ cells and include tissues from all three embryonic germ layers (ectoderm, mesoderm, and endoderm). As a result, these often contain hair, sebaceous material, cartilage, bone, teeth, or neural tissue. On rare occasions, functional thyroid tissue may be present. Dermoids may be found in both ovaries

Table 21.3. Classification of Ovarian Neoplasms

Tumors of coelomic epithelial origin
    Serous tumors
    Mucinous tumors
    Endometrioid tumors
    Mesonephroid (clear cell) tumors
    Mixed mesodermal tumors
    Undifferentiated carcinoma
    Carcinosarcoma
Tumors of germ cell origin
    Teratoma
      Mature teratoma
        Dermoid cyst
        Solid adult teratoma
        Struma ovarii
        Malignant change in mature teratoma
      Immature teratoma
    Choriocarcinoma
    Dysgerminoma
    Embryonal carcinoma (endodermal sinus tumor)
    Gonadoblastoma
Tumors of gonadal stromal origin
    Granulosa-theca tumors
      Granulosa tumor
      Thecoma
    Sertoli-Leydig tumors
      Arrhenoblastoma
      Sertoli tumor
    Gynandroblastoma
    Lipid cell tumors
Tumors of nonspecific mesenchyme
    Fibroma
    Hemangioma
    Leiomyoma
    Lipoma
    Lymphoma
    Sarcoma
Tumors of metastatic to the ovary
    Breast
    Endometrium
    Gastrointestinal tract (Krukenberg's)
    Lymphoma

in between 10% and 20% of cases. Rupture of a dermoid, which can result in an intense chemical peritonitis, is a surgical emergency. Cystic teratomas contain malignant elements in only about 1% of cases.

Few benign or malignant tumors produce sex hormones. Examples of types that do are stromal tumors, such as granulosa-theca cell tumors that produce estrogen and Sertoli-Leydig cell tumors that produce androgen (Table 21.4). The impact of hormone-secreting tumors depends on the type of hormone secreted and the age of the patient. Estrogen-secret-

Table 21.4. Hormone-Producing Ovarian Tumors

Androgen-producing tumors
    Adrenal rest
    Dysgerminoma
    Gonadal-stromal
    Gonadoblastoma
    Granulosa-theca cell
    Gyandroblastoma
    Hilus cell
    Lipoid tumor
    Pregnancy related
      Luteoma
      Theca lutein cyst
      Gestational trophoblastic disease
      Choriocarcinoma
    Sertoli-Leydig cell (arrhenoblastoma, Sertoli cell)
Estrogen/androstenedione-producing tumors
    Granulosa-theca cell
    Thecoma
    Teratoma
    Brenner tumors
    Cystadenoma
    Cystadenocarcinoma

ing tumors in childhood cause isosexual precocious pseudopuberty, whereas during the reproductive years they tend to produce amenorrhea and dysfunctional bleeding. The most clinically noticeable of the metabolically active tumors are those that produce androgen. These will disrupt menstrual cycle function, cause hirsutism, and may produce frank virilization.

Not all stromal tumors secrete hormones. About 10% of ovarian tumors are fibromas, which are stromal in origin but do not secrete hormones. These tumors are generally small and firm, but may be accompanied by ascites or a right unilateral hydrothorax (Meigs' syndrome).

OVARIAN CANCER. Ovarian cancer is one of the most feared gynecologic malignancies a practitioner can encounter. It is a disease of poorly defined, nonspecific symptoms (Table 21.5) that appear late in the course of the disease. As a result, it is difficult to diagnose early, with advanced disease found in two thirds of cases. Cure rates for ovarian cancer are consequently poor. Over 90% of ovarian cancer is of the epithelial cell type, thought to arise from pluripotential mesothelial cells of the visceral peritoneum of the ovarian capsule. Repeated ovulation results in metaplastic transformation of these cells and may account for the association between reduced numbers of lifetime ovulations (oral contraception, parity) and a reduced risk of ovarian cancer (Table 21.6).

Ovarian cancer is the fifth most common of all cancers in women and the third most common gynecologic malignancy, yet it carries the highest mortality of any gynecologic cancer, resulting in more deaths annually than cervical and endometrial cancer combined. Deaths from ovarian cancer have gradually risen, with a rate that is now 2.5 times that re-

Table 21.5. Ovarian Cancer Symptoms

Main symptom	Stage of disease	
	Early (%)	Late (%)
Abdominal swelling	26.8	24.3
Abdominal pain	16.9	10.6
Gastrointestinal symptoms	16.3	24.2
Vaginal bleeding/discharge	12.2	11.6
Dysuria	9.9	4.7
Fatigue and/or fever	4.1	14.6
Other	3.6	7.9
No symptoms	10.2	2.1

After: Flam F, Einhorn N, Sjövall K. Symptomatology of ovarian cancer. Eur J Obstet Gynecol Reprod Biol 1988;27:53.

Table 21.6. Historic Risk Factors for Ovarian Cancer

Factor	Relative Risk
Oral contraception (> 5 y)	0.4–0.65
Parity	0.5–0.8
Excessive intake of dietary fat or coffee	Unknown but slight increase (?)
Age >50 y	2
White race	2
Use of perineal talc	2+ (?)
One first or second degree relative with ovarian cancer	3
Relatives (2 or more) with ovarian cancer (no hereditary pattern)	5
Infertility	6 (?)
Familial cancer syndrome	Up to 50% lifetime risk

ported in 1930. Ovarian cancer is predominantly a disease of the postmenopausal woman: the risk of ovarian cancer is low before menopause and progressively increases with age (Fig. 21.1). The average age for detection of ovarian cancer in the United States is 59 years. Despite this, only one quarter of ovarian tumors in postmenopausal women are malignant. This three-to-one ratio of benign to malignant disease should not create complacency, however, because it still represents a twofold increase in risk compared with that of pre-menopausal women. The strongest risk factor yet established for ovarian cancer is a family history, with the greatest risk in those few women with an inheritable cancer syndrome, such as Lynch II. Over 95% of women with ovarian cancer, however, have no identifiable risk factor. The use of oral contraception and high parity are associated with a reduced risk of epithelial ovarian malignancy. The lifetime risk of developing ovarian cancer is approximately 1%.

As yet, there are no effective screening tools for the early detection of ovarian cancer. Ultrasonography, magnetic resonance imaging, computed tomography, and biochemical markers such as CA 125, which are useful for evaluating a suspicious mass or following the progress of treatment, are not of value for mass screening. Studies have repeatedly shown high costs and unacceptably high false-positive rates for these modalities. For those few pa-

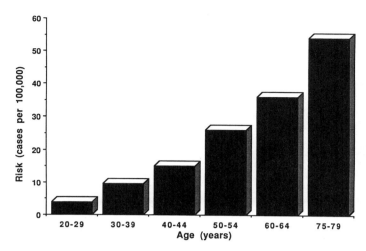

Figure 21.1. Approximate risk of ovarian cancer by age. The risk of ovarian cancer increases progressively with age.

tients at truly high risk (familial cancer syndromes), prophylactic oophorectomy after child-bearing is completed is preferable to any attempt at prolonged surveillance with current technology. Even this aggressive step does not preclude the development of ovarian cancer, as up to 10% of ovarian cancers are found in women who have had bilateral oophorectomies. These cancers are thought to arise from pluripotent celomic epithelial cells of the parietal and visceral peritoneum and are often multicentric in origin.

Other Adnexal Masses

Ectopic pregnancies, tubo-ovarian abscess, and hydrosalpinx are the most commonly encountered nonovarian causes of an adnexal mass. Ectopic pregnancies are seldom detected as an asymptomatic mass, but rather as a part of an acute or catastrophic process. In less acute presentations of ectopic pregnancy, a palpable mass is present only 50% of the time. Although the inflammation involved would suggest otherwise, a walled-off tubo-ovarian infection may be surprisingly asymptomatic, cystic, and mobile. Most often, tubo-ovarian abscesses behave as expected, with pain, fever, and tenderness predominating. Recurrent or chronic infection may be more indolent or may result in a cystic dilatation of the tube (hydrosalpinx), which may present as an adnexal mass. Embryonic remnants, in the form of paratubal or para-ovarian cysts, may reach sizes that make them symptomatic or easily palpated during routine examination.

Extrauterine Gynecologic Masses

Few gynecologic processes involve pelvic structures other than the uterus or adnexa, thus limiting most gynecologic masses to these locations. Two exceptions should be noted: endometriosis and the rare abdominal ectopic pregnancy. Although few clinicians encounter a true abdominal pregnancy, most will encounter patients with endometriosis. Endometriosis, which is a common cause of menstrual pain and dyspareunia, is closely associated with infertility. When advanced, it may be responsible for moderately large pelvic masses and must be considered in any differential diagnosis of a lower abdominal mass.

Endometriosis and its intramural uterine relative, adenomyosis, are relatively common. Many authors cite a prevalence of 10% to 15% for endometriosis in reproductive age women. About 20% of gynecologic laparotomies or laparoscopies, and 30% to 50% of infertility patients undergoing surgical exploration, demonstrate endometriosis. Although endometriosis and adenomyosis are benign, they are progressive and lead to ever-increasing symptoms and damage.

Although endometriosis and adenomyosis may appear at almost any point during the reproductive years, they are most common in the third and fourth decades of life. When endometriosis is found in younger patients, an obstructive anomaly (e.g., an unrecognized double uterus or a cervical and vaginal outflow-tract obstruction) must be considered. Endometriosis generally regresses following menopause.

Endometriosis and adenomyosis are both characterized by endometrial glands and stroma found in locations outside the endometrial lining. Nests of endometrial glands and stroma can occur in many diverse locations throughout the body, although they are most common in the pelvis. In adenomyosis, endometrial implants develop deep within the myometrial wall. Adenomyosis is, therefore, the intramural equivalent of extrauterine endometriosis, although only about 15% of patients with adenomyosis have coexistent endometriosis.

Endometriosis is thought to arise by one of several mechanisms: lymphatic spread, metaplasia of celomic epithelium or müllerian rests, and seeding by retrograde menstruation. Also proposed is direct hematogenous spread. Each of these theories has its proponents and experimental evidence in support. No theory explains all cases and it is likely that many mechanisms may play a part. Once endometrial implants develop, they respond to the hormonal environment in the same manner as the tissues of the endometrium. Under the influence of estrogen, proliferation takes place, which causes pressure on surrounding tissues and peritoneal surfaces. Further thickening happens with the secretory changes induced during the last half of the menstrual cycle. With the withdrawal of estrogen and progesterone at the end of the normal cycle, these ectopic sites of endometrium undergo destabilization and necrosis, which leads to the release of prostaglandins and other products of cellular destruction. These may account for local and systemic effects.

The most common site for endometriosis is on the surfaces of the ovaries, which occurs in about 60% of patients. Other common locations for endometriosis include the posterior cul-de-sac and uterosacral ligaments, fallopian tubes, and rectovaginal septum (Table 21.7). Surfaces of the bowel or the appendix may also be involved, as may episiotomy or cesarean section scars.

Endometrial implants may cause very little damage or may produce extensive damage, including large cystic structures filled with a characteristic thick, dark material. This material gives these "chocolate cysts" their name. When endometriosis involves peritoneal surfaces, it often appears as raised blue to brown spots ("powder burns"). These may range from one to several millimeters in size. Frequently surrounded by fibrosis, they may have a puckered appearance. Near the ovaries, the local inflammatory response engendered by endometriosis can cause dense adhesion formation to the posterior aspect of the broad ligament or the lateral pelvic wall. The resultant mass of tissue and necrotic material may reach

Table 21.7. Common Sites of Endometriosis

Most common site	Frequency (% of patients)
Ovary (frequently bilateral)	60
Pelvic peritoneum over the uterus	
Anterior and posterior cul-de-sacs	
Uterosacral ligaments	
Fallopian tubes	
Pelvic lymph nodes	30
Infrequent	
Rectosigmoid	10–15
Other gastrointestinal tract sites	5
Vagina	
Rare	
Umbilicus	
Episiotomy or surgical scars	
Kidney	
Lungs	
Arms	
Legs	
Nasal mucosa	

15 to 20 cm in diameter. When endometriosis involves the posterior cul-de-sac, retroversion of the uterus, fixation of the rectum, or even rectal damage may result.

Endometriosis does not cause any disruption in the rhythm of menstrual cycles. It may cause midcycle pain when ovarian involvement interferes with ovulation. Midcycle spotting or reduced menstrual flow may occur in patients with endometriosis, although this is not universal. Patients with significant adenomyosis, however, invariably have heavy, painful flow.

Nongynecologic Pelvic Masses

Gynecologists frequently forget that structures other than those of reproduction are found in the pelvis. This oversight is less common in the primary care setting, but the possibility must still be reiterated. Any structure that is normally found in the pelvis or may impinge upon it, including the abdominal wall itself, may be the source of a mass or swelling. This possibility must always be considered in the evaluation of patients with a pelvic mass. Examples of nongynecologic causes of a pelvic mass are shown in Table 21.8.

Abdominal Wall Masses

Although uncommon, the abdominal wall itself may be the source of a mass lesion. Hernias, rectus hematomas, lipomas, cutaneous infections, or enlarged lymph nodes may all present as a swelling or mass. Obese patients may easily have a hernia mistaken for an intra-abdominal mass because of the difficulty in identifying the boundaries of the abdominal wall.

Urologic Masses

Urinary tract structures may be the source of pelvic fullness or a mass, the majority of which will be midline in location. A distended bladder may not cause symptoms of urinary full-

Table 21.8. Nongynecologic Sources of a Pelvic Mass or Distension

Urinary tract
    Bladder carcinoma
    Bladder diverticulum
    Distended bladder (urinary retention)
    Pelvic or horseshoe kidney
    Polycystic kidney
    Urachal cyst
Gastrointestinal tract
    Appendiceal abscess
    Appendiceal tumor
    Carcinoma
    Cecum (distended or redundant)
    Diverticular disease
    Meckel's diverticulum
    Mesenteric cyst
    Sigmoid (distended or redundant)
Musculoskeletal system
    Chondroma
    Ganglioneuroma
    Glioma
    Hernia
    Neurofibroma
    Osteochondroma
    Osteogenic sarcoma
    Sacral meningoceles
Other
    Accessory spleen
    Ascites
    Aneurysm (aorta or pelvic vessels)
    Lymph nodes (Hodgkin's disease, lymphoma, lymphosarcoma)
    Hematoma
    Pancreatic cyst
    Peritoneal inclusion cyst
    Splenic cyst

ness or urgency in a patient who is overdistended owing to a neurogenic bladder or postoperative bladder atony. Congenital abnormalities of the urinary tract, such as a horseshoe kidney, a ptotic normal kidney (unilateral or bilateral), or a urachal cyst may all present as a pelvic mass. Intravenous pyelography or ultrasonography will often establish the diagnosis. The possibility of a bladder tumor must also be considered.

Gastrointestinal Masses

Pathologic processes and normal anatomic variants in the gastrointestinal tract may all account for a palpable pelvic or abdominal mass. A redundant sigmoid, distended cecum, mesenteric cyst, or a stool-filled segment of colon may provide a convincing mass during pelvic examination. Diverticular disease can cause significant perirectal and pelvic scarring, resulting in an indurated, somewhat fixed and tender midline mass. This may at times be difficult to differentiate from carcinoma, except for its more extraluminal location.

Musculoskeletal

As with the abdomenal wall, the musculoskeletal system is an uncommon source for pelvic masses. Predominantly found in the presacral or coccygeal area, congenital or acquired masses (e.g., a meningomyelocele, neurofibroma, or sarcoma) are rarely discovered at the time of pelvic examination. These must be differentiated from more common midline posterior masses caused by endometriosis, diverticular disease, and colon pathology.

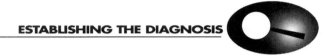

ESTABLISHING THE DIAGNOSIS

Although the classification of pelvic tumors is organized around tissues and pathophysiology, the clinical diagnosis is more often driven by the nature and acuity of any presenting symptoms. As noted, these characteristics are also important in planning therapeutic options.

Acute, Symptomatic Masses

Adnexal masses may invoke symptoms of pain or pressure and may be associated with fever, nausea, vomiting, diarrhea, syncope, or shock. In any reproductive age woman, adnexal pain (with or without a mass) should be considered an ectopic pregnancy until proved otherwise. The availability of rapid, sensitive β-HCG measurements and transvaginal ultrasonography make diagnosing ectopic pregnancy much easier, but only if the possibility has been entertained. There are many other processes that mimic an ectopic pregnancy that must also be considered (see Chapter 5, Complications of Early Pregnancy, Table 5.5).

The assessment of adnexal masses under emergency conditions can try the skill of the clinician but, if anything, is even more important than when time is not such a factor. A history of the character, onset, location, radiation, and alteration of the pain may help to suggest a cause. Acute, sharp pain is more likely to be due to torsion, bleeding, or rupture, whereas gradual growth or inflammation has a more indolent course. On palpation, masses that have undergone torsion will be mobile, cystic, and tender. Masses that have engendered an inflammatory response (abscess, endometriosis, or diverticular disease) will be more fixed and ill-defined.

Torsion of the adnexa is almost always associated with the presence of an ovarian, tubal, or paratubal mass. More common in the less well supported right adnexa, torsion occurs without apparent warning and is often the first indication of an adnexal mass. When torsion occurs, tissue ischemia and frank infarction result. The pain of torsion is generally abrupt, intense, and unilateral. Often accompanied by nausea and vomiting, the pain may wax and wane, with the gastrointestinal symptoms restricted to the peak of discomfort. Torsion must be differentiated from an ectopic pregnancy, generally by a pregnancy test. The absence of fever, leukocytosis, or a high sedimentation rate in the early phases of the process are also helpful in suggesting the diagnosis. Ultrasonography may demonstrate a cystic adnexal mass, but the acute character and intensity of symptoms usually encountered means that the diagnosis is most often made at the time of surgery.

Pelvic inflammatory disease with abscess formation may present acutely with pain and fever. Rupture of these abscesses represents a potentially life-threatening event that must be evaluated and acted upon quickly. Milder cases with abscess formation require aggressive antibiotic therapy and hospitalization (see Chapter 26, Sexually Transmitted Disease and "PID"). Torsion of an adnexal mass or bleeding into a cyst, although inherently less dangerous, nonetheless represents a problem that often necessitates prompt surgical therapy. Stabilization and complete assessment must, of course, be the first priority and carried out while consultation is being arranged and before the patient is taken to the operating room.

In acutely symptomatic patients who are, or may be, pregnant, ultrasonography is of greatest utility. Transvaginal ultrasonography may be diagnostic if extrauterine cardiac activity is detected. When an intrauterine gestation is documented, the chance of an additional ectopic pregnancy is low, but not zero. Detection of free fluid in the peritoneal cavity is of little help in the evaluation of patients suspected of inflammatory processes, as it cannot differentiate reliably between generalized peritoneal irritation, tubo-ovarian abscess (with or without rupture), appendicitis, bleeding, or normal peritoneal fluid occupying the dependent areas of the abdomen. Ancillary information, such as the patient's temperature, pulse, and white blood cell count, may be more helpful.

The management of most acutely symptomatic adnexal masses will be surgical. Exceptions to this include those patients who are thought to have a ruptured benign cyst (follicular or luteal), who are stable, and who have improving symptoms. Here, watchful waiting is appropriate. Certainly, unstable patients, such as those with ectopic pregnancies, torsion, or ruptured abscesses, require rapid stabilization and surgical therapy.

Asymptomatic Masses

The management of asymptomatic masses varies with age; reproductive age patients are much more likely to have benign processes, older patients may have neoplasia or a malignancy. Just as in those with acute symptoms, much of the diagnosis and subsequent therapy will be based on history and physical evaluation. For example, older patients with a history of a change in bowel habits require an evaluation of the colon, whereas a young woman with a small unilateral cyst found near midcycle may only require re-evaluation during the early part of the next menstrual cycle.

There are no laboratory tests that are of specific help in the global diagnosis of pelvic masses. Laboratory investigations may support specific diagnoses. Examples would be the use of an elevated white blood count or erythrocyte sedimentation rate in patients with tubo-ovarian abscesses or a positive pregnancy test in a patient suspected of having an ectopic pregnancy.

Young Patients

Premenarchal patients with pelvic masses require careful and aggressive evaluation. Nongynecologic causes must be evaluated and the possibility of pregnancy (although unlikely) must be considered in adolescent girls, even if menarche has not been demonstrated. Adnexal masses of gynecologic origin must be treated in a manner similar to that applied to women after the menopause: the mass is presumed to be malignant until proved otherwise. Imaging and early consultation are indicated in these patients.

Reproductive Age Patients

Midline pelvic masses are most often due to pregnancy, leiomyomata, or other nongynecologic causes. The possibility of a pregnancy is easily addressed, leaving leiomyomata as the next most likely diagnosis. Asymptomatic adnexal masses in menstrual age women are most often due to functional processes such as those related to pregnancy, pedunculated leiomyomata, and follicular or luteal cysts.

The diagnosis of fibroids is established on clinical findings, based primarily on palpation, uterine sounding and, occasionally, ultrasound in patients who are difficult to examine. Fibroids should be firm, smooth, nontender, and clearly associated with the uterine corpus. Although ultrasonography, tomography, or magnetic resonance imaging often can make the diagnosis of fibroids, these modalities are seldom required for diagnosis.

Masses lateral to the uterus may be adnexal in origin or may be due to nongynecologic processes. The history and physical examination can help narrow the potential diagnoses by suggesting the possibility of an ectopic pregnancy, tubo-ovarian abscess, or musculoskeletal, gastrointestinal, or urologic cause. Ultrasonography is useful in distinguishing solid and cystic masses and can often help identify the approximate origin of the mass in question.

There are a number of factors that may help suggest the likelihood that an adnexal mass is benign or malignant (Table 21.9). These characteristics, along with the size and location of the mass, may be used to guide the diagnosis and management of these patients (Fig. 21.2). Benign adnexal masses should be smooth, round, cystic, mobile, and nontender. When their location and character can be reliably assessed (in a thin, cooperative patient) and the size of the mass is less than 6 cm, observation is appropriate. Re-evaluation of the mass in 2 to 6 weeks to look for regression may be all that is required.

Ultrasonography, computed tomography, and magnetic imaging are of limited value in evaluating asymptomatic masses in young patients. Exceptions to this are those patients in whom clinical assessment is impractical or inadequate (e.g., massive obesity) or those in whom malignancy is suspected. For these patients, ultrasound imaging may help to differentiate cystic and solid masses or to separate uterine from adnexal processes. Computed tomography may help evaluating enlarged lymph nodes, a thickened omental cake, collections of ascitic fluid, or extra-pelvic involvement when a malignancy is suspected.

Prior to making the diagnosis of endometriosis, the clinician must also entertain other processes that could produce the patient's complaints and findings. When pelvic pain is present, pelvic scarring due to surgery or to infection, uterine fibroids, gastrointestinal, urologic, or musculoskeletal problems are all potential considerations. Retroversion or fixation of the uterus should suggest the possibility of endometriosis or pelvic scarring, but does not

Table 21.9. Diagnostic Features Suggestive of Benign or Malignant Processes

Characteristic	Benign processes	Malignant processes
Character	Cystic	Solid or lobulated cystic
Location	Midline	Lateral
Mobility	Mobile	Fixed
Surface	Smooth	Rough or shaggy
Ultrasonography	Thin wall (<3 mm)	Thick wall (>3 mm)
	Smooth inner wall	Papillary inner wall
	Simple cyst	Solid or septated cystic

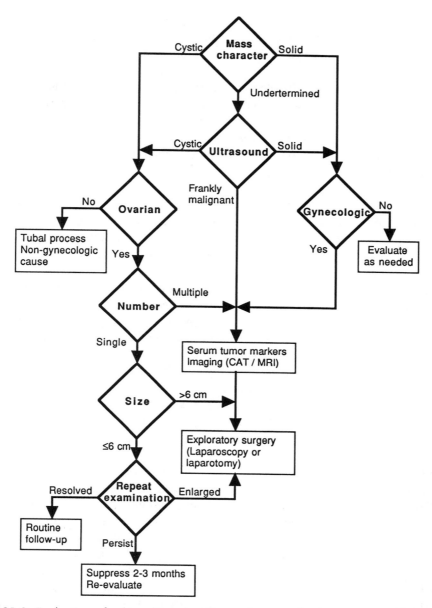

Figure 21.2. Evaluation of adnexal masses. The evaluation of pelvic masses in reproductive age, nonpregnant women depends to a great extent on the character of the mass. Solid masses of gynecologic origin should be considered suggestive of malignancy and evaluated with computed tomography (to look for signs of distant disease) and prepared for surgical exploration and diagnosis. Small, unilocular masses may be followed or suppressed, whereas masses that are multiple, large, grow, or do not suppress also require surgical intervention.

confirm it. Tubal damage and pelvic adhesions are particularly possible in patients with coexisting infertility.

The evaluation of the patient's history and physical examination is extremely important in making the diagnosis of endometriosis or adenomyosis. The patient with endometriosis often presents with symptoms of pelvic pain, dyspareunia, or premenstrual and menstrual pain. The pain and dyspareunia reported by these patients is of the visceral, or "deep thrust" type. This is especially true when endometriosis involves the uterosacral ligaments. Some patients have pain with bowel movements (dyschezia) caused by these uterosacral ligament implants. Involuntary infertility is also a frequent but not invariant presenting complaint. Patients with adenomyosis generally report heavy periods with clots and cramps, although up to 40% of patients may be asymptomatic.

Pelvic examination of patients with endometriosis may reveal tender nodules along the uterosacral ligaments or in the posterior cul-de-sac. When present, these nodules are very helpful in establishing the diagnosis. Large cystic masses caused by endometriosis may be fixed or free, tender or nontender, unilateral or bilateral. They may range from small to large and are not always accompanied by other findings suggestive of endometriosis. Often the pain reported by patients seems inversely proportional to the amount of disease; small implants seem to be exquisitely painful and large endometriomata may be asymptomatic.

Any diagnosis of endometriosis based solely on history or physical findings must be considered provisional. Ultimately, the diagnosis of endometriosis rests on direct inspection of the involved area, supported by histologic confirmation. In the case of adenomyosis, only histology can confirm the diagnosis. Many patients receive presumptive treatment, without laparoscopic confirmation of endometriosis, because of laparoscopy's invasive nature. The patient with probable endometriosis needs little additional evaluation beyond the history and physical prior to considering diagnostic laparoscopy. As technology improves, there may be a place for endovaginal ultrasonography or magnetic resonance imaging, but at present they are of limited utility in establishing the diagnosis.

Adenomyosis may be suspeced clinically, but is ultimately a histologic diagnosis. The characteristic history of painful, heavy periods, accompanied by a generous, symmetric, firm or "woody" uterus suggests, but does not confirm, the diagnosis.

Older Patients

Perimenopausal and postmenopausal patients may still have benign processes causing an adnexal mass, but the likelihood of a malignant process is much increased, thereby altering their management. In these patients, masses larger than 6 cm generally prompt surgical exploration and excision. In some studies, masses larger than 10 cm carried a greater than 60% risk of malignancy, whereas masses smaller than 5 cm had less than a 5% chance of being cancerous. The availability of transvaginal ultrasonography to measure and track masses has meant that smaller masses that once would have required exploration may be followed conservatively. As in younger patients, the size, shape, mobility, and consistency of the mass should be estimated. Irregular, immobile, or mixed character masses (solid and cystic) are more likely to be malignant and deserve immediate consultation and surgical exploration. The final diagnosis of ovarian cancer must be made surgically.

Serum testing for tumor markers, such as CA-125, lipid-associated sialic acid (LSA), carcinoembryonic antigen (CEA), alpha-fetoprotein (AFP), and others, should be reserved for use in following the progress of patients with known malignancies and not used for prognostic evaluation. No combination of serum tests has proved to be a consistent or accurate screening tool. Many nonmalignant processes, such as endometriosis, may lead to moderate elevations of these markers, yielding false-positive results. The absence of elevations in these tests cannot disprove the possibility of cancer. The combination of high false-positive and false-negative rates has left these tests best suited for following the results of surgery, chemotherapy, or radiation treatments. If uncertainty exists, a sample may be drawn prior to surgery and held until the gross or microscopic appearance of the mass is determined. If malignancy is confirmed or strongly suspected, it may be processed at that point to provide a baseline value. If benign disease is found, the sample is discarded.

THERAPEUTIC OPTIONS

Fibroids

The management of patients with uterine leiomyomata has changed somewhat over the past decade. Improved imaging techniques have allowed more conservative therapy to be available for most patients. Despite this change, the mainstay of therapy for fibroids remains surgery. Ultimately, the choice of therapy should be based on the age of the patient and her desire for fertility, the size of the uterine myoma, the presence and severity of symptoms, and ancillary conditions that may affect the patient's care. One possible decision algorithm involving these factors is shown in Figure 21.3.

Surgical Therapy

The traditional indications for surgery for fibroids have been based on three broad considerations (in the absence of acute problems such as prolapse, torsion, or degeneration). These three criteria are: refractory symptoms, size, and rate of growth. Symptoms such as bleeding, pressure, pain, recurrent abortion, infertility, or urinary compromise may indicate the need for surgical therapy if medical options cannot be applied or have failed. It has been recommended that uterine fibroids of greater than 12 to 14 weeks size (or single fibroids greater than 8 cm in women desiring fertility) be removed. This has been based both on the presumption that fibroids of this size will eventually become symptomatic and on the inability to assess the adnexa clinically. When the pelvic examination was the primary modality for diagnosing adnexal pathology, the latter reason was possibly the most compelling. However, the use of ultrasonography to image the adnexa has blunted this indication. When fibroids grow rapidly or show growth after the menopause, exploration and removal is indicated because of the possibility of a malignancy or an incorrect diagnosis. Edema, infection, or carneous degeneration of fibroids may also cause rapid growth in the size of fibroids. The risk of malignant change (sarcoma) in fibroids is extremely low, generally below 0.3%.

Myomectomy is customarily chosen for those who desire continuing fertility, for asymptomatic fibroids greater than 8 cm, and those women with a limited number of fibroids. Myomectomy is contraindicated in the presence of pregnancy, adnexal disease, known malignancy, or in those cases where it would cause a major disruption of the endometrial surface. In those patients who undergo myomectomy, between 25% to 90% will have recurrences and 25% to 60% will undergo hysterectomy or require other therapy in the subsequent 20 years. Term pregnancy rates are generally reported in the range of 40% for those who undergo myomectomy. Both the patient and those providing the counseling

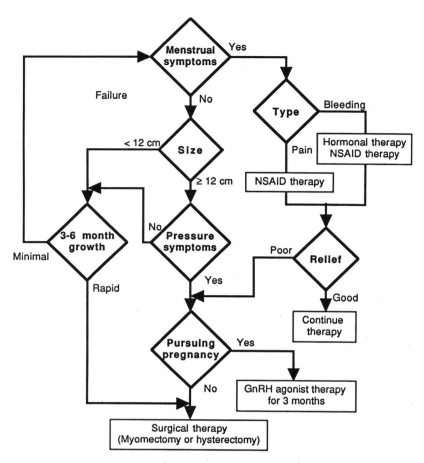

Figure 21.3. Management of premenopausal uterine leiomyomata. Premenopausal women with known leiomyomata can generally be managed in a conservative manner. If rapid growth occurs, the diagnosis must be suspected and the possibility of an adnexal growth mimicking fibroids, degeneration in one or more fibroids, an intrauterine process, or a sarcoma evaluated. NSAID = Nonsteroidal anti-inflammatory drug; GnRH = gonadotropin-releasing hormone.

should be aware that between 10% and 30% of planned myomectomies become hysterectomies at the time of surgery, owing to the number or location of the fibroids encountered. Up to one third of myomectomy patients experience febrile morbidity during the immediate postoperative period.

In addition to pelvic exploration, hysterectomy provides an opportunity to treat ancillary problems, but results in the obvious loss of fertility. Hysterectomy, of course, is major surgery, with 8% to 15% of patients requiring transfusion when fibroids are present.

Nonsurgical Therapy

Surgery is not always the best choice for patients with leiomyomata. Before following a conservative course, it is important to ascertain whether the fibroids are the true cause of the patient's findings and symptomatology. This is especially true in patients with chronic pelvic pain because fibroids are rarely the cause of any long-term discomfort greater than a vague sense of pelvic heaviness. In the case of bleeding or dysmenorrhea, therapies such as non-steroidal anti-inflammatory drugs or oral contraceptives may provide satisfactory results.

Medical therapy with medroxyprogesterone acetate has been advocated to suppress ovulation and decrease circulating estrogen levels slightly. This usually resolves symptoms of pain or bleeding, but the uterine fibroids generally remain unchanged. Danazol sodium can be used to reduce estrogen levels, but it is associated with a number of side effects, making it less desirable. Excellent, but relatively short-term results can be obtained using gonadotropin-releasing hormone (GnRH) agonists. These agents create a reversible medical menopause, during which time uterine volume is often dramatically decreased. Reductions of 50% to 60% in overall uterine volume and 50% in the size of large uterine fibroids are not uncommon. The amenorrhea that accompanies this treatment is often associated with a significant rise in hemoglobin and hematocrit. Maximal uterine response is generally achieved in 3 months of therapy, but unfortunately a return to pretreatment levels is often seen within 6 months of discontinuing the medication. For this reason, the role of GnRH agonist therapy is generally restricted to attempts to increase the possibility of myomectomy, to enable endoscopic or vaginal approaches to therapy, to improve the patient's preoperative condition, or to reduce the operative blood loss and chance of intraoperative transfusion. When intraoperative blood loss has been measured, a reduction by one third or greater has been recorded following GnRH pretreatment. Some patients who are pursuing pregnancy may be treated just prior to conception in an effort to reduce the chance of pregnancy loss or complications due to the size and presence of fibroids.

Adnexal Masses

Some authors favor placing young patients with small, presumably benign, cystic masses on ovulation suppression therapy, such as oral contraceptives, to hasten the process of regression. Regression rates of 65% to 75% are often cited for this approach; however, because definitive studies are lacking, this strategy is largely a matter of personal choice. Physiologic ovarian enlargements, including follicular or corpus luteum cysts, should not be present in oral contraceptive users. For this reason, patients who are already using oral contraceptives and develop adnexal masses are more likely to have pathology that will not regress, increasing the possibility that eventual surgical exploration may be required.

Because the risk of ovarian cancer increases with age and ovarian size decreases after the menopause, it was once felt that any palpable ovary found in a postmenopausal women had to be investigated as a possible cancer. This included surgical exploration for any ovary larger than 4 cm to 6 cm in size. Studies of these women have shown that the risk of surgical intervention is greater than the likelihood of finding malignant disease. The advent of high-quality imaging through ultrasonography, magnetic resonance, or computed tomography has allowed most of these women to be followed clinically. Those without overt evidences of malignancy, such as ascites, adenopathy, complex echo pattern, or fixation of the mass, may be followed as long as no growth of the mass is found. Some authors have suggested that this be restricted to women within 3 years of menopause and to masses less than 5 cm in size.

Masses that are greater than 6 cm and those that enlarge or become symptomatic require surgical evaluation or therapy, no matter what the patient's age. This may be carried out by laparoscopy or laparotomy based on the skill and preference of the surgeon, as well as the proposed pathology and planned intervention. Benign ovarian cysts can generally be treated conservatively by removal of the cyst, preserving as much ovarian tissue as possible for patients of reproductive age. Extensive tubo-ovarian abscesses, endometriosis, or endometriomata of greater than 5 cm generally require more extensive surgical therapy. Total abdominal hysterectomy with bilateral salpingo-oophorectomy is preferable when further fertility is not an issue. Preservation of the ovaries in younger women or estrogen replacement therapy for those with oophorectomy does not introduce significant risk of recurrence for patients with endometriosis. For those patients desiring further fertility, conservative surgery consists of resection of endometriomata, lysis of adhesions, and ablation of implants using electrocautery or laser. Some authors advocate uterine suspension to prevent retroversion and fixation, although the value of this is subject to debate. Ovarian cancer is treated by surgery, supplemented by chemotherapy and/or radiation therapy, and should be managed under the care of a gynecologic oncologist.

Medical therapy is appropriate for patients with minimal to moderate endometriosis. For the patient with minimal disease and tolerable symptoms, therapy with oral progestins or a combination oral contraceptive agent may provide adequate suppression of the endometrial implants. When symptoms are more troublesome, a pseudopregnancy induced using continuous high-dose progestins (e.g., medroxyprogesteron acetate 20 to 30 mg/d) or continuous oral contraceptives in rising doses are often effective. Most patients gain some benefit and up to 40% of patients may eventually conceive with this therapy. Despite this success, many patients do not tolerate this therapy well and endometriosis often returns following treatment cessation.

For patients with more advanced endometriosis, a pseudomenopause may be effective, using either an estrogen agonist (such as danazol sodium) or GnRH agonists (such as luprolide or nafarelin). With either therapy a transient worsening of symptoms may occur at the start of therapy. Both therapeutic approaches are expensive and carry the potential for significant side effects. Neither therapy ensures long-term success. In early studies with danazol, 40% of patients had a recurrence after 3 years.

Re-evaluation of any endometriosis therapy must be at no less than 6-month intervals. History and physical evaluations are usually sufficient. In more complicated cases, or those in which fertility is an issue, consider a follow-up hysterosalpingogram or repeat laparoscopy. Consultation should be obtained as needed.

HINTS AND COMMON QUESTIONS

In reproductive age women, a normal ovary is palpable about half of the time, but less often in postmenopausal women and in those taking oral contraceptive agents.

Women close to menopause are more likely to have residual functional ovarian cysts, making the ovaries slightly larger and more irregular. This enlargement is generally bilateral and roughly symmetric.

Uterine fibroids are extremely rare before the age of 20. As a result, other diagnoses should be entertained in these patients.

Although 5% to 15% of infertility patients have uterine fibroids, most studies suggest that only 2% to 3% have no other cause of infertility. As a result, care must be taken not to mislead patients about the reproductive impact of either their fibroids or of fibroid-directed therapy.

Endometrial biopsy is seldom of help in establishing the diagnosis of fibroids, adenomyosis, or leiomyosarcoma.

Calcification in uterine leiomyomata or dermoids is common and often demonstrated on x-ray studies. The presence of such calcification, however, does not differentiate between benign fibroids and other pathologies.

Some types of uterine fibroids may show some enhancement on computed tomography when iodinated contrast material is used. This may make them difficult to differentiate from intrauterine malignancies.

Ultrasonography is generally of greater value than computed tomography in the evaluation of pelvic masses.

If a functional ovarian cyst is suspected in a woman of reproductive age, the mass should be re-evaluated during the first 10 days of the next menstrual cycle.

Because the contents of cystic teratomas are of low density, they are often found "floating" anterior to the uterus, displacing the uterus posteriorly. Other cystic ovarian tumors, including endometriomas, are more likely to displace the uterus forward.

The pain of adnexal torsion generally comes and goes with a periodicity that varies from hours to days, or longer. This is in contrast to the variable pain caused by obstruction of the bowel, ureter, or common bile duct, which is more regular and frequent.

Pain that is acute, short, and accompanies intercourse or exertion, may be due to rupture of a normal follicle at midcycle or to bleeding into a corpus luteum late in the menstrual cycle, just prior to menses. Only if symptoms progress is intervention required. Follow-up during the first 10 days of the next menstrual cycle is indicated, to check for signs of persistence or other adnexal pathology.

Tubo-ovarian abscesses tend to be bilateral, except in some patients wearing an intrauterine contraceptive device.

The number of pelvic examinations performed on patients suspected of having a tubo-ovarian abscess should be limited to reduce the likelihood of bacteremia, intraperitoneal spill, or outright rupture. Such events are associated with devastating consequences and should be avoided.

Unlike oral contraceptives which reduce the risk, there is no evidence that the use of postmenopausal hormone replacement therapy has any effect, either positive or negative, on the risk of ovarian cancer.

Women with ovarian cancer may report increasing abdominal girth despite constant or reduced caloric intake. Although hepatic, renal, or cardiac disease; benign tumors; ascites; or other nongynecologic processes may cause similar symptoms, the practitioner should be alerted to the possibility of ovarian cancer when confronted with such a history.

Biochemical markers are sometimes useful in monitoring the response of ovarian cancer to surgery, radiation, or chemotherapy. They are not, however, useful in differentiating benign from malignant disease. Only surgical exploration, with cytologic and histologic confirmation, can make that distinction.

In endometriosis, there is a seeming paradox between the extent of disease and the severity of symptoms. As a result, the first indication of disease in asymptomatic patients may be the palpation of an endometrioma or scarred and swollen adnexal structures.

Cervical cytology detects only about 20% of known endometrial carcinomas. When endometrial cancer is a possibility, endometrial sampling must be performed.

SUGGESTED READINGS

General References

Grimes DA, Economy KE. Primary prevention of gynecologic cancers. Am J Obstet Gynecol 1995;172:227.

Jones HW III. Ovarian cysts and tumors. In Jones HW III, Wentz AC, Burnett LS (eds). Novak's Textbook of Gynecology, 11th ed. Baltimore: Williams & Wilkins, 1988;782–783.

Stenchever MA. Approach to the patient. In Herbst AL, Mishell DR, Stenchever MA, Droegemueller WR (eds). Comprehensive Gynecology, 2nd ed. St Louis: CV Mosby, 1992;172–179.

VanNagell JR Jr, Depriest PC, Gallian HH, Pavlik EJ. Ovarian cancer screening. Cancer 1993;71:1523.

Vollenhoven BJ, Lawrence AS, Healy DL. Uterine fibroids: a clinical review. Br J Obstet Gynaecol 1990;97:285.

Wingo PA, Tong T, Bolden S. Cancer statistics 1995. CA Cancer J Clin 1995;45:8.

Specific References

General Diagnosis and Management

Bachmann GA. Hysterectomy: a critical review. J Reprod Med 1990;35:839.

Bayer AI, Wiskind AK. Adnexal torsion: can the adnexa be saved? Am J Obstet Gynecol 1994;171:1506.

Boente MP, Godwin AK, Hogan WM. Screening, imaging and early diagnosis of ovarian cancer. Clin Obstet Gynecol 1994;37:377.

Cane P, Azen C, Lopez E, Platt LD, Karlan BY. Tumor marker trends in asymptomatic women at risk for ovarian cancer: relevance for ovarian cancer screening. Gynecol Oncol 1995;57:240.

Carter JR, Lau M, Fowler JM, Carlson JW, Carson LF, Twiggs LB. Blood flow characteristics or ovarian tumors: implications for ovarian cancer screening. Am J Obstet Gynecol 1995;172:901.

Coddington CC, Collins RC, Shawker TH, et al. Long-acting gonadotropin hormone-releasing hormone analog used to treat uteri. Fertil Steril 1986;45:624.

Fleischer AC. Transabdominal and transvaginal sonography of ovarian masses. Clin Obstet Gynecol 1991;34:433.

Goldstein SR. Conservative management of small postmenopausal cystic masses. Clin Obstet Gynecol 1993;36:395.

Jacobs I, Davies AP, Bringes J, et al. Prevalence screening for ovarian cancer in postmenopausal women by CA 125 measurement and ultrasonography. BMJ 1993;306:1030.

Jain KA. Prospective evaluation of adnexal masses with endovaginal gray-scale and duplex and color Doppler US: correlation with pathologic findings. Radiology. 1994;191:63.

Kroon E, Andolf E. Diagnosis and follow-up of simple ovarian cysts detected by ultrasound in postmenopausal women. Obstet Gynecol 1995;85:211.

Pittaway DE, Fayex JA, Douglas JW. Serum CA 125 in the evaluation of benign adnexal cysts. Am J Obstet Gynecol 1987;157:1426.

Schwartz PE. Ovarian masses: serological markers. Clin Obstet Gynecol 1991;34:423.

Schwartz PE. The role of tumor markers in the preoperative diagnosis of ovarian cysts. Clin Obstet Gynecol 1993;36:384.

Suren A, Osmers R, Kulenkampff D, Kuhn W. Visualization of blood flow in small ovarian tumor vessels by transvaginal color doppler sonography after echo enhancement with injection of Levovist. Gynecol Obstet Invest 1994;38:210.

Weiner Z, Thaler I, Beck D, et al. Differentiating malignant from benign ovarian tumors with transvaginal color flow imaging. Obstet Gynecol 1992;79:159.

Whittemore AS, Harris R, Itnyre J. Characteristics relating to ovarian cancer risk: collaborative analysis of twelve U. S. case-control studies. II. Invasive epithelial ovarian cancers in white women. Am J Epidemiol 1992;136:1184.

Woolas RP, Xu FJ, Jacobs IJ, et al. Elevations of multiple serum markers in patients with stage I ovarian cancer. J Natl Cancer Inst 1993;85:1748.

Yamashita Y, Torashima M, Hatanaka Y, et al. Adnexal masses: accuracy of characterization with transvaginal US and precontrast and postcontrast MR imaging. Radiology 1995;194:557.

Zanetta G, Vergani P, Lissoni A. Color doppler ultrasound in the preoperative assessment of adnexal masses. Acta Obstet Gynecol Scand 1994;73:637.

Fibroids

American Fertility Society. Myomas and reproductive dysfunction: guideline for practice. Birmingham, Alabama: AFS, 1992.

Brown JM, Malkasian GD, Symmonds RE. Abdominal myomectomy. Am J Obstet Gynecol 1967;99:126.

Burton CA, Grimes DA, March CM. Surgical management of leiomyomata during pregnancy. Obstet Gynecol 1989;74:707.

Cramer SF, Horiszny JA, Leppert P. Epidemiology of uterine leiomyomas. J Reprod Med 1995;40:595.

Cramer SF, Patel D. The frequency of uterine leiomyomas. Am J Clin Pathol 1990;94:435.

Friedman AJ, Haas ST. Should uterine size be an indication for surgical intervention in women with myomas? Am J Obstet Gynecol 1993;168:751.

Maheux R, Guilloteau C, Lemay A, Bastido A, Fazekas AT. Regression of leiomata uteri following hypoestrogenism induced by repetitive luteinizing hormone-releasing hormone agonist treatment: preliminary report. Fertil Steril 1984;42:644.

Parazzini F, Negri E, LaVecchia C, et al. Oral contraceptive use and risk of uterine fibroids. Obstet Gynecol 1992;79:430.

Reiter RC, Wagner PL, Gambone JC. Routine hysterectomy for large asymptomatic uterine leiomyomata: a reappraisal. Obstet Gynecol 1992;79:481.

Winer-Muram HT, Muram D, Gillieson MS. Uterine myomas in pregnancy. Journal of the Canadian Association of Radiology 1984;35:168.

Adnexal Masses and Ovarian Cancer

Adami H-O, Hsieh C-C, Lambe M, et al. Parity, age at first childbirth, and risk of ovarian cancer. Lancet 1994;344:1250.

Adamson GD, Pasta DJ. Surgical treatment of endometriosis-associated infertility: meta-analysis compared with survival analysis. Am J Obstet Gynecol 1994;171:1488.

Andolf E. Ultrasound screening in women at risk for ovarian cancer. Clin Obstet Gynecol 1993;36:423.

Averette HE, Nguyen HN. The role of prophylactic oophorectomy in cancer prevention. Gynecol Oncol 1994;55:S38.

Booth M, Beral V, Smith P. Risk factors for ovarian cancer: a case control study. Br J Cancer 1989;60:592.

Carlson KJ, Skates SJ, Singer DE. Screening for ovarian cancer. Ann Intern Med 1994;121:124.

Daly MB, Lerman C. Ovarian cancer risk counseling: a guide for the practitioner. Oncology 1993;7:27.

Herman JR, Locher GW, Goldhirsch A. Sonographic patterns of ovarian tumors: prediction of malignancy. Obstet Gynecol 1987;69:777.

Howard FM. Surgical management of benign cystic teratoma: laparoscopy vs. laparotomy. J Reprod Med 1995;40:495.

Karlan BY, Platt DL. The current status of ultrasound and color doppler imaging in screening for ovarian cancer. Gynecol Oncol 1994;55:S28.

Kerlikowske K, Brown JS, Grady DG. Should women with familial ovarian cancer undergo prophylactic oophorectomy? Obstet Gynecol 1992;80:700.

Lynch HT, Severin MJ, Mooney MJ, Lynch J. Insurance adjudication favoring prophylactic surgery in hereditary breast-ovarian cancer syndrome. Gynecol Oncol 1995;57:23.

Lynch HT, Watson P, Conway T, Lynch J. Hereditary ovarian cancer: Natural history, surveillance, management, and genetic counseling. Hematology-Oncology Annals 1994;2:107.

Mackey SE, Creasman WT. Ovarian cancer screening. J Clin Oncol 1995;13:783.

Mais V, Guerriero S, Ajossa S, Angiolucci M, Paoletti AM, Melis GB. Transvaginal ultrasonography in the diagnosis of cystic teratoma. Obstet Gynecol 1995;85:48.

Rosenberg L, Palmer JR, Zauber AG, et al. A case-control study of oral contraceptive use and invasive epithelial ovarian cancer. Am J Epidemiol 1994;139:654.

Rosenberg L, Shapiro S, Slone D, et al. Epithelial ovarian cancer and combination oral contraceptives. JAMA 1982;247:3210.

Seltzer V, Batson JL, Drukker BH, et al. NIH Consensus Development Panel on Ovarian Cancer. Ovarian cancer: screening, treatment, and follow-up. JAMA 1995;273:491.

Whittemore AS, Harris R, Itnyre J, the Collaborative Ovarian Cancer Group. Characteristics relating to ovarian cancer risk: collaborative analysis of 12 case-controlled studies. Am J Epidemiol 1992;136:1184.

Endometriosis

Barbieri RL. Etiology and epidemiology of endometriosis. Am J Obstet Gynecol 1990;162:565.

Butler L, Wilson E, Belisle S, et al. Collaborative study of pregnancy rates following danazol therapy of stage I endometriosis. Fertil Steril 1984;41:373.

Buttram VC Jr. Evolution of the revised American Fertility Society classification of endometriosis. Fertil Steril 1985;43:347.

Buttram VC. Conservative surgery for endometriosis in the infertile female: a sudy of 206 patients with implications for both medical and surgical therapy. Fertil Steril 1979;31;117.

Cook AS, Rock JA. The role of laparoscopy in the treatment of endometriosis. Fertil Steril 1991;55:663.

Egger H, Weisman P. Clinical and surgical aspects of ovarian endometriotic cysts. Arch Gynecol Obstet 1982;233:37.

Friedman AJ, Hornstein MD. Gonadotropin-releasing hormone agonist plus estogen-progestin "add-back" therapy for endometriosis-related pelvic pain. Fertil Steril 1993;60:236.

Hughes EG, Fedorkow DM, Collins JA. A quantitative overview of controlled trials in endometriosis-associated infertility. Fertil Steril 1993;59:963.

Laube DW, Calderwood GW, Benda JA. Endometriosis causing ureteral obstruction. Obstet Gynecol 1985;65:69S.

Lauerson NH, Wilson KH, Birnbaum S. Danazol: an antigonadotropic agent in the treatment of pelvic endometriosis. Am J Obstet Gynecol 1975;123:742.

Meldrum DR, Chang RJ, Lu J, Vale W, Rivier J, Judd HL. "Medical oophorectomy" using a long-acting GNRH agonist—A possible new approach to the treatment of endometriosis. J Clin Endocrinol Metab 1982;54:1081.

Nicholson SC, Slade RJ, Ahmed AIH, Gillmer MDG. Endometrial resection in Oxford: The first 500 cases—A 5-year follow-up. Br J Obstet Gynaecol 1995;15:38.

Olive DL, Schwartz LB. Endometriosis. N Engl J Med 1993;328:1759.

Pittaway DE. CA-125 in women with endometriosis. Obstet Gynecol Clin N Am 1989;16:227.

Punnonen RH, Kikkanen VP. Endometriosis in young women. Infertility 1980;3:1.

Sampson JA. Peritoneal endometriosis due to dissemination of endometrial tissue into the peritoneal cavity. Am J Obstet Gynecol 1927;14:422.

Schmiidt CL. Endometriosis: a reappraisal of pathogenesis and treatment. Fertil Steril 1985;44:157.

Schriock E, Monroe SE, Henzl M, Jaffe RB. Treatment of endometriosis with a potent agonist of gonadotropin-releasing hormone (nafarelin). Fertil Steril 1985;44:583.

Schweppe KW, Wynn RM. Ultrastructural changes in endometriotic implants during the menstrual cycle. Obstet Gynecol 1981;58:465.

Waller KG, Shaw RW. GnRH analogs in the treatment of endometriosis: long-term follow-up. Fertil Steril 1993;59:511.

Wentz AC. Premenstrual spotting: its association with endometriosis but not luteal phase inadequacy. Fertil Steril 1980;33:605.

Willims TJ, Pratt JH. Endometriosis in 1,000 consecutive celiotomies: Incidence and management. Am J Obstet Gynecol 1977;129:245.

Wright S, Valdes CT, Dunn RC, Franklin RR. Short-term Lupron or Danazol therapy for pelvic endometriosis. Fertil Steril 1995;63:504.

Other Masses

Cady B, Stone MD, Wayne J. Continuing trends in the prevalence of right-sided lesions among colorectal carcinoma. Arch Surg 1993;128:505.

Peipert JF, Wells CK, Schwartz PE, Feinstein AR. Prognostic value of clinical variables in invasive cervical cancer. Obstet Gynecol 1994;84:746.

Simon J. Occult blood screening for colorectal cancer: a critical review. Gastroenterology 1985;88:820.

Winawer SJ, Zauber AG, Stewart E, O'Brien MJ. The natural history of colorectal cancer. Cancer 1991;67:1143.

22

Pelvic Pain

Acute pain is usually a harbinger of physiologic distress. No process that generates the sensation of "pain" is without physiologic risk at some level. Whether it is pressure atrophy of the gums during natural teething or the disruption of the cervix and vagina during childbirth, even "normal" processes that involve pain represent, at least on the cellular level, some element of adversity. Acute pelvic or abdominal pain may be the first sign of a life-threatening process ranging from ectopic pregnancy to appendicitis. In these situations, a rapid, focused examination and prompt diagnosis are necessary to prevent major disability or loss of life.

Chronic pain is a major source of morbidity and disability, costing uncounted billions of dollars annually in both direct and indirect costs. Pelvic pain is by far the most common type of chronic pain complaint suffered by women, accounting for up to 10% of all outpatient gynecology visits. The investigation, diagnosis, and treatment of chronic pelvic pain accounts for one third of laparoscopic procedures and 15% of hysterectomies performed in the United States every year. Every clinician is familiar with the degree of disability (and clinical frustration) caused by chronic pelvic pain. In the face of poorly defined symptoms, secondary agendas, often unrealistic expectations, and a sense of failure (by both doctor and patient), the process of establishing a cause of the patient's complaints is difficult and intimidating. A specific organic cause is often difficult or impossible to establish. Frequently symptoms of depression, fatigue, loss of libido, and disturbances in eating and sleeping accompany the complaints of pain. Ultimately, the pain itself takes on the character of disease, no longer just a symptom. Although a difficult task, identification of the cause of this enigmatic problem is critical to effective therapy. Even in cases of chronic pain, the value of a timely, correct diagnosis cannot be overstressed. Achieving that diagnosis, however, sometimes requires all the skill and talent a clinician can muster.

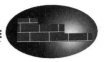

"Pain"

There are no tests to detect or measure pain; pain is a perception, nothing more. Generally, but not always, pain is based on information sent through the nervous system from diverse locations in the body. Four phases are involved in pain: nociception, or the origination and detection of a neural signal caused by a noxious event; pain, or the recognition of the signal or event; suffering, or affective responses to the event; and pain behavior, or adaptive changes (functional or dysfunctional) made based on the pain. Based on this sequence, pain results directly from, and is proportional to, tissue trauma. This model is useful in conditions like appendicitis, but is inadequate to describe what occurs in chronic pain states.

A broader pain theory includes the moderating and compounding effects of psychosocial factors. These factors modify the type and degree of symptoms expressed in response to a given stimulus. This model of pain explains the observation that the perception of pain and reactions to it are based on a complex interaction of individual variability, expectation, culture or rearing, emotion, and mood. As a result, what creates pain, and the impact of that pain, is inconstant and unpredictable from person to person and from time to time. At times there is little or no apparent relationship between the stimulus and the response. Even the characterization of pain as always emotionally unpleasant may not invariably hold (e.g., the interpretation of "painful" stimuli as pleasant or erotic in cases of masochism).

Nociception occurs when a somatic or visceral event activates a peripheral receptor. The physiologic (or pathophysiologic) events that evoke these signals are few: thermal (heat or cold), mechanical (stretch, distention, or muscular contraction), and chemical irritation (arising from the liberation of such diverse componds as acetylcholine, acids, bradykinin, histamines, potassium ions, prostaglandins, proteolytic enzymes and serotonin, released by inflammation, ischemia, or necrosis). To some extent the stimulus that creates pain is tissue or organ specific. For example, thermal injury occurring in the skin is painful, whereas thermal injury to the bowel is not (e.g., opening a colostomy with a hot cautery).

The processes that create chronic or recurrent pain may be lumped into those that are structural (ongoing processes such as arthritis or metastatic cancer), psychophysiologic (such as continuing muscle spasm creating pain after the original insult has passed), and somatizational (as found in those who internalize stress and express it in the form of pain).

Pain signals from the pelvic organs arrive at the spinal cord by way of small afferent fibers that accompany sympathetic nerves. These enter the spinal cord at T10, T11, T12, and the L1 levels. Their course carries them through the uterine, cervical, and pelvic plexuses; the hypogastric nerve; the superior hypogastric plexus (the presacral nerve); as well as the lumbar and lower lumbar sympathetic chains. Exact pathways are difficult to trace with certainty, making any attempt to block pain sensation through interrupting these nerves difficult and likely to fail.

Localization of pain is often difficult. An example of this difficulty is the phenomena of referred pain. Referred pain is especially common with visceral pain transmitted via "slow pain fibers" (type C fibers). Generally characterized as *burning* or *aching* in nature, this pain arises from conditions that affect a wider area, such as inflammation or ischemia. "Fast pain fibers" (type Aδ fibers) transmit pain that is sharp and moderately well localized (e.g., from the skin). This pain originates in processes that are better localized, such as pressure or tissue damage. Neither slow nor fast pain fibers adapt to a stimulus, but rather continue to generate the pain signal as long as the stimulus is present. Under some conditions, the threshold for stimulation may actually decrease, leading to hyperalgesia (as seen in sunburned skin).

Because the visceral and parietal pain fibers travel through different anatomic paths, the different types of pain that these fibers generate may be interpreted as arising from different areas of the body, even though they were generated by the same process. Because visceral structures do not have cortical representations, the sensation of pain is generally referred to superficial areas of the body. These areas are usually those with similar innervation as that of the viscus. A good example of this is appendicitis, where the achelike pain of visceral sensation is localized to the periumbilical area, while the sharp pain of parietal peritoneal irritation is felt directly over the right lower quadrant.

Causes of Acute Pelvic and Abdominal Pain

Assessing the possible causes of acute pelvic and lower abdominal pain can be greatly facilitated by remembering that five common mechanisms account for most pain: perforation, distention, ischemia, inflammation, and hemorrhage. The first three of these involve processes that have abrupt, almost catastrophic, time courses and should give rise to appropriately similar symptoms. The other two processes involve more indolent pathologies, leading to more gradual development of poorly focused symptoms. Using these distinctions, it is often easy to develop a possible list of causes for the pain the patient is experiencing. For example, the patient who reports rapid onset of pain over the course of a few minutes is not likely to have a pelvic infection, but rather could have a ruptured ectopic pregnancy. Pain that gradually increases over several days is unlikely to be due to torsion of an ovarian cyst. Understanding these five mechanisms also makes it easier to understand why ovarian cysts (especially those that are an incidental finding on ultrasonography) are seldom the source of acute pain and rarely the root of chronic pain. (Perforation would lead to the deflation and loss of the cyst; distention is a dynamic process that requires relatively rapid growth of the cyst; ischemia, which requires torsion, would be obvious; inflammation does not occur other than with infection or rupture of some types of cysts; and hemorrhage, which could cause distension, is an abrupt process, like torsion, that should be clinically obvious.)

Acute pain and pain of less than 3 months duration, generally has an identifiable pathophysiologic process as its source. The possible sources for acute pelvic pain are comparatively limited, making the differential diagnosis relatively easy. Care must be taken not to be lulled into the common trap of presuming that any pelvic or lower abdominal pain occurring in a woman must originate in her "female organs." Gastrointestinal, urologic, musculoskeletal, metabolic, infectious, and neurologic sources must also be considered, just as they would in a man. A summary of some of the important causes of acute pain that should be considered are shown in Table 22.1.

Gynecologic Causes of Acute Pain

ADNEXAL PROCESSES. Accidents of pregnancy, such as ectopic pregnancy or spontaneous abortion, are among the most common causes of acute pelvic pain in women. Ectopic pregnancy

Table 22.1. Causes of Acute Pelvic Pain

Cause	Symptoms and signs	Time course	Identifying features
Gynecologic			
Adnexal			
Ectopic pregnancy	Acute lateralized pain, intra-abdominal bleeding, hypovolemia, collapse, death	Minutes to hours	Positive pregnancy test, vaginal ultrasonography showing empty uterus or adnexal cardiac activity
Pelvic infection	Fever, chills, diffuse pain, nausea, rebound tenderness	Hours to days	Elevated temperature, white blood count, sedimentation rate, peritoneal signs including cervical motion tenderness
Torsion	Acute lateralized pain, pain with movement, nausea common	Minutes to hours	Adnexal mass on examination or ultrasonography
Ovulation	Milder lateralized lower quadrant pain	Hours	Occurs midcycle, 14 d prior to menstruation, absent in those using ovulation suppressing contraception (birth control pills, progesterones)
Uterine			
Abortion (spontaneous, incomplete, missed)	Vaginal bleeding, lower abdominal cramping	Hours to days	Menstrual history, positive pregnancy test, gestation with no cardiac activity on ultrasonography, cervical changes
Myoma (fibroids)	Pelvic pressure, acute midline pain with bleeding or ischemia	Days (hours rarely)	Tender mass associated with the uterus, absence of peritoneal signs until late
Other			
Urinary infection	Frequency, dysuria, midline pain/pressure	Hours to days	Urinalysis, urine culture, bladder tenderness
Inflammatory bowel disease	Colicky, diffuse pain, alternating diarrhea and constipation	Days	Sigmoidoscopy
Appendicitis	Colicky, diffuse pain localizing to right lower quadrant, fever, nausea, obstipation	Hours to days	Elevated temperature, high white blood count, sequence of symptoms
Aortic aneurism	Abrupt midabdominal and back pain	Minutes to hours	Pulsatile mass, loss of distal pulses

is one of the most dangerous gynecologic conditions to induce acute pelvic pain. Ectopic pregnancies still account for a significant number of maternal deaths each year. In roughly one third of deaths from ectopic pregnancy, a delay in diagnosis is involved. Because of the degree of risk, the possibility of ectopic pregnancy must be considered in any woman of menstrual age who presents with acute lower abdominal pain. Most tubal pregnancies become symptomatic between 6 and 8 weeks after the last menstrual period, when the tube can no longer stretch enough to accommodate the growing gestation. Stretch of the peritoneum overlying the affected fallopian tube gives rise to lateralized pelvic or lower abdominal pain. Irritation of the posterior cul-de-sac by leaking blood pooling in the dependent portions of the abdominal cavity can cause a bearing down sensation reminiscent of constipation. If frank rupture occurs, intraperitoneal bleeding can be life threatening. (Abortion and ectopic pregnancy are more fully discussed in Chapter 5, Complications of Early Pregnancy.)

Pelvic infections (pelvic inflammatory disease [PID]) accounts for almost 7% of non-traumatic emergency room visits for abdominal pain. This is second only to gastroenteritis as a specific diagnosis. Pain-causing pelvic infections can run the gamut from acute diffuse abdominal pain found in salpingitis to vague symptoms occasioned by a smoldering tubo-ovarian abscess. (For further information about the causative organisms and natural course of pelvic infections, see Chapter 26, Sexually Transmitted Disease and "PID".)

An adnexal or pedunculated pelvic mass, such as a fibroid, may twist on its mesentery compromising its blood supply and resulting in ischemia. The resultant pain is generally strong, precipitate, and worsened by movement. Its onset is occasionally related to a change of body position, although this history is unreliable or absent in most cases. The pain is generally lateralized and directly associated with a tender, painful pelvic mass. With time, peritoneal irritation will lead to more diffuse pain, rebound tenderness, and cervical motion tenderness.

Cystic masses do not generally cause pelvic pain. However, when a cystic mass is suddenly distended (as when bleeding occurs within the mass), pain may be produced. Rupture or torsion of these masses may also cause acute discomfort. Bleeding and torsion produce similar symptoms that are frequently reported as being iliac or inguinal in location. Bleeding, which is self-limited, may cause intermittent symptoms with a period of improvement or even complete, spontaneous resolution.

Although not generally painful, occasionally ovulation can cause discomfort. The pain is frequently described as sharp, with an element of dull aching. It is usually well localized and should occur only at approximately 14 days prior to the next menstrual flow. It should not be present in women taking oral contraceptives or using long-acting progesterone contraception (Norplant, Depo-Provera); or in premenarchal or postmenopausal women. A careful history may elicit similar episodes during previous menstrual cycles.

UTERINE CAUSES. Uterine fibroids only rarely present with the symptoms of abdominal pain. Although fibroids can be a source for menstrual pain (see Chapter 18, Menstrual Pain), they are an uncommon source for acute or subacute pain. Acute pain is only created by distention or ischemia brought about when bleeding or necrosis happen in rapidly growing myomas. Ischemia also occurs should a pedunculated fibroid undergo torsion. History and physical examination generally suggest the diagnosis.

Infection limited to the uterus (endometritis) only occurs after delivery, abortion (spontaneous or induced), or instrumentation, such as biopsy or intrauterine contraceptive device (IUCD) placement. Cervical discharge, signs of ascending infection, or salpingitis often are present at the same time.

Urologic Causes

Urinary tract infections rank third behind pelvic infections as a cause for abdominal pain treated in emergency rooms (accounting for slightly more than 5% of cases of nontraumatic abdominal pain). The discomfort of lower urinary tract infections is generally suprapubic or pelvic, and rarely involves areas outside the lower abdomen. As with other inflammatory processes, the evolution of symptoms before the patient seeks treatment is generally one ranging from a few hours to 1 or 2 days. Upper urinary tract infections will not cause pelvic or lower abdominal symptoms, except when in addition to, or radiating from flank, back, or upper abdominal locations.

Urinary tract stones may cause some of the worst acute pain encountered outside of major trauma. Ureteral caliculi cause abrupt distention of the upper collecting system and severe reactive muscle spasms, leading to flank pain with radiation to the groin. Hematuria (gross or microscopic) is common. Bladder stones may also cause hematuria, but are less likely to cause acute pain. When they do cause pain, it tends to be in midline and suprapubic locations.

As with gynecologic tumors, urinary tract tumors are generally painless unless torsion, bleeding, infarct, or infection occur. Palpation of the bladder may reveal a mass or persistent hematuria may be present, directing the course of further investigation.

Gastrointestinal Causes

The gastrointestinal tract is the most common source of acute abdominal pain, with gastrointestinal inflammatory processes accounting for most of the causes in both men or women. Gastroenteritis, appendicitis, and inflammatory bowel diseases are the gastrointestinal sources for most acute pain. Intussusception, volvulus, bowel obstruction, and infarcts of the bowel wall will cause acute pain, but owing to their rarity will not be discussed in detail.

As with any other inflammatory process in the abdominal cavity, appendicitis begins with diffuse irritation of the local peritoneum, manifested by vague, periumbilical, colicky pain. As the severity of the inflammation increases, better localized right lower quadrant sharp pain develops. Peritoneal irritation initially causes hypermobility of the gut (nausea, vomiting, diarrhea) followed by quiescence or ileus (obstipation). Fever, chills, and an elevated white blood cell count are typical.

Perforation of a gastric or duodenal ulcer generally presents as upper abdominal sharp pain, but the symptoms are not always classic. Diffuse abdominal pain, including the pelvis, associated with nausea and vomiting is common in acute billiary tract and pancreatic disease. These patients most commonly report radiation of their pain to the back or shoulders; however, these disorders can be confused with pelvic causes unless a wider differential diagnosis is considered.

More apt to cause lower abdominal and pelvic pain are events, such as bowel obstruction (including that due to internal herniation, intussusception, or volvulus), enterocolitis, diverticulitis, spasms due to inflammatory bowel disease, or the presence of a neoplasm. Pelvic or abdominal pain accompanied by fever and explosive, voluminous, often bloody diarrhea is the hallmark of infectious enterocolitis. Traction on the bowel mesentery, acute bowel distention, ischemia, or inflammation generally cause a constant, diffuse, noncrampy discomfort. Crampy or colicky pain, which is more typical in bowel lumen distention or increased motor activity of the bowel wall, is typical of small bowel obstruction. Discomfort due to distention of the ascending colon and cecum is generally perceived as periumbilical in location, but may be suprapubic and mimic uterine pain. Although the symptoms of left-sided colonic processes often localize toward the left abdomen, lower colonic and sigmoid distress is frequently bilateral and suprapubic.

In inflammatory bowel disease, the process of inflammation within the bowel wall induces pain, whether the inflammation is from a viral enteritis or from a chronic inflammatory process such as Crohn's disease. Even in chronic processes like the latter, acute, intermittent episodes are generally the complaint that brings the patient to seek treatment and leads to the diagnosis. In addition to inflammation, distention of any hollow abdominal organ can cause acute pain. In the gastrointestinal tract, this can happen gradually, as with constipation, or abruptly, as with herniation and obstruction. History is generally helpful in establishing a differential diagnosis; however, in extreme cases, a diagnosis may not be established without exploratory surgery.

Other, Less Common Causes

The musculoskeletal system may be the source of acute pain mimicking that of pelvic origin. Acute musculoskeletal pain is often sharp in nature and closely associated with an identifiable event, such as trauma, lifting, turning, or the like. The most common examples of this would be acute strain or hematoma formation in the rectus muscle from a sudden cough, prolonged pushing during the second stage of labor, or with heavy lifting. The pain reported is usually well localized and frequently involves point tenderness. A history of trauma or exertion may not be present.

Musculoskeletal pain frequently radiates in, or is referred to, areas quite distant from the source of the nociceptive signal. On occasion, a trigger point is identified that induces or reproduces the patient's complaint. These hypersensitive areas overlying muscles induce muscular spasms and pain. They may be found throughout the body, but are most common in the abdominal wall, back, and pelvic floor when pelvic pain is the complaint.

Acute vascular problems, such as an expanding aneurysm or embolism to a visceral vessel, may also precipitate acute abdominal pain. Although uncommon, pelvic pain can accompany dissection, leakage, or rupture of an abdominal aortic aneurysm. The presence of a pulsatile mass suggests the diagnosis. If the patient's condition permits, ultrasonography may be useful in confirming the diagnosis.

Some less common processes to be considered as sources of abdominal pain are: Sickle-cell crisis, acute intermittent porphyria, heavy metal poisoning, drug use (especially cocaine), and toxins (e.g., black widow spider bite). Neuralgia due to vertebral disk disease, tabes dorsalis, or herpetic radiculopathy (shingles) may cause abdominal pain.

Causes of Chronic Pelvic Pain

Chronic pelvic pain can be produced by gynecologic, urologic, gastrointestinal, musculoskeletal, or other processes, most of which have parallels with the causes of acute pain. Some potential sources of chronic pain are listed in Table 22.2.

Table 22.2. Causes of Chronic Pelvic Pain

Gynecologic	Musculoskeletal
Extrauterine	Ankylosing spondylitis
Adhesions (debated)	Degenerative joint disease
Chronic ectopic pregnancy (rare)	Fibromyocitis
Chronic pelvic infection	Hernias (abdominal, femoral)
Cysts (generally not a cause of pain)	Herniated disk
Endometriosis	Herpes zoster (shingles)
Retained ovary syndrome	"Low back pain"
Uterine	Levator ani syndrome (spasm of pelvic floor)
Chronic endometritis (rare)	Myofascial pain (trigger points)
Fibroids	Nerve entrapment syndromes
Intrauterine polyps	Obesity
Intrauterine contraceptive device	Osteoporosis (fractures)
Pelvic congestive syndrome (?)	"Pain posture"
Pelvic relaxation	Spondylolisthesis
Urologic	Other
Chronic urinary tract infection	Abuse (physical or sexual, prior or current)
Detrusor dyssynergia	Adrenal insufficiency
Interstitial cystitis	Bipolar personality disorders
Stone	Depression
Urethral syndrome	Drug use (especially cocaine)
Gastrointestinal	Heavy metal poisoning
Cholelithiasis	Hyperparathyroidism
Chronic constipation	Mesenteric adenitis
Chronic appendicitis	Pelvic tuberculosis
Diverticular disease	Parasites
Esophagitis	Porphyria
Enterocolitis	Psychosocial stress (marital discord,
Gastric/duodenal ulcer	work stress)
Inflammatory bowel disease	Sickle-cell disease
Crohn's disease	Sleep disturbances
Ulcerative colitis	Somatization
Irritable bowel syndrome	Sympathetic dystrophy
Ischemic bowel disease	Tabes
Neoplasia	
Pancreatitis	

After: American College of Obstetricians and Gynecologists. Pelvic Pain. ACOG Technical Bulletin 223. Washington, DC: ACOG, 1996.

Most subacute (3–6 months duration) and chronic pain states (> 6 months) begin with an acute nociceptive event. That event may go unrecognized or unremembered owing to the passage of time. As time passes, the pain itself begins to take precedence, shifting the focus from the underlying process that initiated the sequence of events. It is during this phase that pain behaviors, both functional and dysfunctional, develop. The evolution of pain behavior and chronic pain syndromes are summarized in Figure 22.1.

Gynecologic Causes

There are many pathologic conditions involving the pelvic viscera that do account for pain complaints. Endometriosis is thought to cause pelvic heaviness and dyspareunia through

Months

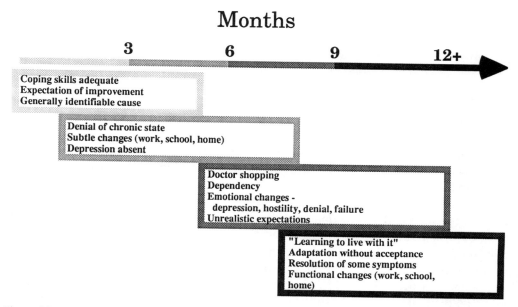

Figure 22.1. Evolution of Pain. Chronic pain and pain behaviors tend to evolve with time.

scarring and chemical irritation. Early studies indicated that intraperitoneal prostaglandin levels might be elevated in women with endometriosis, accounting for the origination of pain and the commonly associated infertility these women experience. Unfortunately, subsequent studies have failed to support these earlier findings. In addition, some studies find the prevalence of endometriosis is the same in women with and without pain, raising questions about causality.

The weight and pressure of uterine fibroids or adnexal tumors (both benign and malignant) can lead to chronic complaints. Pelvic adhesions can cause discomfort when stretched, but this requires a dynamic process. During intercourse or bowel movements such dynamics may occur, but in the activities of day-to-day living the connection is less clear. Uterine prolapse may sometimes produce an achy or crampy discomfort, with frank pain during intercourse or bowel movements. Retroversion of the uterus has been proposed as a source of chronic pain, but the observation that this occurs in roughly 20% of normal women, casts doubt on this theory. It is more plausible that disease processes (e.g., endometriosis) may simultaneously result in fixation of the uterus in a retroverted position and be responsible for the pain encountered.

Gastrointestinal Sources

Gastrointestinal disorders are also common sources of subacute, recurrent, or chronic pelvic pain. The most common of these is irritable bowel syndrome (IBS), which may be responsible for up to half of all cases of chronic pelvic pain. The pain of IBS is usually colicky in character, associated with a sensation of rectal fullness or incomplete emptying. The pain is most often improved with bowel movement but worsens 1 to 2 hours after meals. The pain is usually worse at or around the time of menstruation, and may be associated with dyspareunia, obscuring the diagnosis. The symptoms of IBS often wax and wane, but will remain present for cycles that last from weeks to months in up to one fifth of patients. These symptoms often parallel physical or emotional stress, mimicking somatization. Although IBS can present with pain as its only symptom, constipation, frequently with intermittent diarrhea, is a common complaint in these patients. Bowel movements often occur less than three times a week and are hard or pelletlike. When diarrhea is present (manifest as an increase in frequency or volume of stools, or both), it is independent of osmotic load or food intolerance (e.g., lactose intolerance). Women with IBS have an increased prevalence of somatization disorders, anxiety, depression, hysteria, and hypochondriases. Some reports cite rates of up to 90% for coexistent psychopathology. Adjunctive psychotherapy significantly increases the rate of improvement compared with medical therapy alone, supporting a causative role for psychopathology.

Inflammation of the bowel in Crohn's disease or ulcerative colitis causes visceral pain even in the absence of obstruction or perforation. The symptoms of inflammatory bowel disease are often indistinguishable from those of IBS, although the fever and bloody stools that are common in inflammatory bowel disease are not a part of IBS. The widely separated nature of Crohn's disease lesions, often involving both the large and small bowel, results in diffuse and nonspecific symptoms and findings. Stenosis, obstruction, fibrotic adhesive disease, and internal or perineal fistula formation are common in this process. An indolent low-grade fever lasting for days or weeks is common. Fecal urgency, incontinence, or rectal bleeding are often present. Colonic involvement may present with pain in either or both lower quadrants. When acute, the symptoms of Crohn's disease must be differentiated from those of dysentery and diverticulitis. Cramping that is relieved by voluminous, often bloody diarrhea is typical in ulcerative colitis. Patients with ulcerative colitis are less likely to have acute pain than are those with Crohn's disease.

In older patients, diverticular disease can be a source of significant morbidity. Abdominal pain and diarrhea are the most common symptoms, mimicking irritable bowel syndrome. Bleeding, perforation, and abscess formation may also occur. Patients with diverticular disease generally will not have the psychological overlay seen in IBS and symptoms will not be altered by stress. The pain of diverticular disease is usually in the left lower quadrant and improves with bowel movements or the passage of gas. Although diverticula can be demonstrated on barium enema or tomography, symptoms may occur before radiologic detection is possible.

A recent report suggests that the appendix may be an overlooked source for chronic abdominal pain. In the small number of patients reported so far, 90% of the appendices removed showed pathologic changes, including signs of chronic inflammation. According to this report, most of the patients had undergone surgical exploration (laparoscopy or laparotomy) in the past without diagnosis. At the time of the reported laparoscopic exploration and appendectomy, all had abnormal-appearing appendices. Clearly, the appendix does not represent a common source of chronic pelvic pain, but it does deserve consideration.

Other Causes

There are a number of less common urologic processes that may cause chronic pelvic pain in women. These range from interstitial cystitis and chronic urethral syndrome to detrusor sphincter dyssynergia and urolithiasis. Inflammation is the mechanism responsible for most urologic chronic pain, with muscular spasm accounting for the rest. In some cases this may

Figure 22.2. Several postural changes have been associated with the development of chronic pelvic pain. Exaggerated lordosis, kyphosis-lordosis, and excessive pelvic tilt (as seen when carrying a baby on the hip) may all distort muscle and joint relationships, leading to chronic pain.

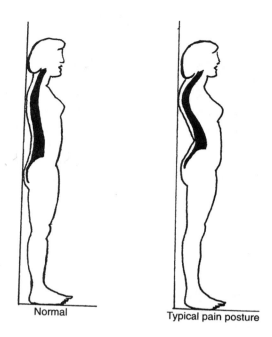

Normal   Typical pain posture

be triggered by an antecedent infection; in others, such as interstitial cystitis, the ultimate causation is unknown.

Chronic pelvic pain can also originate in the musculoskeletal system. Herniation of a disc, spondylolisthesis, exaggerated lumbar lordosis, or "pain postures" that induce abnormal stresses on muscles or ligaments (such as the chronic pelvic tip brought on by carrying a baby on one hip) may all be sources of ongoing pelvic pain(Fig. 22.2). Pain over the distribution of a single nerve root may be found when herniation of a disc occurs, following surgery, in conditions like arthritis, or in obese patients where soft tissue or weight-induced posture change may cause impingement on the nerve.

Chronic Pain Without Obvious Pathology

There has been a great deal written about the enigma of chronic pelvic pain without clinically obvious cause. Much of this literature has been built on speculation or uncontrolled observation. Many early reports emphasized the prevalence of childhood abuse, incest, and other life events in patients with chronic pain. These patients have a higher than average prevalence of physical or sexual abuse, dysfunctional families (in childhood or current), or psychosocial stresses, but causal links are lacking. Recent publications have examined the role of two potential causes of chronic pain states that may be overlooked and thus under diagnosed: depression and sleep disorders. It is well documented that somatic complaints may arise from these sources, making them worthwhile areas to explore in the evaluation of pelvic pain.

In patients with chronic pain, there is often a strong overlay of psychological symptoms. Some studies indicate that a history of depression, prior abuse, or overreaction by spouses are the best predictors of severity in pelvic pain. Although stress and depression are often present in these patients, the clinician should presume that there is an organic cause. Only when other reasonable causes have been eliminated, should the diagnoses of somatization, depression, or sleep or personality disorders be considered. Frequently, listening to the patient often provides clues to a psychological ethiology. Worsening of symptoms during times of stress, inconvenient recurrences that remove the patient from unpleasant situations, excessive dependency, and other signs of an emotional component should be suggestive of this diagnosis.

Patients with sleep disturbances are often identified as ones who internalize psychological disturbances, making somatic complaints more likely. Patients with sleep disturbances are usually below age 40 and describe themselves as tense, anxious, preoccupied, worried, depressed, and they complain of poor mental and physical health. This strongly parallels the classic patient with chronic pelvic pain and is similar to the feelings reported by patients with clinical or subclinical depression. This suggests that both depression and sleep disorders may predispose to somatization (expressed as chronic pelvic pain). While supported by a growing number of papers in the literature, psychological disturbances remain only an attractive hypothesis for the derivation of nonorganic pelvic pain.

One cautionary note is in order: Neither the patient nor the physician should be lulled into the belief that if depression is present there is no organic disease, and vice versa. Clearly, these two conditions can and do coexist. Even in patients with obvious psychosocial stress, organic pathology can and does occur. It is also wise to recall that pain is a perception and that pain arising from psychological sources is no less "real" or less debilitating than that from physiologic processes. Not recognizing the stress that pain can cause or the difficulty in dealing with pain that underlying depression engenders, is to risk failure. Clearly both must be addressed.

Even in patients diagnosed with somatization disorders, care must be taken to watch for intercurrent physical illness. Similarly, the possibility of drug or alcohol dependence should be considered and appropriate detoxification instituted.

ESTABLISHING THE DIAGNOSIS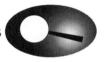

Although often said, it is nonetheless true that effective therapy cannot be implemented without a correct diagnosis. In acute pelvic pain, this can be anticipated for almost all patients using only their history, a careful physical examination, and a few select laboratory or imaging adjuncts.

Noncyclic chronic pelvic pain is another matter. It can be one of the most perplexing complaints. An exact organic cause is often difficult or impossible to establish. Indeed, approximately one third of patients with chronic pelvic pain who undergo laparoscopic evaluation have no identifiable cause determined. (By extension, however, two thirds of these patients will have potential causes recognized where none was apparent clinically.) Using a multidisciplinary approach (in concept or as a team evaluation), common clinical sense, a careful history, and a limited number of diagnostic procedures, will generally yield success.

Acute Pain

The diagnosis and management of acute pain is most often straightforward. Occasionally, establishing a definitive diagnosis may have to be deferred while a patient is stabilized (e.g., an emergency such as ruptured tubal pregnancy with intra-abdominal bleeding). In situations like these, it makes little difference whether the patient's intraperitoneal bleeding is from a ruptured ectopic pregnancy, a bleeding corpus luteum, or a ruptured spleen, the patient must be stabilized rapidly and surgically explored. To an extent, the type of exploration (laparoscopy vs. laparotomy) may be dictated by the presumptive diagnosis, but even this consideration is secondary to the stabilization process. Patients with acute pain who are not in immediate danger still require aggressive evaluation to allow prompt intervention to reduce their discomfort.

History

The information provided by the patient's history can be vital to directing the diagnostic process. Rapid onset processes are more likely to indicate potentially disastrous events and significant jeopardy. Ectopic pregnancy, rupture of a cyst, perforation of an organ, or abrupt ischemia must all be considered. When symptoms evolve in a more controlled fashion, it is easier to establish a plan of investigation. In these cases, inflammation, infection, and organ dysfunction are all more plausible. In either case, the onset, character, and radiation of the pain is important. Factors that modify the pain (better, worse, or different) should be sought. These include posture changes, meals, bowel movements, voiding, and intercourse. Other symptoms, such as nausea, vomiting, diarrhea, constipation, urinary frequency, dysuria, dyspareunia, fever, chills, and others, should be noted. A history of previous surgeries, pelvic infections, infertility, and any obstetric experiences may be of significance.

Of critical importance in the evaluation of women is a menstrual history. The character, timing, duration, rhythmicity, and date of last menses are important. Any contraceptive the patient and her partner use may help to evaluate the risk of pregnancy and other conditions (e.g., pelvic infections).

Patients with ectopic pregnancies may present with acute catastrophic collapse, a history of progressive lower abdominal discomfort, or anything in between. The key to diagnosis in these patients is suspicion. Any patient of childbearing age, even those who have had a tubal sterilization, must be suspected of having an ectopic pregnancy. The pain of an ectopic pregnancy is nonspecific. It is usually lateralized at first and may then become diffuse if there is intraperitoneal bleeding. Cul-de-sac irritation may cause tenesmus, and it is not uncommon for these patients to come to medical attention having passed out in the bathroom while trying to have a bowel movement. Vaginal bleeding may occur in patients with ectopic pregnancies, but its presence is insufficient to differentiate between an ectopic pregnancy and accidents occurring to intrauterine gestations.

The hallmark of pelvic inflammatory disease is lower abdominal and pelvic pain, although this pain may be absent in about 6% of cases. Symptoms are generally gradual in onset, covering a period of from a few hours to several days. In over 80% of cases symptoms will have been present for less than 15 days. It is frequently difficult to differentiate between the symptoms of pelvic infection and appendicitis. The symptoms of appendicitis generally begin around the umbilicus and then become generalized, with a sharp component located in the right lower quadrant. Pelvic infections tend to begin with diffuse pelvic symptoms that stay diffusely centered in the lower abdomen. When pain is present during menstruation and tampons are used, toxic shock syndrome must be considered and the characteristic rash of this disease sought.

Although variable in intensity and duration, crampy, lower abdominal pain is an almost constant finding in spontaneous abortion. Vaginal bleeding (varying from bright red to dark brown), a menstrual history commensurate with pregnancy, and a positive pregnancy test should indicate the possible diagnosis. Because abdominal tenderness is generally not present, any tenderness suggests a re-evaluation of the possibility of ectopic pregnancy, even in the face of a history of tissue having been passed.

In keeping with the multiorgan causes of pain, the history must also include a review of gastrointestinal, urologic, and musculoskeletal functions. This review must be directed toward both the presence of symptoms in these areas and the relationship between these systems and the pain the patient reports. Establishing only that the patient has regular bowel habits may overlook pain that is worse immediately following defecation. The review of other organ systems must also include more subtle symptoms, such as a change in the color or character of urine and stool (as in metabolic and biliary disease or in obstructing colon lesions).

For patients with urinary tract infections, a history of frequency and dysuria is customarily present, and fever (if any) is generally mild. Upper urinary tract infections (pyelitis, nephritis) presents with more generalized signs of infection and tenderness in the costovertebral area. Fever is more common in these patients. Pain may radiate toward the pelvis, but seldom originates there. Urinalysis will separate these causes from others in the differential diagnosis.

The pain of urinary calculi is among the most intense encountered from any cause. Classically originating in the flank and radiating to the groin on the affected side, the pain is abrupt, intense, and unrelieved by the patient's position. Palpation of the abdomen and pelvis does not usually elicit tenderness. Palpation over the kidney on the involved side often causes pain. A urinalysis revealing hematuria, combined with an acute course and lateralized signs and symptoms, helps to differentiate this problem from urinary tract infection.

Most gastrointestinal sources of acute pain induce a similar picture of diffuse, colicky, abdominal pain. Fever is often present. Early nausea and vomiting are frequent. A history of blood or mucus in the stool suggests gastrointestinal disease. The history, progression of symptoms, and physical findings, combined with blood counts, selected serum chemistry studies, and proctoscopic examination (for some patients), will establish a specific diagnosis.

Physical Examination

The physical examination of the patient with abdominal or pelvic pain must begin with a basic assessment of status. Measurement of blood pressure (in two positions if blood loss is suspected), pulse rate, and temperature is imperative. An evaluation of the heart and lungs should also be included, with its priority determined by the patient's history and general condition.

When performing the abdominal examination, it is often useful to begin by asking the patient to indicate "where it hurts" on their exposed belly. The area involved, as well as the way in which the patient points, will be helpful in evaluating the degree of localization. Locations indicated with the whole hand suggest more diffuse processes than those pointed to with a single finger.

Gentle palpation of the entire abdomen for masses or tenderness should be carried out. Palpation should include the epigastrium, flanks, mid- and low back, and inguinal areas.

Deep breathing, muscle contraction-relaxation, or other relaxation techniques may facilitate this examination. Efforts to avoid discomfort, where possible, will be rewarded by a more cooperative patient and ultimately more valuable information. When gentle palpation is used, true rigidity, as opposed to voluntary guarding, can be elicited. The finding of a mass will help to direct further evaluations. A diffuse, doughlike consistency of the abdomen suggests intraperitoneal bleeding and requires further investigation.

Deep palpation and an evaluation of rebound tenderness are next. Peritonitis may be confirmed by having the patient cough or by upward tapping on the patient's heels, both of which will disturb the peritoneum, resulting in pain. When significant peritonitis is present, bowel sounds are absent. Gentle palpation while listening with the stethoscope reduces the patient's expectation of discomfort and provides an opportunity to confirm earlier findings. Auscultation at the same time can disclose altered bowel sounds or vascular bruits.

A pelvic and rectal examination is mandatory for the patient with abdominal or pelvic pain. This should include a speculum examination of the cervix. The presence of blood or discharge should be noted and cultures obtained when appropriate. Finding uterine or adnexal masses or tenderness quickly focuses the diagnostic process. Peritoneal irritation may be indicated by exaggerated discomfort when the cervix and uterus are gently moved by the internal examining hand. (Motion of the peritoneum during rectal examination also causes discomfort when inflammation exists.) Rectal examination may be confirmatory and may also reveal signs of masses and bleeding not previously appreciated, which can change the direction of further investigation. A stool guaiac test should always be performed.

Either culdocentesis or paracentesis can be useful in the evaluation of the patient with pain, although with the advent of high-resolution abdominal and transvaginal ultrasonography these have fallen out of favor somewhat. When nonclotting blood, purulent fluid, or fecal material is found they can contribute significantly to the diagnostic process. It should be remembered that both paracentesis and culdocentesis are invasive procedures and the information gained has limitations. Their use must be reserved for only those patients where the information gained outweighs the discomfort and risk involved.

Laboratory, X-ray, and Ultrasound Studies

The laboratory evaluation of the patient with acute abdominal or pelvic pain is at once straightforward and simple, but vitally important. A complete blood count will help to identify inflammatory processes through elevations in the white blood count, as well as alterations in the differential count. The patient's hemoglobin or hematocrit is helpful in evaluating possible blood loss, although it may be unchanged in acute, uncompensated blood loss. An evaluation of serum chemistries may be useful in evaluating gastrointestinal or billiary sources of pain, as well as general status. These tests should be requested based on specific possible diagnoses rather than general screening. Urinalysis is a very quick and inexpensive way to evaluate the role of the urinary tract in the development of the patient's pain.

Because of the risks that a missed diagnosis entails, virtually all women with acute abdominal or pelvic pain should have a sensitive pregnancy test performed. With the availability of sensitive pregnancy tests, a positive result is generally found even in the early gestations typical of spontaneous abortion or ectopic pregnancy. In patients with an ectopic pregnancy, some elevation of the white blood count is common, and a low-grade fever may be present if leakage of blood has occurred over an extended period. Vaginal bleeding need not be present in patients with ectopic gestations, but will generally be found in those with a miscarriage.

When a purulent cervical discharge is present, a gram stain and culture are appropriate even if pelvic inflammatory disease is not the primary diagnosis. Therapeutic choices are based on the clinical picture and the gram stain, rather than on the results of the culture which can take 48 hours or more to return. Rapid tests for chlamydia and gonorrhea are available, but carry high false-positive and false-negative rates, limiting their utility.

Imaging by x-ray or ultrasonography have only limited value as screening tools for patients with acute pain. An x-ray examination may confirm air-fluid levels, the presence of free air in the peritoneal cavity, or dilated loops of bowel. Ultrasonography can help identify pelvic masses or free fluid when present. When ectopic pregnancy is suspected, ultrasonography may be useful if it demonstrates an intrauterine pregnancy. The absence of an intrauterine gestation strongly suggests an ectopic pregnancy but does not prove it because very early intrauterine gestation can easily be missed. If cardiac activity is found in the adnexa, it is diagnostic.

Chronic Pain

Establishing a credible differential diagnosis for chronic pain suffers is not as difficult as it seems. It does require a wide-ranging approach, because of the nonspecific nature of the symptoms usually reported. For the patient who reports suprapubic pain, the temptation to jump automatically to gynecologic or urologic causes risks missing a referred musculoskeletal or psychosocial cause. A thorough, broad-based evaluation (sometimes including laparoscopy), along with psychological evaluation and support are required. Increasing the likelihood of finding the underlying process simultaneously increases the probability of a successful therapy. Common clinical sense, a careful history, and a limited number of diagnostic procedures, generally yield success.

History

The history is the most important part of the evaluation of any patient with chronic pelvic pain. The character, location and radiation, onset, duration, and evolution of the pain over time must be elicited. Drawings or other aids may be helpful, but are not required (Fig. 22.3).

Attention should be paid to factors that make the symptoms change, not just improve or worsen. The impact of factors such as diet, activity, bowel movements, voiding, bladder filling, and sexual activity must all be explored. The possibility of physical or sexual abuse must be considered. Each of these areas must be explored more fully when they appear to be tied to the patient's pain complaints. This is especially true when a history of painful sexual activity is obtained. There is a natural reluctance to pursue this aspect of a patient's history, but it is very important to ask further questions that may suggest possible causes for the pain. The type of sexual activity involved, the location and character of the discomfort, the frequency of both pain and sexual activity, sexual practices, orgasmic capability, and the ability to have sexual activities that do not cause pain, must all be explored. For example,

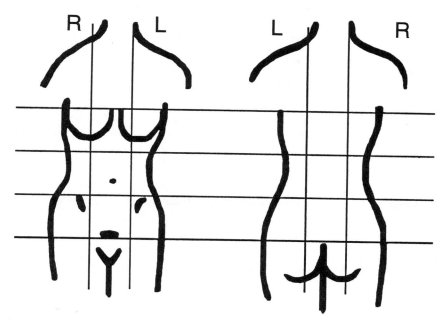

Figure 22.3. Use of a drawing or other visual aids to help assess the location and character of chronic pain often provides an indication of the likelihood of organic disease or somatization. Multiple locations with vague or changing symptoms suggest somatoform disorders, whereas relatively well-focused symptoms are more often due to organic changes. After: Smith RP, Metheny WP, Nolan TE. A tool for the assessment of chronic pelvic pain. Journal of Psychosomatic Obstetrics and Gynaecology 1992;13:281.

pain that is made worse by deep penetration will have different origins than will complaints of sharp vulvar pain accompanied by vaginismus.

Many patients with chronic pain complaints report a worsening of their symptoms at, or near, the time of menstruation. For this reason, much of the evaluation of these patients parallels the evaluations used for patients with dysmenorrhea. Complaints of heavy menstrual flow combined with pain, suggest uterine changes such as adenomyosis, myomas, or polyps. The coexisting complaint of infertility may suggest that endometriosis is a possibility, although this diagnosis can only be established with certainty through laparoscopy. When the patient notes that her symptoms started only after placement of an IUCD, it is appropriate to think of the IUCD as a probable cause. Unfortunately, even the relationship of recurrent pain to menstruation, or the presence of dyspareunia, is no more than suggestive that a gynecologic cause exists.

There are no symptoms that uniquely identify genitourinary structures as the source of the patient's pain. Symptoms arising from the genitourinary system tend to be crampy to sharp in character. They localize to the lower abdomen in the midline, with occasional radiation to the back. Bladder or ureteral pain may radiate to the vagina or groin. As with acute processes, inflammatory conditions are more poorly localized than are focal processes.

When the urinary tract is the root of chronic pain, most patients will note a relationship between the pain and voiding, an increase in frequency, urgency, hesitance, nocturia, or other urinary symptoms, although these may only be found on careful questioning. Although stress urinary incontinence often accompanies pelvic relaxation and a cystourethrocele, stress urinary loss by itself is not diagnostic of either pelvic support problems nor does it help indicate a source of chronic pain. A history of recurrent urinary tract infections, especially if associated with negative urine cultures, should raise the possibility of a urinary pathology.

Musculoskeletal pain of long duration is often ill defined, achy, and can closely mimic that of gynecologic origin, even to the point of variation during the menstrual cycle. Strains, sprains, herniations, and spasms may all play a part in either the origination or the persistence of pain symptoms. Under some conditions, the muscular component of a pathologic process may provide the majority of the symptoms expressed, as in the case of reactive lumbar muscular spasms that occur with ureteral stone passage. The influence of postural changes on the intensity or attributes of the pain may help suggest a musculoskeletal origin. This type of pain is often worse late in the day, or with activity, and rarely wakes the patient at night.

Complaints of back problems, urinary difficulties, gastrointestinal symptoms, or the like should alert the physician to the possibility of nongynecologic causes for chronic pain. Because of shared sensory tracts, it is often very difficult to distinguish between pain sensations arising from the gastrointestinal tract and those from the uterus, tubes, or ovaries. Patients with gastrointestinal conditions causing pelvic pain will note some relationship of the pain to meals or defecation or will report some disturbance in digestive functions, such as anorexia, nausea, vomiting, early satiety, distention or bloating, "gas," diarrhea, or constipation. The patient should be asked about laxative use, fecal urgency, and problems evacuating the rectum (such as excessive straining for a bowel movement). The presence of blood or mucus in the stool suggests gastrointestinal disease. Fever, chills, and malaise should suggest an inflammatory process. Alternating diarrhea and constipation or symptoms that worsen with stress should suggest irritable bowel syndrome or somatization. The presence of pelvic heaviness, change in abdominal contour, or involuntary weight loss should raise the possibility of intra-abdominal neoplasia.

Office screening for the presence of depression, somatization, or sleep disorders can be easily carried out. Clearly, the first step is to recognize the possibility that these may be factors contributing to pelvic pain. The factors evaluated should include psychosocial stress, as well as martial, financial, social, sexual, and other pressures. In the case of sleep disorders, simple questioning regarding problems falling asleep or staying asleep, made in the course of the initial history, will suggest a problem. Special questionnaires or sleep laboratory evaluations are not necessary.

The detection of depression is only slightly more difficult. Vague and changing symptoms, weight loss, change in appetite, loss of libido, and chronic fatigue may all suggest the presence of depression. Attitude and body language (e.g., slumped posture, poor eye contact) may suggest a problem. The Beck Depression Inventory is a quick and simple instrument to take and score. It consists of 21 multiple choice items, scored on a scale of 0 to 3. Scores of greater than 13 indicate the presence of clinical depression. The test can be easily used in the clinical setting to evaluate those patients in whom depression is suspected. Based on the prevalence of depression in chronic pain patients, screening of all patients with chronic pelvic pain should be considered.

The wide range of differential diagnoses possible for patients with chronic pelvic pain suggests a multidisciplinary, holistic approach. This can involve psychiatric evaluation or testing, social workers, physical therapists, gastroenterologists, anesthesiologists, orthopedists, and others. In most settings, this kind of team is impractical. This team is not a requirement to care for these patients; however, because of their complexity, one should consider referral to such a team anytime the diagnosis remains elusive or simple interventions are unsuccessful.

Physical Examination

Although in most cases of chronic pain the correct diagnosis is suggested by the history, a careful physical assessment is still critical to the diagnostic process. The physical examination is directed toward finding possible underlying pathologies or establishing their probable absence.

At the start of the examination, the patient should be asked to indicate the location of the pain. Pain indicated using a single finger is more likely to be caused by organic pathology than when the patient uses a sweeping motion of the whole hand. Actions which duplicate the patient's complaint should be noted. Undue discomfort should be avoided to minimize guarding which would limit a thorough examination.

The examination must include a thorough evaluation of the patient's entire abdomen (upper and lower), mid- and low back, and the pelvic and rectal areas to avoid missing possible nongynecologic causes. Special attention should be paid to those areas most directly involved with the patient's symptoms. The examiner should also note the patient's reactions. Is the pain altered by the examination? Is the pain less when palpation is made with the stethoscope or while the patient is distracted? These observations can be as important as any other finding.

Physical examination of patients with gastrointestinal disease is often nonspecific. Distension of the abdomen is suggestive of gastrointestinal disease, but is nonspecific. Patients with IBS may have diffuse tenderness with greater sensitivity in the left lower quadrant and over the sigmoid. When this tenderness is present without signs of inflammation, it is highly suggestive of IBS. When inflammation is present, diverticulitis should be suspected. Anorectal findings of fistulae or abscesses suggest inflammatory bowel disease, whereas masses forewarn the possibility of neoplasm or endometriosis. Excessive discomfort during rectal examination is common in patients with IBS.

Care should be taken to fully evaluate the low back, abdominal, and pelvic musculoskeletal system as possible sources for the pain. Viewing the patient's spine while she is sitting and standing and watching her walk a few paces may suggest a musculoskeletal problem. Asking the patient to bend at the waist can make a previously overlooked scoliosis apparent. Assessment of leg length, joint range of motion, and muscle strength may reveal an unexpected source for pain referred to the pelvis or lower abdomen. Consultation with a physical therapist for some of these less familiar evaluations may be helpful.

On pelvic examination, asymmetric or irregular enlargement of the uterus should suggest myomas or other tumors. Symmetric enlargement of the uterus is often present in adenomyosis and occasionally when intrauterine polyps are present. The presence of painful posterior cul-de-sac nodules and restricted motion of the uterus suggests endometriosis. Restricted motion of the uterus is also found in patients with pelvic scarring from adhesions or inflammation. Inflammatory processes, past or present, may cause palpable thickening of the adnexal structures. Cultures or Pap smears should be obtained as needed.

Laboratory, X-ray, and Ultrasound Studies

Laboratory tests will not be cost-effective without a specific indication. Some authors recommend a complete blood count, erythrocyte sedimentation rate (ESR) and Venereal Disease Research Laboratory (VDRL) test as general screening measures. These may suggest occult organic disease. Urinalysis and culture, even when the patient has no urinary complaints, may occasionally uncover a chronic cystitis or other urologic disease.

In any patient with chronic pelvic pain, a stool sample for occult blood should be obtained. Measurements of urethral caliber (to assess stenosis) or office cystoscopy may be indicated for some patients. Patients with anemia should be evaluated by flexible sigmoidoscopy to assess the possibility of neoplasia as cause. Anoscopy, colonoscopy, gastroscopy, or consultation with a gastroenterologist may also be indicated for selected patients.

Patients and providers are often anxious to employ ultrasound, computed tomography (CT) scanning, or magnetic resonance imaging (MRI) evaluations in the search for a cause of chronic pain. Except in massively obese patients or those with a strong suspicion of malignancy, these modalities are not much help, although some authors suggest using them to search for ascites, gallstones, masses, or pancreatic enlargement. Barium enema, intravenous pyelography, and other radiologic investigations should be reserved for those patients in whom a specific diagnosis is being considered. They are not good screening tests for chronic pelvic pain patients. Specialized consultation is probably warranted when these tests are considered.

In patients with a significant cyclic component to their complaints, suppression with oral contraceptives or gonadotropin-releasing hormone (GnRH) agonists as a diagnostic trial may be of help in establishing the role of the reproductive system. In selected patients, the evaluation may need to be supplemented by diagnostic laparoscopy.

Diagnostic laparoscopy is appropriate in the evaluation and treatment of patients experiencing chronic pelvic pain with no clinically evident cause. In some studies, over half the patients who had normal pelvic examinations had pathology identified. Unfortunately, the same studies indicate that almost 20% of those thought to have pelvic pathology based on the clinical examination, had normal laparoscopic evaluations. Laparoscopy is of greatest help when the pelvic examination is abnormal, initial therapy fails, or when negative findings are sufficiently significant to justify the operative risks involved (e.g., patients with morbid fears of cancer). Laparoscopy will not identify pathology in up to a third of chronic pain patients. The absence of findings, however, does not exclude the possibility of somatic disease, and may be therapeutic in and of itself. Between 20% and 40% of patients with normal laparoscopic findings report improvement of their pain following laparoscopy even though no therapy was carried out.

Laparoscopy allows the pelvic viscera to be inspected for signs of subclinical endometriosis or pelvic adhesive disease. Ablative therapy or lysis of adhesions may be considered at this time. Inspection of the anterior and posterior cul-de-sacs, the sigmoid, cecum, appendix, and the upper abdomen (the liver edge and gall bladder) may be accomplished. Because laparoscopy is clearly an invasive procedure with the possibility of serious consequences, it should be reserved until other diagnostic avenues have been explored.

Hysteroscopy and colposcopy have little place in the evaluation of either acute or chronic pelvic pain.

THERAPEUTIC OPTIONS

Acute Pain

Every clinician recognizes that the first and foremost therapy for any acute pain, is the effective treatment of its cause. This may vary from emergency surgery to reassurance and simple support. Catastrophic events will require specialized, inpatient care. When the cause of pain is determined to be self-limited and does not threaten the long-term health or safety of the patient, primary, ambulatory care is suitable. For these patients, symptomatic therapy, either directly or as an adjunct to pathology directed therapy, is appropriate. (Specific therapies for the gynecologic antecedents of acute pain mentioned are discussed in other appropriate chapters, and are not repeated here.)

When supportive analgesia is considered, two approaches may be reasonable: direct pain relief by centrally acting analgesics and pain prevention through blocking the origin of the pain signal. Most commonly used pain interventions fall into the first category, whereas nonsteroidal anti-inflammatory agents and transcutaneous electrical nerve stimulation (TENS) fall into the latter group.

When central analgesics are used, they should be instituted early and in sufficient doses to result in reasonable relief. A number of studies have demonstrated that the best result is obtained by overcoming the sensation of pain before it has become well established, rather than trying to suppress the feelings once they have become severe. Side effects are common and care should be taken with any analgesic. Sedation is frequent with moderate to strong analgesics and appropriate warnings must be given to patients about driving and other hazardous activities. A summary of common analgesics is shown in Table 22.3.

The analgesic action of many agents may be enhanced through the use of adjuncts such as butalbital (for example with acetaminophen and caffeine; Fioricet, or aspirin and caffeine; Fiorinal). When musculoskeletal processes are involved, the use of muscle relaxants (e.g., Flexeril, Norflex, Norgesic, Parafon, Robaxin, Soma, Valium) may increase the efficacy of analgesics, or replace them completely.

Nonsteroidal anti-inflammatory drugs (NSAIDs) have little central analgesic action, but instead work to block the origination of the pain signal by interfering with the synthesis of prostaglandins and their action, or both. These agents will be very effective if the antecedent pathology responsible for the pain involves the generation of prostaglandins (as in inflammation, or primary dysmenorrhea). When prostaglandin production is not a major part of the pathophysiology present, these agents will not provide satisfactory pain relief. (These agents are discussed at length in Chapter 18, Menstrual Pain.)

TENS therapy acts to "scramble" the pain signal through direct stimulation of peripheral nerves. The exact mechanism of action is debated, but for many patients TENS provides excellent pain relief. This modality is most effective for musculoskeletal pain, but even visceral pain may be relieved. Although TENS units are moderately expensive (they may be rented as well), the lack of systemic side effects and their degree of efficacy make them attractive for pain syndromes that last more than a few days. Unfortunately, TENS therapy should not be used in patients who are pregnant.

Table 22.3. Commonly Used Analgesics

Drug	Oral dose (mg)	IM* dose (mg)	Comments
Mild Analgesics			
Acetaminophen	650 q3–4 h		Available singly or in multiple combinations
Aspirin	325–500 q3–4 h		Oral or suppository
Nonsteroidal agents	Variable		Only mild central analgesia, best for processes that involve liberation of prostaglandins, Ketorolac available as IM (15–30 mg q6 h)
Intermediate Agents			
Propoxyphene	65 q3–4 h		Related to methadone, may accumulate with repetitive doses, overdose may cause convulsions
Codeine	15–60 q4–6 h	30–60 q4–6 h	Well absorbed orally
Oxycodone	5–30 q4–6 h	5–10 q4–6 h	Short-acting, fewer side effects than codeine, may be combined with other agents
Hydrocodone	5–10 q4–6 h		Has moderate antitussive activity, generally combined with other agents
Pentazocine	50–100 q4–6 h	30–60 q4 h	Mixed agonist, antagonist, may cause withdrawal in narcotic dependent patients
Strong Analgesics			
Meperidine	50–100 q3–4 h	50–100 q2–4 h	Has toxic metabolites, not for use in patients on monoamine oxidase inhibitors or those with renal dysfunction, 75% of oral dose lost in feces, not recommended for chronic use
Butorphanol tartrate		2 q3–4 h	Mixed agonist, antagonist, may cause withdrawal in narcotic-dependent patients, has dose ceiling
Dezocine		10 q3–6 h	Mixed agonist, antagonist, may cause withdrawal in narcotic-dependent patients, has dose ceiling

Table 22.3. (continued)

Nalbuphine HCL		10 q3–6 h	Mixed agonist, antagonist, may cause withdrawal in narcotic-dependent patients, has dose ceiling
Morphine	30–60 q3–4 h 90–120 q12 h	10 q3–4 h	Controlled release form allowing twice a day dosing
Hydromorphone	6 q3–4 h	1.5–2 q4–6 h	Short-acting narcotic
Methadone	10–20 q3–4 h	2.5–10 q3–4 h	Long-acting oral, used for maintenance treatment of addicts, little abuse potential
Levorphanol	4 q6–8 h	2 q6–8 h	Long-acting, good oral absorption, similar to methadone
Oxymorphone		1 q3–4 h	Rectal suppositories 5 mg q4–6 h
Fentanyl			Transdermal 25–50 μg/h q72 h, used only for long-term therapy (e.g., cancer pain)

*IM = intramuscular administration; for short-term use only.
q = every.

Chronic Pain

As with acute pain, successful chronic pain management depends on establishing a working diagnosis. Although analgesics, antispasmodics, and birth control pills may have some temporary benefit, only specific therapy aimed at correcting the cause will ultimately be successful. Because it may not be possible to relieve pain in all cases, it is sometimes necessary to settle for little improvements, enhanced coping strategies, or behavioral modifications. The overall goals of chronic pain management are summarized in Table 22.4.

Medical therapy for pain involves more than analgesics. If an intrauterine contraceptive device is the likely cause of chronic, recurring pain, removal is in order. If the cause of the patient's complaints appears to be pelvic relaxation or retroversion of the uterus, a pessary may be curative. When the definitive therapy is not practical or available (e.g., multiple fibroids in a patient wishing no possibility of hysterectomy or impaired fertility), modifications of the menstrual cycle may be indicated. This may be as simple as the use of oral contraceptives or it may involve more extensive modifications such as cycle suppression with agents like danazol, depo-medroxyprogesterone acetate (DMPA), or GnRH agonists. The GnRH agonists are helpful in evaluating the role of the uterus and ovaries in patients with chronic pain by creating a "medical hysterectomy." If suppression with a GnRH agonist fails to provide improvement, it is unlikely that surgical removal of the organs will give any better results.

Careful consideration must be given before any referral is made for possible surgery in

Table 22.4. Principles of Chronic Pain Management

Treat the underlying disorder
Treat pain promptly and aggressively
Assess psychological factors early
Enlist the help of the patient
Establish reasonable goals
Use multiple treatment modalities for synergy
Use narcotic drugs with caution
Provide positive reinforcement and support at all stages

these patients. Surgical therapy for chronic pelvic pain must be limited and carried out with the full knowledge by both doctor and patient that the pain may not be improved and may even be made worse by the surgical procedure. Only in those few patients in whom a specific, surgically correctable process can be pointed to with some probability as the root of the patient's complaints, can there be a chance for successful surgical therapy.

Hysterectomy or oophorectomy are often carried out for pelvic pain, but long-term success is disappointing. Hysterectomy should be reserved for only those patients with pain that is clearly uterine in origin and known to be from a surgically correctable cause. The ovary is sometimes involved with acute processes, but is seldom the source of chronic pain complaints, making oophorectomy unlikely to provide relief. (The rare exception to this is the retained ovary syndrome that may occur when an ovary left at the time of hysterectomy becomes enmeshed in dense adhesions.) Even in those patients with surgically correctable conditions, both the physician and the patient must understand the possibility (if not the probability) that the pain may be unchanged or even worsened by the procedure. It should be noted that roughly 25% of patients referred for evaluation of chronic pelvic pain have previously undergone hysterectomy without resolution of their complaints.

The possible exceptions to these surgical caveats is the use of laser ablation of the uterosacral ligaments (LUNA) or presacral neurectomy. These are generally reserved for those patients in whom no other therapy has been useful. Although some reports claim up to 85% relief from pain, these procedures are far from innocuous and their use should be severely limited.

Analgesics

Analgesics are an obvious first step when nonspecific therapies must be used. For mild pain, aspirin, acetaminophen, propoxyphene, or their compounds have found wide use and are a resonable starting point in any therapy. Unfortunately, the pain many of these patients experience is of sufficient magnitude that these agents may be less than fully effective, prompting many to move to more potent drugs.

Strong pain, especially pain that does not respond to initial treatment, warrants even stronger agents, such as narcotics. Adjusted to the needs of the individual, these stronger agents may give good pain relief, but side effects (such as sedation) may still render the patient unable to function normally. For most patients, transient use of these drugs is well tolerated and does present a significant abuse potential. Undertreatment of pain is more likely to lead to chronic pain states and drug-seeking behavior. Drug abuse and dependence are more likely when care is fragmented, episodic (such as frequent emergency room visits), or when it is given by multiple providers. This risk diminishes with early, aggressive, time-limited, effective therapies. If abuse or drug-seeking behavior are suspected, drugs such as methadone can provide analgesia with less addicting euphoria and no significant street value for resale.

Combinations of medications (such as combining NSAIDs and opiates) may increase analgesic potency. Care must be exercised to avoid simultaneously compounding side effects. The use of these drugs should be limited and care exercised. Nonsteroidal agents may be used in place of more potent agents, but because the main analgesic action of these drugs is via inhibition of prostaglandin synthesis, they are of little value in pain processes that do not involve prostaglandin release.

When analgesics, especially stronger agents, are utilized care must be taken to avoid secondary gains that may contribute to or worsen the psychosocial aspects of the problem. Watch for direct positive reinforcement (such as special attention, care, or nurturing), indirect positive reinforcement (such as avoidance behaviors), and extinction or negative reinforcement of "well" behaviors. Each of these factors complicates improvement and may prevent total resolution of the patient's symptoms. It is important to involve the patient directly in the process of adaptation and rehabilitation. Having the patient take an active responsibility increases the success in establishing positive adaptive behaviors and decreases dependency and the "need to be ill."

When medications are used, they should be given on a regular basis, not "as needed." The latter requires the patient to have pain and validates the her symptoms, often fueling the social aspects of pain behavior. Just enough medication should be given to get the patient to the next regular appointment. Neither the appointment nor the medication should be altered based on the pain. Both the patient and physician should understand the long-term nature of the illness and its treatment. By minimizing secondary gain and removing the pain as a controlling influence, somatization and psychosocial factors may be separated from other causes and minimized.

Other Modalities

Because some studies have shown a high incidence of sleep disorders in these patients, some centers have reported success with medications such as amitriptyline (Elavil) in doses of 25 to 50 mg at bedtime. Any agent that improves sleep, especially rapid eye movement (REM) sleep patterns may be successful in reducing pain. It is unknown if this success is due to a causal relationship between sleep disturbances and symptoms of pain or merely reflects improved coping from more restful sleep. Although methodologic problems abound in most of the published literature on the use of antidepressants in chronic pain patients, meta-analysis and more recent studies indicate a significant improvement in pain for a high percentage of patients treated with these drugs.

Physical therapy and exercise programs may be of great help in patients with musculoskeletal components to their pain. Massage and tactile stimulation in the area of pain can suppress pain signals and may possibly explain the pain relief obtained by liniments, rubbing, or acupuncture. The application of heat or cold, when not otherwise contraindicated, may provide relief for some patients. The use of TENS therapy can provide excellent pain relief for some patients without the side effects associated with pharmacologic agents. Nerve blocks and trigger point injections may be of significant help in selected patients, whereas psychotherapy, biofeedback, relaxation therapy, acupuncture, or hypnosis may help others. Some patients respond well to anti-inflammatory medications, muscle relaxants, mechanical support, active and passive exercise, stretch, diathermy, and other modalities. Even exercise programs directed toward enhancing strength or mobility can be therapeutic. Postural education may be helpful; it provides a chance for the patient to take responsibility for her pain and recovery and reduces dependency behaviors. Success with these modalities is influenced by patient motivations and the underlying physiology involved.

Pain management for patients with disseminated malignancies or terminal illness poses a unique and challenging problem. Although these problems extend beyond the scope of gynecologic care and the focus of this book, many of the same principles that apply to pelvic pain can be applied to these patients as well. Excellent reviews of this aspect of pain management are contained in the US Department of Health and Human Services publications listed in the general reference section at the end of this chapter.

HINTS AND COMMON QUESTIONS

Many patients anticipate discomfort during examination of the abdomen or pelvis. Asking about the patient's most recent bowel movement provides a good distraction during palpation and results in a more objective examination.

Although most clinicians (and many patients) are familiar with the trick of palpating the abdomen with a stethoscope to provide a more objective evaluation of abdominal tenderness, few know about the trick of "splitting" the hands during pelvic examination. To get a more objective sense of true pelvic tenderness, palpate in one lower quadrant while the internal pelvic hand palpates the opposite adnexa. Patients who anticipate pain or who are amplifying tenderness, tend to follow the abdominal hand and report discomfort based on its actions. Patients with true adnexal tenderness will report pain either in both lower quadrants or will report it on the side of internal palpation.

Having the patient raise her head or lift her legs will result in tightening of the abdominal wall musculature. When pain in increased by this maneuver, the abdominal wall itself is generally the source.

When IBS is suspected, bulk-forming agents, anxiolytics, and low-dose antidepressants are recommended. Anticholinergics have generally fallen out of favor owing to a lack of effectiveness at doses that do not cause significant side effects.

Empiric treatment of chronic pelvic pain patients with antibiotics is inappropriate in the absence of positive cervical cultures, pyuria, or clinical criteria establishing a high likelihood of specific infection.

SUGGESTED READINGS

General References

American College of Obstetricians and Gynecologists. Pelvic Pain. ACOG Technical Bulletin 223. Washington, DC: ACOG, 1996.
American Fertility Society. Management of endometriosis in the presence of pelvic pain. Fertil Steril 1993;60:952.

Bass C, Benjamin S. The management of chronic somatisation. Br J Psychiatry 1993;162:472.

Beck A. Depression inventory. Philadelphia: Center for Cognitive Therapy, 1991.

Bonica JJ, ed. The management of pain, 2nd ed. Philadelphia: Lea & Febiger, 1990.

Budd K. Chronic pain—challenge and response. Drugs 1994;1(suppl):22.

DiGregorio GJ, Barbieri EJ, Ferko AP, et al. Handbook of Pain Management, 4th ed. West Chester, PA: Medical Surveillance Inc., 1994.

Drife JO. The pelvic pain syndrome. Br J Obstet Gynaecol 1993;100:508.

Ford CV. The somatizing disorders. Psychosomatics 1986;27:327.

Gamsa A. The role of psychological factors in chronic pain. I. A half century of study. Pain 1994;57:5.

Gamsa A. The role of psychological factors in chronic pain. II. A critical appraisal. Pain 1994;57:17.

Goldenberg DL. Fibromyalgia syndrome. JAMA 1987;257:2782.

Hodgkiss AD, Watson JP. Psychiatric morbidity and illness behavior in women with chronic pelvic pain. J Psychosom Res 1994;38:3.

International Association for the Study of Pain. Classification of chronic pain, descriptions of chronic pain syndromes and definitions of pain terms. Pain 1986;3(suppl):S1–S225.

Jacox A, Carr DB, Payne R, et al. Management of cancer pain. Clinical Practice Guideline No. 9. AHCPR Publication No. 94–0592. Rockville, MD: Agency for Health Care Policy and Research, US Department of Health and Human Services, March 1994.

King PM, Myers CA, Ling FW, Rosenthal RH. Sociocultural and musculoskeletal factors in chronic pelvic pain. Journal of Psychosomatic Obstetrics and Gynecology 1991;12:87.

Ling FW, ed. Contemporary management of chronic pelvic pain. Obstet Gynecol Clin N Am 1993;20(4):627.

Loeser JD, Egan KJ, eds. Managing the chronic pain patient. New York: Raven Press, 1989.

Lundberg WI, Wall JE, Mathers JE. Laparoscopy in the evaluation of pelvic pain. Obstet Gynecol 1973;42:872.

Pilowsky I, Katsikitis M. A classification of illness behavior in pain clinic patients. Pain 1994;57:91.

Pratt RB. Cancer Pain. Philadelphia: JB Lippincott, 1993.

Rachlin ES. Myofacial Pain and Fibromyalgia: Trigger Point Management. St. Louis: Mosby, 1994.

Rapkin AJ, Kames LD. The pain management approach to chronic pelvic pain. J Reprod Med 1987;32:323.

Rapkin AJ, Kames LD. History of physical and sexual abuse in women with chronic pelvic pain. Obstet Gynecol 1990;76:92.

Rapkin AJ, Reading AE. Chronic pelvic pain. Current Problems in Obstetrics Gynecology Fertility 1991;14:102.

Reidenberg MM, Portenoy RK. The need for an open mind about the treatment of chronic nonmalignant pain. Clin Pharmacol Ther 1994;55:367.

Reiter RC, Gambone JC. Nongynecologic somatic pathology in women with chronic pelvic pain and negative laparoscopy. J Reprod Med 1991;36:253.

Renaer M. Chronic pelvic pain without obvious pathology in women. Eur J Obstet Gynec Reprod Biol 1980;10:415.

Schmidt RE, Babock DS, Farrell MK. Use of abdominal and pelvic ultrasound in the evaluation of chronic abdominal pain. Clin Pediatr 1993;32:147.

Slocumb JC. Chronic somatic, myofacial, and neurogenic abdominal pelvic pain. Clin Obstet Gynecol 1990;33:145.

Smith RP. Somatization. In Ling FW, Laube DM, Nolan TE, Smith RP (eds). Primary Care in Gynecology. Baltimore: Williams & Wilkins, 1995.

Steege JF, Stout AL, Somkuti SG. Chronic pelvic pain in women: toward an integrative model. Obstet Gynecol Surv 1991;12:95.

Travell JG. Chronic myofascial pain syndromes. Advances in Pain Research and Therapy 1990;17:129–137.

Williamson HA JR, Williamson MT. The Beck depression inventory: normative data and problems with generalizability. Fam Med 1989;21:58.

Specific References

Applegate WV. Abdominal cutaneous nerve entrapment syndrome. Surgery 1972;71:118.

Bates MS, Edwards WT, Anderson KO. Ethnocultural influences on variation in chronic pain perception. Pain 1993;52:101.

Beard RW, Pearce S, Highman JH, Reginald RW. Diagnosis of pelvic vericosities in women with chronic pelvic pain. Lancet 1984;2:946.

Benson RC, Hanson KHJ, Matarazzo JD. Atypical pelvic pain in women: gynecologic-psychiatric considerations. Am J Obstet Gynecol 1959;77:806.

Carleson KJ, Miller BA, Fowler FJ Jr. The Maine Women's Health Study: II. Outcomes of nonsurgical management of leiomyomas, abnormal bleeding, and chronic pelvic pain. Obstet Gynecol 1994;83:566.

Covington EC. Depression and chronic fatigue in the patient with chronic pain. Prim Care 1991;18:341.

Cox GB, Chapman CR, Black RG. The MMPI and chronic pain: the diagnosis of psychogenic pain. J Behav Med 1978;1:437.

Creed F, Craig T, Farmer R. Functional abdominal pain, psychiatric illness, and life events. Gut 1988;29:235.

Cunanan RG, Couren NG, Lippes J. Laparoscopic findings in patients with pelvic pain. Am J Obstet Gynecol 1983;146:589.

Dalton JA, Feuerstein M, Carlson J, Roghman K. Biobehavioral pain profile: development and psychometric properties. Pain 1994;57:95.

Deardorff WW, Chino AF, Scott DW. Characteristics of chronic pain patients: factor analysis of the MMPI-2. Pain 1993;54:153.

Deathe AB, Helmes E. Evaluation of a chronic pain programme by referring physicians. Pain 1993;52:113.

Dellemijn PL, Fields HL. Do benzodiazepines have a role in chronic pain management? Pain 1994;57:137.

Fayes JA, Toy NJ, Flanagan TM. The appendix as the cause of chronic lower abdominal pain. Am J Obstet Gynecol 1995;172:122.

Flor H, Fydrich T, Turk DC. Efficacy of multidisciplinary pain treatment centers: a meta-analytic flow. Pain 1992;49:221.

Fukaya T, Hoshiai H, Yajima A. Is pelvic endometrtiosis always associated with chronic pain? A retrospective study of 618 cases diagnosed by laparoscopy. Am J Obstet Gynecol 1993;169:719.

Gambone JC, Reiter RC. Nonsurgical management of chronic pelvic pain: a multidisciplinary approach. Clin Obstet Gynecol 1990;33:205.

Gangar KF, Stones RW, Saunders D, et al. Br J Obstet Gynaecol 1993;100:360.

Gershon S. Chronic pain: hypothesized mechanism and rationale for treatment. Neuropsychobiology 1986;15:22.

Goetsch MF. Vulvar vestibulitis: prevalence and histologic features in a general gynecologic practice population. Am J Obstet Gynecol 1991;164:1609.

Gross RJ, Doerr H, Caldirola D, Guzinski GM, Ripley HS. Borderline syndrome and incest in chronic pelvic pain patients. Int J Psychiatry Med 1981;10:79.

Harrop-Griffiths J, Katon W, Walker E, Holm L, Russo J, Hickok L. The association between chronic pelvic pain, psychiatric diagnoses, and childhood sexual abuse. Obstet Gynecol 1988;71:589.

Heisterberg L. Factors influencing spontaneous abortion, dyspareunia, dysmenorrhea, and pelvic pain. Obstet Gynecol 1993;81:594.

Hogston P. Irritable bowel syndrome as a cause of chronic pain in women attending a gynecology clinic. BMJ 1987;294:934.

Jensen MP, McFarland CA. Increasing the reliability and validity of pain intensity measurement in chronic pain patients. Pain 1993;55:195.

Jensen MP, Turner JA, Romana JM. Correlates of improvement in multidisciplinary treatment of chronic pain. J Consult Clin Psychol 1994;62:172.

Kresch A, Seifer DB, Sachs LD, Varrese I. Laparoscopy in 100 women with chronic pelvic pain. Obstet Gynecol 1984;64:672.

Landau B, Levy RM. Neuromodulation techniques for medically refractory chronic pain. Annu Rev Med 1993;44:279.

Longstreth GF, Preskill DB, Youkeles L. Irritable bowel syndrome in women having diagnostic paparoscopy or hysterectomy: relation to gynecologic features and outcome. Dig Dis Sci 1990;35:1285.

Malone MD, Strube MJ. Meta-analysis of non-medical treatments for chronic pain. Pain 1988;34:231.

Magni G, Moreschi C, Rigatti-Luchini S, Merskey H. Prospective study on the relationship between depressive symptoms and chronic musculoskeletal pain. Pain 1994;56:289.

Maruta T, Swanson DW, McHardy WO Jr, et al. Three year follow-up of patients with chronic pain who were treated in a multidisciplinary pain management center. Pain 1990;41:47.

McClaflin RR. Myofascial pain syndrome. Primary care strategies for early intervention. Postgrad Med 1994;96:56.

McFadden IJ, Witalla VF. Differing reports of pain perception by different personalities in a patient with chronic pain and multiple personality disorder. Pain 1993;55:379.

Nolan TE, Elkins TE, Chronic pelvic pain. Differentiating anatomic from functional causes. Postgrad Med 1993;94:125.

Nolan TE, Metheny WP, Smith RP. The unrecognized association of sleep disorders and depression in chronic pelvic pain. South Med J 1992;85:1181.

Pérez-Stable EJ, Miranda J, Muñoz RF, Ying YW. Depression in medical outpatients: underrecognition and misdiagnosis. Arch Intern Med 1990;150:1083.

Peters AAW, van Dorst E, Jellis B, et al. A randomized clinical trial to compare two different approaches in women with chronic pelvic pain. Obstet Gynecol 1991;77:740.

Rapkin AJ. Adhesions and pelvic pain: a retrospective study. Obstet Gynecol 1986;68:13.

Rapkin AJ, Kames LD, Darke LL, Stampler FM, Naliboff BD. History of physical and sexual abuse in women with chronic pelvic pain. Obstet Gynecol 1990;76:92.

Reading AE. A comparison of the McGill Pain Questionnaire in chronic and acute pain. Pain 1982;13:185.

Reading AE. A critical analysis of psychological factors in the management and treatment of chronic pelvic pain. Int J Psychiatry Med 1982;12:129.

Reiter RC, Gambone JC. Demographic and historic variables in women with idiopathic chronic pelvic pain. Obstet Gynecol 1990;75:428.

Reiter RC. Occult somatic pathology in women with chronic pelvic pain. Clin Obstet Gynecol 1990;33:154.

Renaer M, Vertommen H, Nijs P, Wagemans L, Van Hemerlijck T. Psychological aspects of chronic pelvic pain in women. Am J Obstet Gynecol 1979;134:75.

Renaer MJ, Vertommen H, Mijs P, et al. Psychic aspects of pelvic pain in women. Am J Obstet Gynecol 1979;134:75.

Roseff SJ, Murphy AA. Laparoscopy in the diagnosis and therapy of chronic pelvic pain. Clin Obstet Gynecol 1990;33:137.

Schmidt RE, Babcock DS, Farrell MK. Use of abdominal and pelvic ultrasound in the evaluation of chronic abdominal pain. Clin Pediatr 1993;32:147.

Slocumb JC. Neurologic factors in chronic pelvic pain: trigger points and the adbominal pelvic pain syndrome. Am J Obstet Gynecol 1984;149:536.

Smith RP, Metheny WP, Nolan TE. A tool for the assessment of chronic pelvic pain. Journal of Psychosomatic Obstetrics and Gynecology 1992;13:281.

Smith WB, Safer MA. Effects of present pain level on recall of chronic pain and mecication use. Pain 1993;55:355.

Soellner W. Huter O, Wurm B, Kanter J, Rumplmair W. Longitudinal follow-up of chronic pelvic pain and occurrence of new symptoms 5 to 7 years after laparoscopy. Am J Obstet Gynecol 1993;168:1645.

Steege JF, Stout AL. Resolution of chronic pelvic pain in women after laparoscopic lysis of adhesions. Am J Obstet Gynecol 1991;165:278.

Stenchever MA. Symptomatic retrodisplacement, pelvic congestion, universal joint, and peritoneal defects: fact or fiction? Clin Obstet Gynecol 1990;33:161.

Stoval TG, Ling FW, Crawford DA. Hysterectomy for chronic pelvic pain of presumed uterine etiology. Obstet Gynecol 1990;75:676.

Summitt RL, Ling FW. Urethral syndrome presenting as chronic pelvic pain. Journal of Psychosomatic Obstetrics and Gynecology 1991;12:77.

Taylor HC. Vascular congestion and hyperemia. I. Physiologic basis in history of the concept. Am J Obstet Gynecol 1949;57:211.

Taylor HC. Vascular congestion and hyperemia. II. The clinical aspects of congestion-fibrosis syndrome. Am J Obstet Gynecol 1949;57:637.

Toomey TC, Hernandez JT, Gittelman DF, Hulka JF. Relationship of sexual and physical abuse to pain and psychological assessment variables in chronic pelvic pain patients. Pain 1993;53:105.

Turk DD, Okifuji A. Detecting depression in chronic pain patients: adequacy of self-reports. Behav Res Ther 1994;32:9.

Turk DC, Rudy TE, Sorkin BA. Neglected topics in chronic pain treatment outcome studies: determination of success. Pain 1993;53:3.

Vercellini P, Bocciolone L, Vendola N, Colombo A, Rognoni M, Fedele L. Peritoneal endometriosis: morphologic appearance in women with chronic pelvic pain. J Reprod Med 1991;36:533.

Von Korff M, Le Resche L, Dworkin SF. First onset of common pain symptoms: a prospective study of depression. Pain 1993;55:251.

Walker EA, Katon WJ, Jemelka R, et al. The prevalence of chronic pelvic pain and irritable bowel syndrome in two university clinics. Journal of Psychosomatic Obstetrics and Gynecology 1991;12(suppl):65.

Walling MK, O'Hara MW, Reiter RC, et al. Abuse history and chronic pain in women: I. Prevalences of sexual abuse and physical abuse. Obstet Gynecol 1994;84:193.

Walling MK, O'Hara MW, Reiter RC, et al. Abuse history and chronic pain in women: II. A multivariate analysis of abuse and psychological morbidity. Obstet Gynecol 1994;84:200.

Williams AC, Richardson PH. What does the BDI measure in chronic pain? Pain 1993;55:259.

Woodforde JM, Merskey H. Personality traits of patients with chronic pain. J Psychosom Res 1972;16:167.

23

Sexual Assault and Abuse

Women are, and always have been, the disproportionate victims of violence in all societies. In the United States it is estimated that a woman is abused, battered, or assaulted every 9 seconds. This amounts to over 3.5 million episodes a year. Studies report that 20% to 40% of adults report abuse or sexual victimization before the age of 18, and 10% to 25% of wives experience sexual violence at the hands of their husbands at some time in their marriage. Although the rate of increase has slowed somewhat, forcible rapes in the United States increased over 35% between 1975 and 1984. Rape now makes up 5% to 10% of violent crime in this country. As protectors of women's health, we must be familiar with and watchful for the manifestations of abuse and sexual mistreatment.

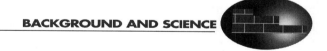

BACKGROUND AND SCIENCE

Definitions

The word rape is derived from the Latin word "rapere," meaning "to seize." Rape is a crime of violence. All victims are harmed psychologically, one third sustain minor genital or nongenital injuries, almost 10% sustain major trauma, and 0.5% die. Rape and sexual assault encompass manual, oral, or genital contact by one person without the consent of the other in a way that would be considered sexual in a consensual situation. It does not require penetration, ejaculation, force, or evidence of resistance, only the lack of consent. The legal definition varies slightly by location, but often includes elements of fear, fraud, coercion, or threat. In some areas, the mentally incompetent, those under the influence of drugs or alcohol, or those underage are deemed incapable of giving consent for any otherwise consensual sexual activity, resulting in "statutory rape." In many locales, changing laws now recognize the possibility of rape within marriage as a part of spousal abuse or as a separate legal entity.

Domestic violence and spousal abuse are terms used to describe violence between partners in an ongoing relationship. Almost universally, women are the victims of domestic violence, accounting for almost 95% of incidents. While the definition of battering requires only one episode of physical abuse, a pattern of escalating violence is more typical. In the typical battering relationship three phases are usually present; a tension-building phase that gradually escalates; the battering incident, which may be triggered by almost any event; and a period of contrition during which the batterer apologizes and asks for forgiveness. Despite the apparent remorse, this cycle tends to repeat, with each episode involving greater physical harm and risk and less remorse. Over one half of men who abuse their wives abuse their children as well.

Elder abuse is a newly publicized form of physical abuse that affects women. This abuse involves older women, most often past the age of 75, occurring at the hands of adult children. These patients are frequently disabled, widowed, and living with relatives. White patients are more frequently the victims of elder abuse than are patients of other races.

The National Center on Child Abuse and Neglect defines child sexual abuse as "contact or interactions between a child and an adult, when the child is being used for the sexual stimulation of that adult or another person. Sexual abuse may be committed by a person under the age of 18 years, when that person is either significantly older than the victim, or when the abuser is in a position of power, or control over that child." Sexual abuse includes, but is not limited to, disrobing, exposure, photography or posing, oral-genital contact, insertion of foreign bodies, and vaginal or rectal intercourse. Genital penetration is not a part of the definition and is, therefore, not required for the activity to constitute abuse. Less than 10% of childhood sexual assault involves penetration.

The risk of sexual abuse is greatest for children living in single-parent homes or those living with stepparents or in the homes of substance abusers. Adolescents are at higher risk for sexual assault by acquaintances or strangers.

Incest is the term applied when there is sexual activity inappropriate to a normal family relationship. Relatives may be of any degree or gender, including stepchildren or stepparents. Ninety percent of incest victims are female. Most perpetrators of child abuse are known to the child, with only about 10% to 15% of cases involving strangers. When a stranger is involved, the event is usually a solitary episode and is reported promptly, whereas family abuse is more likely to be ongoing and unreported. Brief or episodic occurrences are the rule, but once abuse occurs, it tends to be repeated, often with successive daughters. Only about 0.2% to 0.3% of children are involved in persistent incestuous relationships. For these children, the average duration before detection is more than 5 years.

Most incest involves fathers and daughters and begins gradually, without violence. These secret "games" progress from hugs and kisses to nudity, fondling, and overt sexual acts. Forced sexual behavior may extend outside of the father-daughter relationship, as the child may be enticed to perform for other members of the family or strangers. Secrecy is maintained by threats that the victim, not the abuser, will be punished if the behavior is discovered. The father is often characterized as rigid, patriarchal, and immature. Often he is an alcohol abuser. He brings to the relationship a sexual need, but is unlikely to have an extramarital affair. When a mother is present, she is often chronically depressed, debilitated, or sexually unavailable. The mother is often aware of the abuse, but chooses to ignore or deny it. One or both of the parents may themselves have been the victims of abuse. From external appearances, the family appears close knit but socially withdrawn, shy, or isolated.

Fewer than 10% of children and adult survivors of incest have normal psychological profiles at the time of evaluation. Guilt, anger, behavior problems, somatic complaints and illness, lying, stealing, school or employment failure, running away, divorce, and sleep disturbances are common in these patients. Altered or dysfunctional sexual development, including promiscuity, homosexuality, and prostitution, are common findings.

Incidence and Prevalence

Although no group of women is immune from the threat of rape, the highest proportion occurs to young, single women of low socioeconomic status (Table 23.1). The incidence of rape has been estimated to be 60 per 100,000 women, but there may be three to ten times as many rapes committed as are reported to authorities. Of those who report a rape, only 60% to 80% wish to prosecute the attacker. This reticence to prosecute is based on mistrust

Table 23.1. Demographics of Reported Sexual Assaults

	Total (%)
Age	
<10	7
10–15	16
16–20	27
21–30	35
31–40	9
>40	6
Race	
Black	36
White	59
Other	5
Marital status	
Single	75
Married	14
Other	11
Assailant	
Stranger	50
Casual acquaintance	30
Well known to victim	20
Location of attack	
Victim's home	26
Automobile	18
Assailant's home	15
Other	41

After: Cartwright PS. Sexual violence. In Jones HW III, Wentz AC, Burnett LS (eds). Novak's Textbook of Gynecology, 11th ed. Baltimore: Williams & Wilkins, 1988;527.

of the judicial system, a sense of futility, unfamiliarity with the options available, or fear of reprisal, and should not be interpreted as reflecting on the validity of the allegation.

One quarter to one half of all rapes occur at home (either the victim's or the attacker's), but only one third of these involve a male intruder. Most attackers are known to the victims. Up to one fifth of rape victims have been victims previously. Of these women, about 25% have been raped by someone well known to them, such as an ex-lover, employer, coworker, neighbor, or relative. Two thirds of recurrent rape victims are vulnerable owing to mental impairment, substance abuse, or psychiatric disorder.

Weapons are used in 30% to 50% of sexual assaults. Although handguns are the most common weapon, physical injury is twice as likely to occur when a knife or club is used (60% to 80% vs. 35% to 40%). Multiple attackers are involved in only 15% of sexual assaults.

"Date rape" represents a subset of sexual assault. Approximately 50% of campus rapes occur during dates. Estimates of sexual violence occurring in the setting of a dating relationship indicate that 10% to 25% of high school students and 20% to 50% of college students have experienced some form of sexual violence. One survey found that over 25% of college women and almost 10% of college men had experienced or committed an act that met the legal definition of rape. Date rape is less often reported than other sexual assaults because of a feeling of guilt or complicity. Other than the setting and degree of familiarity with the assailant, date rape differs little from any other form of sexual assault. "No" means "no" in any setting.

Current estimates suggest that there are over 1.5 million cases of domestic violence each year in the United States, almost all of which involve women as the victim. In as least one fourth of these cases, there have been three or more episodes of violence in the 6 months preceding the report of abuse. It is estimated that between 5% and 25% of women treated for injuries in emergency rooms receive these injuries as a result of domestic violence. Unfortunately, the correct diagnosis is rendered in less than 5% of cases. Between one third and one half of all female homicides occur at the hands of a male partner.

When physical abuse is reported, it is often only when injury occurs. In almost 85% of reported cases, the injuries sustained are sufficient to require medical treatment. Although battering most often involves fists or kicking, lacerations and fractures are not uncommon. The most frequent locations for injuries include the head, neck, chest, abdomen, and breasts. Upper extremity injuries often result from defensive efforts. Ten to twenty percent of pregnant women report physical abuse during pregnancy. For these women, injuries to the breast and abdomen are more frequent.

Elder abuse is estimated to have a prevalence of between 500,000 and 2.5 million cases per year in the United States. These estimates suggest that it is as common as child abuse, but less well recognized.

Childhood sexual abuse is thought to go unreported in 50% to 95% of cases. Roughly one of every four girls and one of every seven boys, will be sexually abused before the age of 18. Sexual abuse represents only about 10% to 15% of childhood abuse cases, although both physical and sexual abuse often coexist. One recent report suggested that the incidence of child abuse has risen by over 300% in the past few years, but this fails to take into account the effects of increased awareness and reporting. Even with increasing awareness, the possibility of childhood sexual abuse is often overlooked. In one study of adults reporting sexual abuse, only one quarter of those who reported the abuse were believed.

The Rape-trauma Syndrome

There is a well-recognized set of behaviors that occur after a sexual assault. These responses are organized into three phases: the acute phase, lasting from hours to days; a middle or readjustment phase that lasts from days to weeks; and a final, reorganization or resolution phase that involves life-long changes.

In the initial hours or days after a sexual assault, the victim may be unable to cope with the events that have occurred. This decompensation may or may not be evident by the time the patient seeks care. During this period emotions are volatile, with the patient moving from one extreme to another, from calm composure to tears or rage. Fear, guilt, anger, depression, and problems concentrating are common. Flashbacks to the assault are frequently experienced. Ideation is often disturbed to the point that the patient may mistakenly be presumed to be under the influence of drugs or alcohol. Even simple tasks such as recalling a home telephone number can be difficult. This cognitive dysfunction may itself be very distressing. Physical complaints may be vague and general. The patient may complain of generalized soreness, problems eating or sleeping, and headaches. These are involuntary reactions and the patient should be reassured that they are common reactions and not a sign of "going crazy."

During the initial phase of the rape-trauma syndrome, patients may mechanically perform routine tasks, including those that are inappropriate or that actually hinder the process of evaluation and evidence collection. These include showering, cleaning, vacuuming, or shopping. These behaviors are referred to as a "retreat into routine activities." This behavior pattern is motivated by a desire to regain control; it does not indicate the depth of psychological stress the patient is under and is definitely not proof that the assault did not occur, was invited, or was any less traumatic.

The middle or readjustment phase of the syndrome is marked by what appears to be the resolution of many of the issues about the assault. This resolution may not be completely functional, as the patient often rationalizes the events, unrealistically blames herself for the attack, or makes inappropriate plans to avoid similar situations in the future. Flashbacks and nightmares may continue and phobias may develop. These phobias may be directed toward consensual sex and sexuality or they may be unrelated, such as claustrophobia, acrophobia, and the like. During this phase the patient often attempts to find or fabricate reasons why the attack occurred or ways it could have been prevented. These give way to the late phase of the syndrome as a more realistic view of her victimization takes place.

In the late phase of the rape-trauma syndrome, the patient recognizes that her assault was just that, an assault, and she comes to grips with the fact that she could have had no control over the events. This phase is often accompanied by painful transitions, often involving significant changes in lifestyles, work, or friends. Insomnia, depression, somatic complaints, and poor self-esteem are common during this phase. For some, this phase can be extremely disruptive and prolonged.

Roughly one third of rape victims suffer long-term psychiatric problems. The risk of this is greatest for those over age 40, those assaulted in their homes by a stranger, and those with a history of previous mental illness. Whites are more likely to suffer long-term consequences than are blacks, but all women deserve intensive follow-up and counseling.

The health care provider has three basic responsibilities in the care of someone who may have been raped or abused: the detection and treatment of serious injuries, the preservation of evidence, and protection against sequelae. The first of these deals with establishing the diagnosis, the other two with interventions specific to rape. Fortunately, most patients who seek care do so within the first 6 hours after the assault, improving the chances of obtaining valuable forensic evidence and allowing early intervention into the emotional and physical sequellae of sexual assault and abuse (Fig. 23.1).

Almost any primary care provider is capable of obtaining the history and performing the physical assessments necessary in cases of suspected abuse or sexual assault. The most important factor is a willingness to do so with compassion, care, and sensitivity. Anyone who is unable or unwilling to bring these skills to the encounter should not place themselves in the situation, and must provide referral or supplementary coverage by someone who can.

History

Any patient who states that she has been the victim of a sexual offense should be treated as if it has occurred. Sometimes the history will not be this clear cut. The longer it has been since an assault or when abuse is ongoing, the more likely it is for the presenting complaints to be unrelated to the underlying concerns generated by the attack. Somatic complaints and subtle behavioral changes may suggest the possibility of domestic violence or abuse (Table 23.2).

Even though it is difficult, all patients must be encouraged to discuss the details of the attack or attacks. This not only establishes important details that will help to direct further investigation, it provides legal evidence and also helps the process of resolution to begin. In ad-

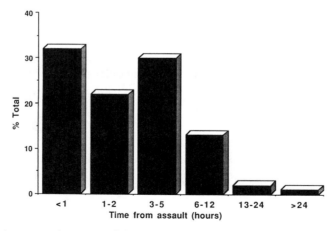

Figure 23.1. Delay in seeking care following sexual assault. Most victims of sexual assault seek care within 6 hours of the assault, offering an opportunity to collect good forensic evidence to aid prosecution.

Table 23.2. Adult Behaviors Suggestive of Abuse

Behavioral changes
    Dependency (often accompanied by male partner)
    Evasiveness
    Excessive embarrassment
    Fear or fright
    Frequent crying (often without reason)
    History of overdose
    Jumpiness
    Passivity
    Shyness
    Substance abuse
Somatic complaints
    Back pain
    Chest pain
    Choking sensation (globus hystericus)
    Generalized cryptic or chronic pain
    Headaches
    Hyperventilation
    Insomnia
    Pelvic pain
    Unexplained injuries or injuries of various ages

dition to details of the specific offense, it is important to establish background information such as the date and time of the last consensual intercourse, methods of contraception, and last menstrual period. Any actions taken since the event, such as bathing, douching, changing clothes, urinating, defecating, cleaning of nails, tooth brushing, or gargling, should be noted.

Often the diagnosis of physical or sexual abuse, especially in children, is made based on suspicion and careful follow-up. Behaviors that should suggest the possibility of abuse are listed in Table 23.3. In adults, multiple injuries of different ages, injuries that are poorly explained, or signs of trauma that are covered up should suggest the possibility of abuse. The patient who seems excessively intimidated, has vague complaints, or maintains poor eye contact may have a hidden agenda that may include abuse. The patient who hides a black eye with sunglasses and refuses to remove them in the office should be suspected of being an abuse victim and directly questioned whether "someone did this to you?" A structured screening tool, such as the five-question Abuse Assessment Screen, increases the likelihood of detecting abuse, but any method that raises awareness and opens discussion improves the chances of detection.

The diagnosis of child sexual abuse is based on suspicion and the history obtained from the child. The physical examination is seldom diagnostic. The initial history should be obtained from the parent or caregiver apart from the child, then obtained separately from the child. Some authors have suggested that these interviews be taped for later reference, but this is better suited to the emergency room or rape evaluation center, and not the primary care setting. Both the history and the subsequent physical examination must be recorded in detail. Dictation of these findings, which facilitates legibility and detail that may not be found in handwritten notes, should be seriously considered for any setting.

Table 23.3. Behaviors Suggestive of Childhood Sexual Abuse

Advanced or inappropriate sexual or anatomic knowledge
Appetite or eating disorders
Behavioral regression
Depression and introversion
Deterioration (sudden) of school performance
Enuresis
Genital or rectal itching
Hypochondriasis
Illegal acts or antisocial behaviors
Perineal warts
Posttraumatic stress disorder
Prostitution
Psychosomatic disorders
Recurrent abortions or pregnancies, especially in very young adolescents
Recurrent sexually transmitted disease
Recurrent urinary tract infection
Runaways
School truancy or attachment (fear of home)
Self-destructive behavior
Sexual acting out
Sleep disorders
Somatization
Substance abuse
Suicide attempts

Physical Examination

The first priority is always the management of any life-threatening injuries or processes. Although uncommon, this aspect cannot be overlooked. Victims of sexual assault should receive a complete examination, including pelvic and rectal examinations, and focused evaluations of any area involved in trauma (Table 23.4).

Because one of the pivotal aspects of sexual assault is the loss of control, every effort should be made to allow the patient control over even the most trivial aspect of the physical examination. All physical contacts should be preceded with a comment or a request for permission: "I need to look at your abdomen, if that is all right with you?" The presence of a chaperone is an absolute necessity, but a friend or support person of the patient's choosing may also be included.

The physical examination is normal in one half of rape victims and in over two thirds of children who have been sodomized. Despite this frequent lack of collaborating evidence, the physical examination is vital for documentation and to detect potentially life-threatening injuries that the patient may not be aware of or may have overlooked. Wherever possible, the physical examination should be performed within 72 hours of the presumed event. Special rape evaluation kits are available in many jurisdictions and should be used if available. Whether such a kit is used or not, there are some samples that should be obtained in all cases (Table 23.5). These samples should be obtained in all patients, even if they do not wish to report or prosecute the case.

Table 23.4. Evaluation of a Rape Victim

Demographics	Coercion history
Past medical history	Weapon
Allergies	Restraints
Medications	Threats
Surgeries	Altered consciousness/diminished capacity
Contraception	Drugs
Gynecologic history	Alcohol
Last menses	Medications
Consensual intercourse past 72 h	Sexual acts
Infection	Penetration
Medications	Where
Procedures	With what
Assault history	Ejaculation
Date	Foreign bodies
Time	Condoms
Place	Lubricants/other substances
Surroundings	Oral acts
Assailant identification	Post assault activities
Number	Bathing
Race (for forensics)	Douching
What each did	Change of clothes
	Gargling

Table 23.5. Forensic Specimens in Purported Rape or Sexual Abuse*

Specimen	Site	Comments
Wet preparation	Vagina	Examined for sperm, note motility
		May be taken from any site alleged to be involved
Dry swab (2–3 each site)	Vagina, mouth, throat, rectum, (mons)	To be examined for sperm, acid phosphatase, blood group antigens
		Mouth specimen from buccal pouch or upper molars
		Rectal swab must be from more than 1–2 cm from anus
		Moistened swab or gauze may be used to take samples from other areas, then dried
Saliva		Used to determine antigen secretion status
		May be obtained on 2 × 2 gauze and dried
Hair combings	Head and pubic area	Hairs obtained and comb used should be submitted separately
Nail scrapings and clippings		Some localities require separate right and left samples
Clothing		Clothing that is torn, bloody, or suspected of carrying semen
		Includes tampons, pads, and diapers
Documentation of trauma		Photographs or detailed drawings of abrasions, bruises, bites, pinch marks, and so forth

*Specimens may vary with locality and the availability of a rape evidence kit. Familiarity with local requirements is mandatory.

For any rape victim were blood is found in the vagina, great care must be taken to identify the source. Common sites of lacerations are the vaginal wall, the lateral fornices, and cul-de-sac. These areas must be adequately visualized, even if general anesthesia is required. Lacerations that perforate the peritoneal cavity require surgical exploration. Examination under general anesthesia is also indicated anytime the patient is unable to urinate, or there is hematuria, lower abdominal tenderness, or signs of occult blood loss, such as hypovolemia.

It is critical that any forensic samples or specimens obtained be handled in such a way that they can be used as evidence. If there are specific instructions on the handling of evidence as a part of a rape evaluation kit, it should be followed explicitly. In the absence of such instructions, the most important factor in the value of the evidence is the "chain of evidence." This is the provenance of each piece of evidence that documents the passage of the specimen from the patient, to the forensic laboratory, and eventually to a court. This chain must be unbroken and well documented. Once a specimen is obtained it must be kept in the custody of the person obtaining it until it can be directly, and personally, handed over to a superior, administrator, or law enforcement official. When the specimen is transferred, it should be noted when and to whom it was entrusted. Any break in this chain can result in the loss of that item as evidence and may jeopardize the possibility of a conviction.

Especially when examining children, it must be recognized that many anatomic and pathologic processes may be confused with signs of sexual abuse. Vaginal or vulvar hemangiomas, urethral caruncles or eversion, and vulvar skin changes such as lichen sclerosis may all be present and can be confused with signs of trauma. Even frank genital trauma may not be abuse related. Straddle injuries, such as falling on the crossbar of a boy's bicycle, will generally cause symmetric trauma and usually involve the anterior and posterior portions of the

Table 23.6. Strength of Findings in Presumed Abuse

Normal (Nonsupportive)
    No abnormalities
    Variations of normal
Nonspecific (Nonsupportive)
    Irritation, redness, abrasions
    Friability of posterior fourchette
    Healed lacerations of hymen, vagina, or anus
    Labial adhesions
    Hymeneal tags, bumps, and clefts
    Bruising
    Nonspecific infections
Suspicious
    Anal gaping ($\geq$ 1 cm when buttocks separated)
    Hymeneal-vaginal tears
    Hymeneal-perineal tears
    Hymeneal opening $\geq$ 1 cm
    Presence of foreign pubic hair
    Sexually transmitted disease
    Bite marks, pinches, burns
Definitive
    Presence of sperm
    Pregnancy

vulva and surrounding perineum. Trauma restricted to the 3 to 9 o'clock portions of the vulva are suggestive of abuse. Signs of bites, pinch marks, burns, or grip marks anywhere on the body suggest abuse, even if sexual impropriety has not been involved.

Very frequently, abused children will not have specific findings that support the diagnosis. Between 30% and 50% of children who are the victims of sexual abuse have normal vulvar findings. Between 65% and 85% of children with anal penetration will have a normal perineum when examined. At best, most physical findings only support a diagnosis of abuse, they cannot establish it (Table 23.6).

Children who are being evaluated for possible sexual abuse may be difficult or impossible to examine vaginally. In the absence of bleeding or overt trauma, specimens can be obtained by blindly passing a swab into the vagina. Speculum examination is always preferred, and is mandatory when penetration is presumed. In some, examination under anesthesia may be required.

CLINICAL INTERVENTION

Medical Concerns

Laboratory studies performed outside the needs of forensics should include cultures for chlamydia and gonorrhea, a screening serologic test for syphilis and human immunodeficiency virus (HIV), hepatitis antigens, a urinalysis (often with culture), and a pregnancy test for all menstrual-aged women, even those sterilized or using contraception. Cultures should be obtained from the vagina, cervix, anus, and oropharynx. These studies, and follow-up assessments for serologic change, are directed toward safeguarding the patient.

Antibiotic prophylaxis should be offered to all adults and children who are the victims of acute assaults. The risk of acquiring a sexually transmitted disease is uncertain but is estimated to be 3% to 5%, or less. The risk of becoming infected with HIV is unknown. Studies do indicate that women who are raped have a higher rate of pre-existing sexually transmitted diseases, further supporting the value of antibiotic treatment. The choice of antibiotics should be based on local prevalence of disease, drug allergies, and the presence of a known pregnancy. These are summarized in the flow chart shown in Figure 23.2. Tetanus toxoid should be given if indicated.

For patients at risk for pregnancy, postcoital contraception should be offered. If the patient chooses prophylaxis (Table 23.7), she must be counseled that if interdiction is unsuccessful, the agents used are teratogenic and a therapeutic abortion is recommended. These strategies are generally not effective if begun more than 48 hours after exposure. When they are begun promptly, failure is estimated to be in the range of 1 in 500 to 1 in 1000. For women who are not otherwise protected from pregnancy by virtue of contraception, sterilization, hysterectomy, or menopause, the risk of pregnancy with a single midcycle unprotected act of intercourse is estimated to be between 1 in 10 and 1 in 50.

Emotional Support

In the initial phase of clinical interaction, the primary goal is to provide reassurance and a return of control. Despite what might seem to be an unnecessarily traumatic reliving of the

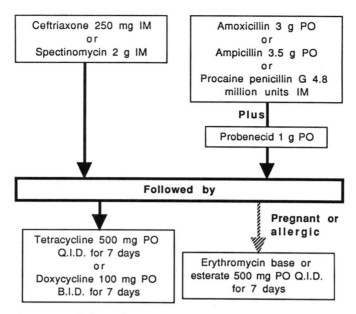

Figure 23.2. Antibiotic prophylaxis for sexual assault victims (adults). In localities with penicillin-resistant gonorrhea, ceftriaxone is recommended. This also provides coverage for rectal and pharyngeal infections that older regimens, including spectinomycin do not. (B.I.D. = Twice daily; Q.I.D. = Four times daily; PO = by mouth; IM = intramuscular injection)

Table 23.7. Pregnancy Interdiction for Sexual Assault Victims

Diethylstilbestrol, 25 mg orally, twice daily for 5 d with prochlorperazine (Compazine) 10 mg orally every 8 h
OR
Ethinyl estradiol, 0.05 mg plus norgestrel, 0.5 mg (Ovral), two tablets orally twice daily for 2–5 d (usually 3 d)
OR
Ethinyl estradiol, 5 mg orally once daily for 5 d
OR
Conjugated estrogen, 10 mg orally four time daily for 5 d

event, the patient should be encouraged to talk about the assault, the events surrounding it, and her feelings. This begins the process of working through the trauma, as the patient gains an understanding of her victimization. For similar reasons, the patient should be encouraged to work with law enforcement agencies and support groups. Both actions will improve the emotional outcome of the process.

Follow-up contacts by the health care provider, social service agencies, or support groups should be early and often. Many suggest that these may be as simple as a telephone call the next day to check up on the patient. Additional contacts at 1 or 2 weeks, a month, and periodically thereafter help provide support and identify evolving problems. Physical re-evaluation should be performed at 1 and 6 weeks to check for delayed symptoms or signs of pelvic infection, bleeding abnormalities, delayed menses, suicidal ideation, or other possible sequellae of the attack. Retesting for HIV and hepatitis B status should be scheduled for 12 to 18 weeks after the assault.

During the latter portions of the initial reaction to sexual assault and during the readjustment phase, patients characteristically transfer blame for the assault to themselves. Although the patient may have exercised poor judgment in her actions, location, dress, or behavior, this does not justify her assault. While the poor judgment should not be condoned, fault for the attack should be placed where it truely belongs, with the attacker.

Legal Considerations

Legal definitions of physical abuse and sexual assault vary from location to location, and health care providers should be familiar with those in effect in their area. In many locations, suspected sexual assault must be reported to law enforcement authorities. In all locations, suspected abuse, sexual or otherwise, occuring to a minor must be reported.

Medical records involving possible abuse or sexual assault must be carefully made, legible, and unambiguous. These records must only record objective findings and must not attempt to draw conclusions or identify the perpetrator. In all jurisdictions, rape and assault are legally determined and are not a medical diagnosis.

Great care must be taken with the phrases used in the medical records of patients who may have been victims of abuse or sexual assault. Off-hand medical phrases that seem innocent may present legal problems later. For example, it is best to avoid the phrase "normal examination," substituting instead phrases such as "unable to rule out abuse," or "sexual assault is neither confirmed nor denied." Final impressions that avoid legally defined terminology, such as "findings consistent with sexual abuse," are more appropriate than "Impression: rape." On the other side of the coin, some authors have suggested that the term "alleged rape" implies disbelief which may weaken an eventual legal case. Phrases that are less open to interpretation might include "history of sexual assault," or "possible rape." Clearly, great care in the initial crafting of the record will save a great deal of time later with explanation and possible testimony.

HINTS AND COMMON QUESTIONS

Most sexual assaults occur between 6 PM and 6 AM.

The rate of sexual assault decreases during the winter months in the northern United States.

The best advice one can give to young women to decrease the risk of date rape is to limit or avoid the use of alcohol. Studies indicate that alcohol use is involved in over half of all college rapes.

In 55% of rapes where the victim prosecutes, an arrest is made, and in 70% of cases the arrest is made within a week of the attack.

The term "molestation" is nonspecific. It is often used as a euphemism for abuse or assault, often of a less violent or nongenital nature.

Sexual abuse dose not usually include infantile sex games, such as "playing doctor," when acted out between children of roughly the same age.

Because child abuse is generally an ongoing process, delaying a detailed history or examination while obtaining expert assistance is not inappropriate.

If a support person, such as a spouse, friend, or companion, is available for the victim of a rape, it is helpful if they bring a change of clothing for the patient. This helps provide a separation from the assault and replaces any clothing kept in evidence.

The use of a Wood's lamp (ultraviolet light) will cause semen stains on skin or clothing to fluoresce, aiding in their identification and sampling.

When performing the speculum examination, only water should be used to lubricate the speculum because other lubricants can interfere with or destroy evidence.

All sexual assault victims should have saline and potassium hydroxide wet mounts of vaginal secretions obtained and examined for the presence of *Trichomonas* or *Candida* organisms.

The location and character of bites, bruises, pinch or grip marks, burns, or other signs of trauma should be carefully documented in any case of possible abuse or sexual assault. Photographing these findings will provide the best documentation, but care must be taken to allow the patient control by obtaining her consent and acquiescence.

Victims of repeated sodomy may loose normal anal sphincter tone, resulting in gaping or an anus that can easily admit two to four fingers. These patients may also display a relaxation phase to the normal anal wink reflex elicited by gently stroking the perineum with a cotton tip swab.

It is not unusual for a victim to be raped during menstruation. When the patient is a tampon user, extra care must be exercised to check for vaginal trauma and to be sure the tampon has been removed. If a tampon is recovered, it should be submitted along with other evidence for forensic evaluation.

Evidentiary specimens such as clothing should not be placed in plastic bags. They should be placed either in evidence containers provided by law enforcement agencies or in a sealed and labeled paper bag. Plastic bags retain moisture and promote bacterial and fungal growth that may materially alter the value of the evidence collected.

The absence of sperm does not rule out the possibility of sexual assault. Azoospermia, oligospermia, vasectomies, male sexual dysfunction, and the estimate that 30% of assault victims douche before seeking care, all contribute to the absence of sperm in one third to two thirds of cases.

If a child or adult has been involved in a long-standing abusive relationship, acute antibiotic prophylaxis is not necessary. Treatment may be based on the results of cultures. Empiric treatment is appropriate if the assailant is known to be infected or if compliance is in doubt.

Just as in sexual assault involving adults, childhood sexual abuse patients should be reassured that they were the victims of a wrongful act for which they have no responsibility or blame.

Syphilis may not be adequately treated by some of the antibiotic combinations commonly given as prophylaxis to victims of sexual assault. Therefore, it is very important to obtain initial and follow-up serology to screen for infection so that additional antibiotic coverage can be provided if needed.

Because of the real risk of increasingly violent episodes of spousal abuse, every effort should be made to help patients exit an abusive relationship or, at the very least, provide contacts to agencies who can provide guidance, support, or shelter as needed.

SUGGESTED READINGS

General References

AMA Council on Scientific Affairs. Violence against women: relevance for medical practitioners. JAMA 1992; 267:3184.

American College of Obstetricians and Gynecologists. Adolescent acquaintance rape. ACOG Committee Opinion 122. Washington, DC: ACOG, 1993.

American College of Obstetricians and Gynecologists. The battered woman. ACOG Technical Bulletin 124. Washington, DC: ACOG, 1989.

American College of Obstetricians and Gynecologists. Sexual assault. ACOG Technical Bulletin 172. Washington, DC: ACOG, 1992.

American Medical Association. Diagnostic and treatment guidelines on domestic violence. Chicago: American Medical Association, 1992.

Batten DA. Incest: a review of the literature. Med Sci Law 1983;23:245.

Burgess WA, Holmstrom LL. Rape trauma syndrome. Am J Psychiatry 1974;131:981.

Burgess WA, Holmstrom LL. Adaptive strategies and recovery from rape. Am J Psychiatry 1979;136:1278.

Cartwright PS. Sexual violence. In Jones HW III, Wentz AC, Burnett LS (eds). Novak's Textbook of Gynecology, 11th ed. Baltimore: Williams & Wilkins, 1988;525.

Chez RA. Woman battering. Am J Obstet Gynecol 1988;158:1.

Goodwin J. Sexual Abuse: incest Victims and Their Families. Chicago: Year Book Medical Publishers, 1989.

Helton A. Battering during pregnancy. Am J Nurs 1986;86:910.

Hilberman E. Overview: the "wife-beater's wife" reconsidered. Am J Psychiatry 1980;137:1336.

Hillard PJ. Physical abuse in pregnancy. Obstet Gynecol 1985;66:185.

Maltz W. The Sexual Healing Journey: a Guide for Survivors of Sexual Abuse. New York: Harper Collins, 1991.

McFarlane J, Parker V, Soeken K, Vullock L. Assessing for abuse during pregnancy. Severity and frequency of injuries and associated entry to prenatal care. JAMA 1992;267:3176.

Muram D. Child sexual abuse. In Sanfilippo JS, Muram D, Lee PA, Dewhurst J (eds). Pediatric and Adolescent Gynecology. Philadelphia: WB Saunders, 1994;365.

National Center on Child Abuse and Neglect (NCCAN). Child sexual abuse: incest, assault and exploitation. Special Report. Washington, DC: HEW, Children's Bureau, 1978.

Paddington PL, ed. Treatment of Adult Survivors of Incest. Washington, DC: American Psychiatric Press, 1993.

Peipert JF, Domagalski LR. Epidemiology of adolescent sexaul assault. Obstet Gynecol 1994;84:867.

Reece RM. Child Abuse. Baltimore: Williams & Wilkins, 1994.

Sugg NK, Inui T. Primary care physicians' response to domestic violence: opening Pandora's box. JAMA 1992; 267:3157.

Walch AG, Broadhead WE. Prevalence of lifetime sexual victimization among female patients. J Fam Pract 1992; 35:511.

Specific References

Child Abuse and Incest

Bays J, Chadwick D. Medical diagnosis of the sexually abused child. Child Abuse Negl 1993;17:91.

Enos WF. Forensic evaluation of the sexually abused child. Pediatrics 1986;78:385.

Finkelhor D, Hotaling G, Lewis IA, et al. Sexual abuse in a national survey of adult men and women: prevalence characteristics and risk factors. Child Abuse Negl 1990;14:19.

Green AH. Child maltreatment and its victims: a comparison of physical and sexaul abuse. Psychiatr Clin North Am 1988;11:591.

Herjanic B. Sexual abuse of children. JAMA 1978;239:331.

Hobbs CJ, Wayne JM. Sexual abuse of English boys and girls: the importance of anal examination. Child Abuse Negl 1989;13:2.

Kendall-Tackett KA, Williams LM, Finkelhor D. Impact of sexual abuse on children: a review and synthesis of recent empirical studies. Psychol Bull 1993;113:164.

Lindberg FH, Distad LJ. Posttraumatic stress disorders in women who experienced childhood incest. Child Abuse Negl 1985;9:329.

Muram D. Child sexual abuse—genital tract findings in prepubertal girls. I. The unaided medical examination. Am J Obstet Gynecol 1989;160:328.

Muram D. Child sexual abuse: relationship between sexual acts and genital findings. Child Abuse Negl 1989:13: 211.

Muram D, Elias S. Child sexual abuse—genital tract findings in prepubertal girls. II. Comparison of colposcopic and unaided examinations. Am J Obstet Gynecol 1989;160:333.

Muram D. Rape, incest, trauma: the molested child. Clin Obstet Gynecol 1987;30:754.

Pokorny SF, Kozinetz CA. Configuration and other anatomic detail of the prepubertal hymen. Adolescent and Pediatric Gynecology 1988;1:97.

Rimsza ME, Miggerman MS. Medical evaluation of sexually abused children: a review of 311 cases. Pediatriacs 1982;69:8.

Russell DEH. The incidence and prevalence of intrafamilial and extrafamilial sexual abuse of female children. Child Abuse Negl 1983;7:133.

Springs FE, Friedrich WN. Health risk behaviors and medical sequelae of childhood sexual abuse. Mayo Clin Proc 1992;67:527.

Tilelli JA, Turek D, Jaffe AC. Sexual abuse of children: clinical findings and implications for management. N Engl J Med 1980;302:319.

Rape and Rape Evaluation

Binder R. Why women don't report sexual assault. J Clin Psychiatry 1981;42:437.

Cartwright PS, Sexual Assault Study Group. Reported sexual assault in Nashville-Davidson County, Tennessee 1980–1982. Am J Obstet Gynecol 1986;154:1064.

Everett R.B. The rape victim: a review of 117 consecutive cases. Obstet Gynecol 1977;50:88.

Hampton HL. Care of the woman who has been raped. N Engl J Med 1995;332:234.

Hicks DJ. Rape: sexual assault. Am J Obstet Gynecol 1980;137:931.

Irwin KL, Edlin BR, Wong L, et al. Urban rape survivors: characteristics and prevalence of human immunodeficiency virus and other sexually transmitted infections. Obstet Gynecol 1995;85:330.

Jenny C, Hooton TM, Bowers A, et al. Sexually transmitted diseases in vicitms of rape. N Engl J Med 1990;322:713.

Nagy S, Adcock AG, Nagy MC. A comparison of risky behaviors of sexually active, sexually abused, and abstaining adolescents. Pediatrics 1994;93:570.

Norton LB, Peipert JF, Zierler S, Lima B, Hume L. Battering in pregnancy: an assessment of two screening methods. Obstet Gynecol 1995;85:321.

Parrot A. Acquaintance rape among adolescents: identifying risk groups and intervention strategies. Journal of Social Work and Human Sexuality 1989;8:47.

Solola A, Scott C, Severs H, Howell J. Rape: management in a noninstitutional setting. Obstet Gynecol 1983; 61:373.

Soules MR. The forensic laboratory evaluation of evidence in alleged rape. Am J Obstet Gynecol 1978;130:142.

Abuse

Chez RA. Woman battering. Am J Obstet Gynecol 1988;158:1.

Giordano NH, Giordano JA. Elder abuse: a review of the literature. Soc Work 1984;29:232.

Goldberg WG, Tomlanovich MC. Domestic violence, victims and emergency departments: new findings. JAMA 1984;251:3259.

Helton A. Battering during pregnancy. Am J Nurs 1986;86:910.

Hillard PJ. Physical abuse in pregnancy. Obstet Gynecol 1985;66:185.

Klause PA, Rand MR. Family Violence. Washington, DC: US Department of Justice, Bureau of Justice Statistics, 1984.

Mayer L. The severely abused woman in obstetrics and gynecologic care. J Reprod Med 1995;40:13.

Parsons LH, Zaccaro D, Wells B, Stovall TG. Methods of and attitudes toward screening obstetric and gynecology patients for domestic violence. Am J Obstet Gynecol 1995;173:381.

Richwals GA, McCluskey TC. Family violence during pregnancy. Advances in International Maternal Child Health 1985;5:87.

US Department of Health and Human Services; Public Health Service: Health Resources and Services Administration. Surgeon General's Workshop on Violence and Public Health: Report. DHHS Publication No. HRS-D-MC 86–1. Washington, DC: Government Printing Office, 1986.

24

Sexual Dysfunction

Despite the pervasive nature of sexuality in our culture, media, and lives, a large proportion of our patients have, or will have, problems involving their sexuality. Notwithstanding a greater openness about all sexual matters, the fast pace of life, the realities of dual income families, and a push to live up to perceived standards set by the mass media have left many couples grappling with real or imagined sexual dysfunction. Most adults are sexually active, and 92% of American women will have children. Nonetheless, sexual expression, for many, is still problematic. Many studies report that even in "happy" or "very happy" marriages, sexual dysfunction occurs in almost two thirds of women, with three quarters reporting sexual difficulties that fall short of true dysfunction (e.g., lack of interest or inability to relax). Almost half the women reported trouble becoming sexually excited, one third had trouble maintaining excitement, and one third were completely disinterested in sex. Almost half of the women in one study reported difficulties in achieving orgasm and 15% had never been able to have an orgasm at all.

A survey of 2365 single people published in Mademoiselle found that 55% of men had had erectile problems, 20% had never performed oral sex, and only 12% reported that they knew where the clitoris is located. This same study found that 70% of women and a surprising 25% of men had faked an orgasm at some time. Many studies show that even among well adjusted, happily married couples, over 50% have sexual problems and 10% to 30% of women have never achieved orgasm. It is reasonable to estimate that roughly 25% of the general population has either a sexual dysfunction or significant concern. With sexual dysfunction this prevalent, we must be sensitive to our patient's concerns and be prepared to provide support, counsel, and intervention.

Because of both the nature of the problem and the prevailing views of sexuality, this is an area in which we cannot passively wait for our patients to raise the issue, but rather we must include it in our routine review of health issues. Patients are bombarded by images, lay publications, and TV talk shows that suggest that they may be the only ones who are not sexually ecstatic. Even the patient's sexual partner may presume that if the woman neither complains nor refuses intercourse, no problem could possibly exist. In this environment, it is little wonder that patients are reluctant to initiate discussions of sexual matters owing to uncertainty, embarrassment, or a sense of propriety.

Notwithstanding the logic of discussing and treating sexual dysfunction as a part of the office care of women, many health care providers are reluctant to take on the task. The topic is sensitive, specific training is often lacking, and there may be concern about the time this type of counseling may require. The reality is that we are ideally suited (and adequately prepared) to provide the type of counseling required by most patients. Most patients are relieved to find that the subject is one that is not out of bounds. Our patients do not want to become "sexual athletes," but rather to be comfortable with their sexual expression and relationships. It is as logical a part of our practice as for a proctologist to inquire about a patient's bowel habits. With some simple techniques, the evaluation of sexual dysfunction as an aspect of our care will be easier and much more natural and will occupy no more time than the evaluation and treatment of any other gynecologic concern. As a result, simple office sexual counseling can provide a rewarding and valuable addition to the total care of the patient.

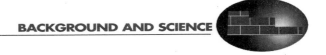

BACKGROUND AND SCIENCE

Types of Dysfunction

As noted in Chapter 8, Sexuality, successful sexual expression may be broken down in three phases: proximation, preparation, and consummation. Problems can occur in any or all of these phases.

Difficulties in the proximation phase of sexual response are expressed as inhibited desire. This is the most common female sexual dysfunction, occurring in between 10% and 50% of women (and probably an equally number of men, although less commonly reported). Inhibited desire may present as an absolute lack of interest or as a relative imbalance between the perceived levels of interest between two sexual partners. This must be carefully differentiated from an inequity in the frequency of initiation of sexual activity by each partner. There is no standard by which inhibited sexual desire can be measured; rather, it is a subjective determination and cannot be based on the frequency of intercourse. True inhibited desire is a diminished or absent ability to achieve arousal, a lack of interest in sexual activities, or, in the extreme, revulsion. Complaints of inhibited desire are often how problems with relationships, previous failures or conditioning, fatigue, fear, repression, or depression first present. Although some of these patients have orgasmic dysfunctions, most are fully capable of sexual response and orgasm, but have no interest in starting or carrying through the process.

Some authors have divided inhibited sexual desire into classifications of primary and secondary: primary for those who never experience sexual desire and secondary for those who lose interest that previously existed. Patients who never experience sexual desire are more likely to have deep-seated social or emotional problems such as childhood trauma (abuse, incest, rape), dysfunctional families (alcohol, drugs, divorce) or exceptionally strong negative family or religious attitudes about sex. Patients who experience loss of sexual desire are more likely to have experienced a change in life situation (birth of a child, marriage, marital discord, change in job status). Exploring the onset, evolution, and the environment in which the problem exists will generally indicate the root of the difficulty.

Difficulties in the preparation phase are manifest by problems such as a lack of arousal, inadequate lubrication, or vaginismus. Both physiologic and psychologic arousal are necessary for successful sexual expression. Organic conditions such as diabetes, vaginitis, pregnancy, vestibulitis, or medications may all cause or complicate problems with this phase of sexuality. Similarly, anger, fear, guilt, poor self-image, or distraction can prevent normal arousal. When evaluating patients with preparation phase problems, remember that arousal (and eventually orgasm) require sufficient and effective stimulation given in the proper environment. A failure of any of these elements will result in dysfunction.

Dyspareunia and orgasmic failure characterize dysfunctions of the consummation phase. Dyspareunia is often caused by physical conditions such as endometriosis, pelvic adhesions, fibroids, irritable bowel syndrome, vestibulitis, and others, which require careful history and physical assessment (Chapter 25, Sexual Pain).

The causes of orgasmic dysfunction are less clear cut. Most studies indicate that only 30% to 40% of women are able to experience orgasm during intercourse. Many women require additional, supplemental, or alternate forms of stimulation to be orgasmic. Many patients who do not achieve orgasm during intercourse are fully orgasmic with additional manual stimulation, oral-genital stimulation, a vibrator, or through masturbation. (About 30% to 40% of women require concurrent clitoral stimulation during intercourse to achieve orgasm.) This is common enough that it should be viewed as a problem only if it is a source of concern for the patient or her partner. Foreplay, masturbation, and receiving oral sex were listed as the best part of sex by over 30% of the subjects in one study and over 40% in another; therefore, patients requiring such stimulation can be reassured that they are "normal."

Perversion, or altered forms of sexual expression, are beyond the scope of this discussion, except to say that sexual expression is highly variable and as long as the forms it takes are acceptable to the couple and are not dangerous or illegal, they should be viewed as variants, not as pathologies. Roughly 70% of men will at some time in their life perform some form of "perverse" act, with 60% doing so on a regular basis. The authors reporting these figures seldom define "perverse," which leaves a great deal to the imagination, both scientifically and otherwise.

Sources of Dysfunction

The most common causes of sexual dysfunction are relationship problems, intrapsychic factors, and medical factors. Problems in any or all of these areas can be the source of dysfunction and each should be kept in mind during discussions with the patient.

Relationship problems are an obvious source for sexual problems, but they are often overlooked by both the patient and her clinician. Marital or relationship stresses may be acted out by sexual distancing, orgasmic failure, or exploitation. Anger, hidden agendas, lack of trust or infidelity may be expressed through the withdrawal of intimacy. Libidinal mismatches are common, but when combined with poor communication, lead to dysfunction. Dual income families may not realize the impact fatigue and a fast-paced lifestyle may be having on their ability to express warmth and be sexually expressive. Even in this era of widely available information and sexually explicit materials, sexual ignorance and inexperience can still be a source of concern, which adds embarrassment to ignorance of an already touchy topic. Each of these factors must be considered and can be easily investigated with a few simple questions.

Trauma, negative sexual experiences, and mental illness (including depression) can all play a part in the development of sexual dysfunction. Childhood or adolescent conditioning can set moral or ethical boundaries that are restrictive or unrealistic. Family or societal mixed messages about sex and sexuality can create ambiguities that result in inhibited desire or orgasmic failure. These types of experiences can set the stage for later dysfunction. Roughly 90% of men and 75% of women enter marriage with "eager anticipation." This means that 10% of men and 25% of women have problems from the start with anger, disgust, aversion, or indifference. It is sad to say, but evidence shows that physical abuse, in childhood or ongoing in adults, must be considered as a potential cause of sexual dysfunction. Sexual concerns are often the first indication of abuse.

Once proximation and arousal have occurred, orgasmic success requires effective stimulation, of a sufficient quality over a sufficient time, provided in a supportive environment. Failures in any of these areas may present as orgasmic problems.

Medical Factors

Medical factors that influence sexual performance include drugs and alcohol, depression, anxiety, chronic illness, pregnancy, untreated menopause, and the effects of surgical therapies. The sexual impact of drugs and alcohol are generally well known and are shown in Table 24.1. Despite the negative physiologic effects of even small amounts of alcohol, approximately half of women (and 60% of men) report having had sex because they had too much to drink.

Table 24.1. Common Classes of Drugs that Affect Sexuality

Agent or class	Sexual effect
Alcohol	Reduced arousal, vaginal dryness, oligomenorrhea (chronic use)
Antihypertensives (with sympathetic effects)	Reduced libido and arousal, (impotence*) anorgasmia
Anticholinergics	Reduced libido, arousal, (impotence)
Antihistamines	Sedation, vaginal dryness
Amphetamines	Reduced libido, vaginal dryness, (impotence), anorgasmia
Barbiturates	Reduced libido, (impotence)
Clonidine	(Impotence), anorgasmia
Cocaine	Reduced libido, arousal, and orgasm
Diazepam	Reduced libido, anorgasmia
Narcotics	Reduced testosterone and libido
Phenytoin	Reduced libido, (impotence)
Sedatives	Reduced arousal
Thiazide diuretics	(Impotence)

*Impotence in men; may result in vaginal dryness or reduced vaginal, labial, and clitoral engorgement in women.

Less frequently appreciated are the effects of some of our own interventions, such as surgery. In one study of women who had undergone mastectomy, 38% of their sexual partners had not seen the surgical scar by 3 months after the procedure and 33% of the women had not resumed sexual activity by 6 months after surgery. In another study, it was found that the best predictor of postoperative sexual function was the patient's preoperative sexual happiness. Those with active and satisfying sex lives returned to more active and fulfilling sexual expression after hysterectomy. Scarring and sore muscles may cause either short- or longterm inhibitions to full sexual expression. Despite the significance of sexuality in most of our patients' lives, we are often reluctant to discuss the potential impact (positive or negative) of our interventions, despite the positive impact that those discussions may have.

Chronic illness, deforming injuries, or congenital anomalies can adversely affect sexual development or expression. Chronic illness often can cause stress in relationships, with that stress expressed through sexual distancing and orgasmic dysfunction. Many diseases can directly affect sexual performance or desire. For example, diabetics may experience lubrication or orgasmic problems due to small vessel or neural damage. Multiple sclerosis, traumatic paraplegia, and muscular dystrophy are other obvious examples of medical conditions with profound sexual impact. Sexually transmitted diseases such as *Trichomonas vaginitis,* genital herpes, or human immunodeficiency virus infections also may affect sexuality and sexual expression.

Depression and affective disorders may be difficult to separate from desire and orgasmic dysfunction. In depression there is global anhedonia extending to all aspects of the patient's life. Sleep disturbances, loss of appetite, and altered mood are commonly present. These patients tend to be reluctant to pursue therapy directed toward their sexual problems and response to treatment is poor. Paradoxically, many of the medications used to treat depression may contribute to further libido, arousal, or orgasmic dysfunction.

Pregnancy

The profound impact of pregnancy on sexuality and sexual behavior is often overlooked or ignored by both the patient and her doctor. During pregnancy sexual interest and expressiveness both decline and change as the pregnancy progresses. The frequency of intercourse drops to roughly half of that experienced in early pregnancy. (An average of over two times per week in the first trimester to approximately once a week or less near term.) About 50% of this reduction is due to discomfort; 25% of couples decrease their activity out of fear of causing harm; and 25% attribute the decline to a loss of interest.

Most studies find that during the third trimester women prefer holding or hugging rather than direct sexual stimulation. Orgasmic capabilities also decline during pregnancy. In some studies, of the 45% of couples who used manual stimulation before pregnancy, only 57% were successfully orgasmic at least once during pregnancy. The orgasm rate for oral-genital sex also declined, from a rate of 16% who were nonorgasmic by this route before pregnancy, to 58% by the ninth month of pregnancy. These changes are normal and require only reassurance for the patient and her partner. For the most part, studies indicate that sexual frequency and satisfaction during pregnancy are most closely related to frequency and degree of satisfaction prior to conception.

Even though the general effect of pregnancy is often negative, nursing mothers report a higher level of sexual interest than do non-nursing mothers. Even orgasm from nursing is occasionally reported. Nursing may interfere with vaginal intercourse because of the vaginal dryness most nursing mothers experience. Without the use of additional lubricants this may lead to insertional dyspareunia or discomfort with prolonged thrusting.

Patients who are infertile or those who have recently lost a pregnancy are also at high risk for sexual difficulties. The change in self-image and the mechanization of conception often required by infertile couples, results in sexual dysfunction for the majority of these patients. Similarly, those couples who attain pregnancy after a prolonged period of trying often have great ambivalence or a fear of losing the pregnancy, which result in withdrawal of intimacy or abstinence. Fertile couples who lose an early pregnancy may have the same reaction due to their grief.

MENOPAUSE. With the loss of ovarian steroids at menopause (natural, premature, or surgical), there is a loss of vaginal wall thickness and an increased incidence of vaginal dryness. If untreated with estrogen replacement, this can lead to painful insertion and penetration, abrasions, trauma, and dyspareunia. Once established, these problems can further inhibit desire and lubrication, create muscle spasms, and begin a cycle that may end in complete abstinence. With estrogen maintenance (or replacement) these problems can be avoided. Loss of vaginal tone or laxity may occur with aging, leading to decreased sensation for the patient and her partner, but the use of Kegel exercises or changes in coital positions may lead to improvement.

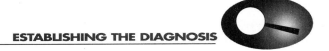

ESTABLISHING THE DIAGNOSIS

History

It has been said that the foundation of all medical therapy is the history. In office sexual counseling this is certainly the case. Many health care providers are intimidated by the nature of the subject or by a feeling of inadequate background or training that creates enough discomfort that they are tempted to skip the subject altogether. The problem of discomfort, for both the patient and the interviewer, may be dealt with simply by assuming the same matter-of-fact air that we all have when we run through a review of systems ("Have you had any nausea, vomiting, diarrhea, or constipation?"). The demeanor and language used should reflect a routine and natural attitude toward the subject. Factors that facilitate sexual counseling and communication are shown in Table 24.2.

The feeling of inadequacy is almost as easy to handle. Studies have shown that a completely adequate way of uncovering sexual problems can be embodied in as few as three questions:

- Are you sexually active? (Are you sexually involved? Are you having sexual relations?)

- Do you have any pain? (Are you satisfied with your sexual activity? Is it satisfactory? Are you happy with it?)

- Do you have any sexual problems or question?

With these three questions, or ones based on these three, one can uncover as many sexual problems as with much more elaborate and lengthy questionnaires. In one study, when

Table 24.2. Sexual Counseling and Communication Guidelines

- Do no harm
  - Disinterest, boredom, silence
  - Misinformation
  - Imposing personal values
- Provide a setting for communications
  - Privacy
  - Confidentiality
  - Defined time limits
- Employ an effective attitude
  - Permission
  - Warmth, support
  - Active listening
  - Observation
  - Professional
  - Be nonjudgmental
- Use effective communication skills
  - Establish commonality of terms
    - Level
    - Sexual words
  - Open-ended questions
  - Use of silence
  - Move from less to more sensitive issues
- Establish expectaions
  - Explore myths
  - Determine goals
  - Set realistic time lines

these questions were given to a group of sexually active patients visiting a clinic for routine care, it was found that almost 50% of patients has sexual complaints and one third were interested in medical referral or intervention when it was offered. These three questions found 100% of the problems identified by a much longer and more involved questionnaire used as a control. More involved assessments of sexual behavior have been advocated, but these three simple questions touch on the most common areas of sexual difficulty and open the subject up as an area of acceptable discussion.

Once it is determined that there is an area of sexual concern, the history evolves in much the same way that it would for any other medical problem: begin with a description of the problem, evaluate the course or evolution of the problem, determine the patient's assessment of the cause behind the problem, find out what interventions have been attempted and their result, and establish the patient's expectation and goals. It is no accident that this pattern of assessment parallels that taken for other medical histories. It is exactly that similarity, and the familiarity that it imparts, that should provide one less reason for not taking a good sexual history. Using this model, it becomes natural to follow-up a patient's complaint of pain with intercourse with questions about sexual practices, preferences, positions, and use of sexual aids. These questions are no longer foreign, stilted, or embarrassing, but are just part of a routine investigation of a medical concern. This familiarity makes the process more relaxed and natural for both the patient and the interviewer.

In addition to having an air of acceptance, gentle progression from the nonthreatening to more sensitive issues can help both the interviewer and the patient to be more comfortable and open. For example, begin discussions about pleasure and sensuality with what types of foods or music the patient enjoys or what her favorite movie is. Move on to a discussion of physical pleasures such as sunbathing, warm baths, hair combing, or a back rub, progressing to lovemaking (in the global sense, romance), and concluding with sexuality and intercourse. It is easy to understand that if one's first question is "do you like leather underwear?" that will be an impediment to communication, whereas the same information gained after establishing a patient's preference for bondage, combined with a history of recurrent yeast infections, will seem natural and will be answered openly and honestly.

Frequently, a problem may spill over from one area into another. Performance anxiety and spectatoring may affect both desire and ability to respond successfully. Previous orgasmic failures may lead to a defeatist attitude, suppressing libido. Loss of communications and stereotypic behaviors can lead to disinterest as well as to orgasmic failure. Because of these overlaps, the evaluation of sexual problems must be global.

Sexual problems require that one expands the basic screening history by exploring such things as the forms of sexual expression used, number and type(s) of sexual partners, problems with vaginal lubrication, and orgasmic success. As with other histories, it is important to allow the patient free rein through the use of open-ended questions. One word of warning: In the area of sexuality euphemisms abound and it is critically important that both you and the patient are talking about the same thing. If the patient complains that "my husband always wants to kiss me on my button," be very sure that both of your meanings of "button" are the same.

Just as in cases of physical abuse, the patient may be reluctant to express an intimate problem or ask a question even though it is the main reason for her visit. The physician should be watchful for signs of a hidden agenda any time the patient's reason for making the appointment seems vague or overly trivial. Examples would include the young woman who complains of a "vaginal odor," but who has physiologic secretions or the new bride with complaints of being "tired all the time." In these situations, the patient may feel that some pretext is necessary to make the visit, rather than admitting the real (sexual) reason. It is easier to tell your receptionist, their spouse, or mother that they have a medical problem than it is to say "I can't have an orgasm." These patients require a slower, more delicate, approach that uses very open-ended questions and multiple, varied opportunities to discuss the underlying problem. Phrases such as "is there anything else I can do for you" sound open-ended but carry the connotation of a last opportunity. More neutral phrases such as "what else can I answer for you" do not set a time limit and lead to a greater freedom of exchange. For some patients it may even take multiple visits. Alertness and caring will generally uncover the true agenda.

Sometimes opening up the question of sexuality can lead to an outpouring of history, questions, or complaints. Two things should be remembered: 1) Occasionally patients will report information in an effort to shock, provoke, surprise, or unnerve the interviewer. This is a form of testing and sometimes a way of shifting control of an uncomfortable situation to the patient herself. This is best handled by remaining detached, objective, and nonjudgmental. 2) As in other areas of medical care, things are a problem only if they are a problem. The patient who says she is a lesbian does not automatically require any special help unless her being a lesbian presents a problem to her. If the patient likes to use vibrators it may not be a problem unless she likes to use them while on city buses. Unless the patient's situation presents a medical, social, or psychological problem, no intervention is required or should be attempted.

Investigation

Once a problem has been discovered, the focus becomes one of investigation aimed at gathering enough information to establish a working diagnosis.

Generally, the patient will take the lead when there is a problem, allowing the history and its details to follow a natural progression, as it does with most other types of complaints. The same details of onset, character, development, and change that would be important in the history of any other complaint are just as important in the history of a sexual dysfunction. Were there any events that surrounded the onset of the problem (like the discovery of an infidelity, the use of drugs or alcohol, the birth of a child, the loss of a pregnancy)? Was its onset abrupt or gradual? How have the symptoms evolved over time? (Gradual onset problems are more likely to be organic than are those with a sudden appearance.) Are the patient's complaints based on physical changes (lubrication, pain) or on emotional functions (libido, arousal, orgasm)? Does the problem occur with every sexual encounter? Do other forms of pleasuring cause the same complaint? Is there anything that makes the problem better, worse, or different?

In addition to specifics surrounding the patient's complaint, a general sexual history should be explored. This should range from age at first intercourse and number of life-time partners, to current sexual patterns. Questions about the frequency (achieved and that desired by both partners, time of day, day of week), forms of sexual expression (setting, privacy, sex play, special modes of expression, partners), and degree of communication (verbalization of needs and likes, unspoken fantasies) will all help to indicate problem areas or direct further inquiries. Many times the patient will respond vaguely, necessitating prompting. For example when exploring foreplay, it may be helpful to assist with questions such as, "When you and your husband are romantic, is there much kissing?" "Does he caress or kiss the skin of your body?" "Is that pleasurable?" "How long does that last?" and so forth.

When evaluating patients with orgasmic difficulties, it is important to differentiate between situational dysfunction and complete orgasmic failure. This may help to differentiate between those with relationship problems, intrapsychic factors, and medical factors. Those with global difficulties (inability to achieve orgasm with any form of stimulation under any conditions) are more likely to have intrapsychic or medical factors than are those who become anorgasmic with an abusive partner but can still achieve orgasm with fantasy or self-stimulation.

Patients with orgasmic dysfunction should also be questioned about the types of simulation the couple uses and enjoys. Exploring the acceptability and previous experience, degree of arousal created, and orgasmic success (if any) with various types of stimulation may help direct both further diagnostics paths and possible future recommendations. Look for trials and effects of pelvic movement, other positions, altered breathing patterns, adjunctive stimulation, and note their effects. It is important to ask about other forms of stimulation, and how "active" is the patient (e.g., involved, communicative, participatory, demonstrative, and so forth). Some authors suggest compiling this information in the form of a grid, although this level of formality is seldom required for the type of counseling encountered in the primary care setting.

Patients with dyspareunia represent a special form of both sexual dysfunction and pelvic pain. This particular problem is discussed in Chapter 25, Sexual Pain.

Medical factors that affect sexuality must be included in any investigation of sexual dysfunction. This begins with a simple review of current medications and alcohol use. Popular culture aside, even small amounts of alcohol can significantly decrease vaginal lubrication. It is easy to understand how the patient with a sexual concerns can get into a self-defeating spiral of alcohol use to relax, attempting to overcome a sexual problem that is itself made worse by the use of alcohol. Following assessment of drug and substance use, a general review of health is appropriate. Hypothyroidism, diabetes, arthritis, hypertension, migraine headaches, and the like can all have impacts on sexuality that may be overlooked by the patient.

Physical Evaluation

All patients with sexual concerns should have a careful general evaluation of their physical status. General measures, such as weight and blood pressure, may be just as important in establishing the root of sexual problems as is the pelvic examination. The patient's state of sexual development (Tanner stage), hormonal function, and structural integrity should be noted. Musculoskeletal problems (back pain, scoliosis, arthritis) may limit sexual expression or bring about sexual problems without the patient's knowledge. Metabolic disease may interfere with sexual functioning. As with any other relatively strenuous physical activity, sexual functioning involves all of the body systems, demanding that an assessment of their function be made.

The pelvic evaluation of a patient with sexual concerns or dysfunction is similar to any gynecologic evaluation, except for a slight shift in focus toward those physical factors that influence sexual success. The estrogen state of the vulva, the size of the clitoris, the size and condition of the vaginal introitus are often noted in a cursory manner, but take on more significance in the patient with sexual dysfunction. The patient who reports dyspareunia requires a careful evaluation of those structures that may relate to her complaints. This might range from the size, position, and mobility of the uterus for the patient with deep thrust, internal pain, to a colposcopic examination of the vulva to look for vestibulitis in the patient with insertional pain.

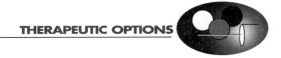

THERAPEUTIC OPTIONS

It is not the establishment of a diagnosis, which is often merely a restatement of the patient's complaint, that is the stumbling block for most practitioners. How to treat is the puzzle that keeps many practitioners from acknowledging sexual dysfunction. Masters and Johnson pioneered the idea that most sexual problems are derived from sociocultural deprivation and sexual ignorance and not from deep psychosexual conflicts. This change in think-

Table 24.3. Goals of Sexual Counseling or Therapy

Sex is more than intercourse
    Look at larger picture of sensuality
Leave each encounter feeling good
    Feel good—don't ask for orgasm
Give and receive pleasure
    Enjoy giving *and* accepting pleasure
Open good communications
    Listen without feeling criticized, provide cooperative communications
Learn to say "yes" instead of "no" (or at least "maybe")
    Learn to suggest alternatives, break rejection cycle
Improve the quality, not necessarily the quantity
    Better sex is better than more sex
Have fun, not work
    Sex shouldn't be work; it requires interesting and interested partners
Allow "space" for each other
    Allow distance without abandonment
Go slowly, provide reassurance
    Take your time

ing opened up the possibility that sexual problems were amenable to successful intervention by counseling outside the realm of intensive psychotherapy. Learning theory replaced psychiatric insight and behavior therapy supplanted psychotherapy.

To be effective as a counselor for most simple sexual concerns does not require extensive, specialized training. More important than a psychoanalytic background or extensive therapeutic experience, is common sense, a degree of sensitivity, and a willingness to listen. Some of this is innate; some can be learned, although opportunities in most formal medical training programs are often lacking. Many short refresher courses are available that may be helpful for reviewing current concepts, increasing personal comfort with the subject, and exploring one's personal feelings and biases.

Sexual counseling by the nonspecialist is aimed at reducing anxiety and demands for performance, removing impediments to responsiveness, and providing guidance to the physical and psychological behaviors that will enhance sexual expression. The ultimate goals of sexual counseling or therapy are simple and are shown in Table 24.3. With these simple goals in mind, it should be apparent that at least rudimentary diagnosis and therapy is well within the purview of all health care providers.

An extremely simple, but very effective approach to therapy is the PLISSIT model suggested by Annon. This model is made up of four levels of intervention: **P**ermission, **Li**mited Information, **S**pecific **S**uggestions, and **I**ntensive **T**herapy. These steps are applied in order. At each step a large number of dysfunctions will be resolved leaving few patients who require referral for intensive or specialized therapy.

Permission

The permission stage of this appraoch is as simple as it sounds: giving permission. Many patients only need permission for what they are doing or want to do.

"I have always wanted to have sex first thing in the morning when I am rested. Is this normal?" "Yes, it is perfectly OK."

"I feel like we are getting in a rut. Is it OK to try some different positions?" "Yes."

"I seem more interested in girls than in boys." "Is that a problem for you?" "No." "Then it is perfectly all right."

If a sexual behavior is realistic, something both partners are comfortable with, involves no danger or coercion, and causes no harm, "go ahead." The patient should be given permission to explore and take an active role in her own sexual pleasure. This can include permission for such things as self-exploration (masturbation), the initiation of sexual encounters, and the use of fantasy, erotica, and sexual aids (oils, feathers, vibrators, and so forth).

Limited Information

When permission is not enough, providing limited information often is the solution to the problem. The information given at this stage need not constitute a medical lecture on the topic, but rather a small tidbit specific to the patient's concerns.

"My husband and I like to have anal sex. Are we weird or something?" "A large number of couples try anal sex at sometime or another, and a small number use it as a consistent part of their lovemaking."

For limited information to work, the physician should be generally familiar with a range of sexual behaviors—norms and forms of expression. Most clinicians have already gleaned this information from popular publications. A collection of such "handy facts" is provided in Table 24.4.

Sometimes a combination of permission and limited information is useful.

"I have always wanted to have sex first thing in the morning when I am rested. Is this normal?" "Yes, it is perfectly OK." "But doesn't that make me over-sexed or something?" "No, many couples find sex better when they are rested."

"My husband and I like to have anal sex. Are we weird or something?" "As long as you are careful, both of you are comfortable with it, and it isn't causing any problems, it is perfectly all right to enjoy anal stimulation. A large number of couples try anal sex at sometime or another, and a small number use it as a consistent part of their lovemaking."

The principles of permission and limited information can also be applied in a preventative manner to minimize the impact of changes or processes that might be expected to have a sexual impact.

"It looks like the you and the baby are doing fine. You may have noticed that as your pregnancy has progressed, marital relations have been a bit more difficult. Most couples can continue to be sexually active, but they find that they either have to experiment with different sexual positions or substitute other things like holding and caressing to show their love. See what seems to work best for you."

Table 24.4. Useful Statistics*

Sexual dysfunction
    Up to 50% of married couples
    25% to 35% of women have trouble reaching orgasm
    10% to 15+ % of women have never had an orgasm
    63% of women and 40% of men have had dysfunction at some time
Effects of pregnancy
    By the 9th month, almost 60% of couples abstain and frequency of sexual activity drops to half prepregnancy rate for the rest.

Reasons	
Discomfort	46%
Fear	27%
Loss of interest	23%
Awkwardness	17%
Advice of physician	8%

Foreplay
    Amount and variety are related to age and education
    Two thirds of couples use adjuncts (oils, vibrators, feathers).
    Women (55%) and men (30%) say foreplay is better than intercourse.

Frequency of intercourse
    Varies with age and education

Median	8.5/mo
Married	
Age 16–20	4/wk
Married couples in their 20s	45% report 3–4/wk
Age 60	1/wk

Sexual practices
    Three fourths of women like to vary the location and setting of sex

Average duration of intromission	10 min
Male superior	70
(exclusively)	9%
Female superior	75%
Side to side	50%
Rear entry (vaginal)	40%
Sitting	25%
Anal	
Tried once	43%
Use regularly	2%
Cunnilingus	
Often or occasional	87%
Very/somewhat enjoyable	90%
Fellatio	
Often or occasional	85%
Very/somewhat enjoyable	51%

Premarital intercourse

Sex by age 15	13–15%
Age 13–19 who have had sex	41%
Median age of first intercourse	16.2
Average lifetime partners	1.6
Married women with premarital sex	80%
age <20	96%

Table 24.4. (continued)

Extramarital relations	
Males	23–37%
Females by age 40 (1948)	26%
Females by age 40 (1977)	40%
Employed wives	53%
Unemployed wives	24%
Mate swapping	2%
Masturbation	
Women (to orgasm)	60%–80%
Men (to orgasm)	70%–95+ %
Married women	
Often or occasional	68%
Unsatisfying	20%
Age 80–102	
Men	72%
Women	40%
Likelihood of orgasm vs intercourse	3 ×
Men unaware of partner's masturbation	92%
Homosexuality	
Same sex contact	
Men	50%
Women	28%
Exclusively	
Men	5%–22%
Women	2%–6%

*A compilation from various sources, to be used as "ballpark" or "thumbnail" statistics for patient counseling and reference.

An adjunct to limited information is the educational pelvic examination. Because of cultural and anatomic differences, many women have little or no knowledge of their genital anatomy. It is not uncommon for women to have either no image or a negative image (dark, dirty, smelly) of the vulva and vaginal area. A gentle, slow pelvic examination, with descriptions of the structures (assisted by a hand mirror in many cases), can begin a process of improved self-image and provide information needed for later suggestions. This examination provides an opportunity to talk about sensitive structures, the role of muscles, and how to do Kegel exercises. This also provide tacit permission for further exploration by the patient or her partner.

Specific Suggestions

When permission and limited information fail to improve the problem, specific suggestions may be called for. These do not have to be exotic, complex, or imaginative. In most cases, they will be obvious and suggested by the situation. They require only some simple understanding of sexuality, physiology, or just plain common sense.

"It feels like my husband is bumping into something up inside of me when he pushes in deeply." "That is not uncommon and as long as it is not causing you pain, it is probably not anything to worry about." "It isn't causing pain, but I don't like the feeling."

"You might try switching to a position that gives you more control over the depth of his penetration, such as one with you on the top."

"My husband thinks I am 'frigid' because I don't want sex the moment he walks in the door." "Many times lovemaking must take a back seat to other things in life. It is understandable that in the middle of cooking dinner, with the spaghetti boiling over and the kids running around the house, you may feel less than amorous. Let your husband know that your 'not now' means 'not now' but also may mean 'maybe later.' Try to make time for each other, even if it is only to be able to talk over how each other's day went. Look for ways to relax and enjoy both your own sensuality and sexuality and your husband's as well. Consider altering your routines to keep your enjoyment of each other fresh. This can vary from a surprise dinner out to sending the children off to a sitter and arranging an intimate evening. The change from your routines will make the time together more enjoyable and your lovemaking much more exciting for both of you (and he will no longer think you are uninterested)."

Simple suggestions may be augmented by specific suggestions for self-exploration, change in positions used for intercourse, desensitizing, or pleasuring exercises, when needed.

Some of the simplest yet most important suggestions that we can provide are those that allow the patient to relax and those that enhance communication between partners. Suggestions that facilitate relaxation help to avoid becoming a goal-oriented outside observer intent on achieving some preset objective ("spectatoring"). Because it is not possible for the patient to will an orgasm anymore than her partner can "make her" have one, it is better to focus on the process and not the end. This relieves pressure (permission), reduces anxiety, and decreases distractions caused by being their own observer, trying to analyze and predict outcomes. This allows the most sexually responsive organ (the brain) to be brought to bear through enjoyment, visualization, communication, or fantasy.

Keeping communications open between partners is vital when sexual issues are at stake. It is paradoxic that in the era of the information highway and talk radio, we conduct lovemaking with more secrecy than a spy mission. We have no hesitation in asking someone (even a stranger) to scratch our back, in a certain location and in a certain way, but will not tell our spouse to "move a little to the left" during sex. This idea may be conveyed to patients through illustrations.

"Imagine you are at dinner. You have a roll and your husband has the butter. It would not make sense to feel mad or disappointed because he did not pass the butter, even though he clearly can see you have a roll and he knows you always like the butter. You would say "please pass the butter" and everything would be fine. On the other hand, if he passed you the butter, but you are trying to cut down on dietary fat, you would say "No, thanks, I am trying to cut down." Once again, everything would be fine. What you like and want sexually at any given time is much the same, and without hints, comments, request, and suggestions neither of you will automatically know what each other wants. This can take the form of messages like "gently," "a little faster," "higher," or "oh, that's great" or with simple signs like guiding his hand with yours. It is also OK to ask what he would like, to encourage him to tell you about his likes and dislikes as well."

One way of facilitating communication is a technique called "bookmarking." In this technique, the patient takes a book or magazine (romance novels, women's magazines, *National Geographic, Cosmopolitan, Playboy, Playgirl,* how-to or self-help books, erotica, pornography, or whatever) and finds a passage or picture containing an activity, setting, or mood that the patient likes or would like to explore as part of lovemaking. She then marks the spot in some way (bookmark, corner folded over, sticky note) and leaves the material (with varying degrees of subtlety) where her partner will find it. He then may either act on this new knowledge or may move the bookmark to something either more acceptable or more interesting, and "sends" the message back. In this way, the first steps toward both communication and expression of unspoken fantasies may be taken.

In addition to bookmarking, self-help and erotic materials may serve other purposes as well. Erotic material, in one form or another, is widely available in almost all locations throughout the country. Although often clandestine, most adults have had at least some exposure to erotic matter, and studies indicate that women are just as interested and aroused by erotic material as are men. Sixty percent of women have been to a pornographic movie (most with their husbands) and 70% of wives like to dress in erotic clothes for their husbands. Sales and rentals of X-rated videos have increased almost 30% in the past few years and over 20% of American women have used video tapes in their lovemaking. Recent studies indicate that over 15% of women report having purchased erotic material over the past year. (For comparison, 90% of American men under 50 have read *Playboy* or *Penthouse.*) Suggestions regarding the use of oils, feathers, vibrators, costumes, and the like (also used by more than 20% of women) may also be appropriate. Erotica provides information, arousal, safety, escapism, and empowerment. Erotica is fantasy in tangible form. Most erotica involves intercourse to only a limited degree, concentrating most on foreplay and noncoital stimulation, which can be instructive to many couples. Erotica can provide a way to explore interests, discover likes and dislikes, or open communications. The type, depth, and character of these materials may vary from the clinical to the prurient, from innocent romantic diversion to the frankly "kinky." The extent to which these elements are used in counseling and education will be dictated by the comfort and experience of both the clinician and the patient. A brief list of printed materials that may be used as adjuncts to counseling (with a description of type and content) is shown in the reference lists at the end of this chapter.

When self-awareness and exploration seem appropriate, it is often wise to work through the process in steps, because many patients have emotional, cultural, or religious concerns about self-pleasuring or masturbation. Successive awareness and sensation exercises are graded to allow comfort with the process and increase the likelihood of success. This may begin with a hot bath with special perfumes, incense, bubbles, and the like, moving to self-examination in a mirror (the whole body progressing to genitals), followed by genital exploration, and finally to genital stimulation (by self and then partner). When this is done with the expressed instruction to not have an orgasm, the true focus of sensual exploration can be maintained and performance anxiety reduced.

Intensive Therapy

When the problem is more complex or is deep seated, the intensive, specialized therapy of a trained sexual therapist, psychiatrist, psychologist, or other specialist should be considered. Examples might include vaginismus or orgasmic dysfunction. Some consider suggestions such as sensate focus exercises, foreplay techniques, specific coital positions, the use of fantasy, and the like as a part of intensive therapy. The designation of "specific suggestion" versus "intensive therapy" has more to do with the comfort and experience of the provider involved than it does with any formal guidelines. Clearly, such interventions as psychotherapy, marital counseling, the use of sexual surrogates, or clinical measurement of arousal are well beyond the realm of most of us and referral is generally in order.

Expected Outcomes

The ultimate goal of office sexual counseling is to allow the patient and her partner to be comfortable with their sexuality. Ideally, the patient should be able to leave every sexual encounter feeling good. We strive to make the patient comfortable in both giving and receiving pleasure and to appreciate that good sex is more than just intercourse. Sexual expression should be fun, not work. Successful counseling should open communications between the patient and her partner as well as with the physician. A better self-image should be fostered. Finally, we strive to improve the quality of sex, not necessarily the quantity. In most cases, we can reach these goals through simple office counseling.

HINTS AND COMMON QUESTIONS

Hints

Be careful about labeling, especially self-labels such as "frigidity" or "oversexed." Although these are most often incorrect, they may signal underlying concerns, frustrations, or inaccuracies that should be addressed. Explore classifications of this type with questions like: "What do you mean by that?" "How did you decide that?" "What makes you feel that way?" In doing this, try to avoid "why" questions which can often be interpreted as critical or accusatory.

When asking specific sexual questions, be extra mindful of phrases that carry unwanted connotations or unspoken emotion. An open-ended question that presumes normality, like "How often do you masturbate?" is better than "Do you masturbate?" The latter question places the patient on the defensive. The former suggests a normal behavior that may be discussed, quantitated, or denied.

When suggestions are offered to couples with sexual problems, be careful not to set semantic traps that may contribute to the problem. Using common phrases such as "pleasuring" or "foreplay" imply some goal or outcome (in this case achieving pleasure or leading to intercourse). Terms that are more neutral (such as sensation [sensate] focusing), have little additional implication; because they are directly related to the process itself and are less outcome based, they are better.

When making specific sexual suggestions to a couple be careful to avoid separating sex and lovemaking. Although it is true that a desire to be close, to be held or caressed, and to have sex may exist independently or in any order, separating them (as may happen with the timed intercourse an infertility therapy may demand) risks further eroding communication and creating toiletlike mechanical actions devoid of those things that make lovemaking so much more than sex.

Patients who are reluctant to use self-exploration or masturbation may be reassured by shifting the focus from the sexual to sensual. When this type of suggestion is couched in the overall context of learning about one's self (what provides pleasure, gives comfort, empowers responsibility, and so forth) it may be seen as less threatening or unnatural.

Having a "wet dream," for either a woman or a man, is not a sign of anything abnormal. It does not mean a person is oversexed or under served. Although more common in men, arousal and orgasm does occur in women and is entirely normal.

When you refer a patient for possible hysterectomy, it is common for the patient to wonder (aloud or not) what the impact on sexual function will be. The patient (and her partner) should be reassured that the loss of the uterus will not automatically change the patient in any sexual way. She will not be more or less desirable, more or less able to be sexually responsive, and will not have a change in libido or interest. Although some patients do experience changes, they are based more on expectation and the preoperative process than on the hysterectomy directly. For example, a patient who has been bleeding continuously or who has had a terrible fear of pregnancy, may now be more sexually expressive after her surgery than she was before it.

"How do I know if I have had an orgasm?" is a common question patients ask or an implicit part of the answers involved in an investigation of orgasmic capability. While we can go into long discussions of physiology with the patient, one of the best descriptions (for counseling purposes) is: "It is somewhat like a sneeze. You can't really describe it, but when it is over, it was the right thing" or "was exactly what was needed." Descriptions of this sort help break the pulp fiction image of fireworks and bare-chested he-men and provide a more realistic, approachable standard. Many patients will discover that they have been orgasmic, but just in a different subjective way than they thought they should be.

Patients may ask about simultaneous orgasms. Many counselors suggest that this goal-oriented, outcome-based expectation may actually get in the way, making orgasmic success impossible or losing an opportunity to enjoy each other's pleasure. (Simultaneous orgasms are a waste of one orgasm.) Failure to achieve simultaneous orgasms is not a failure at all, but fortuitous.

SUGGESTED READINGS

General References

American College of Obstetricians and Gynecologists. Précis V. 1994;97.

American College of Obstetricians and Gynecologists. Sexual Dysfunction. ACOG Technical Bulletin 211. Washington, DC: 1995.

Annon JS. The behavioral treatment of sexual problems. Honolulu: Enabling Systems, 1974.

Annon JS. The behavioral treatment of sexual problems: brief therapy. New York: Harper and Row, 1976.

Bancroft J. Human sexuality and its problems. New York: Churchill, Livingstone, 1983.

Butler RN, Lewis MI, Hoffman E, Whitehead ED. Love and sex after 60: how to evaluate and treat the sexually active woman. Geriatrics 1994;49:33.

Duddle M, Brown ADG. The clinical management of sexual dysfunction. Clin Obstet Gynecol 1980;7:293.

Frank E, Anderson C, Rubinstein D. Frequency of sexual dysfunction in "normal couples." N Engl J Med 1978;299:111.

Hite S. The Hite Report. New York: Macmillan Publishers, 1976.

Janus SS, Janus CL. The Janus Report on Sexual Behavior. New York: John Wiley & Sons, Inc, 1993.

Kaplan HS. Disorders of Sexual Desire. New York: Brunner-Mazel, 1979.

Kaplan HS. The Illustrated Manual of Sex Therapy. New York: Brunner-Mazel, 1987.

Kenyon FE. Homosexuality in gynecologic practice. Clin Obstet Gynecol 1980;7:363.

Lechtenberg R, Ohl DA. Sexual Dysfunction: Neurolgic, Urologic, and Gynecologic Aspects. Philadelphia: Lea & Febiger, 1994.

Masters W, Johnson V. Human Sexual Inadequacy. Boston: Little, Brown, and Co, 1970.

Meyer JK. The treatment of sexual disorders. Med Clin North Am 1977;61:811.

Moore JT, Goldstein Y. Sexual problems among family medicine patients. J Fam Pract 1980;10:243.

Murphy WD, Coleman E, Hoon E, Scott C. Sexual dysfunction and treatment in alcoholic women. Sexuality and Disability 1980;3:240.

Schover LR, Jensen SB. Sexuality and chronic illness: a comprehensive approach. New York: Guilford Press, 1988.

Tavris C, Sadd S. The Redbook Report on Female Sexuality. New York: Delacorte Press, 1977.

Wabrek AJ. Sex counseling in office practice. In Glass RH (ed). Office Gynecology, 4th ed. Baltimore: Williams & Wilkins, 1993;189.

Specific References

Alexander B. Disorders of sexual desire: diagnosis and treatment of decreased libido. Am Fam Physician 1993;47:832.

Comfort A. Sexual Consequences of Disability. Philadelphia: George F Stickley Co., 1978.

Corney RH, Crowther ME, Everett H, Howells A, Shepherd JH. Psychosexual dysfunction in women with gynaecological cancer following radical pelvic surgery. Br J Obstet Gynaecol 1993;100:73.

Dameron GW Jr. Helping couples cope with sexual changes pregnancy brings. Contemporary OB/GYN 1983;21:23.

Gross M. Reversal by bethanechol of sexual dysfunction caused by anticholinergic antidepressants. Am J Psychiatry 1982;139:1193.

Hatch J. Psychophysiological aspects of sexual dysfunction. Arch Sex Behav 1981;10:49.

Maypole J. Medical students learn about sexuality and sensitivity. JAMA. 1994;272:1069.

Morokof P, Heiman J. Effects of erotic stimuli on sexually functional and dysfunctional women: multiple measures before and after sex therapy. Behav Res Ther 1980;18:127.

Nadelson CC, Marcotte DB, eds. Treatment Interventions in Human Sexuality. New York: Plenum Press, 1983.

Plouffe L. Screening for sexual problems through a simple questionnaire. Am J Obstet Gynecol 1985;151:166.

Post LL. Sexual side effects of psychiatric medications in women [letter]. Am J Psychiatry 1994;151:1247.

Psychological Aspects of Breast Cancer Study Group. Psychological response to mastectomy. Cancer 1987;59:189.

Riley AJ, Riley EJ. A controlled study to evaluate directed masturbation in the management of primary orgasmic failure in women. Br J Psychiatry 1978;133:404.

Rubenstein C. Sex Generation. Mademoiselle, 1993;(June):129.

Semmens J, Wagner G. Estrogen deprivation and vaginal function in postmenopausal women. JAMA 1982;248:445.

Shen WW, Sata LS. Inhibited female orgasm resulting from psychotropic drugs. J Reprod Med 1983;28:497.

Sipski ML, Alexander CJ. Sexual activities, response and satisfaction in women pre- and post-spinal cord injury. Arch Phys Med Rehabil 1993;74:1025.

Solberg DA, Butler J, Wagner NN. Sexual behavior in pregnancy. N Engl J Med 1973;288:1098.

Weber AM, Walters MD, Schover LR, Mitchinson A. Sexual function in women with uterovaginal prolapse and urinary incontinence. Obstet Gynecol 1995;85:483.

Wilson G, Lawson D. The effect of alcohol on sexual arousal in women. J Abnorm Psychol 1976;85:489.

Zeiss AM, Rosen GM, Zeiss RA. Orgasm during intercourse: a treatment strategy for women. J Consult Clin Psychol 1977;45:891.

Patient Resources and Counseling Aids

(To be used as adjuncts to evaluation and treatment, not as a substitute.)

Banks C. Tart Tales: Elegant Erotic Stories. New York: Carroll & Graf Publishers, Inc., 1994. (A compilation of well written short stories with mildly erotic themes that may be used to open communications and give permission.)

Barbach L. Pleasures: Women Write Erotica. New York: Harper & Row, 1984. (A collection of short stories written by women that contain explorations of sensuality and erotic situations. Soft-core in nature, this may be used to give permission and explore likes and dislikes.)

Borrelli J, ed. Letters to Penthouse IV. New York: Warner Books, 1994. (A collection of variable quality letters that explore various forms of sexual expression and experiences. This book, and others like it, may be used to explore interests and dislikes, identify areas of interest or discomfort, and open communication through permission to fantasize or verbalize.)

Comfort A. The New Joy of Sex. New York: Crown Publishers, Inc, 1993. (An updated version of the standard, this book provides an excellent guide not only to the organs (plumbing) of sex, but also explores intimacy, love, and health issues.)

Comfort A. More Joy of Sex. New York: Simon and Schuster, Inc, 1973. (A part of the original standard and a companion to The Joy of Sex, this volume explores more of the lovemaking aspects of sex. It also has good discussion of problems such as alcohol, disability, and special forms of expression.)

Hill C, Wallace W. Erotica. An Illustrated Anthology of Sexual Art and Literature. New York: Carroll & Graf Publishers, Inc., 1992. (A "coffee-table" book that provides a somewhat scholarly exploration of erotic art and literature through the ages.)

Hill C, Wallace W. Erotica II. An Illustrated Anthology of Sexual Art and Literature. New York: Carroll & Graf Publishers, Inc., 1992. (A sequel, this volume provides additional examples and discussion.)

Lloyd JE. Nice Couples Do. How to Turn Your Secret Dreams into Sensational Sex. New York: Warner Books, 1991. (Explores the role of fantasy and communication in sex, with examples of the use of fantasy to broaden horizons. This volume also discusses the use of "bookmarking.")

Lloyd JE. If It Feels Good. New York: Warner Books, 1992. (Shows how to enhance lovemaking by exploring the five senses.)

Lloyd JE. Come Play With Me. New York: Warner Books, 1994. (The most current of the three Lloyd books, this volume looks at games and role playing as a way of enhancing communication. It also contains a good discussion of "bookmarking." This volume duplicates, at least conceptually, much of what is contained in Nice Couples Do, so for most couples one or the other is probably adequate.)

Milonas R. Fantasex. A Book of Erotic Games for the Adult Couple, revised ed. New York: Perigee Books, 1983. (A collection of fantasies, role playing, and games to facilitate expanding horizons and experimentation.)

Slung M. Slow Hand. Women Writing Erotica. New York: Harper Collins Publishers, 1992. (Erotica, by women for women, providing permission and fantasy by exploring the idea that erotica is more than flesh on flesh.)

Tisdale S. Talk Dirty to Me: An Intimate Philosophy of Sex. New York: Doubleday, 1994. (One woman's personal discussion of sex and sexuality. An interesting exploration of psychology and sociology.)

25

Sexual Pain

Dyspareunia (painful intercourse) is a special form of both chronic pelvic pain and sexual dysfunction. Although inhibited sexual desire is statistically more common, dyspareunia is far more likely to be the source of spontaneous complaint. Occasional discomfort for one or both partners during intercourse is common (about 15% of women each year) and requires no special investigation or treatment. When recurrent or severe (less than 2% of women), it represents not only a warning sign of possible trouble, but may itself become the source of escalating dysfunction.

Dyspareunia is derived from roots that literally mean bad or difficult mating. Some limit "dyspareunia" to patients with vaginal or lower abdominal pain due to penetration or thrusting of the penis in the vagina in the absence of organic disease. While pain is the manifestation, the diagnosis and treatment of dyspareunia encompasses much more than the pain itself. Attention must also be focused on the impact of sexual dysfunction on the patient's life as well as outside factors that may contribute to the dysfunction itself. Most cases of dyspareunia can be successfully diagnosed and treated in a primary care setting without specialized techniques or training. Referral is necessary for only a small percent of these patients.

BACKGROUND AND SCIENCE

Dyspareunia can be classified according to two different, complimentary schemes: Primary versus secondary and insertional versus deep-thrust. The separation into primary or secondary types is based on the temporal development of the problem. Women who experience difficulty dating from their first attempt at intercourse are classified as having primary dyspareunia. Those women who develop problems with previously successful sexual expression are said to have secondary dyspareunia. (This classification is also used for male sexual pain, which is beyond the scope of this discussion.)

The distinction between insertional and deep-thrust dyspareunia is intuitive but important in helping identify potential causes. Some authors add a third type of dyspareunia, vaginal. This is characterized as vaginal barrel discomfort, tightness, or fullness. The causes and treatment of this type closely parallel that of insertional pain, and they will be discussed as one.

Statistics about the prevalence of dyspareunia are generally lacking. Some recent surveys suggest that most couples experience one or more mild, transient episodes with only minor disruption in sexual function. Almost 15% of women experience one or more episodes of painful intercourse per year and about 20% experience lubrication problems per year.

No matter what the classification, dyspareunia is ultimately a symptom that may have many disparate sources, acting singly or in concert. As a result, the evaluation of patients with this complaint must be careful and wide ranging. It also requires that an open mind be kept for possible additional factors that may be acting in addition to the first cause uncovered.

Primary Dyspareunia

While uncommon anatomic conditions such as vaginal agenesis, hymeneal stenosis, duplication of the vagina, or a vaginal septum will cause difficulty with a woman's first attempt at intercourse, problems dating from first attempts at intercourse may also be psychogenic. Fear of intercourse may arise from many sources, real or imagined, but may result in failure of lubrication and vaginal muscle spasms that may be sufficient to make intromission impossible.

When either anatomic or emotional factors result in sexual failure, anxiety, fear, altered self-image, and a failure mentality may result. The stage is then set both for psychologic propagation of the problem and for a continuing circle of failure (Fig. 25.1). Clearly, both emotional and physical factors must be identified, as either the cause or the result of sexual pain, and promptly addressed.

Secondary Dyspareunia

Secondary dyspareunia is sexual pain that arises in women who have previously been able to perform sexually, although, paradoxically, orgasmic success is not a part of this definition. The onset of dysfunction may be either abrupt or insidious and the problem may be mild or debilitating.

Although secondary dyspareunia can arise from physical or emotional sources, a physical process is most common. (Acquired emotional sexual dysfunction tends to present with anorgasmia, libidinal dysfunction, or insertional pain due to arousal problems.) As in primary dyspareunia, no matter what the originating event, emotional overlays may quickly develop and must also be considered.

Clinically, the separation of dyspareunia into primary and secondary types is not as use-

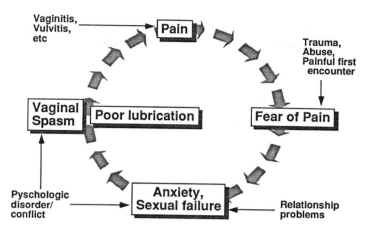

Figure 25.1. Cycle of self-perpetuating sexual pain.

ful in establishing a cause or directing therapy, as is the classification of insertional versus deep-thrust pain.

Insertional Pain and Vaginismus

Insertional dyspareunia is pain that occurs with sexual penetration. This may be in the form of mild discomfort which may be tolerated, pain that completely prevents intromission, or anything in between. In severe cases, this may extend to severe vaginal spasms that interfere with penetration. Insertional pain is often described as sharp, burning, or pinching. The discomfort is generally localized to the vulva, perineum, or outer portion of the vagina. Potential causes of insertional pain (Table 25.1) are many, but most can be identified through careful history and physical examination.

Vaginismus is a special case of insertional dyspareunia in which intense vaginal muscle spasms in the pelvic floor and vaginal wall virtually prevent intromission. There is no evidence that the vaginal canal is structurally different in these women, but rather a spasm of the pelvic floor results in functional narrowing. Vaginismus can be primary or secondary, transient or persistent; it may be a mild problem that aggravates other sexual dysfunction but still allows intercourse or a major dysfunction that impacts on all aspects of the patient's life. These patients may continue to be orgasmic, but most cannot tolerate penetration. For some, this may extend to any vaginal penetration by their partner (e.g., fingers, tongue), self-penetration (e.g., masturbation, tampons), or clinical examination.

Vaginismus has often been described as a manifestation of significant phobic reactions, anxiety, hostility, hysteria, or aversion. In severe cases this may be so, but in milder forms it may also be a learned behavior or protective reaction based on previous negative experiences. Some authors report that up to 80% of vaginismus is situational, suggesting the latter explanation is more common. Others contend that most vaginismus is primary, and results

Table 25.1. Possible causes of Insertional Dyspareunia

Congenital factors
    Duplication of the vagina
    Hymeneal stenosis
    Vaginal agenesis
    Vaginal septum
Cystitis (acute or chronic)
Hemorrhoids
Inadequate lubrication
    Abuse (current or past)
    Arousal disorders
    Insufficient foreplay
    Medication
    Phobias
Pelvic (levator) muscle spasm
Pelvic scarring
    Episiotomy
    Surgical repairs (colporrhaphy)
Proctitis
Trauma (acute or chronic sequella)
Urethral diverticula
Urethral syndrome
Urethritis (bacterial or Chlamydial)
Vaginismus
Vulvar
    Atrophic vulvitis
    Chancroid
    Chemical irritation (deodorants, adjuncts, lubricants)
    Herpes vulvitis
    Hypertrophic vulvar dystrophy
    Lichen sclerosis
    Lymphogranuloma venereum
    Vestibulitis
    Vulvitis (infectious)
    Vulvodynia

from phobia or aversion. All possibilities must be considered when vaginismus is suspected or apparent.

Deep-thrust Dyspareunia

Abdominal, pelvic, or vaginal pain that arises during thrusting, especially with deep penetration, is often described as ache-like, burning, a sense of fullness, or like something being bumped. This form of sexual pain is often dependent on the type of sexual activity involved or the positions used. Positions or practices that result in particularly deep or forceful penetration, such as male superior or rear entry positions, are more likely to result in this type of pain. Conditions that can potentially give rise to deep-thrust dyspareunia are shown in Table 25.2.

Sometimes included with deep-thrust pain is discomfort that occurs at or after orgasm.

Table 25.2. Possible Causes of Deep-thrust Dyspareunia

Gynecologic
    Extrauterine
      Adhesions
      Chronic pelvic infection
      Cysts
      Endometriosis
      Pelvic relaxation
        Cystocele, urethrocele, rectocele, enterocele
      Prolapsed adnexa or adnexa adherent to vaginal apex
      Retained ovary syndrome
    Uterine
      Adenomyosis
      Fibroids
      Malposition (retroversion)
Urologic
    Chronic urinary tract infection
    Detrusor dyssynergia
    Interstitial cystitis
    Urethral syndrome
Gastrointestinal
    Chronic constipation
    Diverticular disease
    Inflammatory bowel disease
      Crohn's disease
      Ulcerative colitis
    Irritable bowel syndrome
Musculoskeletal
    Fibromyocitis
    Hernias (abdominal, femoral)
    Herniated disk
Other
    Inadequate arousal (failure of vaginal apex expansion)
    Pelvic tumors
      Benign or malignant, gynecologic or otherwise

This is generally described as crampy or laborlike. It may occur owing to pelvic congestion or the strong uterine contractions that accompany orgasm. There has been some suggestion that this is more common in women with primary dysmenorrhea because of the similarity of mechanism, although this has not been adequately studied.

ESTABLISHING THE DIAGNOSIS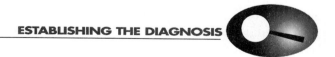

The diagnosis of dyspareunia is really one of patient self-reporting. More important is the establishment of causation and the implementation of effective therapy. Care must be taken to avoid labeling any dyspareunia as purely physical or only emotional in origin. Most often a mixture of factors is present that causes or contributes to the problem. Probable causation is established based on both a careful history and the results of physical examination.

History

Dyspareunia may be a presenting complaint or a more indolent problem that is only apparent if the interviewer raises the topic. For this reason, it is important that every review of systems include questions that open up the topic of sexuality and sexual function. Dyspareunia will be quickly identified by the commonly used screening question "Do you have any discomfort or problems with intercourse?" Some authors emphasize the use of "discomfort" rather than "pain" to allow a broader set of complaints to be addressed. This may be a matter of personal preference. The most important part is to ask questions about sexuality and sexual function.

When obtaining a detailed history from patients with dyspareunia, special attention must be paid to several specific areas: the character and location of the complaints, the situations and actions that precipitate the discomfort, the chronology of the complaint, the impact of the problem, and any solutions that have been attempted (and their results). Each of these areas makes specific contributions to the evaluation process.

As with any complaint of discomfort, the character, severity, location, and radiation of symptoms are important in directing the course of the investigation. This information also provides the classification of the patient's dyspareunia into insertional or deep-thrust types. Pain that is sharp and well defined (e.g., vulvar pain) can be expected to come from a different cause than that characterized by a dull, achy, or crampy pain (e.g., pelvic relaxation). Lateralized pain probably has a different source than that reported to be diffusely located in the midline (e.g., ovarian cyst vs. uterine fibroids). The presence of other, nonsexual symptoms (e.g., menstrual pain, vaginal discharge, or vulvar lesions) may be particularly meaningful.

With sexual pain it is very important to establish the frequency of the complaint and the specific situations in which it occurs. Pain that happens with every attempt at intercourse may have a very different root than discomfort that occurs with only one sexual activity. Symptoms that occur only in specific situations or only with certain activities may suggest emotional conflicts or concerns (aversion, fear, coercion) or a physical process that is only affected by that activity (urethritis made manifest by rear-entry positions). Coexistent libidinal, arousal, or orgasmic dysfunction may become apparent during this discussion, suggesting additional diagnostics or interventions beyond the issue of pain.

The evolution of symptoms over time is also potentially significant. Pain that is gradual in onset suggests different antecedents than do symptoms that gradually worsen with time. New or changing symptoms not only point to evolving pathologies but also suggest other impacts the dysfunction may have manifest in symptoms of emotional withdrawal, libidinal dysfunction, or premature ejaculation. In addition, this may serve to alert the clinician to other issues (including global ones such as anxiety or personality disorders) that need to be addressed by any treatment programs suggested.

Information about what actions the couple have taken, on their own or under the advice of others, may indicate their level of comfort and sophistication in sexual matters. This line of inquiry will indicate areas or therapy that have been unsuccessful in the past, thus avoiding repeating a failure.

Physical Examination

The physical examination of patients with dyspareunia is focused on the possibility of organic contributors to the patient's complaints. This is true even when a significant emotional component is present, for this does not preclude the possibility of a physical or disease process as provoking or perpetuating the problem.

Although it is natural to focus on the pelvic examination in patients with sexual pain, a general evaluation of the patient cannot be overlooked. Musculoskeletal, gastroenterologic, urologic, or neurologic conditions may all precipitate or contribute to pain with intercourse. For example, a hernia that becomes symptomatic during abdominal wall contraction and the muscular exertion of intercourse may easily be overlooked if only a pelvic examination is performed.

The pelvic examination of patients with dyspareunia must be performed with care if maximal information is to be obtained. The need to allow the patient a sense of control (that should be a part of every pelvic examination) is even more acute in these patients. The patient should be alerted to every touch and maneuver before it takes place to avoid surprise or guarding. For those patients with significant apprehension, allowing the woman to indicate the source of pain, to guide inspection, or assist speculum insertion with her own hands results in a more informative and comfortable examination. Giving a patient with vaginismus an opportunity to learn that slow, gentle penetration of the vagina can be accomplished without pain will not only allow the pelvic examination to be performed, but may begin the process of therapy that leads to satisfactory intercourse. As in patients with other sexual dysfunction, allowing the patient to watch the examination through a hand mirror may also facilitate the examination, promote communication, and provide education.

Inspection of the vulva begins the pelvic examination. When insertional complaints are prominent, care should be given to a search for lesions, thickenings, skin or pigment changes, and hyperesthetic areas such as those found with vestibulitis. The size and configuration of the vaginal introitus should be noted, along with any traumatic, surgical, or obstetric (episiotomy) scars. A brief assessment of neurologic function should be performed (gross sensation, sphincter reflex). Gentle palpation of the vulvar tissues using a moist cotton-tipped applicator may help delineate specific areas of tenderness or hypersensitivity.

A "monomanual" (one-handed) examination follows, with special care and attention being paid to those areas that the patient reports as symptomatic. Using gentle pressure, assess the tone of the pelvic floor muscles, along with the degree of voluntary control over these muscles. Roughly 25% of patients with muscular spasm during sexual activity will not manifest the spasm during clinical examination. Therefore, the absence of spasm does not rule out vaginismus as a possible diagnosis.

Pressure along the back wall of the vagina may suggest proctitis even before the rectal examination is performed. Gentle pressure under the urethra may indicate chronic urethritis or urethral syndrome. Milking the urethra may demonstrate a discharge in patients with a urethral diverticulum, urethritis, or a Skene's gland infection. Gentle motion of the cervix may suggest both the degree of mobility present and the role of the uterus and adjacent structures in the pain process.

A speculum evaluation is performed next. Based on the findings of the monomanual examination, the size and type of speculum used may be chosen to allow the procedure to be performed with less patient discomfort. For some patients a small Peterson, a virginal, or even a nasal speculum may be required (Fig. 25.2). Inspection of the vaginal walls for lesions, signs of trauma or infection, presence of congenital anomalies, and the patient's estrogen status should all be carried out. Papanicolaou smear and cervical cultures should be obtained.

Lastly, a traditional bimanual examination is performed to confirm those findings suggested earlier. This portion of the examination will be more sensitive for identifying changes in uterine size or mobility, adnexal pathology, and changes in the posterior cul-de-sac (suggestive of scarring or endometriosis). The latter is also addressed by the rectovaginal examination that concludes the procedure.

Laboratory studies are of limited value in the evaluation of dyspareunia with the exception of urinalysis, microscopic examination of vaginal secretions, and cultures (cervical and urethral). Colposcopic evaluation of the vulva or introitus may reveal acetowhite areas, punctation, or early papillary changes, although the application of acetic acid solution may be exquisitely painful for many of these patients.

It would be unlikely for imaging studies to identify a cause of dyspareunia that was not clinically apparent, except in the case of a completely uncooperative patient for whom an adequate examination is impossible. Laparoscopic examination of the pelvic structures may confirm adhesions or endometriosis, but the invasive nature of this procedure limits it to those patients with additional concerns sufficient to justify the associated risks.

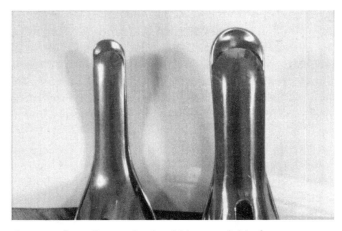

Figure 25.2. A selection of small specula should be available for use in vaginismus patients. Shown are a small Peterson and a narrower "virginal" (left) version. A nasal speculum (see Fig. 7.1) may also be used.

THERAPEUTIC OPTIONS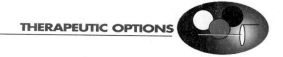

Specific Therapy

Because dyspareunia is ultimately a symptom, the specific therapy for any form of sexual pain is directed toward the underlying cause. This may be as simple as therapy for vaginitis or vulvitis or as intensive as hysterectomy for severe pelvic scarring due to endometriosis or pelvic infections. The majority of conditions that result in dyspareunia are amenable to outpatient management, and hence may be addressed in a primary care setting.

Adjunctive therapy in the form of vaginal lubricants (water-soluble or long-acting agents like Astro-Glide, Replens, Lubrin, K-Y Jelly, and others), local anesthetics (for vulvar lesions), or pelvic relaxation exercises may be appropriate while more specific therapy is underway. The judicious use of anxiolytics or antidepressant medications for selected patients, such as those with vulvodynia or vaginismus, may also be appropriate. This should not be considered first-line therapy, but employed for a limited time only, while efforts are directed toward the underlying physical or emotional pathologies present.

Modifying sexual techniques used by the couple may reduce pain with intercourse. Delaying penetration until maximal arousal has been achieved improves vaginal lubrication, ensures vaginal apex expansion, and provides an element of control for the female partner. Sexual positions that allow the women to control the direction and depth of penetration (such as woman astride) may also be of help. The extent to which these have been tried by the couple or their willingness to try them at your suggestion may indicate the psychodynamics that may be present.

Vaginismus

Patients with vaginismus require special therapeutic support. Although many techniques, including hypnosis, have been suggested, therapy generally takes a three-pronged approach that consists of behavior modification, vaginal dilatation, and emotional counseling. The first two of these may easily be begun in a primary care setting. Depending on the severity of the emotional component and the comfort of the provider, successful counseling may also take place in the primary care setting with referral as necessary.

Behavior modification therapy for vaginismus consists of muscle awareness and training exercises, the most common of which mimic the Kegel exercises used in mild forms of incontinence (Chapter 27, Urinary Infection, Incontinence, and Pelvic Relaxation). In this form of the exercise, the examiner places a finger just inside the introitus and the patient is asked to contract the same muscles she would use to stop the flow of urine. The examiner can judge the degree of contraction and provide feedback so that the patient can identify the actions that result in contraction of the pelvic floor. The patient is then instructed to place her own finger in the vaginal opening and identify the muscles that are being contracted. With this increased awareness, practice is continued in a effort to actively relax these muscles. Once some facility is attained, the contraction/relaxation exercises can be continued without the use of the finger.

Vaginal "dilatation" exercises are primarily directed toward learning that something can be contained in the vagina without resulting in pain. This can be carried out using plastic syringe covers or specially made vaginal dilators. Therapy begins by having the patient insert the smallest size (roughly the size of the fifth finger) into the vagina. This should be attempted in a relaxed, comfortable setting, such as a warm bath. Once comfort is consistently attained, the size is gradually increased. It is the process of control, insertion, and muscle relaxation that occasions symptom improvement, not a mechanical dilatation. Once a larger size can be comfortably inserted, intercourse is reintroduced. This may begin with the patient continuing her own insertions with her partner present, progressing to partner introduction of the dilator, patient-controlled insertion of the penis, and lastly normal intercourse. As comfort improves, attention may then be directed toward pleasure.

The third avenue of treatment for vaginitis is counseling. In its simplest form, this is directed toward reassurance, education, and identification of causative factors. The use of a hand mirror during pelvic examination or Kegel exercise instruction may improve awareness and important knowledge of the anatomy. Reassurance that an anatomic abnormality is not present may go a long way toward acquiring a cooperative, positive attitude. Significant phobias, major personality disorders, and signs of abuse (physical, sexual, or emotional) require specialized intervention.

Emotional Support

As previously noted, it is rare for dyspareunia to exist without significant emotional components that either contribute to the development of the complaint or arise because of it. Early, aggressive management of this aspect of the patient's problem is necessary to avoid the development or propagation of even more recalcitrant sexual dysfunction.

The emotional care of these couples centers around support and specific treatment. These two lines are often intertwined, with support and permission providing the cornerstone of both. Wherever possible, the patient should be reassured about the normality of her anatomy, the frequency of this problem in others, the likelihood of successful therapy, and the probable source of the complaint. Information and specific suggestions to reduce or eliminate the pain can also be used to address the emotional aspects of the problem. The role of each of these is discussed at length in Chapter 24, Sexual Dysfunction.

HINTS AND COMMON QUESTIONS

It is not uncommon for dyspareunia to present as a complaint of vaginal discharge. This occurs because it is easier to tell office personnel "I have an infection" than "I have pain with sex." Many patients also assume that sexual pain must be an indication of infection and seek evaluation and treatment based on their presumption of cause. Anytime the complaint of vaginitis appears to be out of proportion to the clinical findings, suspect a sexual dysfunction.

Patients often presume that sexual pain is evidence of infertility, a lack of love, punishment for some past transgression, or bad technique. Although bad technique may occasionally play a role, care must be taken to identify and quickly address the emotional overlay and misconceptions that often coexist. This is most simply done through reassurance, timely diagnosis, and treatment.

Be wary of the patient who says "everything is perfect" except for their dyspareunia. Dyspareunia sufficient to prompt the patient to seek care seldom exists in a vacuum. For most couples, dyspareunia is accompanied by, or will cause, other stresses that have to be addressed. When the couple reports no other problems, it may reflect a lack of awareness of other conflicts or a denial state in which the complaint of pain substitutes for the actual, most serious, problem.

Many couples feel that if they could only "relax a bit" during sex the pain would be improved. They then resort to alcohol or drugs to accomplish this self-directed "goal," actually making the problem worse through the adverse effect these agents have on sexual performance (see Chapter 24, Sexual Dysfunction). Patients should be warned about this possibility early in the diagnostic and therapeutic process.

When searching for a cause of dyspareunia during a pelvic examination, be careful to establish that any pain elicited is the same as that experienced during intercourse. Most pelvic examinations engender some discomfort, but that discomfort may be different than what the patient experiences during sexual activities. For example, the patient may report a sharp sensation followed by aching when the ovary is palpated, but when deep penetration occurs experiences midline, deep pelvic pain, owing to endometriosis. Asking "Is that the pain you are having during sex?" may help to relieve this potential confusion.

When vestibulitis is suspected, pelvic examination may still be carried out if the clinician uses a single finger, a virginal speculum, and all pressure is kept toward the anterior vaginal wall, avoiding the perineum as much as possible. Care must be taken to avoid excessive pressure on the urethra as this will be uncomfortable, although not to the degree caused by manipulation of the posterior fourchette.

Use caution in the diagnosis and management of vulvar dystropies. These may present as a source of insertional pain, but may also harbor areas of precancerous changes. When in doubt, biopsy can make the distinction.

Vaginismus may be present even if there is no sign of muscular spasm during pelvic examination. In mild forms, vaginal spasms occur only in the setting of attempted penile penetration. Clinical examination, tampon insertion, masturbation, and occasionally digital insertion by a partner may be tolerated. In the absence of clinically identified spasm, the diagnosis may still be provisionally made while further investigation is initiated and empiric therapy is begun.

If atrophy is the cause of insertional dyspareunia, estrogen therapy will restore tissue elasticity and the ability to lubricate normally, but this may take up to 6 months to accomplish. To speed the process, topical estrogen facilitates the tissue changes and provides a soothing adjunct at the same time.

Do not overlook the role of the male partner in couples with dyspareunia. It is not uncommon to find the development of erectile dysfunction in male partners of women with vaginismus or dyspareunia. (Some authors report a rate as high as 15% to 20% of these men.) The man may also be the source of unrealistic expectation, misinformation, stress, or trauma (physical, emotional, or sexual). Including these aspects in your evaluation may speed diagnosis and therapy, or both.

SUGGESTED READINGS

General References

American College of Obstetricians and Gynecologists. Précis V. 1994;101.

Fink P. Dyspareunia: Current concepts. Medical Aspects of Human Sexuality 1972;6:28.

Fordney DS. Dyspareunia and vaginismus. Clin Obstet Gynecol 1978;21:205.

Fullerton W. Dyspareunia. BMJ 1971;2:31.

Kaplan HS. Disorders of Sexual Desire. New York: Brunner-Mazel, 1979.

Lamont JA. Vaginismus. Am J Obstet Gynecol 1978;131:632.

Lamont JA. Female dyspareunia. Am J Obstet Gynecol 1980;136:282.

Michael RT, Gagnon JH, Laumann EO, Kolata G. Sex in America: A Definitive Survey. Boston: Little, Brown and Company, 1994.

Steege JF. Dyspareunia and vaginismus. Clin Obstet Gynecol 1984;27:750.

Steege JF, Ling FW. Dyspareunia. A special type of chronic pelvic pain. Obstet Gynecol Clin North Am 1993;20:779.

Specific References

Carson CC III, Segura JW, Keyes TW. Psychologic characteristics of patients with female urethral syndrome. J Clin Psychol 1979;35:312.

Fuchs K. Therapy of vaginismus by hypnotic desensitization. Am J Obstet Gynecol 1980;137:1.

Goetsch MF. Vulvar vestibulitis: prevalence and histologic features in a general gynecologic practice population. Am J Obstet Gynecol 1991;164:1609.

Kent HL, Wisniewski PM. Interferon for vulvar vestibulitis. J Reprod Med 1990;87:1138.

Peckham BM, Make DG, Patterson JJ, et al. Focal vulvitis: a characteristic syndrome and a cause of dyspareunia. Am J Obstet Gynecol 1986;154:855.

Reamy K. The treatment of vaginismus by the gynecologists: an eclectic approach. Obstet Gynecol 1982;59:58.

Sarrel PM, Steege JF, Maltzer M, et al. Pain during sex response due to occlusion of the Bartholin's gland duct. Obstet Gynecol 1983;62:261.

Schover LR, Youngs DD, Cannata R. Psychosexual aspects of the evaluation and management of vulvar vestibulitis. Am J Obstet Gynecol 1992;167:630.

26

Sexually Transmitted Disease and "PID"

Changing behavior patterns and the emergence of fatal sexually transmitted diseases (STDs), have made it even more imperative that we are familiar with this aspect of gynecologic care. If we are to reduce the prevalence and minimize the impact of STDs, it is necessary to understand their epidemiology, diagnosis, and management strategies. We must be familiar with the organisms responsible, their modes of transmission, and the signs, symptoms, and physical findings associated with the disease, as well as screening and diagnostic methods. Lastly, we must understand the potential sequelae of these diseases in terms of long-term fertility and general health. It is essential that we be alert to the possibility of sexually transmitted disease in all patients, perform diagnostic evaluations, and be prepared to institute appropriate treatments promptly. We must also educate our patients about the risks involved in today's sexually open society.

The impact of changing sexuality has had wide-reaching implications, not the least of which has been the explosive increase in the number and types of sexually transmitted diseases—from acquired immune deficiency syndromes (AIDS) to vaginitis—seen by the practitioner. They range from a minor inconvenience to those that may lead to loss of fertility, create long-term disability, or result in life-threatening illness. Although many of these diseases can be acquired by nonsexual means, sexual transmission represents the major route by which they are transmitted.

In the United States there are approximately 13 million cases of sexually transmitted diseases annually, excluding human immunodeficiency virus (HIV) infections. Far from the success of declining rates reported a number of years ago, there has been a new upsurge of infections. In the last few years, this country has seen an increase of approximately 75% in the number of cases of syphilis reported. Steady or increased rates of gonococcal infections, herpes vulvitis, and other STDs are the rule. Over 85% of sexually transmitted infections occur to young people aged 15 to 29, often with life-long consequences. It is, therefore, incumbent on all who provide health care for women to be aware of the risks, facile in the diagnosis, and vigorous in the therapy of sexually transmitted disease.

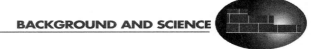

BACKGROUND AND SCIENCE

Bacterial Infections

Chlamydia Trachomatis

The second most common sexually transmitted disease and most common bacterial STD is *Chlamydia trachomatis*. More common than *Neisseria gonorrhoeae* by as much as 10 to 1 in some studies, infections by *Chlamydia trachomatis* can be the source of significant complications and infertility. This organism may be found in between 4% and 20% of pregnant patients and 30% of sexually active adolescent women. Up to 40% of sexually active women have antibodies to chlamydia, suggesting prior infection. The risk of contracting chlamydia is five times greater with three or more sexual partners and four times higher for patients using no contraception or nonbarrier methods of birth control.

The high prevalence of chlamydial infections is due to several factors: The infection is frequently asymptomatic and thus many women do not seek treatment unless their partner develops symptoms or their infection progresses. Chlamydia has a long incubation period (average, 10 days) and may persist in the cervix as a carrier state for many years.

An infection by this obligate intracellular organism may manifest itself as cervicitis, pelvic inflammatory disease, or as the much less common, lymphogranuloma venereum. Because this infection tends to involve the mucosal layers and not the entire structure, mild cases of cervicitis or tubal infections caused by Chlamydia may be virtually asymptomatic, allowing continuing damage and culminating in a high risk for subsequent infertility or ectopic pregnancy. Chlamydial infections are also responsible for nongonococcal urethritis and inclusion conjunctivitis.

Neisseria Gonorrhoeae (Gonorrhea)

This gram-negative intracellular diplococcus remains a common infectious agent, accounting for about 1 million cases of infection annually in the United States. A rate of penicillin-resistance that approaches 50%, an increased frequency of asymptomatic or minimally symptomatic infections, and changing patterns of sexual behavior have all contributed to its continuing prevalence. It is highly contagious. It is estimated that one episode of intercourse with an infected partner carries a 20% chance of infection for men but a 60% to 80% chance of infection for women. This rate rises to 60% to 80% for both sexes with four or more exposures. Roughly 3 of 1000 sexually active women have the disease. Co-infection with other STDs is common, with roughly 25% to 45% of patients with gonococcal infections having concomitant chlamydial infection.

Damage caused by *N. gonorrhoeae* infection causes an increased risk of recurrent pelvic infection, chronic pelvic pain, or infertility due to tubal damage or hydrosalpinx formation.

The impact of a gonorrheal infection is much greater for women than it is for men. For every three men infected, two women will undergo one or more days of hospitalization. For every 18 men infected, one woman undergoes surgery. It is estimated that one episode of gonorrhea carries a 15% infertility rate and this rises to 75% for three or more infections. The risk of an ectopic pregnancy is increased 7 to 10 times in women with a history of salpingitis.

Infections with *N. gonorrhoeae* may be found in numerous sites, many of which have few if any symptoms; however, many do carry significant long-term effects (e.g. gonococcal conjunctivitis can rapidly lead to blindness). Most commonly, the first signs or symptoms of genital tract infection occur 3 to 5 days after exposure. Between 40% and 60% of patients will have symptoms, although they are often mild enough to be overlooked. Infection in the lower genital tract is characterized by a malodorous, purulent discharge from the urethra, Skene's duct, cervix, vagina, or anus (even without rectal intercourse). The presence of greenish or yellow discharge from the cervix should suggest the possibility of either *N. gonorrhoeae* or *C. trachomatis* infections. Infection of the Bartholin's gland occurs frequently and can progress to secondary infections, abscesses, or chronic cyst formation. Urethral infections occur simultaneously in 70% to 90% of women with cervical infections. Infection of the pharynx is found in 10% to 20% of heterosexual women with gonorrhea. Because roughly one half of patients with oral gonorrhea have no symptoms, this site should not be overlooked when cultures are taken from patients suspected with gonorrhoeal infections.

Although *N. gonorrhoeae* infections tend to cause more severe symptoms than chlamydial infections, up to 50% of patients may be asymptomatic. This indolent course may result in delayed or missed diagnosis. Disseminated infections are infrequent (approximately 1% of patients) but can lead to significant arthritis or conjunctivitis. Untreated gonorrheal conjunctivitis can rapidly cause blindness. Neonatal infections acquired from an infected mother may result in conjunctivitis or pneumonia.

Syphilis

Since antiquity, syphilis has been the prototypic venereal disease. The number of syphilis cases has dramatically risen, with a 75% increase between 1985 and 1990 (Fig. 26.1). The net result is that over 50,000 new cases were reported in 1990. This rapid increase is due, in part, to the same social changes that have led to rising rates of other venereal diseases and to the increased use of newer antibiotics to treat penicillin-resistant gonorrhea. (In the past, penicillin treatment of gonorrhea provided protection against coexisting syphilis.) Although more common in younger patients (Fig. 26.2), the possibility of syphilis must be entertained in patients of any age.

Treponema pallidum is one of a very small group of spirochetes that are virulent for humans. Despite the poor virulence of other members of this family, *T. pallidum* is virulent. It is estimated that roughly one third of patients exposed to early syphilis will acquire the disease. This is because this motile anaerobic spirochete can rapidly invade even intact moist mucosa. For this reason, the most common sites of entry for women are those directly exposed to infected semen: the vulva, vagina and cervix. Chancres may also be found in or near the anus, rectum, pharynx, tongue, lips, fingers, or the skin of almost any part of the body.

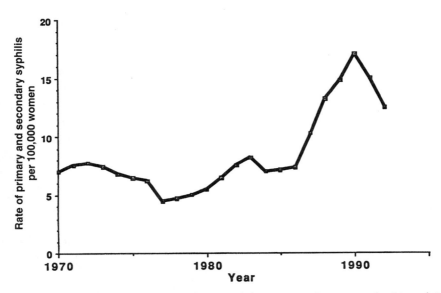

Figure 26.1. Rate of Primary and Secondary Syphilis Among Women in the United States, 1970–1992. After: Centers for Disease Control and Prevention. Sexually transmitted disease surveillance, 1992. Atlanta: Division of STD/HIV Prevention 1993;10.

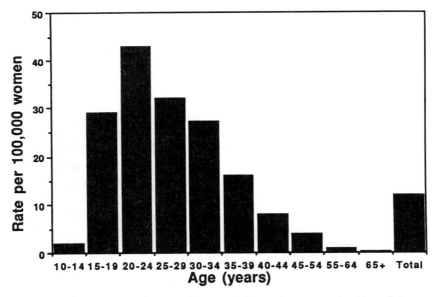

Figure 26.2. Age of Primary and Secondary Syphilis in Women in the United States. After: Centers for Disease Control and Prevention. Sexually transmitted disease surveillance, 1992. Atlanta: Division of STD/HIV Prevention 1993;10.

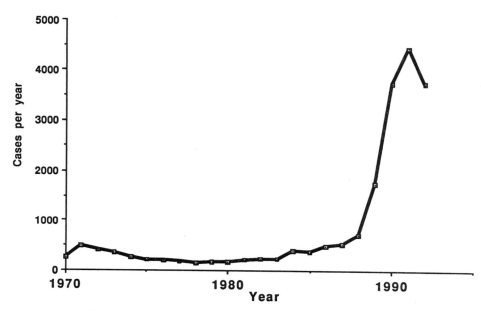

Figure 26.3. Rate of Congenital Syphilis in the United States, 1970–1992. After: Centers for Disease Control and Prevention. Sexually transmitted disease surveillance, 1992. Atlanta: Division of STD/HIV Prevention 1993;10.

Transplacental spread of syphilis occurs at any time during pregnancy and can result in congenital syphilis, which has shown an alarming rise in the past few years(Fig. 26.3). Transplacental infection occurs in roughly 50% of patients with untreated primary or secondary disease. Half of these patients will have premature deliveries or stillbirths. Tertiary and late syphilis are associated with lower transmission rates and less perinatal morbidity.

About 10 to 60 days (average, 21 days) after inoculation with *T. pallidum,* a painless ulcer (chancre) appears. The chancre is shallow, firm, punched out, with a smooth base and rolled edges. Even though it is often accompanied by adenopathy, the chancre is most often overlooked. Serologic testing based on the presence of antibodies will generally be negative at this stage. Spontaneous healing of the chancre occurs in 3 to 9 weeks.

If untreated, 4 to 8 weeks after the primary chancre appears, secondary syphilis develops. This is typically characterized by low-grade fever, headache, malaise, sore throat, anorexia, generalized lymphadenopathy, and a diffuse, symmetric, asymptomatic maculopapular rash over the palm and soles (sometimes referred to as "money spots" due to the coinlike character of the rash). Highly contagious secondary eruptions, called mucous patches, occur in 30% of patients during this phase. In moist areas of the body, flat-topped papules may coalesce, forming condylomata lata, which are distinguished from venereal warts by their broader base and flatter surface. In untreated individuals, this stage will resolve spontaneously in 2 to 6 weeks, evolving into the latent phase in 15% to 40% of patients.

Even though transmission of the infection is unlikely in the latent phase (except via blood transfusion or placental transfer), crippling damage to the central nervous or skeletal systems, heart, or great vessels often ensues in the form of destructive, necrotic, granulomatous lesions (gummas) that develop from 1 to 10 years after the initial infection. Serious cardiovascular or neurologic complications occur in between 5% and 20% of patients.

Viral Infections

Herpes Genitalis

Office visits for herpes simplex infections have increased tenfold in the past 10 years. It is estimated that there are over 20 million recurrent cases and between 300,000 and 500,000 new cases of herpes in the United States each year. Up to 150 million people in the United States may harbor the virus. Studies suggest that 1 of every 200 asymptomatic women are shedding herpes virus. Over 70% of American women have antibody evidence of exposure to one or both types of herpes virus.

Roughly 80% of genital herpes infections are caused by herpes simplex virus type 2, with the remaining 20% caused by the type 1 virus. Exposure to type 1 virus often happens in childhood and is responsible for oral "cold sores." Previous infection with type 1 virus appears to provide some immunity to type 2 infections.

Herpes infections during pregnancy pose a special risk. Herpes has been blamed for as many as 30% of spontaneous abortions. Babies born to mothers with active herpes virus have a 50% risk of acquiring the infection—an infection that carries an 80% mortality rate. Despite this distressing figure, 40% to 70% of all neonates with herpes are born to asymptomatic mothers making the significance of this STD all the greater.

Herpes simplex infections are highly contagious. Roughly 75% of sexual partners of infected individuals will themselves contract the disease if intercourse occurs during viral shedding. The incubation period from infection to symptoms is generally about 6 days (range 3–9), with first episodes lasting from 10 to 12 days. The virus replicates in the parabasal and intermediate cells of the skin. It passes from cell to cell until it encounters nerve cell endings that provide access to local ganglia. Of those patients who do develop symptoms (not all do), the development of the classic vesicular lesions is often preceded by a prodromal phase of mild paresthesia and burning, beginning approximately 2 to 5 days after infection. This will progress to very painful vesicular and ulcerated lesions 3 to 7 days after exposure. Initial episodes of herpes infections are notable for these painful vesicular lesions which may prompt hospitalization in up to 10% of cases. Dysuria due to vulvar lesions, urethral and bladder involvement, or autonomic dysfunction may lead to urinary retention.

Primary infections are characterized by malaise, low-grade fever, and inguinal adenopathy in 40% of patients. Inguinal adenopathy may persist for several weeks after the resolution of the vulvar lesions. Suppuration is uncommon. Systemic symptoms, including aseptic meningitis, fever, headache, and meningismus, can be found in 70% of patients 5 to 7 days after the appearance of the genital lesions. This generally resolves over a period of 7 to 10 days. Healing of the lesions is generally complete. Cervical infections may produce only a profuse, watery discharge and systemic symptoms.

Following initial infection, the virus may become established in sacral root ganglia, which acts as a reservoir for future recurrences. Between 60% and 90% of patients have recurrences of the herpetic lesions in the first 6 months after initial infection. Although generally shorter and milder, these recurrent attacks are no less virulent. Patients are infectious during the period from first prodrome through crusting of the lesions. Viral shedding may also occur asymptomatically, making steps to prevent further transmission mandatory.

Human Papilloma Virus

Human papilloma virus (HPV) infection is the most common viral sexually transmitted disease in the United States. This DNA virus is found in 2% to 4% of all women and up to 60% of patients have evidence of the virus when polymerase chain reaction techniques are used. Over the past 15 years the number of infected individuals has increased almost sevenfold. It has recently been estimated that 4% of all clinic visits by women are for the treatment of condyloma acuminata caused by HPV infections. Subclinical infections may be as much as eight times more common, with less than 2% of patients with HPV having clinical condyloma.

The highest incidence of HPV infections is among women age 16 to 25, with the most common presentation of symptomatic infection being genital warts (condyloma acuminata). The virus is hardy and may resist even drying, making transmission and autoinoculation common. There is some evidence that fomite transmission rarely occurs. This virus is easily spread. Fifty percent of sexual partners of women with HPV have visible lesions and 25% have subclinical infections. The use of condoms has not been shown to reduce the spread of HPV, but use should still be encouraged to reduce the spread of other sexually transmitted diseases.

The usual incubation period from infection to clinical manifestation is 2 months, but may vary from 1 to 6 months. Active viral replication in condyloma may last 6 to 9 months. The immune system apparently plays a role in suppressing the clinical impact of this infection. As a result, those who are immunocompromised (e.g., transplant, AIDS, or pregnant patients) may experience rapid and exuberant growth of condyloma. External factors that suppress the immune system (steroids, cigarette smoking, metabolic deficiencies, and other viruses such as herpes) may have similar effects. When HPV is identified in one area of the genital tract, subclinical evidence of the virus may be found in other areas in between one third and one half of cases. Therefore, patients with vulvar or vaginal condyloma must be carefully screened and followed for the cervical abnormalities associated with this virus.

Unlike many STDs, long-term complications of HPV infection may take years to develop. For example, several subtypes (16, 18, 31, 33, 35, and others) are associated with the development of cervical neoplasia. Roughly 90% of patients with cervical squamous cell carcinoma have evidence of HPV DNA present in their cervical tissues. It is currently thought that it requires a cocarcinogen (e.g., smoking, other viruses, or nutritional factors) before malignant transformation can take place. Because these patients are at higher risk for cervical neoplasia, close follow-up with Pap smears and/or colposcopy at 6- to 12-month intervals is recommended. As noted in Chapter 13, Abnormal Pap Smears, HPV serotyping is not currently indicated for either the management of HPV as a sexually transmitted disease or for the assessment of cervical neoplasia risk.

HIV and AIDS

Recent data show that AIDS has become the number one killer of Americans aged 25 to 44. It is estimated that as many as 2 million Americans, or 0.7% of the entire population, may be infected with HIV. Although transmission of HIV can occur via blood transfusion, pregnancy, or the drug-associated use of contaminated needles, the exchange of body fluids during sexual activity represents a major mode of spread, making HIV infection and AIDS sexually transmitted diseases. There is no evidence that HIV can be transmitted by casual contact, immune globulin preparations, hepatitis B vaccine, or contact with insects. This virtually uniformly fatal disease is generally diagnosed either through screening of individuals at high risk, or based on the presence of suspicious secondary infections or rare tumors (e.g., Kaposi's sarcoma).

Women have the fastest growing rate of HIV infection in the United States. In 1993, AIDS was the fourth leading cause of death for women between the ages of 25 and 44 and it is anticipated that at the current rate of spread, by the year 2000 it will rank second behind heart disease as an overall cause of death for women. In 1994, there were 14,081 cases of AIDS in women, representing 18% of all cases, with these numbers rapidly rising from year to year (Fig. 26.4). Although HIV affects a disproportionate proportion of black and Hispanic women (77%), any sexually active woman is potentially at risk. The largest risk for HIV infections is via drug use (41% in 1994), but heterosexual transmission ranks a very close second, accounting for roughly 37% of all infections (Table 26.1). The median age of women with AIDS in the United States is 35, with 84% of cases occurring in women between the ages of 15 and 44 years.

It is important to recognize that, for women, HIV infection is often closely linked to social factors such as drug use, physical or sexual abuse, and domestic violence. These factors often make it even more difficult for the woman to take steps to protect herself from disease exposure or to seek help and counseling. (See also Chapter 23, Sexual Assault and Abuse.)

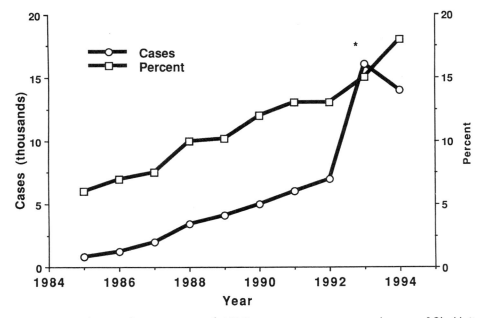

Figure 26.4. Number and percentage of AIDS cases among women (age ≥ 13), United States, 1985–1994. *AIDS surveillance case definition was expanded in 1993. After: Centers for Disease Control and Surveillance. Update: AIDS among women—United States, 1994. MMWR 1994;44:881.

Table 26.1. Exposure Source for Adult and Adolescent AIDS Cases in the United States.

Exposure category	October 1992–September 1993	No. %	Cumulative total	No.%
Injecting drugs	6,891	47	19,878	49
Heterosexual contact	5,545	43	14,997	37
Transfusion/tissue recipient	496	3	2,388	6
Hemophilia	27	0	73	0
Unknown	1,833	12	3,366	8
Total	14,792		40,702	

After: Centers for Disease Control and Prevention. Sexually transmitted disease surveillance, 1992. Atlanta: Division of STD/HIV Prevention, 1993:10.

In 1993, roughly 7000 HIV-infected women gave birth, resulting in an estimated 1000 to 2000 or more infected infants. The generally accepted prevalence of HIV infections is between 1.6 and 1.7 per 1000 live births, although this rate varies regionally (e.g., 3.4 per 1000 births in the Northeast) and is rising annually. Because the risk of transmission of AIDS to a fetus is high despite new prophylactic therapies (30% to 50%) and the fact that maternal AIDS often worsens during pregnancy, pregnancy should be postponed until more is known about transmission to infants or effective therapies become available.

In 90% of patients, infection by the human immunodeficiency virus produces only nonspecific symptoms, often mimicking mononucleosis. Febrile pharyngitis is most common, with fever, sweats, lethargy, arthralgia, myalgia, headache, photophobia, and lymphadenopathy seen soon after infection and lasting up to 2 weeks. Incubation from infection to clinical symptoms ranges from 5 days to 3 months, with an average of 2 to 4 weeks.

Following recovery from the initial infection, the patient enters a carrier state during which symptoms are absent, but viral shedding occurs. Immune dysfunction generally becomes apparent roughly 10 years after the initial infection. The development of immunocompromise is rare before 3 years after infection; less than 35% develop symptoms of AIDS before 5 years.

Minor Sexually Transmitted Diseases

Chancroid, granuloma inguinale, lymphogranuloma venereum (LGV), molluscum contagiosum, parasites (pediculosis pubis or scabies), enteric infections, and some vaginal infections (trichomonas) may all be spread through sexual activities. Pertinent information about these less-frequent infections are summarized in Table 26.2.

Chancroid

Chancroid is more common than syphilis in some areas of Africa or Southeast Asia, but uncommon in the United States, with only about 1500 cases per year reported. *Hemophilus ducreyi*, the causative agent of chancroid, is not capable of infecting intact skin, thus the lesions of chancroid tend to be found in areas traumatized by sexual activity. *H. ducreyi* infection typically causes one to three painful "soft chancres" to appear 3 to 10 days after exposure. Although ten times more common in men than in women, these vulvar chancres

Table 26.2. Minor Sexually Transmitted Diseases

Disease	Causative agent	Main symptom	Diagnosis	Treatment
Chancroid	*Hemophilus ducreyi*	Painful, "soft chancres," adenopathy	Clinical, smears, culture	Erythromycin: 500 mg. qid for 10 d
Granuloma inguinale	*Calymmato-bacterium granulomatis*	Raised, red lesions	Clinical, smears	Tetracycline 500 mg. q6h for 3 wk
Lymphogranuloma venereum (LGV)	*Chlamydia trachomatis*	Vesicle, progressing to bubo	Clinical complement fixation test	Tetracycline 500 mg q6h for 3 weeks
Molluscum contagiosum	Molluscum contagiosum (DNA virus)	Raised papule with waxy core	Clinical, inclusion bodies	Desiccation, cryotherapy, curettage
Parasites	Pediculosis pubis, scabies	Itching	Inspection	Lindane 1%
Enteric infections	*Neisseria gonorrhoeae, Chlamydia trachomatis, Shigella sp, Salmonella,* protozoa	Diarrhea	Culture	Based on agent
Vaginitis (sexually transmitted)*	*trichomonas*	Odor, irritation	Microscopic examination of secretions	Metronidazole 500 mg bid for 7 d

*Debate persists about the sexual transmission of bacterial vaginosis.
After: Sexually Transmitted Disease. In: Beckman CRB, Ling FW, Barzansky BM et al. (eds). Obsterics and Gynecology, 2nd ed. Baltimore: Williams & Wilkins, 1995;309.
qid = four times a day; q6h = every 6 hours; bid = twice a day.

break down over about a 2-week period to form shallow, progressive ulcers with red, ragged, undermined edges, with little surrounding inflammation. Material from these ulcers is virulent and can infect other body sites.

In approximately 50% of patients, the unilateral adenopathy caused by chancroid progresses to massive enlargement and inflammation, called "buboes." These may rupture and drain causing extensive soft tissue and skin damage. The diagnosis is established on the basis of clinical findings, gram-negative coccobacillus on smears from the primary lesion, or, rarely, on culture of aspirates of the bubo. Biopsy is also diagnostic, although not often performed. Treatment is with erythromycin (500 mg) four times a day or trimethoprim (160 mg) plus sulfamethoxazole (800 mg) twice a day. Both treatments must continue for no less than 10 days or until the lesions heal. Fluctuant nodes may be drained by aspiration through adjacent normal tissue, but incision and drainage delays healing and should not be attempted.

Granuloma Inguinale

Granuloma inguinale (also called donovanosis) is relatively common in the tropics, New Guinea, and the Caribbean areas, but accounts for fewer than 100 cases per year in the United States. This infection is caused by the bipolar, gram-negative bacterium *Calymma-*

tobacterium granulomatis. With an incubation period of 1 to 12 weeks, this mildly contagious infection first presents with single or multiple subcutaneous papules. These evolve to form raised, red, granulomatous lesions that bleed on contact, undergo ulceration, necrosis, and extremely slow healing. These lesions are confined to the genitalia in 80% of cases. Unlike other ulcer-producing venereal diseases, granuloma inguinale does not produce marked adenopathy. Pseudoadenopathy is noted when granulomatous involvement of subcutaneous tissue mimics bubo formation. Diagnosis is established clinically or through the identification of intracytoplasmic bacteria (Donovan bodies) in mononuclear cells. Treatment consists of tetracycline (500 mg) every 6 hours for a 3-week period. Secondary infection or significant scarring may occur in untreated cases. Because of relapse and late scarring, these patients should be followed carefully for several weeks.

Lymphogranuloma Venereum

Like other minor STDs, lymphogranuloma venereum (LGV) is seen only sporadically in North America and Europe, but is prevalent in other parts of the world. Although 20 times more common in men than in women, LGV can still present both a diagnostic problem and a source of considerable morbidity for those patients with the disease. Clinically, LGV evolves through several stages. The primary lesion is an often overlooked painless vesicle of 2 to 3 mm in size that appears 1 to 4 weeks after inoculation. A mild low-grade fever or malaise is often present. The lesions heal rapidly over the course of several days, leaving no scar. The secondary stage begins about 1 month later and is characterized by bubo formation, which is unilateral in two thirds of cases. In 10% to 20% of patients, the accompanying edema and fibrosis may cause a linear depression parallel to the inguinal ligament, referred to as a "groove sign." In one third of patients, abscess formation, rupture, and fistula formation occur. Chronic progressive lymphangitis with chronic edema and sclerosing fibrosis may occur causing extensive destruction of the vulva. Rectal stenosis may occur as well.

Lymphogranuloma venereum, which is caused by several serotypes of *Chlamydia trachomatis,* can be diagnosed by complement fixation testing. Eighty percent of patients will have a titer of 1:16 or greater. Approximately 20% of patients with LGV will have false-positive Venereal Disease Research Laboratory (VDRL) tests. Biopsy of the lesions is not diagnostic because of the nonspecific damage caused. Clinically, LGV may be mistaken for cancer. Treatment should be begun even before confirmatory tests have returned. Treatment with tetracycline (500 mg) four times a day, for 3 weeks is recommended. Erythromycin or doxycycline may also be substituted.

Molluscum Contagiosum

Molluscum contagiosum is caused by the largest member of the pox virus group. This mildly contagious DNA virus infects epithelial tissues and, after several weeks incubation, causes a round, umbilicated papule, 2 to 5 mm in size. These papules contain a yellow, waxy core of cheesy material. Generally asymptomatic, these lesions may grow slowly for months. The diagnosis may be suggested by the clinical picture and established by finding inclusion bodies in material from the core of the lesion. Treatment is based on obliterating the lesion. This is done by desiccation, cryotherapy, curettage, laser ablation, or chemical cautery ($AgNO_3$). Follow-up should be in 1 month to look for new lesions.

Parasites (Pediculosis Pubis, Scabies)

Phthirus humanus (pubic or crab lice) and *Sarcoptes scabiei* (scabies or itch mite) are parasitic insects that may be transferred through sexual activity or through contact with contaminated clothing or bedding. Infestations occur most frequently in the pubic hair area. Spread to other hairy areas can and does take place. Scabies infections are not confined to hairy areas, but may be found in any area of the body. The bites of these insects produce intense itching. In scabies, this itching is greatest at night. Close inspection of the affected area will generally reveal nits, feces, burrows, or the insects themselves. These organisms are treated with local cleansing and topical applications of lindane 1% (Kwell). Other family members should be treated and the home disinfected at the same time.

Enteric Infections

Once only the province of gay males, sexually transmitted enteric infections now may appear in almost any patient. In patients who engage in anal intercourse, *N. gonorrhoeae, C. trachomatis,* herpes, and syphilis may cause proctitis. Fecal-oral contamination may lead to infection with *Shigella* sp., *Salmonella* sp., or protozoa. Suspicion, anoscopy or proctoscopy, and laboratory evaluations may all be indispensable in establishing the diagnosis.

Vaginitis

Sexual activity is a major route of spread, or precipitating factor, for some forms of vaginitis (notably trichomonas). The coexistence of vaginal infections and other more serious sexually transmitted diseases, dictates that appropriate additional screening should be considered for these patients. A more extensive discussion is found in Chapter 28, Vulvitis and Vaginal Infections.

Pelvic Inflammatory Disease ("PID")

Pelvic inflammatory disease represents the most serious infection in women aged 16 to 25. Eighty-five percent of cases of this ascending infection are associated with sexually active women of menstrual age. The remaining 15% of cases follow instrumentation such as endometrial biopsy, hysterosalpingography, intrauterine contraceptive device (IUCD) placement, or the like. In roughly one third of cases, the causative organism is *N. gonorrhoeae* by itself. One third of cases involve infection with *N. gonorrhoeae* and additional "mixed" infections with other organisms. The other third of infections are due to mixed aerobic and anaerobic bacteria, including respiratory pathogens such as *Haemophilus influenzae, Streptococcus pneumoniae,* and *Streptococcus pyogenes* found in up to 5% of cases. Polymicrobial infections are present in more than 40% of laparoscopically proved cases of salpingitis, with one study reporting an average of 6.8 bacterial types per patient. Chlamydia is involved in roughly 20% of cases, with this rate rising to about 40% among hospitalized patients. Because many of the anaerobic bacteria found in mixed infections mimic those found in the vagina of patients with bacterial vaginosis, bacterial vaginosis is considered a risk factor for the development of pelvic infections. Death from pelivic infections or their complications (for women 15 to 45) is reported to be 0.29 per 100,000.

Although pelvic inflammatory disease is an ascending infection, only about 15% of women with cervical *N. gonorrhoeae* infections develop acute pelvic infections. Evidence

Table 26.3.   Comparative Symptoms of Gonorrhea and Chlamydia Infections

	Gonorrhea	Chlamydia
Onset	Rapid	Slow
Location	General	Mucosa
Inflammatory response	Strong	Mild
Impact	Cytotoxic	Immunologic

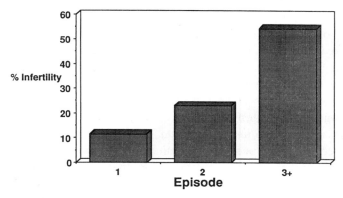

Figure 26.5. Infertility after "PID". (After: Weström L. Am J Obstet Gynecol 1980;138).

suggests that orgasmic uterine contractions or the attachment of *N. gonorrhoeae* to sperm can provide transportation to the upper genital tract. *N. gonorrhoeae* infection of the fallopian tubes, adnexa, or pelvic peritoneum causes complaints of pain and tenderness, development of fever or chills, and elevated white blood count. Peritoneal involvement may spread to include perihepatitis (Fitz-Hugh-Curtis syndrome). Infection of the upper genital tract by *Chlamydia* causes a milder form of salpingitis with more insidious symptoms. Once a chlamydial infection is established, it may remain active for many months, furthering the tubal damage. Characteristics of these two similar, but different, infections are summarized in Table 26.3.

Pelvic inflammatory disease leads to tubal factor infertility, ectopic pregnancy, and chronic abdominal pain in a high percentage of patients. The risk of infertility roughly doubles with each subsequent episode, resulting in a 40% rate of infertility after only three episodes (Fig. 26.5). Women with documented salpingitis have a fourfold increase in their rate of ectopic pregnancy. Prevention of these sequellae is based on prevention of infection (barrier contraception, "safe sex"), screening for those at risk, and aggressive treatment.

ESTABLISHING THE DIAGNOSIS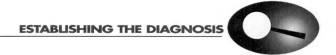

The sexual habits and modes of expression that an individual chooses will affect her risk of infection, as well as the site and presentation by which an infection may manifest itself.

Therefore, a detailed sexual history must be obtained from all patients, and is invaluable for any patient in whom a STD is either likely or suspected. Most sexually transmitted infections require skin-to-skin contact or the exchange of body fluids for transmission. Other activities that meet these criteria may also put the patient at risk.

All patients who are (or might be) sexually active should be examined for the possibility of sexually transmitted disease. This is not a condemnation of lifestyle or personal choices, but rather a simple necessity of good medical care. As noted in Chapter 3, Secrets of the Gynecologic History and Physical Examination, every patient deserves a speedy, gentle, compassionate, and thorough evaluation. When evaluating for the possibility of STD, the inguinal region should be inspected for rashes, lesions, and adenopathy. The vulva should be checked for lesions, ulceration, or abnormal discharge, and palpated for thickening or swelling (Table 26.4). The Bartholin's glands, Skene's ducts, and urethra must be checked. Patients with urinary symptoms should have the urethra gently "milked" to express any discharge. The vagina and cervix must be inspected for lesions and abnormal discharges using a warmed speculum. When STD is suspected or risk is high, cultures for gonorrhea, chlamydia, or other infections should be obtained from the cervix. Lastly, the perineum and perianal areas must also be evaluated for signs of sexually transmitted diseases. Gonorrhea cultures of the rectum should be obtained in those patients who engage in anal intercourse. In addition, the oral cavity, as well as cervical and other lymph nodes, must be evaluated. Clinical findings, combined with suspicion and the patient's history, generally establish the diagnosis. Evaluation of the patient's partner should be encouraged anytime a STD is diagnosed or suspected. Because 20% to 50% of patients with a sexually transmitted disease have more than one coexisting infection, one venereal disease found is suggestive of others.

Bacterial Infections

Chlamydia Trachomatis

The most common sites of chlamydial infection are the cervix and fallopian tubes. Physical findings in chlamydial infections are often subtle and nonspecific. Eversion of the cervix with mucopurulent cervicitis supports the diagnosis but is not pathognomic. Any patient with acute PID, a suspicion of gonorrhea, or trichomonas vaginitis, should also be suspected of having *Chlamydia*.

The diagnosis of *Chlamydia* infection is generally made on clinical suspicion. Cultures on cycloheximide-treated McCoy cells are very specific and may be used to confirm the diagnosis, but these cultures are expensive, difficult to perform, and often not available. Two clinical screening tests have gained popularity: an enzyme-linked immunoassay (ELISA) performed on cervical secretions and a monoclonal antibody test carried out on dried smears. The ELISA technique is easy to do and carries a 97% specificity, but cannot be completed rapidly. The monoclonal technique is faster, but requires precision in making the slide and the use of a fluorescent microscope for interpretation. In low prevalence populations, screening with either technique is associated with unacceptably high false-positive rates, which limits their use. Because of these limitations, final diagnosis is usually lacking and empiric therapy the norm.

Pregnant women who are at high risk (age < 25, multiple sexual partners, new partner within the preceding 3 months, other STDs) should be screened for chlamydial infections

Table 26.4. Genital Lesions in Sexually Transmitted Diseases*

	Herpes	Genital warts	Syphilis	Chancroid	LGV†	Granuloma inguinale
Organism	Herpes simplex virus	Human papilloma virus	Treponema pallidum	Hemophilus ducreyi	Chlamydia trachomatis	Calymmatobacterium granulomatis
Incubation	3–7 d	1–8 mo	10–60 d	2–6 d	1–4 wk	8–12 wk
Primary lesion	**Vesicle**	Papule/polypoid	Papule	Papule/pustule	Papule/pustule vesicle	Papule
Number	**Multiple, coalesce**	Variable	One	One – three	Single	Single or multiple
Pain	**Yes**	No	**Rare**	**Often**	No	**Rare**
Shape	Regular	Irregular	Regular	Irregular	Regular	Regular
Margins	Flat	Raised	Raised	**Red, undermined**	Flat	**Rolled, elevated**
Depth	Superficial	Raised	Superficial	**Excavated**	Superficial	Elevated
Base	Red, smooth	Normal, pink, white	Red, smooth	**Yellow, gray**	Variable	Red, **rough**
Induration	None	None	**Firm**	Rare, soft	None	**Firm**
Secretions	Serous	None	Serous	**Purulent, hemorrhagic**	Variable	Rare, hemorrhagic
Lymph nodes	Firm, tender	**Normal**	Firm, nontender	Tender, suppurative	Tender, suppurative	Pseudoadenopathy
Duration	5–10 d, **recurrent**	Months	Weeks	Weeks	Days	Weeks

Boldfaced items are of particular help in making a differential diagnosis.
*Scabies, Molluscum contagiosum, Candida species, and other dermatologic conditions (e.g., hidradenitis suppurativa) may also cause genital lesions.
†Lymphogranuloma venereum
After: Sexually Transmitted Disease. In Beckman CRB, Ling FW, Barzansky BM, et al. (eds). Obstetrics and Gynecology. 2nd ed. Baltimore: Williams & Wilkins, 1995; 310.

within the preceding 3 months, other STDs) should be screened for chlamydial infections during the third trimester.

Neisseria Gonorrhoeae (Gonorrhea)

The possibility of gonorrheal infections must be considered in virtually any patient who presents for care. In one recent study, up to 30% of adolescents presenting for prenatal care had cervical cultures positive for gonorrhea. Although suspected in any patient with a purlent cervical discharge, the diagnosis of *N. gonorrhoeae* infection is still established by culture on Thayer-Martin agar plates kept in a CO_2-rich environment. Cervical cultures provide 80% to 95% diagnostic sensitivity. Cultures should also be obtained from the urethra and anus, although these additional cultures do not significantly increase the sensitivity of testing.

A gram stain of any cervical discharge for the presence of gram-negative intracellular diplococcus supports the presumptive diagnosis, but does not establish it. This often overlooked test carries fair sensitivity (50% to 70%) but excellent specificity (97%). A solid phase enzyme immunoassay for the detection of *N. gonorrhoeae* antigen is available and may provide a rapid screening test for those at risk. All cases of gonorrhea should have cultures obtained to assess antibiotic susceptibility, although therapy should not be delayed pending the results. Other co-existing sexually transmitted diseases, especially syphilis, *C. trachomatis,* and HIV, should be suspected and tested for at the same time.

Syphilis

Although the diagnosis of syphilis may be made by identifying motile spirochetes on dark-field microscopic examination of material from primary or secondary lesions or from lymph node aspirates, for most patients, the diagnosis will be established on the basis of serologic testing (Table 26.5). The VDRL or Rapid Plasma Reagin (RPR) are good non-specific screening tests because they are rapid and inexpensive. These tests may become unreactive in up to 25% of patients in late-stage syphilis. The fluorescent treponemal antibody absorption (FTA-ABS) or microhemagglutination assay for antibodies to *T. pallidum* (MHA-TP) tests are confirmatory or diagnostic, but are not used for routine screening. These tests are useful to rule out false-positive screening tests caused by such diverse conditions as atypical pneumonia, malaria, or some vaccinations. They are also useful in early infections before antibodies have been elaborated. The sensitivity and specificity of these tests are shown in Table 26.6. When screening tests are positive, a follow-up with a treponemal-specific serologic test is indicated (Fig. 26.6). If neurosyphilis is suspected, a lumbar puncture with a VDRL performed on the spinal fluid is required.

Table 26.5. Commonly Used Serologic Tests for Syphilis

Nontreponemal	
Veneral Disease Research Laboratory	VDRL
Rapid Plasma Reagin (card test)	RPR
Automated Reagin Test	ART
Treponemal	
Fluorescent Treponemal Antibody Absorption Test	FTA–ABS
Microhemagglutination Assay for antibodies to *T. pallidum*	MHA–TP

Table 26.6. Sensitivity and Specificity of Serologic Test for Syphilis

Test	Sensitivity				Specificity
	1 °	2 °	Latent		
			Early	Late	Nonsyphilis
VDRL	78	100	96	71	98
RPR	86	100	98	73	98
FTA–ABS	84	100	100	96	97
MHA–TP	76	100	97	94	99

After: Larsen S, Hunter E, Kraus S, eds. A Manual of Tests for Syphilis. Washington, DC: American Public Health Association, 1990.

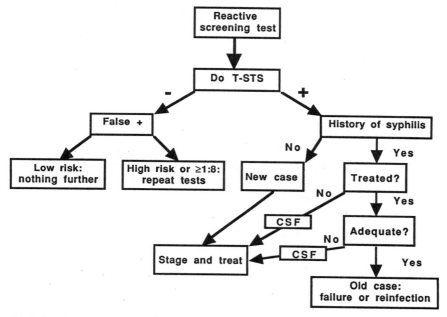

Figure 26.6. Evaluation Strategy for Positive Syphilis Screening Tests.

Viral Infections

Herpes Genitalis

The diagnosis of *Herpes genitalis* is made on the basis of suspicion and clinical findings. Lesions consist of clear vesicles that lyse, progressing to shallow, painful ulcers with a red border. These may coalesce, becoming secondarily infected and necrotic. Lesions may be found on the vulva, vagina, cervix, or perineal and perianal skin, often extending to the buttocks. Recurrences are similar in character, although milder in severity and shorter in duration. The lesions of herpes infections should be easily distinguished by their character and extreme tenderness from the ulcers found in chancroid, syphilis, or granuloma inguinale.

The diagnosis of herpetic infection can be confirmed by viral cultures of material taken by swab from the lesions. This is the most sensitive method of diagnosis and allows confirmation in as little as 48 hours. Scrapings from the base of vesicles may be stained using immunofluorescence techniques to detect the presence of viral particles. Immunofluorescence evaluation is faster than culture techniques and carries approximately 65% to 80% agreement with culture. Smears of vesicular material may also be stained with Wright's stain to visualize giant multinucleated cells with characteristic eosinophilic intranuclear inclusions. Rapid diagnostic kits are available, but current experience suggests that these kits are associated with poor sensitivity and specificity in clinical application and should not be used.

Human Papilloma Virus

Approximately 30% of patients infected by the HPV virus develop soft, fleshy growths (condyloma acuminata) on the vulva, vagina, cervix, urethral meatus, perineum, and anus. They may also be found on the tongue or in the oral cavity. These distinctive lesions may be single or multiple and are generally asymptomatic except for their presence. HPV infections are often accompanied by *Trichomonas* infection or bacterial vaginosis, and these should be screened for in any patient with condyloma. Human papilloma virus is most easily spread by direct skin to skin contact, with autoinoculation resulting in symmetric lesions across the midline.

The diagnosis of condyloma acuminata is made by physical examination, but may be confirmed through biopsy of the warts. Although cytologic changes typical of HPV are often found on Pap smears, Pap smears of the cervix will diagnose only about 5% of patients with the virus. Acetowhite areas can be demonstrated by applying 3% to 5% acetic acid during colposcopy of the cervix, vagina, or vulva. Because the condyloma lata of syphilis may be confused with venereal warts, some care must be taken in making the diagnosis in patients at high risk for both infections. Venereal warts are usually characterized by their narrower base and more heaped-up appearance, although biopsy or serology testing may be required to establish a final diagnosis.

Table 26.7. Baseline Diagnostic Test for HIV-positive Patients

Laboratory
    CD4 and T-cell count and percentage
    Complete blood count, with differential white count
    Electrolytes
    Glucose 6-phosphate dehydrogenase
    Hepatitis B screen
    Liver and renal function tests
    Platelet count
    VDRL or RPR
Other tests
    Cervical culture for gonorrhea and chlamydia
    Pap smear
    Tuberculin skin test with control (*Candida*, mumps, tetanus)

After: American Medical Association Advisory Group on HIV Early Intervention. HIV early intervention. Physician guidelines, 2nd ed. Chicago: American Medical Association, 1994;8.

HIV and AIDS

The diagnosis of HIV is made on the basis of serum screening tests (enzyme immunoassay) and confirmed through repeated testing and the use of Western blot or immunofluorescence assays. Intermediate Western blot results may be obtained owing to incomplete antibody response to HIV in sera or to nonspecific reaction in sera from uninfected persons. Recent infection may not be reflected by these technologies, which require the elaboration of antibodies for detection. False-positive Western blot tests are uncommon and are on the order of less than one in 130,000. Virus culture or polymerase chain reaction testing is reserved for testing in infants in whom maternal antibodies would cloud results.

Once the diagnosis of HIV infections is made, baseline diagnostic testing is essential for the eventual management of these patients. Current recommendations for baseline diagnostic tests for these patients is outlined in Table 26.7.

Current Centers for Disease Control and Prevention guidelines suggest that aggressive screening be offered to all women who are at risk and all women who are pregnant. The latter is especially important even for patients who are perceived as being low risk because recent trials with zidovudine suggest that vertical transmission to the fetus may be reduced by as much as two thirds if early treatment is instituted. As with other sexually transmitted diseases, suspicion is the most important part of establishing the diagnosis.

Pelvic Inflammatory Disease

Establishing the diagnosis of pelvic inflammatory disease is often a difficult clinical challenge. On one hand, we must be aggressive in making this diagnosis and implementing treatment if we are to decrease the likelihood of long-term sequelae, such as infertility and ectopic pregnancy. On the other hand, once the diagnosis of PID is made it tends to follow the patient for the rest of her life. All future abdominal pains will be diagnosed as recurrences or the result of "adhesions," resulting in incorrect diagnosis of other conditions and over-treatment of trivial processes with agents that are not always innocuous. For these reasons, the practitioner must use all the information available to arrive at a working diagnosis.

Traditionally, the diagnosis of PID has been based on the clinical triad of fever, increased erythrocyte sedimentation rate (ESR), and adnexal mass or tenderness. Unfortunately, only about 17% of patients have this triad. There is a high prevalence of confused diagnoses (Table 26.8) and nonspecific symptoms commonly encountered (Fig. 26.7). Even cultures

Table 26.8. Common Conditions Confused with Pelvic Inflammatory Disease

Acute appendicits	25%
Endometriosis	17%
Corpus luteum bleeding	12%
Ectopic pregnancy	11%
Adhesions	7%
"Other"	28%

(After: Jacobson LJ. Differential diagnosis of acute pelvic inflammatory disease. Am J Obstet Gynecol 1980;138:1006.)

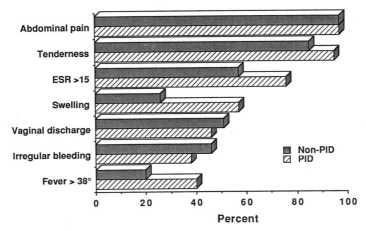

Figure 26.7. Symptom Frequency. ESR = erythrocyte sedimentation rate; Abd Pain = abdominal pain. (After: Jacobson LJ. Am J Obstet Gynecol 1980;138:1006.)

Table 26.9. Diagnostic Criteria for Pelvic Inflammatory Disease

Must have all three
    Tenderness
        Abdominal
        Adnexal
        Cervical
Must have at least one
    Positive gram stain (of cervical secretions)
    Temperature >38° C
    White blood count > 10,000/mL
    Pus on culdocentesis or laparoscopy
    Tubo-ovarian abscess (TOA)

of the cervix are of little help in unequivocally establishing the diagnosis. There is only a 50% correlation between cervical culture and upper tract organisms, and patients with positive cultures for *N. Gonorrhea* have only a 15% attack rate for upper genital tract infection. For these reasons, more specific diagnostic criteria have been established (Table 26.9) and should be rigorously applied.

Patients with pelvic inflammatory disease are usually acutely ill, with fevers of up to 39.5°C, tachycardia, severe bilbateral pelvic and abdominal pain, nausea, and vomiting. These patients may exhibit muscular guarding or rebound tenderness. A purulent cervical discharge is often demonstrated and should be sampled for Gram staining and culture. Palpation of the adnexa generally causes exquisite pain and a mass or fullness may be felt. The differential diagnosis of patients with these symptoms must include septic incomplete abortion, acute appendicitis, diverticular abscess, and adnexal torsion. Confirmation by laparoscopy should be considered for any patient who does not respond in a timely manner or for whom the diagnosis is uncertain.

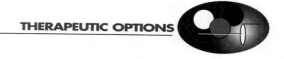

THERAPEUTIC OPTIONS

Bacterial Infections

Chlamydia Trachomatis

In choosing a treatment for patients with *Chlamydia* infections, it is important to consider that 45% of patients with chlamydia have coexisting gonorrhea. Oral doses of tetracycline (500 mg) four times a day for 7 days or doxycycline (100 mg) twice a day for 7 days may be used for most patients. Oral doses of erythromycin base (500 mg) four times a day for 7 days, or erythromycin ethylsuccinate (800 mg four times a day for 7 days) may be substituted for tetracycline in tetracycline-sensitive or pregnant patients. Both treatments carry roughly 95% cure rates. A single 1 gm oral dose of azithromycin also compares favorably with the standard 7-day course of doxycycline, while providing better compliance and fewer side effects.

Pregnant patients with chlamydial infections should be treated with azithromycin, erythromycin base, or erythromycin ethylsuccinate. Quinolones (Ofloxacin), tetracyclines (including doxycycline), and erythromycin estolate are contraindicated in pregnancy and should not be used. For patients who cannot tolerate erythromycin, oral amoxicillin (500 mg) twice a day for 7 to 10 days may be substituted.

Follow-up evaluation for cure with culture or other tests should be carried out, as well as screening for other STDs. (As with all STDs, all sexual partners within the preceding 30 days should be screened and treated for probable infections as well.)

Neisseria Gonorrhoeae (Gonorrhea)

Therapy for patients with suspected or confirmed *N. gonorrhoeae* infections should be based on the site of infection. Initiation of treatment should not be predicated on the results of cultures, but rather on clinical suspicion. Guidelines for treatment are shown in Table 26.10. When patients are treated with the currently recommended ceftriaxone-doxycycline therapy, failure is rare and a follow-up culture is not necessary. Re-examination of the patient in 1 to 2 months for the possibility of reinfection may be warranted in high-risk patients.

Pregnant patients should be treated with a single intramuscular dose of ceftriaxone (250 mg). Oral erythromycin (erythromycin base [500 mg]) four times a day for 7 days may be added to cover the possibility of a coexisting chlamydial infections as noted above. (Tetracycline and the quinolones are contraindicated in pregnancy.) Patients who are sensitive to β-lactam antibiotics can be treated with intramuscular spectinomycin (2 g) once followed by erythromycin. Because of higher failure rates, these patients should have a follow-up culture obtained 3 to 7 days after the completion of therapy.

Any patient exposed to gonorrhea within the preceding month should be cultured and treated presumptively.

Syphilis

The treatment of choice for syphilis remains benzathine penicillin G as outlined in Table 26.10. Patients who are allergic to penicillin can be treated with doxycycline, but oral therapy is associated with a greater risk of failure owing to noncompliance. The patient should

Table 26.10.   Gonorrhea and Syphilis Therapy

	Preferred treatment	Alternative treatment
Gonorrhea: mucosal (all sites)	Ceftriaxone 250 mg IM + (either doxycycline 100 IM bid × 7 days **or** tetracycline 500 mg po qid × 7d) **or** ceftriaxone 250 mg IM + azithromycin 1.0 g po	Doxycycline 100 IM bid + (Spectinomycin 2 gm IM **or** ciprofloxacin 500 gm po **or** cefotaxime 1 gm IV **or** cefixime 400 mg po **or** ofloxacin 400 mg po **or** ampicillin/sulbactam 1.5 gm IM + probenecid 1 g po)
Arthritis	Crystalline penicillin G 12–16 MU/d IV until improved, then ampicillin 500 mg po qid to 7–10 d total, **or** ampicillin 3.5 g, **or** amoxicillin 3 g, + probenecid 1 g po + ampicillin 500 mg po qid × 10–14 d	Cefoxitin, 2 g IV q8h until improved, then tetracycline 500 mg po qid to 7–10 d total
Penicillinase +	Spectinomycin, 2g IM	Cefoxitin 2g IM + probenecid 1g po
Syphilis 1°/2°	Benzathine penicillin G, 2.4 MU IM **or** aqueous procaine penicillin G 600,000 U IM every other day × 8 d	Tetracycline 500 mg po qid × 15 d Erythromycin 500 mg po qid × 15 d in pregnant patients
Cardiovascular/ latent	Benzathine penicillin G, 2.4 MU IM weekly × 3 wk **or** aqueous procaine penicillin G 600,000 U IM every other day × 15 d	Tetracycline 500 mg po qid × 30 d Erythromycin 500 mg po qid × 15 d in pregnant patients
Neurosyphilis	Crystalline penicillin G 3–4 MU IM q4h for at least 10 d	Penicillin G procaine 2–4 MU IM daily + probenecid, 500 mg po qid × 10–14 d

be followed by quantitative VDRL titers and examinations at 3, 6, and 12 months after treatment. A fourfold decline at 6 months or an eightfold decrease by 12 months should be anticipated if cure has been accomplished. Evaluation for the possibility of other STDs is always appropriate.

Pregnant patients should be treated with penicillin. Tetracycline is contraindicated in pregnancy and treatment with erythromycin does not give adequate therapy for the fetus. Therefore, patients who are allergic to penicillin should be admitted to the hospital for penicillin desensitization and therapy.

Viral Infections

Herpes Genitalis

The management of genital herpes infections is directed toward the local lesions and the patient's symptoms. In initial infections, the affected area should be kept clean and dry. Sitz baths, followed by drying with a heat lamp or hair dryer, work well for this purpose. A topical anesthetic (2% xylocaine jelly) may be required if symptoms are severe. If secondary infections occur, therapy with a local antibacterial cream (e.g., neosporin) is appropriate. Acyclovir ointment (5%, applied locally every 3 h, begun within 48 h of onset) will decrease the duration of symptoms and viral shedding, but this therapy has not been shown to decrease the likelihood of recurrence and the shortened symptom duration is often minimal. For patients who have frequent recurrences, oral acyclovir (200 mg) twice a day increased to five times per day (with lesions) is effective in decreasing both frequency and severity of flare-ups, but should be limited to less than 6 months of use.

Vaginal delivery is associated with roughly a 50% chance of fetal infection when active herpes lesions are present. In infants, this infection is associated with significant morbidity and an almost 80% mortality rate. Therefore, patients with active herpes infections should be considered for cesarean section delivery. When there has been prolonged rupture of the amniotic membranes infection may have already taken place, blunting the value of cesarean delivery.

Human Papilloma Virus

The treatment of small, uncomplicated venereal warts is generally by cytolytic topical agents, such as podophyllin (podophyllum resin), bichloracetic or trichloroacetic acid (TCA), or physical ablative methods such as laser, cryotherapy, or electrodesiccation. Podophyllin acts to poison the miotic spindle of dividing cells and also produces local vasospasm resulting in limited ischemia. This is carefully applied to the warts, protecting the adjacent skin, and allowed to remain for between 30 minutes and 4 hours before being washed off the lesions. Treatment can be repeated every 7 to 10 days as needed. Podophyllin may not be used during pregnancy owing to absorption, potentially resulting in neural or myelotoxicity. Success is generally in the range of 75% resolution of overt warts, with a recurrence rate of 65% to 80%. If lesions persist or continually recur, cryosurgery, electrodesiccation, surgical excision, or laser vaporization may be required.

Trichloroacetic acid (85% solution) acts by precipitating surface proteins and must be applied carefully to avoid injury to adjacent tissues. Treatment with TCA produces a white slough that peels off in several days. If necessary, therapy can be repeated every 2 to 3 weeks.

Treatment with 5-fluorouracil (5-FU) 1% or 5% cream is often used as primary therapy or as an adjunct for cervical or vaginal lesions. 5-FU is a pyrimidine antimetabolite that causes necrosis and slough of the rapidly growing tissue found in condyloma. Response is generally better with lesions on nonkeratinized surfaces such as the cervix or vagina. The 5-FU cream is generally applied daily until edema, erythema, or vesiculation occurs, which generally takes place after 7 to 10 days of treatment. Because this results in significant discomfort, many have advocated weekly applications of 5-FU repeated over the course of 10 to 12 weeks. Control rates of approximately 80% can be anticipated, but care should be taken to watch for the possibility of ulcer formation in vaginal tissues during or after therapy.

Physical ablative therapy with laser excision or ablation, cryotherapy, or electrodesiccation can also be used to treat condyloma. If cryotherapy is chosen, three to six treatments are often required, but cure rates are higher than for podophyllin and comparable to laser ablation (60% to 80%). Even with laser ablation, recurrence rates are reported to vary from 25% to 100%.

Therapy with autologous vaccine, dinitrochlorobenzene, and interferon have been advocated but have yet to gain a significant place in clinical practice.

Lesions are more resistant to therapy during pregnancy, in diabetic patients, or in those who are immunosuppressed. Some patients with extensive vaginal or vulvar lesions may require delivery via cesarean section to avoid extensive lacerations and suturing problems in the presence of these lesions. Cesarean delivery decreases the possibility of transmission to the infant and subsequent development of laryngeal papillomata.

Any patient with a history of condyloma should have at least yearly cytologic evaluations of the cervix. The sexual partners of patients with HPV should also be screened for genital warts. Currently, no therapy is indicated for patients with subclinical HPV infections

HIV and AIDS

The results of long-term therapy for HIV infection or AIDS are not available and the development of improved treatment options is incomplete. Therapy with antimetabolites such as zidovudine (Retrovir) have been successful in delaying the progress of the HIV infections for some patients. The treatment of both HIV infection and AIDS is continually evolving, the details of which lay beyond the scope of this discussion. However, it is well within the purview of all practitioners to encourage practices that reduce the risk of acquiring this infection. This should include consistent use of condoms, substance abuse prevention and treatment programs, and counseling programs. For the foreseeable future, prevention is the only meaningful therapeutic intervention available.

Pelvic Inflammatory Disease

Because pelvic inflammatory diease is often polymicrobial, therapy must be aggressive and broad spectrum. Patients with mild disease can be treated as outpatients; however, many patients with pelvic inflammatory disease require hospitalization for adequate care (Table 26.11). Severe cases or patients with one or more prior episodes of PID require careful monitoring because tubo-ovarian abscess formation is likely. These patients require aggres-

Table 26.11. Factors Suggesting Hospitalization for Patients with Pelvic Inflammatory Disease

Differential diagnosis including ectopic pregnancy or appendicitis
HIV-infected patients
Immunosuppressed patients
Intrauterine contraceptive device use
Nulliparity
Paralytic ileus
Peritonitis or toxicity
Pregnancy
Previous treatment failure
Significant gastrointestinal symptoms
Significant morbidity
Temperature >39°C
Tubo-ovarian abscess
Uncertain or complicated differential diagnosis
Unreliable patient
White blood count >20,000 or <4,000

sive intravenous antibiotic therapy and may need surgical drainage. For some, hysterectomy may be required. Rupture of a tubo-ovarian abscess, with subsequent septic shock, may be life threatening.

Ambulatory patients can be treated with either intramuscular cefoxitin (2 g) plus oral probenecid (1 g) combined with a 14-day course of doxycycline (100 mg) twice a day, or a combination of intramuscular ceftriaxone (250 mg) plus the 14-day course of doxycycline. These regimens provide good coverage for gonocorrhea and chlamydia but do not give good coverage for anaerobic infections. An alternative regimen using oral ofloxacin (400 mg) twice a day for 14 days, combined with either oral clindamycin (450 mg) four times a day or oral metronidazole (500 mg) twice a day has also been proposed. Augmentin (500 mg) twice a day for 10 days may also be used with similar results.

For hospitalized patients, the combination of intravenous cefoxitin (2 g) every 6 hours or intravenous cefotetan (2 g) every 12 hours with doxycycline (100 mg) every 12 hours (orally or IV) is recommended. For mixed infections, intravenous clindamycin (900 mg) every 8 hours plus an aminoglycoside such as gentamycin (2 mg/Kg loading doses, followed by 1.5 mg/Kg every 8 hours) will give better coverage. Excellent results have been reported with the combination of clindamycin and aztreonam (2 g) given intramuscularly every 8 hours; this combination may supplant cefoxitin or cefotetan combinations as more experience accumulates. Piperacillin (4 g) combined with tazobactam (500 mg) given every 8 hours by the intravenous route may also be used, but has given cure rates of only 90% (with an additional 5% improved). Following discharge from the hospital, the patient should be maintained on oral doxycycline (100 mg) twice a day or clindamycin (450 mg) four times a day for 14 days.

It should be noted that strains of *N. gonorrhoeae* that cause PID are relatively more resistant to penicillin than those that cause disseminated or lower genital tract (cervical) infections.

As with most sexually transmitted disease, the partners of patients with pelvic inflammatory disease should be screened for gonococcal or chlamydial infections and treated accordingly.

HINTS AND COMMON QUESTIONS

The trading of sex for drugs has been responsible, in part, for the resurgence of sexually transmitted diseases in recent years. For this reason, the possibility of associated problems such as drug abuse, alcoholism, sexual exploitation or abuse, and others should be strongly considered and evaluated in any patient with a STD.

Because pelvic inflammatory disease is an ascending infection, new cases are unlikely in patients who have undergone a tubal sterilization procedure. A recurrence of old disease or a pelvic infection of nongynecologic origin is possible, but far less likely.

Persistent vaginal spotting while on oral contraceptives or following an elective termination of pregnancy may indicate endometritis, placing the patient at increased risk of salpingitis or pelvic infection. Empiric treatment with antibiotics may be justified in those at high risk, or the diagnosis may be confirmed by office endometrial biopsy.

When trying to obtain cervical cultures for *Chlamydia*, plastic- or metal-shafted rayon-

or cotton-tipped swabs are preferred. Wood-shafted or calcium alginate swabs reduce the yield of material when transport media is used owing to leeching of toxic products into the media.

To reduce the discomfort of intermuscular ceftriaxone treatment, 1% lidocaine (without epinephrine) may be used as the diluent.

Pregnant patients who are treated for gonococcal infections during pregnancy should be presumed to have chlamydial infections and be treated empirically.

If spectinomycin or a quinolone antibiotic (ciprofloxacin or norfloxacin) are used to treat gonococcal infections, adequate coverage for possible coexistent early syphilis is not provided. These patients should have a serologic test for syphilis rechecked at 1 month after therapy.

Tetracycline may be substituted for doxycycline in most treatment regimens, but compliance may less because of the need to take tetracycline between meals and a greater incidence of stomach upset. Cost savings are generally minimal.

To limit toxicity with podophyllin, treatments should be limited to less than 0.5 mL total volume and less than 10 cm^2 in area.

To protect areas adjacent to condyloma that are being treated with trichloroacetic acid, the skin may be dusted with talc or sodium bicarbonate powder to neutralized the acid. Petrolatum also protects the tissues, but is messier.

Herpetic vulvitis and the inflammatory response associated with the treatment of condyloma acuminata often produce intense discomfort. Sitz-baths or cool compresses with aluminum acetate (Burrow's solution) may be helpful. The area should be thoroughly dried after the soaks, which may be done with a hair dryer set on cool. Care must be taken to avoid autoinoculation through contact with open lesions or the solutions used in the soaks.

SUGGESTED READINGS

General References

American College of Obstetricians and Gynecologists. Genital human papillomavirus infections. ACOG Technical Bulletin 193. Washington, DC: ACOG, 1994.

Centers for Disease Control and Prevention. 1993 sexually transmitted diseases treatment guidelines. MMWR 1993;42:1.

Centers for Disease Control and Prevention. Sexually transmitted diseases: treatment guidelines. MMWR 1989;38:31.

Centers for Disease Control and Prevention. Sexually transmitted disease surveillance, 1992. Atlanta: Division of STD/HIV Prevention, 1993:10.

Centers for Disease Control and Prevention. Update: barrier protection against HIV infection and other sexually transmitted diseases. MMWR 1993;42:589.

Dodson MG. Antibiotic regimens for treating acute pelvic inflammatory disease. An evaluation. J Reprod Med 1994;39:285.

Droegemueller WR. Infections of the upper genital tract. In Herbst AL, Mishell DR, Stenchever MA, Droegemueller WR (eds). Comprehensive Gynecology, 2nd ed. St Louis: CV Mosby, 1992;691.

Fiumara NJ. Treatment of primary and secondary syphilis: serological response. JAMA 1980;243:2500.

Landers DV, Sweet RL. Sexually transmitted infection. In Glass RH (ed). Office Gynecology. Baltimore: Williams & Wilkins, 1993;1.

Larsen S, Hunter E, Kraus S, eds. A Manual of Tests for Syphilis. Washington, DC: American Public Health Association, 1990.

Jacobson LJ. Differntial diagnosis of acute pelvic inflammatory disease. Am J Obstet Gynecol 1980;138:1006.

Marx R, Aral SO, Rolfs RT, Sterk CE, Kahn JG. Crack, sex, and STD. Sex Transm Dis 1991;18:92.

Sexually transmitted disease. In Beckman CRB, Ling FW, Barzansky BM, et al. (eds). Obstetrics and Gynecology, 2nd ed. Baltimore: Williams & Wilkins, 1995;299.

Specific References

Bacterial Diseases

Berry MC, Dajani AS. Resurgence of congenital syphilis. Infect Dis Clin North Am 1992;6:19.

Centers for Disease Control and Surveillance. Antibiotic-resistant strains of *Neisseria gonorrhoeae:* policy guidelines for detection, management, and control. MMWR 1987;36(suppl 5):1s.

Centers for Disease Control and Surveillance. Recommendations for the prevention and management of Chlamydia trachomatic infections, 1993. MMWR 1993;42(RR-12):1.

Centers for Disease Control and Surveillance. Decreased susceptibility of *Neisseria gonorrhoeae* to Fluoroquinolones—Ohio and Hawaii, 1992–1994. MMWR 1994;43:325.

Crombleholme W, Landers D, Ohm-Smith M, et al. Sulbactam/ampicillin versus metronidazole/gentamicin in the treatment of severe pelvic infections. Drugs 1986;31(suppl 2):11.

Dodson MG. Antibiotic regimens for treating acute pelvic inflammatory disease: an evaluation. J Reprod Med 1994;39:285.

Dodson MG, Faro S, Gentry LO. Treatment of acute pelvic inflammatory disease with aztreonam, a new monocyclic β-lactam antibiotic, and clindamycin. Obstet Gynecol 1986;67:657.

El-Zaatari MM, Martens MG, Anderson GD. Incidence of the prozone phenomenon in syphilis serology. Obstet Gynecol 1994;84:609.

Hammerschlag MR, Golden NH, Oh MK, et al. Single dose of azithromycin for the treatment of genital chlamydial infections in adolescents. J Pediatr 1993;122:961.

Martin DH, Mroczkowski TF, Dalu ZA, et al. A controlled trial of a single dose of azithromycin for the treatment of chlamydial urethritis and cervicitis: The Azithromycin for Chlamydial Infections Study Group. N Engl J Med 1992;327:921.

Matson SC, Pomeranz AJ, Kamps KA. Early detection and treatment of sexually transmitted disease in pregnant adolescents of low socioeconomic status. Clin Pediatr (Phila) 1993;32:609.

Pastorek JG II, Cole C, Aldridge KE, et al. Aztreonam plus clindamycin as therapy for pelvic infections in women. Am J Med 1985;78 (suppl 2A):47.

Pearlman MD, McNeeley SG. A review of the microbiology, immunology and clinical implications of Chlamydia trachomatis infections. Obstet Gynecol Surv 1992;47:448.

Phillips RS, Hanff PA, Wertheimer A, Aronson MD. Gonorrhea in women seen for routine gynecologic care: Criteria for testing. Am J Med 1988;85:177.

Romanowski B, Sutherland R, Fick GH, Mooney D, Love EJ. Serologic response to treatment of infectious syphilis. Ann Intern Med 1991;114:1005.

Sweet RL, Roy S, Faro S, et al. Piperacillin and taxobactam versus clindamycin and gentamicin in the treatment of hospitalized women with pelvic infection. Obstet Gynecol 1994;83:280.

Tapp A, Wise B, Cardozo L. Efficacy and safety of piperacillin/tazobactam in gynecologic infections. J Antimicrob Chemother 1993; (suppl B):61.

Washington AE, Cates W, Zaidi AA. Hospitalization for pelvic inflammatory disease. JAMA 1984;25:2529.

Viral Diseases

American Medical Association Advisory Group on HIV Early Intervention. HIV early intervention. Physician Guidelines, 2nd ed. Chicago: American Medical Association, 1994;8.

Bauer HM, Ting Y, Greer CE, Chambers JC, et al. Genital human papillomavirus infection in female university students as determined by a PCR-based method. JAMA 1991;265:472.

Centers for Disease Control and Surveillance. Update: AIDS amoung women—United States, 1994. MMWR 1994;44:881.

Douglas GC, King BF. Maternal-fetal transmission of human immunodeficiency virus: a review of possible routes and cellular mechanism of infection. Clin Infect Dis 1992;15:678.

Gibbs RS Amstey MS, Sweet RL, Mead PB, Sever JL. Management of genital herpes infection in pregnancy. Obstet Gynecol 1988;71:779.

Jha PK, Beral V, Peto J, et al. Antibodies to human papillomavirus and to other genital infectious agents and invasive cervical cancer risk. Lancet 1993;341:1116.

Koutsky LA, Stevens CE, Holmes KK, et al. Underdiagnosis of genital herpes by current clinical and viral-isolation procedures. N Engl J Med 1992;326:1533.

National Institute of Allergy and Infectious Diseases. Clinical alert: important therapeutic information on the benefit of zidovudine (AZT) for the prevention of the transmission of HIV from mother to infant. Bethesda, Maryland: NIAID, 1994.

Selwyn PA, Schoenbaum EE, Davenny K, et al. Prospective study of human immunodeficiency virus infection and pregnancy outcomes in intravenous drug users. JAMA 1989;261:1289.

Waller SC. A meta-analysis of condom effectiveness in reducing sexually transmitted HIV. Soc Sci Med 1993;36:1635.

27

Urinary Infection, Incontinence, Pelvic Relaxation

Urinary tract function is an integral part of health care for women. Chief among the urinary concerns found in the primary care setting are infections, urinary incontinence, and the effects of the loss of pelvic organ support. Each of these is common, and many aspects of these fall well within the purview of the primary care provider. For example, urinary tract infections are roughly ten times more common for women than for men. The prevalence of bacteriuria in women has been reported as 3% to 8%, with roughly 45% of women aged 15 to 60 experiencing at least one urinary tract infection. Some authors report that up to 75% of women develop an acute urinary tract infection each year.

As more and more patients move into their later years, more women will experience pelvic relaxation and its attendant problems. Although not exclusively the province of the older patient, pelvic relaxation becomes more common as tissues become less resilient and the accumulated stresses of life take their toll. Age, vaginal childbirth, and the effects of lifting, straining, chronic coughs, and the stresses of everyday life may result in the loss of pelvic organ support. Pelvic pressure and pain, dyspareunia, urinary incontinence, and problems passing stools may all result from a loss of pelvic support. Almost half of all women will have involuntary loss of a few drops of urine at some time in their lifetime, with 10% to 15% of women suffering significant, recurrent loss. It has been estimated that more than 25% of women of reproductive age suffer from some degree of urinary incontinence. This number increases to 30% to 40% of women after the age of menopause.

The high prevalence of urinary infections, incontinence, and loss of pelvic support necessitates a familiarity with the diagnosis and treatment of these disorders. Although pelvic relaxation, infection, or other urinary tract disorders are often symptomatic, patients are frequently reluctant to voice these complaints. The health care provider must be sensitive to these complaints as well as to the physical findings that suggest a problem or warrant further exploration.

BACKGROUND AND SCIENCE

Infection

Urinary tract infections can be broadly classified as urethritis, cystitis (including trigonitis), and pyelonephritis based on the involved portion of the urinary tract infected. In 95% of those affected, the urinary tract infections are symptomatic, uncomplicated, affect only the bladder or urethra (do not ascend to the kidneys), and produce no permanent damage. Coliform organisms, especially *Escherichia coli,* are the most common organisms responsible for asymptomatic bacteriuria, cystitis, and pyelonephritis. Ninety percent of first infections and 80% of recurrent infections are caused by *E. coli,* with between 10% and 20% due to *Staphylococcus saprophyticus.* Infection with other pathogens such as *Klebsiella* species (5%) and *Proteus* species (2%) account for most of the remaining infections. Anaerobic bacteria, *Trichomonas,* and yeasts are rare sources of infections except in diabetics, immunosuppressed patients, or those requiring chronic catheterization.

The relatively short female urethra, and exposure of the external meatus to vestibular and rectal pathogens, increase the risk of infection for women. Most urinary tract infections in women ascend from contamination of the urethra, acquired via instrumentation, trauma, or sexual intercourse. Except for the rare exception of tuberculosis infection or infections in immunosuppressed patients, urinary tract infections are rarely acquired by hematogenous or lymphatic spread. Once bacterial seeding of the lower urinary tract occurs, infection may or may not follow. Infection is most likely with more virulent pathogens, altered host defenses, and factors such as infrequent or incomplete voiding, foreign body or stone, obstruction, or biochemical changes in the urine (diabetes, pregnancy, hemoglobinopathies). Estrogen deficiency causes a decrease in urethral infection resistance that contributes to ascending contamination in menopausal women who are not receiving hormone replacement therapy. This altered resistance accounts for the almost 10% prevalence of asymptomatic bacteriuria found in these women.

Intercourse and some contraceptive methods may increase the risk of infection for women. More frequent or especially vigorous coitus may lead to trauma or to urethral massage, propelling pathogens into the upper urethra and bladder. A history of intercourse within the preceding 24 to 48 hours is present in up to 75% of cases of acute urinary tract infection. The use of diaphragm or vaginal spermicides has been implicated as a risk factor for infection. In the case of the diaphragm, partial obstruction of the urethra or urethral trauma induced by the rim of the diaphragm has been postulated as possible mechanisms for this increased risk. Spermicides alter both vaginal pH and normal bacterial flora, potentially increasing the risk of infection.

Asymptomatic bacteriuria is common among older women. Estimates for the prevalence of asymptomatic bacteriuria range from 3% to 50% for women over the age of 65, and 20% to 50% or more for women over the age of 80. Ambulatory, nonhospitalized patients require no treatment because the condition is usually transient. Debilitated or hospitalized patients or those about to undergo genitourinary surgery do require treatment of asymptomatic bacteriuria because of the possibility of bacterial dissemination.

Patients with chronic indwelling urinary catheters have an extremely high incidence of bacteriuria. As with asymptomatic bacteriuria, no treatment is required unless symptoms are present.

Two conditions thought to arise from antecedent urinary tract infections deserve mention: urethral syndrome and interstitial cystitis. Urethral syndrome is a chronic condition characterized by urinary urgency, daytime frequency, a sense of incomplete voiding, variable dysuria, suprapubic fullness, pelvic pain, or dyspareunia. Despite the similarity to cystitis or urethritis, urine cultures are consistently negative, and these patients often have a history of multiple treatments for infection without success. The cause of urethral syndrome is unclear, but infection, trauma, hypoestrogenism, and psychogenic factors have all been postulated. Urethral syndrome must be differentiated from intrinsic bladder pathology such as bladder tumors.

Interstitial cystitis is a progressive, debilitating chronic inflammatory condition affecting the bladder wall that causes severe suprapubic pain with bladder filling, dramatic reduction in bladder capacity, urgency, and frequency. Although interstitial cystitis is ten times more common in women than in men, it is estimated that this condition affects only about 1 of 350 to 415 women. As with urethral syndrome, no specific cause for interstitial cystitis is known, although infection, and allergic, autoimmune, neurologic, and biochemical causes have been proposed.

Pelvic Relaxation

The female pelvic organs are supported by a complex system of muscles, fascias, and ligaments which include the levator muscles, the urogenital diaphragm, endopelvic fascia, and the uterosacral and cardinal ligaments (see Chapter 1, Pelvic Anatomy and Embryology). These structures can lose their ability to provide support through birth trauma, chronic intra-abdominal pressure elevation (such as obesity, chronic cough, or heavy lifting), intrinsic tissue weakness, or atrophic changes due to estrogen loss. Loss of support for the anterior vagina, through rupture or attenuation of the pubovesical cervical fascia, is manifest by descent or prolapse of the urethra (urethrocele), bladder (cystocele), or rectum (rectocele). These are illustrated in Figure 27.1. Cystoceles, urethroceles, or their combination (cystourethrocele) are classically found in patients with true stress incontinence. When these defects are exaggerated, paradoxic continence or even urinary retention may occur. Compromise of ureteral drainage may be found in cases of significant downward displacement of the trigone.

Herniation at the top of the vagina (enterocele) and prolapse of the vagina itself can occur in patients who have had a hysterectomy. Loss of uterine support can lead to descent or prolapse of the uterus. Although pelvic relaxation can affect any of the pelvic structures individually, multiple involvement is most common.

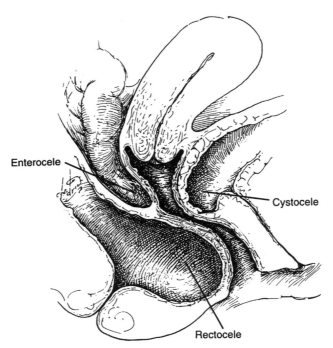

Enterocele

Cystocele

Rectocele

Figure 27.1. Relaxation of pelvic support. (From Beckmann RB, Ling FW, Barzansky BM, et al. Obstetrics and gynecology. 2nd ed. Baltimore: Williams & Wilkins, 1995:334.)

Incontinence

"Urinary incontinence" may be a sign, a symptom, or a condition. It is defined as a condition in which involuntary loss of urine may be objectively demonstrated and such loss presents a social or hygienic problem. The volume of the loss in not as important as the impact it has on the patient and her life.

Incontinence can be classified into three types: 1. Stress incontinence, which involves the immediate loss of small spurts of urine in response to increases in intra-abdominal pressure, as with a cough or sneeze (also called genuine stress incontinence). 2. Urgency incontinence, caused by sensory or motor abnormalities, which result in large volume urinary loss associated with an intense, uncontrolled urge to void, or unanticipated bladder emptying that may occur with provocations, such as a change of position or the sound of running water. 3. Overflow incontinence may occur when the bladder becomes massively over distended and unable to empty, yielding a constant dribble of uncontrollable urinary leakage. Anomalies of the urinary tract, such as fistulae, may also result in continuous urine loss (sometimes referred to as by-pass loss).

A careful history that notes the associated symptoms and events, amount and duration of urine loss, and the position in which urine losses occur is important to establishing the correct diagnosis. Often these characteristics of the patient's complaint suggest a diagnosis (Table 27.1).

Table 27.1. Characteristics of Urinary Incontinence

	Stress	Urge	Overflow/fistula
Associated symptoms	None (occasional pelvic pressure or heaviness)	Urgency, frequency, nocturia	None, fullness, pressure frequency, incomplete emptying
Amount of loss	Small, drops, spurt	Large, complete bladder emptying	Small, dribbling
Duration of loss (episode)	Brief, corresponds to stress	Moderate, several seconds	Often continuous
Ability to inhibit loss	Minimal	None	None
Associated event	Cough, laugh, sneeze, physical activity	None, change in position, running water	None
Position	Upright, sitting; rare supine or asleep	Any	Any
Cause	Structural (cystocele, urethrocele)	Loss of bladder inhibition, increased bladder sensitivity, bladder irritability	Obstruction, loss of neurologic control, fistulae

Genuine Stress Incontinence

Urine passes from the body anytime the pressure inside the bladder exceeds the pressure in the urethra. This is the physiologic mechanism of voluntary voiding, when urethral relaxation and bladder contraction occur. Involuntary urinary loss can take place when there is unequal transmission of intra-abdominal pressure to the bladder and urethra. Stress incontinence is a passive loss and, therefore, notable for urine loss in the absence of bladder muscle contraction. This may happen with the loss of pelvic support and, as a result, stress incontinence is a common complaint of patients with a cystocele or urethrocele.

Incontinence does not occur in all patients with poor anterior vaginal wall support, and the degree of incontinence is often not correlated with the scale of pelvic relaxation. Indeed, paradoxic return of continence or even urinary retention, may occur when a significant cystocele produces acute flexion of the vesicourethral junction. Despite the beguiling simplicity of a history of urine loss with a cough or sneeze, history alone is only 75% accurate in establishing the diagnosis. Additional history, careful physical examination, and often more extensive urodynamic testing are required to establish the diagnosis.

Urgency Incontinence and Retention

Loss of normal enervation and control of bladder function may result in involuntary bladder contraction or bladder atony, leading to urgency and overflow incontinence, respectively. Urgency incontinence occurs in approximately 35% of patients with incontinence. For most of these patients, no specific cause is found for their bladder irritability and they are referred to as having "idiopathic detrusor instability." Neurologic disease must be considered as a possible cause, with multiple sclerosis a major concern for younger patients. Trauma, spinal cord tumors, radical pelvic surgery, stroke, radiation therapy, chronic irrita-

Table 27.2.   Potential Causes of Urgency Incontinence

Allergy
Bladder stone
Bladder tumor
Caffeinism
Central nervous system tumors
Detrusor muscle instability
Interstitial cystitis
Multiple sclerosis
Parkinson's disease
Radiation cystitis
Radical pelvic surgery
Spinal cord injury
Urinary tract infections (acute or chronic)

tion, and the effects of diabetes may also affect bladder sensation and motor control. A partial list of causes of urgency incontinence is shown in Table 27.2.

Patients with detrusor instability, from whatever cause, tend to have reduced bladder capacity and early, intense sensations of bladder fullness. Spontaneous and uninhibitable contractions of the bladder muscles occur, resulting in large volume, uncontrolled urine loss. These contractions, and their accompanying urinary loss, may occur with normal bladder filling or with minimal provocation, such as a change in position, the sounds of water running, or sudden change in intra-abdominal pressure. This occasional association with a sudden change in intra-abdominal pressure often leads to confusion with true stress urine loss. Patients with urgency-type loss will note the loss of large volumes (to the point of bladder emptying) that shortly follow the cough or sneeze. In contrast, patients with stress incontinence have small volume loss that exactly matches the rise and fall of intra-abdominal pressure.

Patients with loss of bladder motor control, or those with outlet obstruction, develop a distended, atonic bladder that may result in episodic overflow of urine. This loss may appear or be exacerbated by intra-abdominal pressure change, mimicking stress incontinence. This condition is referred to as a "neurogenic bladder." Patients in whom a neurogenic bladder is suspected require a thorough neurologic evaluation. Pharmacologic therapy for these patients is often unsatisfactory and many require long-term catheter drainage or intermittent self-catheterization to manage their problem.

Acute urinary retention and bladder distention may follow surgery, epidural or general anesthesia, trauma, or herpetic vulvitis. Rarely, these conditions occur with pelvic masses, marked prolapse of the bladder, or with retroversion of the uterus (causing pressure on the base of the bladder). Acute urinary retention requires prompt and continuous drainage for 24 to 48 hours.

Fistulae

Continuous incontinence will occur when the normal continence mechanism is bypassed, as with fistulae from the vagina to the bladder (vesicovaginal), urethra (urethrovaginal), or the ureter (ureterovaginal). Rarely, communication between the bladder and the uterus (vesicouterine) may also occur through the same mechanisms. Common fistulae are shown in Figure 27.2. Multiple fistulae are present in up to 15% of patients.

Fistulae may result from surgical or obstetric trauma, irradiation, or malignancy, although the most common cause by far is unrecognized surgical trauma. Roughly 75% of fistulae occur after abdominal hysterectomy. Although it is estimated that urinary tract injury occurs in about 8000 of the estimated 700,000 hysterectomies performed each year in the United States, fistulae occur in only about 0.05% of all hysterectomies. Surgical exposure and operator experience appear to be the most significant factors leading to fistulae (only one third of cases occur in procedures performed by gynecologists) rather than the type or degree of disease that prompts the procedure. Signs of a urinary fistula (watery discharge) usually occur from 5 to 30 days after surgery, although they may be present in the immediate postoperative period.

Fistulae between the gastrointestinal tract and vagina may be precipitated by the same injuries that cause genitourinary fistulae. Foul vaginal discharge, with marked vaginal and vulvar irritation, fecal incontinence and soiling, along with the passage of fecal matter or gas from the vagina, are pathognomonic.

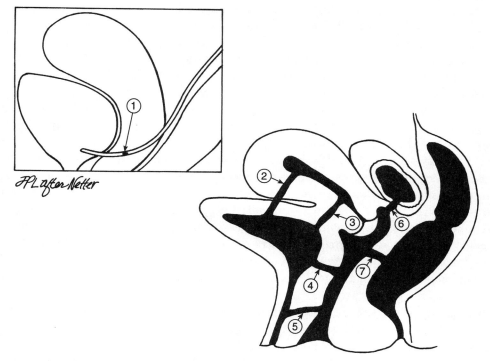

Figure 27.2. Types of genitourinary tract fistulae. 1, Ureterovaginal; 2, Vesicouterovaginal; 3, Vesicocervicovaginal; 4, Vesicovaginal; 5, Urethrovaginal; 6, Enterovaginal; 7, Rectovaginal. (From Beckmann RB, Ling FW, Barzansky BM, et al. Obstetrics and gynecology. 2nd ed. Baltimore: Williams & Wilkins, 1995:337.)

Symptoms of frequency, urgency, nocturia, or dysuria should suggest a urinary tract infection. The symptoms experienced by the individual patient varies with the site of the infection. Irritation of the urethra gives rise to symptoms of dysuria, but frequency and urgency are generally absent. When the bladder wall or trigone is irritated, frequency, urgency, and nocturia emerge. Because cystitis and urethritis generally coexist, most patients will experience most of these symptoms.

Urethritis, by itself, is relatively uncommon. These patients have symptoms of dysuria and pelvic pressure, but most often lack frequency or urgency. Infection with *Neisseria gonorrhoeae, Chlamydia trachomatis,* and *Mycoplasma* and *Ureaplasma* organisms should all be considered when urethritis is suspected. The last two organisms are associated with a more indolent clinical course than when the infecting organism is *N. gonorrhoeae, E. coli* or *Staphylococcus saprophyticus.* A swab inserted into the urethra may be used to obtain material for culture and Gram stain to establish the diagnosis.

Patients with urethral syndrome (also uncommon) will have the symptoms of urethritis, plus daytime frequency, pelvic pain, and dyspareunia, but will have no microscopic or culture findings to support a diagnosis of urethritis. Urethroscopy or cystoscopy should be considered to differentiate this syndrome from intrinsic bladder pathology, such as bladder tumors. Referral or consultation is generally recommended for these patients.

Recurrent lower urinary tract infections require prompt a re-evaluation. Possible causes that must be considered include incorrect or incomplete (e.g., noncompliant) therapy, mechanical factors (e.g., obstruction or stone), or compromised host defenses.

The symptoms engendered by a loss of pelvic support vary based on the structure or structures involved and on the degree of prolapse. Most often these patients report symptoms that are characterized as a diffuse "pressure" or "heaviness," low in the abdomen or pelvis that is worse late in the day, after lifting, or when standing for long periods. Low backache and deep thrust dyspareunia are also frequently reported symptoms. A cystourethrocele can result in stress incontinence, frequency, hesitancy, incomplete voiding, or recurrent infections. When there is complete disruption of support, the patient may be paradoxically asymptomatic and only note the protrusion of tissue from the vagina. Vaginal ulceration, bleeding, infection, or pain frequently accompany complete prolapse. Loss of rectal support may lead to complaints of constipation, painful or incomplete defecation, and a need for vaginal splinting (with the fingers) to permit bowel movements.

The pivotal importance of the history and pretreatment evaluation of urinary incontinence cannot be overstressed. Most surgical failures are the result of a failure of proper diagnosis. Because no single historical factor, physical finding, or test is diagnostic by itself, a great deal of thought and care must go into the evaluation process. To aid in this process, the patient should keep a voiding diary, recording fluid intake, the time and volume of each voiding, and the presence and amount of urinary loss, 3 to 7 days prior to physical evaluation. This often give clues to unexpected causes of urinary complaints (such as excessive fluid intake or unusual voiding patterns).

Physical Findings

The physical examination of women with urinary tract infections are generally nonspecific, although some patients may experience suprapubic tenderness during bimanual examination. Other conditions that can mimic urinary tract infections may be excluded at the time of physical examination. Vulvitis and vaginitis, which may give rise to external dysuria, may be suspected and diagnosed by observation, supplemented by microscopic evaluation of the vaginal secretions. Urethritis, a urethral diverticulum, or infection in the Skene's glands may also be suspected based on physical findings. When palpation of the urethra or bladder elicits significant discomfort, urethral syndrome or interstitial cystitis should be suspected. Costovertebral angle tenderness, fever, or chills suggests the possibility of pyelonephritis.

Pelvic relaxation is best demonstrated by having the patient strain or cough while observing the vaginal opening through the separated labia (Fig. 27.3). This can be done either in the supine or standing positions or both, although the supine examination is often sufficient to establish the diagnosis. When a urethrocele or cystocele is present, a downward movement and forward rotation of the vaginal wall toward the introitus will be demonstrated. A single-bladed speculum (a Sim's speculum or the lower half of a Grave's specu-

Figure 27.3. Patient with cysto-urethrocele. From: Jones (From Jones HW, Wentz AC, Burnett LS. Novak's textbook of gynecology. 11th ed. Baltimore: Williams & Wilkins, 1988:456.)

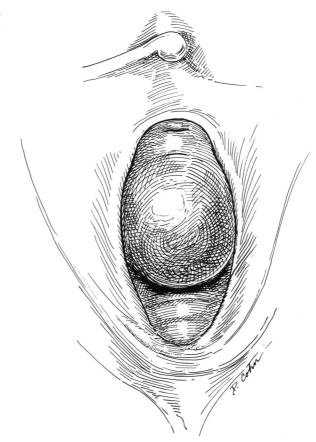

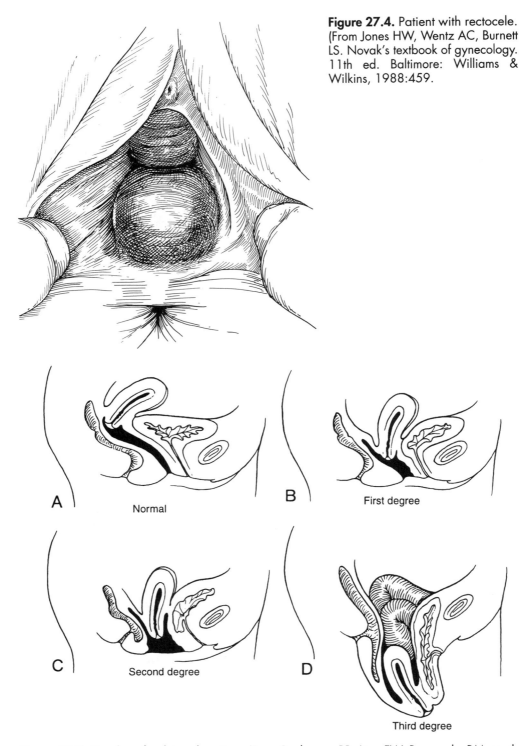

Figure 27.4. Patient with rectocele. (From Jones HW, Wentz AC, Burnett LS. Novak's textbook of gynecology. 11th ed. Baltimore: Williams & Wilkins, 1988:459.

A   Normal

B   First degree

C   Second degree

D   Third degree

Figure 27.5. Grades of pelvic relaxation. (From Beckmann RB, Ling FW, Barzansky BM, et al. Obstetrics and gynecology. 2nd ed. Baltimore: Williams & Wilkins, 1995:336.)

lum) will facilitate the identification a cystocele, rectocele, or enterocele. This allows the separate inspection of the anterior and posterior vaginal walls to differentiate the structures involved. Descent of the uterus may be demonstrated in this way or through palpation. A rectocele may be confirmed by rectovaginal examination. Vaginal outlet relaxation often, but not always, accompanies a rectocele. An example of this is shown in Figure 27.4.

Pelvic relaxation is often quantitated on a 1 to 3 scale based on the descent of the structure involved (Fig. 27.5). Descent limited to the upper two thirds of the vagina, is classed as first-degree. Second-degree prolapse is present when the involved structure reaches the vaginal introitus. Descent beyond the vaginal opening (such as the body of the uterus in procidentia) is classed as a third-degree defect. An example of third-degree vaginal wall prolapse is shown in Figure 27.6.

Cystourethroceles can be quantitated using the "Q-tip test." To perform this test, a sterile cotton swab, dipped in 2% xylocaine, is placed in the urethra (up to the urethrovesical junction) and the angle of upward rotation present when the patient strains is measured. Rotation of greater than 30 degrees from the starting point is generally associated with stress incontinence.

Physical examination of patients with incontinence should be performed with the bladder full. The patient should be examined in both the supine (lithotomy) and standing

Figure 27.6. Patient with vaginal prolapse. (From Jones HW, Wentz AC, Burnett LS. Novak's textbook of gynecology. 11th ed. Baltimore: Williams & Wilkins, 1988:458.)

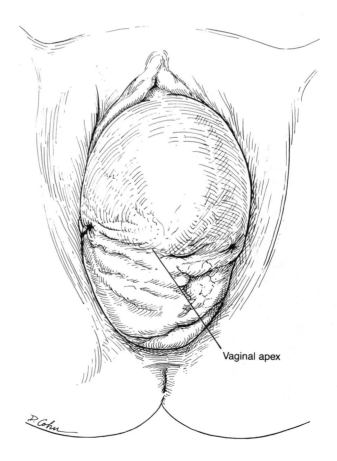

Vaginal apex

positions in an effort to assess pelvic support and to attempt to document incontinence through stress (cough) or provocation (heel drop, running water). Simple neurologic screening tests specifically covering T10 to S4 nerve root function, such as external anal sphincter reflex or perineal sensation, are important parts of the assessment of these patients.

Special Evaluations

Infection

Nonpregnant women with a first episode of classic symptoms suggestive of urinary tract infection do not need laboratory confirmation of the diagnosis, but may be treated empirically. Older patients, pregnant women, those with recurrent infections, or debilitated patients who are suspected of having a urinary tract infection should have the diagnosis confirmed with a urinalysis or a urine culture and sensitivity.

Most often urine for evaluation is collected through a "clean catch midstream" urine sample obtained by cleansing the vulva and recovering a portion of urine passed during the middle of uninterrupted voiding. Urine from urethral catheterization or suprapubic aspiration may also be used. A catheterized specimen or one obtained by suprapubic needle aspiration, should be considered for patients who cannot obtain an uncontaminated specimen (the very young, infirm, or unconscious patients) or when repeated samples show vaginal contamination.

Laboratory urinalysis can be performed or the sample can be examined microscopically by the clinician using a single drop of urine or the precipitate from a centrifuged specimen. For uncentrifuged samples, the presence of more than one white blood cell per high-power field is 90% accurate in detecting infection. Centrifuged specimens may be scanned under low power for the presence of large numbers of white cells. Pyuria is defined as the presence of more than five white cells per high-power field in the centrifuged specimen. Gram stain of urine samples or sediments may be helpful in establishing the diagnosis of infection and may suggest a possible pathogen. "Dip-stick" tests for infection based on the presence of leukocyte esterase are also useful but will be a false-positive in the presence of vaginal contamination and will be a false-negative in infections caused by enterococci (which do not convert nitrate to nitrite). Microscopic examination will reveal the presence of squamous epithelial cells indicating contamination by vaginal secretions. This contamination will not be apparent with "dip-stick" methods.

When the specimen is sent to a laboratory for examination, urinalysis should confirm the presence of white blood cells in moderate numbers. Microscopic hematuria may be present in up to 50% of women with acute cystitis. As with the office examination of a urine specimen, the presence of squamous epithelial cells suggests contamination by vaginal secretions.

If a urine culture is obtained, growth of a single pathogen in levels of greater than 10^5 colony-forming units (CFU) per milliliter of urine confirms the diagnosis of infection and establishes the causative agent. Between 20% and 25% of women with urinary tract infections will have less than 10^5 CFU/mL. For this reason, as few as 10^2 CFU to 10^4 CFU/mL of *E. coli, S. saprophyticus,* or *Proteus* species will confirm infection by these organisms when symptoms are present. Cultures that find multiple pathogens reflect contamination rather than infection.

Patients suspected of having urethral syndrome or interstitial cystitis should undergo urethroscopy and cystoscopy to evaluate other possible causes and to establish the diagnosis. Cystoscopy may demonstrate inflammation of the urethra, a diverticulum, or other abnormality in patients with urethral syndrome. Patients with interstitial cystitis may be unable to tolerate even the most minimal bladder filling. If the bladder is distended, drained, and re-distended for cystoscopy, patients with interstitial cystitis will develop petechial hemorrhages or fissures, which are pathognomic. Biopsy will confirm the diagnosis and rule out other possibilities such as tuberculosis or tumor.

Incontinence and Pelvic Relaxation

When a significant cystocele or urethrocele is present, an evaluation of urinary function is advisable. This is particularly true when the patient's symptoms do not agree with the physical findings. Because of the frequent association of more than one cause of urinary incontinence, patients with incontinence should be considered for urodynamics testing. Although the content of urodynamics testing varies based on the needs of the patient and the preferences of the consultant, at a minimum it includes cystometrics and provocative tests (such as coughing or straining while the bladder is full). Most centers include sophisticated evaluation of bladder compliance and contractility, cystoscopy, and evaluations of the voiding process itself. Pressure profiles of the bladder and urethra, electromyography, and fluoroscopic examinations may also be included. These tests are useful in the evaluation of patients in whom "mixed" causes are suspected. They should also be performed prior to any invasive therapy. Indications for referral and multichannel urodynamics testing are shown in Table 27.3. A summary of normal values often reported in a formal urodynamics consultation are shown in Table 27.4.

A rough indication of the functional significance of a cystourethrocele can be gauged by elevating the bladder neck (using fingers or an instrument) and asking the patient to strain (referred to as a Bonney or Marshall-Marchetti test). If the patient is rendered continent (with at least 200 mL of urine or saline in the bladder), this test may suggest the effect of a pessary or surgical repair. Care must be taken that the results accurately reflect the

Table 27.3. Indications for Multichannel Urodynamics Testing

Historic factors
    Age >65
    Continuous urinary loss
    Failed medical therapy
    Mixed stress and urgency incontinence
    Neurologic disease
    Previous urinary tract surgery
    Recurrent urinary tract infections
    Suspected urethral diverticulum
Physical factors or findings
    Abnormal simple cystometrics
    Incontinence with negative Q-tip test
    Maximal bladder capacity <350 mL or >800 mL
    Neurologic abnormality
    Normal examination with significant incontinence
    Residual volume >100

Table 27.4. Normal Findings During Urodynamics Testing

Cystometrics	
Residual urine	<50 mL
Resting pressure	20–30 cm H_2O
Maximal capacity	300–500 mL
Compliance (rise in pressure)	<10 cm H_2O
First urge (sensation of fullness)	150–200 mL
Profilometry	
Maximal urethral pressure	50–100 cm H_2O
Maximal closure pressure	50–80 cm H_2O
Functional urethral length	>3 cm
Uroflowmetry—(200 mL voided volume)	
Voiding time	<20 s
Peak flow rate	>15 mL/s
Average flow rate	>10 mL/s
Flow pressure (range)	20–60 cm H_2O
Mean maximal flow pressure	58 cm H_2O

effects of elevation of the structures and not mechanical obstruction of the urethra. Because of this uncertainty, this test should not be the sole means of evaluating or selecting therapy. Some centers have abandoned its use completely.

In the primary care setting, patients with incontinence should have a urinalysis and urine culture obtained. (In one study, one third of women with stress incontinence and asymptomatic bacteriuria had resolution of their symptoms with antibiotic treatment.) Pelvic examination, Q-tip testing, and a Bonney test may all be performed. Patients with urgency or overflow incontinence patterns should also have their residual urine volume measured. This is performed by catheterizing the bladder within 15 minutes of the time the patient has a normal void (at least 150 mL). A volume of less than 50 mL is normal.

Chronic constipation and difficulty passing stool may be symptoms of obstructive lesions as well as a rectocele. Screening tests for occult fecal blood should be considered, along with anoscopy or sigmoidoscopy, based on the needs of the individual patient.

Fistulae

Documenting the presence of a genitourinary fistula can be very difficult. Patients suspected of having a fistula must be carefully examined for signs of it, but direct inspection often will not document small openings. The installation of a dilute solution of methylene blue (1 mL/100 mL sterile water or saline) into the bladder, while a tampon is in place in the vagina, will document a vesicovaginal fistula. If staining of the tampon does not occur, a ureterovaginal fistula must be considered. This may then be documented in a similar fashion, using intravenous indigo carmine (5 mL of a 0.8% solution).

If a vesicovaginal fistula is found, cystoscopy is required both to evaluate the location of the fistula in relation to the ureteral opening and bladder trigone and to exclude the possibility of multiple fistulae. Ureterovaginal fistulae should be evaluated by excretory urography to evaluate possible ureteral dilation or obstruction. Retrograde urography may also be required, with the passage of ureteral stents to aid in visualization or as supportive therapy.

Differential Diagnosis

Urinary frequency, urgency, and dysuria most often herald a lower urinary tract infection, but consideration must also be given to other possible diagnoses. The diagnosis of urethral syndrome is often missed because it may be confused with infection. Irritation of the urethra by allergies, atrophy, or the effects of irritating components of the urine (e.g., caffeine) may all imitate lower tract infection. Detrusor instability, interstitial cystitis, and bladder tumors may mimic the urgency and frequency of an infection and must also be considered.

Although the differential diagnosis of pelvic relaxation is generally simple, other processes must be entertained. A moderate sized urethral diverticulum or Skene's gland abscesses may mimic a cystourethrocele. These may be suspected through symptoms, identified by gentle "milking" of the urethra that yields pus, or by cystoscopic examination. It is occasionally difficult to differentiate between a high rectocele and an enterocele, although rectal examination or the identification of small bowel in the hernia sac may demonstrate the distinction. (The presence of an enterocele is often not verified until surgical repair is undertaken.)

Pelvic relaxation is the result of structural failure of tissue, but contributing factors must be considered for the complete care of the patient. Has there been a change in intra-abdominal pressure? Does the patient have a chronic cough that has precipitated her symp-

Table 27.5. Medications with Lower Urinary Tract Side Effects

Class (Examples)	Action	Impact
Antihistamines (Ornade)	Inhibit bladder contraction	Urinary retention
Antihypertensives (Reserpine, Methyldopa, Hydralazine)	Deplete catecholamines resulting in pharmacologic sympathectomy (sympathetic blocker)	Incontinence
Appetite suppressants (Phenylpropanolamine)	Stimulation of urethral muscles	Urinary retention
β-Adrenergic agents (Isoxsuprine, terbutaline, Ritodrine)	Inhibit bladder muscle contractility	Urinary retention
Cholinergic agents (Digitalis)	Increase bladder wall tension and contractility	Decreased capacity, increase intravesical pressure
Dopaminergic agonists (bromocriptine, levodopa)	Increase urethral resistance, decrease bladder contractility	Bladder neck obstruction, urinary retention
Methylxanthines (caffeine)	Decrease urethral closure pressure, increase bladder wall irritability	Incontinence, frequency, urgency
Neuroleptic (major tranquilizers: diazepam, prochlorperazine, promethazine, trifluoperazine, Chlorpromazine, haloperidol)	Internal sphincter relaxation, dopamine receptor blockade	Incontinence
Parasympathetic blockers (atropine, scopolamine)	Inhibit bladder contraction, increases urethral tone	Urinary retention

toms? Is a neurologic process (such as diabetic neuropathy) responsible for the patient's present complaint? Each must be considered prior to the selection of a diagnostic or therapeutic plan.

Urinary incontinence may stem from structural factors, irritation (mechanical or inflammatory trigonitis), neurologic causes (such as diabetes or detrusor instability), or through the effects of medications (Table 27.5). Loss of urine can also take place if there is a breakdown of the social or emotional competence of the patient (e.g., psychosis, neurosis, and so forth). Patients with incontinence should be considered for glucose tolerance, thryroid function screening, and Venereal Disease Research Laboratory (VDRL) testing. A vesicovaginal or ureterovaginal fistula must also be considered, especially in postoperative patients or in those who have received radiation therapy. The possibility of a urethral diverticula must be considered in patients with postvoid dribbling or recurrent urinary tract infections.

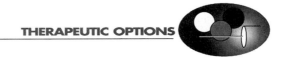

THERAPEUTIC OPTIONS

Urinary Tract Infections

Once a urinary tract infection is diagnosed, antibiotic therapy should be instituted. For most patients, single-dose therapy is roughly as effective for both treatment and recurrence prevention as the traditional 7- to 10-day regimens. Patients who are pregnant, have had symptoms for more than 5 days, do not empty their bladder well, have known urinary tract anomalies, or an indwelling urinary catheter should receive a longer course of antibiotics. Debate persists as to the merits of 3-day therapy and the traditional 10-day courses used in the past for these patients.

Acute cystitis or asymptomatic bacteriuria in pregnant patients can be treated with a number of antibiotic agents. Nitrofurantoin (Macrodantin) produces good urinary antibiosis without undue alteration of the flora of other areas such as the gastrointestinal tract and vaginal canal. Nitrofurantoin is not effective against *Proteus* infections and should not be used when this organism is suspected. Ampicillin, tetracycline, and trimethoprim-sulfamethoxazole (Septra, Bactrim) provide good coverage in the urinary tract, but risk more alteration of intestinal and vaginal flora. Therapy for urinary tract infection should be augmented by hydration and frequent voiding. Urinary acidification (with ascorbic acid, ammonium chloride, or acidic fruit juices) and urinary analgesics (Pyridium) may also be added based on the needs of the individual patient. A summary of commonly used antibiotics for acute cystitis is shown in Table 27.6.

For most patients, symptoms should resolve within 2 to 3 days of the initiation of therapy. No follow-up is necessary after single-dose treatment or multiday treatment for nonpregnant women who experience resolution of their symptoms. Confirmation of cure for all other patients should be carried out by way of urinalysis and culture.

Isolated urethritis caused by *N. gonorrhoeae, C. trachomatis,* or *Mycoplasma* and *Ureaplasma* organisms may be treated with ofloxacin (300 mg twice a day for 7 days) or ciprofloxacin (250 mg twice a day for 7 days). Patients not treated with one of these agents

Table 27.6.   Antibiotic Therapy for Acute Cystitis

Nonpregnant patients—single dose therapy	
Amoxicillin	3 g
Ampicillin	3.5 g
Cephalosporin (first generation)	2 g
Nitrofurantoin	200 mg
Sulfisoxazole	2 g
Trimethoprim (TMP)	400 mg
TMP/sulfamethoxazole	320 (1600) mg
3- to 7-day therapy	
Amoxicillin	500 mg every 8 h
Cephalosporin (first generation)	500 mg 8 h
Ciprofloxacin	250 mg 12 h
Nitrofurantoin	100 mg 12 h
Norfloxacin	400 mg 12 h
Ofloxacin	200 mg 12 h
Sulfisoxazole	500 mg 6 h
Tetracycline	500 mg 6 h
TMP/sulfamethoxazole	160/800 mg 12h
TMP	100 (200) mg 12 h
Pregnant patients—7-day therapy	
Amoxicillin	500 mg 8 h
Cephalosporin (first generation)	500 mg 6 h
Nitrofurantoin	100 mg 12 h

should receive doxycycline (100 mg twice a day for 7 days) plus intramuscular ceftriaxone (250 mg). Pregnant patients should be given erythromycin (500 mg four times a day for 7 days) substituted for the doxycycline.

When pyelonephritis is suspected, aggressive antibiotic therapy is required. Because of the severity of these infections and the possibility of bacteremia, septic shock, adult respiratory distress syndrome, and other serious sequelae, these patients must be hospitalized and cannot be treated in the ambulatory setting.

Treatment of urethral syndrome is imprecise and associated with poor cure rates. Reversible causes (such as irritants, caffeinism, or an estrogen deficit) should be addressed first. Urethral dilatation and massage have been used in some studies with fair results. When simple measures fail, periurethral injections of steroids have been used, but this should be reserved for only a few selected patients. Chronic antibiotic therapy, tranquilizers, smooth muscle relaxants, urethral cryotherapy, and others have been advocated, but with only mixed success.

Interstitial cystitis is difficult to treat and generally requires referral to a urologist. Treatments such as hydrodistention (forcible overfilling of the bladder done under anesthesia) or dimethyl sulfoxide (DMSO) installations are used, but success rates vary from 50% to 90%, and recurrences are common.

Pelvic Relaxation and Incontinence

Because pelvic relaxation involves one or more mechanical defects, therapy is mechanical as well. Therapies range from simple support provided by pessaries and pelvic muscle exercises to surgical repair of tissue defects. For postmenopausal patients, estrogen replacement is often strongly suggested as an important adjunct to other therapies.

Patients who have urgency incontinence may improve with bladder training, biofeedback, or medical therapy. Bladder training is directed toward increasing the patient's bladder control and capacity by gradually increasing the amount of time between voidings. Patients are asked to void on a set schedule based on their shortest normal voiding interval. Once this has been practiced for several days, the interval is lengthened by 10 to 15 minutes each day or so until intervals of 1 1/2 to 2 1/2 hours can be comfortably attained. Often successful by itself (up to 80%), bladder training may be augmented by biofeedback (when available). A log of fluid intake may suggest patterns of intake that can be altered to reduce the risk of urgency during active parts of the day.

Beta-sympathetic activity in the body and dome of the bladder leads to muscle relaxation, whereas alpha-adrenergic activity causes urethral contraction. This difference allows both bladder and urethral function to be manipulated pharmacologically. The pharmacologic treatment of urgency incontinence may take many forms, such as anticholinergic drugs (Pro-Banthine, Ditropan), beta sympathomimetic agonists (Alupent), musculotropic drugs (Urispas, Valium), antidepressants (Tofranil), or dopamine agonists (Parlodel). Because the bladder is parasympathetically innervated, anticholinergic drugs are most commonly used to treat bladder instability of any cause. A summary of the pharmacologic treatment of urgency incontinence is presented in Table 27.7.

Stress incontinence is, for the most part, a surgical disease. Pharmacologic agents may provide some improvement (Table 27.8) but definitive therapy requires mechanical support that is only available through the use of a pessary or surgical repair. The exception to this pessimistic picture is estrogen, which gives improvement rates of up to 70% for postmenopausal women not previously receiving replacement therapy.

Table 27.7. Pharmacologic Agents for Urgency Incontinence

Drug	Dose (mg)	Frequency	Notes
Dicyclomine hydrochloride (Bentyl)	20 (IM)	qid	Requires parental use
Flavoxate hydrochloride (Urispas)	100–200	tid–qid	Fewer side effects, more expensive than some
Imipramine hydrochloride (Tofranil)	25–50	bid–tid	Good for mixed incontinence and enuresis, 60%–75% effective
Oxybutynin hydrochloride (Ditropan)	5–10	tid–qid	Side effects common (75%), 60%–80% effective
Phenylpropanolamine hydrochloride (Propadrine)	50	bid	Alpha-adrenergic sympathomimetic
Propantheline bromide (Pro-Banthin)	15–30	tid–qid	Few side effects, variable absorption, 60%–80% effective
Terodiline hyrochloride (Micturin)	12.5–25	bid	Available outside of United States

qid = 4 times daily; tid = 3 times daily; bid = twice daily.

Table 27.8. Pharmacologic Agents for Stress Incontinence

Drug	Dose (mg)	Frequency	Notes
Phenylpropanolamine	75–150	Every day	May improve mild stress incontinence
Phenylpropanolamine plus chlorpheniramine (Ornade)	75/12	Every 6 h	Better tolerated than phenylpropanolamine alone
Imipramine hydrochloride (Tofranil)	50–150	Every day	Good for mixed incontinence and enuresis, use with care in the elderly
Topical estrogen cream (Premarin)	1–2 (gm)	Every other day	Up to 70% of patients report improvement

The pelvic musculature can be strengthened to some degree through the use of Kegel exercises. This exercise program consists of the repetitive contraction of the pelvic floor muscles as if trying to stop bladder emptying. These muscles are contracted for 3 to 5 seconds, relaxed and recontracted. This cycle is repeated 30 to 40 times throughout the day. These exercises may be helpful for some patients with mild incontinence and they may help provide stronger tissues should surgical repair be attempted. Electrical devices to stimulate the muscles of the pelvic floor (similar to Kegel exercises) are available and provide success at rates comparable to Kegel exercises alone.

Pessaries

Mechanical support for the pelvic organs can be provided by pessaries Figure 27.7). Available in a variety of types and sizes, these are worn in the vagina to replace the missing structural support and to diffuse the forces of descent over a wide area. The most commonly used forms of pessary for pelvic relaxation are the ring (or donut), the ball, and the cube. For occasional use, a large tampon may serve the same purpose. Pessaries are fitted and placed in the vagina in much the same way as a contraceptive diaphragm. To varying degrees, the pessary occludes the vagina and holds the pelvic organs in a relatively normal position. Pessaries offer an excellent alternative to surgical repair, but their use requires the cooperation and involvement of the patient. Patients who are unable or unwilling to manage the periodic insertion and removal of the device are poor candidates for their use. Pessaries will not be well tolerated or provide optimal support in the poorly estrogenized patient. For this reason, many suggest a minimum of 30 days of topical estrogen therapy (for those not already on estrogen replacement) prior to a trial of pessary therapy.

Patients fitted with a pessary need careful initial monitoring. Examination 5 to 7 days after initial fitting is required to confirm proper placement, hygiene, and the absence of pressure-related problems (vaginal trauma or necrosis). Earlier evaluation (in 24 to 48 hours) may be advisable for patients who are debilitated or require additional assistance. Because pessaries come in a large number of sizes, shapes, and materials, many primary care providers prefer to refer these patients for fitting and initial choice of type and then have the patient return for continuing care.

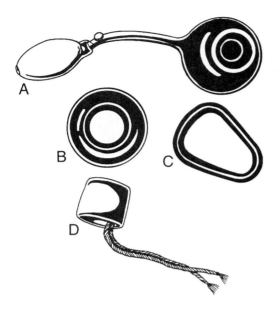

Figure 27.7. Pessaries commonly used for pelvic support. **A**, Inflatable; **B**, Doughnut; **C**, Smith-Hodge; **D**, Cube. (From Beckmann RB, Ling FW, Barzansky BM, et al. Obstetrics and gynecology. 2nd ed. Baltimore: Williams & Wilkins, 1995: 338.)

Surgical Therapy

Surgical repair of pelvic relaxation ranges from hysterectomy to the creation of supportive slings, occlusion of the vagina to plastic repairs (Table 27.9). Surgical repair is almost always reserved for those who have completed childbearing. Repair may be approached from either the vaginal or abdominal routes and each procedure has its own indications, advantages, disadvantages, complications, and failures. No one procedure is best, and every choice of therapy must be individualized. Success is based not only on the procedure chosen, but also on the skill of the surgeon, the degree of pelvic relaxation, and patient risk factors for both the surgery and for recurrence (such as quality of tissues, obesity, and lifestyle).

Because of the frequent concurrence of pelvic relaxation, prolapse, and uterine descent, hysterectomy is often performed simultaneously with other surgical repairs. This combined approach corrects symptoms referable to the descensus, provides access to the uterine support mechanism to reinforce other repairs, and prevents the weight of the uterus from tearing down surgical repairs should further descent occur. Recent reappraisals have cast doubt on the merits of this traditional combination in the absence of other indications for hysterectomy.

Surgical therapy for anterior vaginal support defects and stress incontinence is varied. Each of the surgical techniques advocated attempts to provide renewed support to the pelvic organs by repairing the known or postulated anatomic defects responsible or by creating a compensatory change in the pelvic structures through surgical alteration or reconstruction. Although a complete discussion of the various surgical techniques used goes beyond what is needed in the primary care setting, for counseling purposes, an overview of common procedures is shown in Table 27.9.

Failure of posterior vaginal support, resulting in a rectocele, is surgically treated by reconstructing or reinforcing the rectovaginal septum (posterior colporrhaphy). Prolapse of

Table 27.9.   Surgical Therapy for Urinary Incontinence

Type	Intent	Approach
Anterior vaginal wall repair (anterior colporrhaphy, Kelly plication)	Support the bladder and urethra by reinforcing the endopelvic fascia and vaginal epithelium	Vaginal
Retropubic suspension (Marshall-Marchetti-Krantz, Burch, Richardson para-vaginal repair)	Repair defects in the endopelvic fascia and its attachments	Abdominal
Sling procedure (Goebell-Frangenheim-Stoeckel, Pereya, Stamey)	Supplement or replace the support of the bladder neck and urethra using suture or fascial slings	Combined abdominal and vaginal
Vaginal obliteration (LeFort, colpocleisis)	Provide support by obliterating the vaginal space	Vaginal

(After Beckman RB, Ling FW, Barzansky BM, et al. Obstetrics and gynecology. 2nd ed. Baltimore: Williams & Wilkins, 1995.)

the vagina, with or without a high enterocele, may require suspending the vaginal vault to either the sacrospinous ligament (vaginal or abdominal approach) or to presacral tissues (abdominal sacrocolpopexy). Obliteration of the rectovaginal space (Moschcowitz procedure) is used to treat or prevent future vaginal prolapse or enterocele formation. This may be performed at the time of hysterectomy or as an independent procedure. An enterocele by itself is treated like other hernias, by disection and high ligation of the hernia sac.

Patients who cannot endure long procedures and are not sexually active, may be treated with partial or complete obliteration of the vaginal canal (LeFort procedure, colpocleisis) to provide pelvic organ support.

Patients treated surgically require normal postoperative care and follow-up. Special care is given to avoid coughing, lifting, or straining to protect the surgical repairs until healing can take place. Stool softeners are often advisable as well.

Fistulae

Vesicovaginal fistulae that occur in the immediate postoperative period should be treated by large caliber transurethral catheter drainage. For many patients, this drainage will allow the spontaneous closure of the fistula, obviating the need for further therapy. Spontaneous healing will be evident within 2 to 4 weeks. Drainage beyond this time is unlikely to result in further healing and surgical repair will be required. Similarly, in patients with a ureterovaginal fistula, prompt placement of a ureteral stent, left in place for 2 weeks, allows spontaneous healing for about 25% of patients. Diversion of the fecal flow, provided by a loop colostomy is sometimes successful in allowing small rectovaginal fistulae to heal.

Surgical repair of genitourinary fistulae is generally delayed 2 to 4 months, to allow complete healing of the original insult. In all cases, successful surgical repair consists of meticulous disection of the fistulous tract and careful reapproximation of tissues. Recurrence after surgical repair is common, especially in patients who have undergone radiation therapy for malignancies.

HINTS AND COMMON QUESTIONS

Sexually active women are more likely to have cervicitis, vaginitis, or vulvitis than urethritis (which is relatively uncommon). Because of the similarity of symptoms, patients treated for urethritis with urinary antiseptics, nitrofurantoin, a cephalosporin, or ampicillin, whose symptoms persist should be evaluated for these possibilities. Physical examination and examination of vaginal secretions should assist in the diagnosis. Urinalysis of patients with urethritis will show pyuria but no bacteria. A urine Gram stain or culture may also be of help.

Dipstick screening for hematuria is based on the peroxidase activity of hemoglobin or myoglobin to react with substrate to form a colored product. As a result, free hemoglobin derived from hemolytic anemia or trauma, myoglobin liberated by trauma, extended exercise, or rhabdomyolysis may give false-positive results. Other sources of oxidants, such as residues on poorly washed glassware or bacterial peroxidases, may also confuse the results. High levels of ascorbic acid may inhibit the peroxidase reaction, providing a source of false-negative results as well. There are a number of agents that can produce a red color to urine that may mimic hematuria (Table 27.10). These must be considered in the differential diagnosis before bleeding is presumed.

Routine urine culture is not necessary for most patients suspected of having a urinary tract infection. It should be performed if initial therapy fails, and if the patient experiences recurrent infections, has a debilitating disease, is immunocompromised, or has recently received antibiotics for another infection.

Urinary tract infection often precipitates incontinence in older patients. Therefore, abrupt onset incontinence in these patients should suggest infection, which may be confirmed through urinalysis or culture.

Patients who experience repeated or persistent urinary tract infections with the same organism, especially those with *Proteus mirabilis,* should be considered for cystoscopy or intravenous pyelography because of an increased prevalence of renal stones. Others who should be considered for this type of evaluation include those suspected of renal anomalies, women with a history of childhood infections, or those with painless hematuria.

Anticholinergic drugs must be used with caution in patients with obstructive gastrointestinal disease or tachycardia.

Table 27.10.   Common Medications that may Cause Red Urine

Cascara-containing laxatives
Chloroquine hydrochloride (Aralen)
Ibuprofen
Levodopa
Methyldopa
Nitrofurantoin (Furadantin, Macrodantin)
Phaenacetin
Phenazopyridine hydrochloride (Pyridium)
Phenytoin (Dilantin)
Quinine
Rifampin
Sulfamethoxazole

The abrupt onset of either stress or urgency incontinence suggests either an infectious or allergic cause. Gradual onset of stress incontinence in a recently menopausal woman suggests the effects of estrogen loss. A history of enuresis (bed wetting) suggests an unstable bladder.

The term "nocturia" is defined as being awakened to void two or more times per night. Frequency is defined as voiding more than seven times in a 24-hour period or more often than every 2 hours. These presume a normal pattern and amount of fluid intake.

Finding a cystourethrocele on physical examination does not establish the diagnosis of genuine stress incontinence, it merely supports the clinical suspicion.

Most patients with early symptoms of true stress incontinence will not experience urinary loss while supine. Therefore, if a patient reports urinary loss while recumbent, suspect the possibility of a mixed incontinence or severe anatomic defect. These patients should be strongly considered for referral and sophisticated urodynamics testing.

Patients with urgency incontinence should be warned to avoid caffeine-containing products, which will tend to make their symptoms worse.

A simple office approach to fistula identification that does not require the use of catheters and intravenous medications makes use of oral phenazopyridine hydrochloride (Pyridium). This urinary analgesic will turn the urine an orange-red color. By placing a tampon in the vagina prior to ingesting the medication and then, at a later time, examining the tampon for the presence and location of staining, a fistula may be confirmed.

Patients with complete prolapse of the uterus to outside the vaginal opening (procidentia) are at risk for ureteral obstruction as these structures are brought with the anterior wall of the vagina to an exterior position. Replacement of the prolapse into the vaginal canal and consultation regarding long-term options is recommended.

SUGGESTED READINGS

General References

Abrams P, Blaivas JG, Stanton SL, Andersen JT. The standardization of terminology of lower urinary tract function produced by the International Continence Society Committee on Standardization of Terminiology. Scand J Urol Nephrol 1988;114:5.

American College of Obstetricians and Gyneologists. Urinary incontinence. ACOG Technical Bulletin 213. Washington, DC: ACOG, 1995.

American College of Obstetricians and Gyneologists. Pelvic organ prolapse. ACOG Technical Bulletin 214. Washington, DC: ACOG, 1995.

American College of Obstetricians and Gyneologists. Antimicrobial therapy for obstetric patients. ACOG Technical Bulletin 117. Washington, DC: ACOG, 1988.

Beecham CT. Classification of vaginal relaxation. Am J Obstet Gynecol 1980;136:957.

Consensus Conference. Unrinary incontinence in adults. JAMA 1989;261:2685.

Norton PA, ed. Urinary incontinence. Clin Obstet Gynecol 1990;33:293.

Urinary Incontinence Guideline Panel. Urinary incontinence in adults: Clinical practice guidelines. Rockville, Maryland: Agency for Health Care Policy and Research, Public Health Service, US Department of Health and Human Services, 1992; AHCPR publication No. 92–0038.

Specific References

Infections

Bergman A, Karram M, Bhatia N. Urethral syndrome: a comparison of different treatment modalities. J Reprod Med 1989;34:157.

Buckley RM, McGuckin M, MacGregor RR. Urine bacterial counts after sexual intercourse. N Engl J Med 1978; 298:321.

Bump RC. Urinary tract infection in women. Current role of single-dose therapy. J Repro Med 1990;35:785.

Dunn M, Ramsden PD, Roberts JBM, Smith JC, Smith PJB. Interstitial cystitis treated by prolonged bladder distention. Br J Urol 1977;49:641.

Greenberg RN, Reilly PM, Luppen KL, et al. Randomized study of single-dose, three-day, and seven-day treatment of cystitis in women. J Infect Dis 1986;153:277.

Kaplan W, Firlit CF, Schoenberg HW. The female urethral syndrome: external sphincter spasm as etiology. J Urol 1980;124:48.

Messing EM, Stamey TA. Interstitial cystitis: early diagnosis, pathology and treatment. Urology 1987;12:29.

Pappas P. Laboratory in the diagnosis and management of urinary tract infections. Med Clin North Am 1991;75:313.

Perez-Marrero R, Emerson LE, Feltis JT. A controlled study of dimethyl sulfoxide in interstitial cystitis. J Urol 1988; 140:36.

Powers R. New directions in the diagnosis and therapy of urinary tract infections. Am J Obstet Gynecol 1991; 164:1387.

Stamm WE, Counts GW, Running KR, et al. Diagnosis of coliform infections in acutely dysuric women. N Engl J Med 1982;137:213.

Woolhandler S, Pels RJ, Bor DH, Himmelstein DU, Lawrence RS. Dipstick urinalysis screening of asymtomatic adults for urinary tract disorders. I. Hematuria and proteinuria. JAMA 1989;262:1214.

Pelvic Relaxation and Incontinence

Allen RE, Smith ARB, Hosker GL, Warrell DW. Pelvic floor damage and childbirth: a neurophysiological study. Br J Obstet Gynaecol 1990;97:770.

Bergman A, Bhatia NN. Urodynamics: The effect of urinary tract infection on urethral and bladder function. Obstet Gynecol 1985;66:366.

Bhatia NN, Bergman A. Urodynamic appraisal of the Bonney test in women with stress urinary incontinence. Obstet Gynecol 1983;62:696.

Bhatia NN, Bergman A, Karram MM. Effects of estrogen on urethral function in women with urinary incontinence. Am J Obstet Gynecol 1989;160:176.

Brown ADG. Postmenopausal urinary problems. Clin Obstet Gynecol 1987;4:181.

Crystle CD, Charme LS, Copeland WE. Q-tip test in stress urinary incontinence. Obstet Gynecol 1971;38:313.

Fischer-Rasmussen W, Hansen RI, Stage P. Predictive values of diagnostic test in the evaluation of female urinary stress incontinence. Acta Obstet Gynecol Scand 1986;65:291.

Federkiw DM, Sand PK, Retzky SS, Johnson DC. The cotton swab test. Receiver-operating characteristic curves. J Reprod Med 1995;40:42.

Hodgkinson CP. Stress urinary incontinence. Am J Obstet Gynecol 1970;108:1141.

Hodgkinson CP. Recurrent stress urinary incontinence. Clin Obstet Gynecol 1978;21:787.

Kinn AC, Lindskog M. Estrogens and phenylpropanolamine in combination for stress urinary incontinence in postmenopausal women. Urology 1988;32:273.

Marshall UF, Marchetti DA, Krantz KE. The correction of stress incontinence by simple vesicourethral suspension. Surg Gynecol Obstet 1949;88:509.

Massey A, Abrams P. Urodynamic of the female lower urinary tract. Urol Clin North Am 1985;12:231.

Migliorini GD, Blenning PP. Bonney's test—fact or fiction. Br J Obstet Gynaecol 1987;94:157.

Sutherst JR, Brown MC. Comparison of single and mulitchannel cystometry in diagnosing bladder instability. BMJ 1984;288:1720.

Tchou DC, Adams C, Varner RE. Pelvic floor musculature exercise in treatment of anatomical stress incontinence. Phys Ther 1988;68:652.

Wall LL. Diagnosis and management of urinary incontinence due to detrusor instability. Obstet Gynecol Surv 1990;45:1s.

Walters MD, Diaz K. Q-tip test: a study of continent and incontinent women. Obstet Gynecol 1987;70:208.

Walters MD, Realini JP. The evaluation and treatment of urinary incontinence in women: a primary care approach. J Am Board Fam Pract 1992;5:289.

Weber AM, Walters MD, Schover LR, Mitchinson A. Sexual function in women with uterovaginal prolapse and urinary incontinence. Obstet Gynecol 1995;85:483.

Wyman J, Hawkins S, Choi S, Taylor J, Fantl JA. Psychosocial impact of urinary incontinence in women. Obstet Gynecol 1987;70:378.

Fistulae

American College of Obstetricians and Gyneologists. Genitourinary fistulas. ACOG Technical Bulletin 83. Washington, DC: ACOG, 1985.

Holley RL, Kilgore LC. Urologic complications. In Orr JW JR, Shingleton HM (eds). Complications in Gynecologic Surgery: Prevention, Recognition, and Management. Philadelphia: JB Lippincott, 1994;149.

Symmonds RE. Incontinence: vesical and urethral fistulas. Clin Obstet Gynecol 1984;27:499.

28

Vulvitis and Vaginal Infections

Vulvar irritations and vaginal infections are among the most common gynecologic ailments seen in primary care. Patients with complaints of vulvar irritation and itching constitute approximately 10% of all outpatient visits to gynecologists; patients with "vaginal infections," signaled by vaginal discharge and irritation, are even more common. In gynecologic practices, two to five or more patients a day are commonly seen with these concerns. Anyone who cares for women will encounter these complaints and must be prepared to provide necessary care. The diagnosis and the institution of prompt treatment for vulvitis or vaginitis is appropriate in almost all primary care settings, with referral for specialized evaluations rarely necessary.

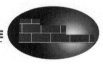

BACKGROUND AND SCIENCE

The tissues of the vulva and vagina represent a rich ecosystem, with many interactions between tissues, fluids, hormones, and microbes. This system is delicately balanced and a disturbance in any element can result in discharge, irritation, odor, or discomfort. Because some element of discharge and aroma (odor in the nonoffensive sense) is always present, it is sometimes difficult to differentiate physiologic from pathologic.

Physiology of the Vulva and Vagina

The skin of the vulva is like that of other areas of the body with stratified squamous epithelium, hair follicles, and sebaceous, sweat, and apocrine glands. The epithelium of the vagina is similar, but is nonkeratinized and lacks these specialized elements. For this reason, the frequently used term vaginal "mucosa" is inaccurate for there are no glands present in this epithelium.

Just as in other areas of the body, the vulva is susceptible to inflammatory and dermatologic diseases. Intertrigo, hidradenitis suppurativa, psoriasis, seborrheic dermatitis, Fox-Fordyce disease, fourth disease, changes caused by Behçet's or Crohn's diseases, viral infections, and parasites may all affect the skin of the vulva. The skin of the vulva is also vulnerable to irritation from vaginal secretions, recurrent urinary loss, or contact with external irritants (e.g., soap residue, perfumes, fabric softeners, or infestation by pinworms). Changes can occur because of the effects of diabetes or hormonal alterations as well as dermatoses such as hypertrophic dystrophy, lichen sclerosis, psoriasis, and others.

The vaginal canal lacks some of the histologic variety of the vulva, but makes up for it with a rich bacterial flora and unique fluid dynamic that creates physiologic vaginal moisture and discharge. A healthy women of reproductive age will make approximately 1.6 to 4.8 g of vaginal secretions a day. These arise from shed vaginal epithelium, which produces the creamy white, slightly curdy character; cervical mucus and vaginal transudate which provides the moisture; and small amounts of material from accessory sex glands such as the Skene's and Bartholin's glands. These components go together to make the normal vaginal secretions that provide physiologic lubrication, which prevents drying and irritation (Figure 28.1). The

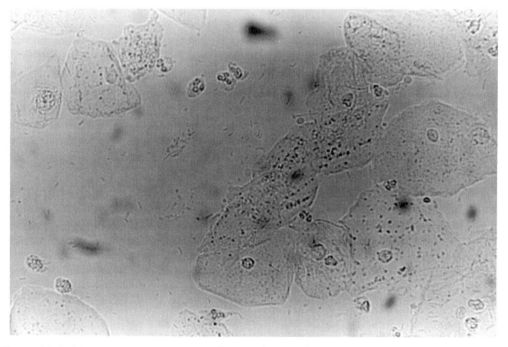

Figure 28.1. Microscopic appearance of normal vaginal secretions. Flat polygonal epithelial cells, occasional white blood cells, and rod-shaped bacteria are normal findings in vaginal secretions. A slight "ground glass" appearance to the epithelia cells is normal and can be distinguished from "clue cells" by the sharp border seen here.

amount and character of this mixture varies under the influence of many factors, including hormonal and fluid status, pregnancy, immunosuppression, and inflammation. Normal vaginal secretions have no "odor," although some slight aroma may be detected on careful examination.

The action of the rich indigenous vaginal flora also contributes to vaginal secretions. There are a great number and variety of organisms that are found in the normal healthy vagina (Table 28.1). These include many, which under other circumstances would be considered pathologic. Normally bacteria are found in concentrations of 10^8 to 10^9 colonies per milliliter of vaginal fluid. Because the vagina is not an open tube, but rather a potential space, a ratio of 5 to 1 anaerobic to aerobic bacteria is normal. This profusion of organisms means that cultures of the vaginal canal are rarely of any help clinically.

Although many bacterial strains are present in the vagina, the predominant organism is *Lactobacillus*. Lactobacilli break down the glycogen present in healthy, well-estrogenized vaginal tissues, liberating hydrogen peroxide and lactic acid and giving the vagina an acidic pH. The normal pH of the vagina is between 3.5 and 4.5. This value is higher (6–8) in premenarchial girls and postmenopausal women who have lower levels of glycogen present. When either the absolute or relative number of lactobacilli decline, changes in pH, chemical irritation, and overgrowth by other organisms may occur.

Multiple pathogens can give rise to vaginal "infections," most common of which are *Candida, Trichomonas vaginalis,* and shifts in microbiologic flora (generally an increase in anaerobic bacteria) associated with bacterial vaginosis and vaginitis. The thicker, more robust vaginal tissues found during the reproductive years are more resistant to infection than are those of premenarchial girls and postmenopausal women. In these groups, direct infection can occur from agents such as gonococcus, which would be rare in menstrual age women.

Table 28.1. Microbiologic Flora of the Normal Vaginal tract

Organism	Range* (%)
Lactobacillus	60–90
Staphyloccus epidermidis	30–60
Diphtheroids	30–60
Alpha-hemolytic *Streptococcus*	15–50
Beta-hemolytic *Streptococcus*	10–20
Nonhemolytic *Streptococcus*	5–30
Group D *Streptococcus*	10–40
Escheria coli	10–25
Bacteroids fragilis	5–15
Bacteroides species	1–40
Peptococcus	5–60
Peptostreptococcus	5–40
Fusobacterium	5–25
Clostridium	5–20
Veillonella	10–30
Candida species	10–15

*Range of normal women with organism present.

A number of factors can predispose to the development of vaginal infections. Systemic processes such as diabetes, pregnancy, and debilitating disease may all increase the risks. Anything that alters the normal vaginal flora can result in overgrowth or infection. This includes smoking, numbers of sexual partners, vaginal contraceptives used, some forms of sexual expression such as oral sex, antibiotic use, hygiene practices and douching, menstruation, and immunologic status.

Foreign bodies can cause significant infection and discharge. These can be found at any age, although we tend to think of them as occurring in the young and the elderly. Foreign bodies may range from innocent objects such as bits of toilet paper, condoms, diaphragms, or retained tampons, to iatrogenic items such as pessaries, to more sinister objects suggesting abuse, neglect, or psychopathology.

ESTABLISHING THE DIAGNOSIS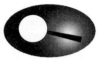

Patients with vulvitis or vaginitis may present with acute, subacute, or indolent symptoms that range from minimal to incapacitating, well localized to those that involve the entire perineal area. In 80% to 90% of cases of increased vaginal discharge, a microbiologic process can be identified. Although generally nonspecific, the patient's history and symptoms may suggest chemical, allergic, or other sources that warrant investigation.

Vulvar Conditions

Infections

SWELLINGS AND RAISED LESIONS. Cystic, painful swelling of the labia in the area of the Bartholin's gland suggests infection. Abscesses in this gland develop rapidly over the course of 2 to 4 days, and are a source of extreme discomfort and disability (Fig. 28.2). These cysts can grow to 8 cm or greater, necessitating surgical drainage. Smaller, more chronic cysts, due to obstruction of the Bartholin's duct, may be identified by gentle palpation at the base of the labia majora. These cysts are smooth, firm, and tender with varying degrees of induration and overlying erythema. The cysts may be clear, yellow, or bluish in color. Over 80% of cultures of material from Bartholin's gland cysts are sterile. Because Bartholinitis or Bartholin's gland abscess may be gonococcal in origin, further evaluation for other sexually transmitted disease is prudent. Most often, culture-positive cysts are secondarily infected by coliform organisms or they are polymicrobial. Mesonephric cysts of the vagina, lipomas, fibromas, hernias, hydroceles, and epithelial inclusion cysts may be confused with Bartholin's gland cysts. Malignancy of the Bartholin's gland is rare, but should be suspected in women over the age of 45 because benign cyst formation and infection is less common in the later reproductive years and after menopause.

The most common raised lesion of the vulva encountered in office practice is condyloma acuminata, accounting for more than 500,000 cases a year, and earning it the distinction of most common sexually transmitted disease (other than pregnancy itself). Also called "venereal warts," these raised lesions are caused by infection by human papilloma virus (HPV, most frequently serotypes 6 and 11) resulting in soft, fleshy, painless growths

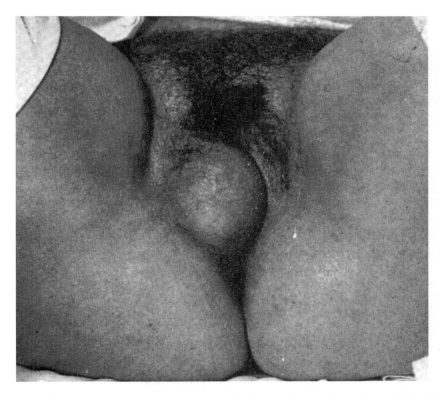

Figure 28.2. Clinical appearance of a Bartholin's gland abscess. (From Jones HW, Wentz AC, Burnett LS. Novak's textbook of gynecology. 11th ed. Baltimore: Williams & Wilkins, 1988:590.)

on the vulva, vagina, cervix, urethral meatus, perineum, and anus (Fig. 28.3). Symmetric lesions across the midline of the genital area are common. Condyloma may also be found on the tongue or within the oral cavity, or on the urethra, bladder, or rectum. These distinctive lesions may be single or multiple and generally provide few symptoms by their presence, although mild irritation or discharge may accompany secondary infections. The virus is spread by skin-to-skin (generally sexual) contact and has an incubation period of from 3 weeks to 8 months, with an average of 3 months. It is thought that the presence of other vaginal infections such as candidiasis, trichomoniasis, or bacterial vaginosis, increases the likelihood of infection by altering normal defense mechanisms, although co-infection is by no means required. Roughly 65% of patients will acquire the infection following intercourse with an infected partner.

Infection of the vaginal epithelium by HPV tends to give rise to more sessile (keratotic) lesions, whereas the condyloma formed in other areas tend to be soft, pink, polypoid, and fleshy. Roughly one third of women with vulvar lesions also have vaginal warts or intraepithelial neoplasia (VAIN), and approximately 40% will have cervical involvement. Cervical condyloma are generally flatter and may be identified through colposcopic examination, Pap smear, or through the application of 3% to 5% acetic acid to make apparent the raised, white, shiny plaques. Exuberant growth and frequent recurrences of condyloma are common in patients who are immunocompromised, diabetic, pregnant, or cigarette smokers.

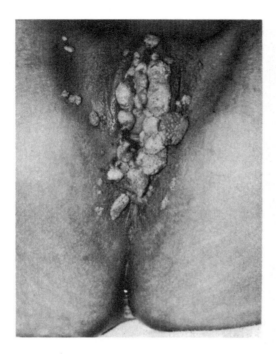

Figure 28.3. Clinical appearance of condyloma acuminata. (From Jones HW, Wentz AC, Burnett LS. Novak's textbook of gynecology. 11th ed. Baltimore: Williams & Wilkins, 1988:583.)

Condyloma may grow during pregnancy only to resolve when the pregnancy ends. Finding condyloma acuminata in a child should suggest the possibility of sexual abuse, but because close nonsexual contact can also result in infection, this is not sufficient evidence, by itself, to establish abuse.

Condyloma are accompanied by *Trichomonas* or *Gardnerella* vaginal infections or other sexually transmitted disease in more than 10% of patients, making further screening of both the patient and her partner important to consider. (See Chapter 26, Sexually Transmitted Disease and "PID".) The diagnosis of condyloma acuminata is made based on physical examination, but may be confirmed through biopsy of the warts. Care must be taken to differentiate these from the smooth topped condyloma lata of secondary syphilis, vulvar intraepithelial neoplasia (VIN), or dysplastic lesions. HPV infections (serotypes 16, 18, 31, 33, 35, 39, 45, 51, and 52) are also associated with cervical changes and an increased risk of cervical atypia and cancer, especially in smokers, requiring careful surveillance (see Chapter 13, Abnormal Pap Smear). Serotyping of HPV infections is currently of little clinical value because all patients, regardless of serotype, require careful follow-up, and Pap smears.

Small, raised, umbilicated lesions are typical of molluscum contagiosum (Fig. 28.4). These asymptomatic lesions are caused by the poxvirus, a mildly contagious sexually transmitted disease. It takes several weeks to months for the lesions to develop after initial infections and autoinfection is common. The lesions begin as domed papules and progress to mature lesions, 1 to 5 mm in diameter, with a umbilicated center filled with a caseous material. The papules may be found anywhere on the body except for mucous membranes. The diagnosis may be made clinically or confirmed by expressing some of the waxy material from the lesion and examining it microscopically for intracytoplasmic molluscum bodies.

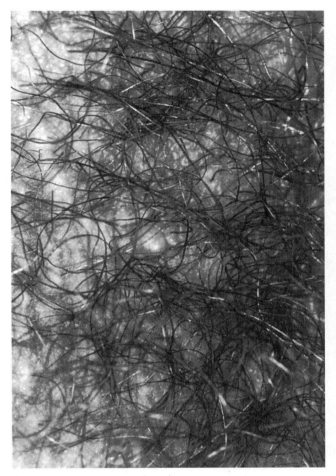

Figure 28.4. Clinical appearance of molluscum contageosum. (From Wilkinson EJ, Stone IK. Atlas of vulvar disease. Baltimore: Williams & Wilkins, 1995:58.)

As with skin elsewhere in the body, fibromas, lipomas, papillomas, hemangiomas, inclusion or sebaceous cysts, and pigmented nevi may all be found in the tissues of the vulva and perineum. Although usually benign, pigmented lesions on the vulva or vagina are uncommon and warrant biopsy to rule out malignancy.

ULCERS AND SORES. The most commonly encountered ulcerative lesion of the vulva is that of herpes simplex infection. The prevalence of herpes infections is estimated to be between 10 and 30 million cases in the United States. Sixty to ninety percent of these infections are caused by the herpes simplex virus (HSV, type II), which is related to the herpes simplex (type I) that causes "cold sores" of the lips. The lesions of a herpes infection appear in 3 to 7 days after initial contact and begin as a vague prodromal tingling or hyperesthesia, followed by vesicular lesions that become ulcerated; they may coalesce into running sores and are extremely painful (Fig. 28.5). These patients are often notable for their painful, "duck waddle" gait when they present to the office for treatment. Dysuria due to vulvar lesions,

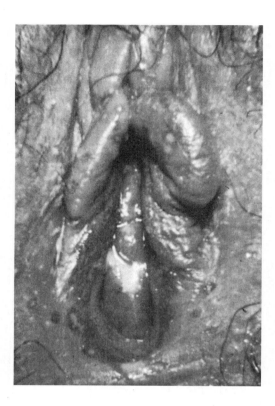

Figure 28.5. Gross appearance of herpes vulvar lesions. (From Jones HW, Wentz AC, Burnett LS. Novak's textbook of gynecology. 11th ed. Baltimore: Williams & Wilkins, 1988:585.)

urethral, or bladder involvement is common and may lead to acute urinary retention. Secondary infection of the ulcerated lesions is common. Primary herpes infections are also characterized by malaise, low-grade fever, and inguinal adenopathy in 40% to 70% of patients. Aseptic meningitis with fever, headache, and meningismus affects some patients 5 to 7 days after the appearance of the genital lesions. This generally resolves over the period of a week. Symptoms of the initial episode generally last 10 to 14 days, but may last up to 6 weeks. In the absence of secondary infection, the lesion will heal without scaring.

Recurrent episodes of herpes vulvitis are milder, with fewer systemic symptoms and lesions that last 5 to 7 days. Recurrences take place in up to 80% of patients with HSV-II infections. The average patient will have four episodes in the first year. Recurrences are fewer (55%) when the vulvar infection is by HSV type I, although these account for fewer than 25% of vulvar infections. Prior "cold sore" infections with HSV-I provide only partial immunity to vulvar infection. Although flare-ups of herpes appear timed to menstruation or emotional stress, scientific proof is lacking. Because viral shedding occurs for a variable period both before recurrent episodes and after lesions have healed, patients should be instructed to avoid intercourse from the first prodrome to until after all lesions have completely re-epithelialized.

Viral cultures from suspected herpes vesicles or from the base of the ulcerated lesions, can recover the virus and confirm the clinical diagnosis, although care in the transport and storage of specimens is required. Culture success is inversely related to the duration of symptoms, with the best results obtained from cultures of the vesicles. Serologic typing of the virus is not necessary. Material scraped from the base of the lesions may also be smeared, fixed, and stained to show multinucleated giant cells and cells with intracellular inclusions (collections of virus particles). Antibody titers are of limited value because 30% to 100% of the sexually active groups studied have an elevated titer. Enzyme-linked immunosorbent assay (ELISA) antigen detection test kits have been marketed, although a thorough evaluation of their sensitivity, specificity, and positive and negative predictive values is lacking. Preliminary studies indicate that false-negative rates of 30% are common. Other lesions that may be mistaken for herpes include primary chancres of syphilis, chancroid, lymphogranuloma venereum, granuloma inguinale, early condyloma, vaccinia, and Behçet's syndrome. (For more information on herpes infections, see Chapter 26, Sexually Transmitted Disease and "PID.")

Herpes infections in pregnancy deserve special mention. When herpes lesions are present near term or during labor significant risk of neonatal herpes infection exists. Roughly 50% of neonates delivered vaginally in the presence of herpes will develop infection. This infection carries a 80% mortality rate and significant risk of permanent ocular or central nervous system sequella. To minimize this risk, cesarean delivery is often recommended for these patients.

Ulcerative lesions are a common presenting symptom for many veneral diseases ranging from the painless ulcers of primary syphilis to symptomatic lesions of chancroid or lymphogranuloma venereum. These must always be considered in the differential diagnosis. A complete discussion of these and a table of characteristics of their lesions may be found in Chapter 26, Sexually Transmitted Diseases and "PID", Table 26.4.

One ulcerative condition that requires special mention is necrotizing fasciitis. Although this process is not unique to the vulvar region, necrotizing fasciitis may begin in, or be mistaken for, secondary infections of other vulvar lesions or Bartholin's gland abscesses. Any patient who is debilitated or is at increased risk (such as diabetics, alcoholics, or nutritionally compromised patients) should be carefully monitored for the possibility of this life-threatening condition.

General Irritation and Allergy

CONTACT DERMATITIS. Diffuse reddening of the vulvar skin accompanied by itching or burning, should suggest a secondary or allergic vulvitis. The list of potential irritants can be extensive, including "feminine hygiene" sprays, deodorants and deodorant soaps, tampons or pads (especially those with deodorants or perfumes), tight-fitting or synthetic undergarments, colored or scented toilet paper, and laundry soap or fabric softener residues. Even topical contraceptives, latex condoms, lubricants, sexual aids, or semen can be a source of irritation. Soiling of the vulva by urine or feces can also create significant symptoms. Severe dermatitis of the vulva due to contact with poison ivy or poison oak is occasionally found.

Contact dermatitis of the vulva results in a symmetric, red, edematous change in the tissues (Fig. 28.6). Ulceration with weeping sores and secondary infection may occur. A careful history, combined with the withdrawal of the suspected cause, usually both confirms the diagnosis and constitutes the needed therapy. In rare cases, the use of hydrocortisone cream may be needed. The possibility of a local *Candida* infection, which can mimic topical irritations, should be ruled out, especially in cases that do not respond or in patients with risk factors such as immunosuppression or diabetes.

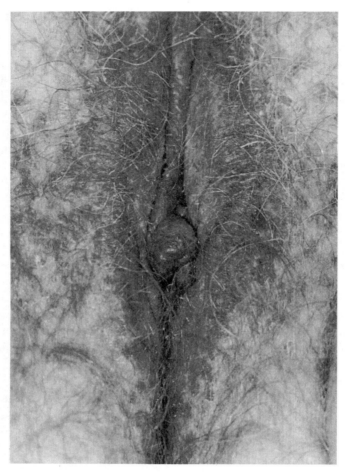

Figure 28.6. Appearance of contact dermatitis. (From Wilkinson EJ, Stone IK. Atlas of vulvar disease. Baltimore: Williams & Wilkins, 1995:81.)

Allergic causes are also frequently found in the occasional pediatric patient who presents with vaginal itching; however, the investigation in these cases must also consider foreign bodies (especially with an accompanying vaginitis or discharge), sexual abuse, and pin worms. Once again, careful history and gentle physical examination will generally provide the diagnosis. Vaginal examination is mandatory for any patient with bleeding or a foul discharge.

INFESTATIONS. In the absence of other obvious findings, vulvar itching may be caused by infestation with *Phthirus pubis* (the crab louse) or *Sarcoptes scabiei* (the itch mite). This is especially true when itching of the mons is part of the patient's complaint. Embarrassment or guilt often delays the diagnosis of these conditions. Pediculosis pubis is caused by close contact with a person already infected by the crab louse. Bedding or towels are a less common source of infection. Highly contagious, a single sexual encounter with an infected partner results in transmission in 90% of cases. Infection generally occurs in hairy areas of the vulva and mons, although other hairy portions of the body may also be affected. The diagnosis is generally made by looking for small black specks (excreta) on the skin or nits (eggs) at the base of hair shafts (Fig. 28.7). The slow moving louse itself may sometimes be directly observed.

Similar to the louse, the itch mite is transmitted by close contact. Unlike pediculosis, scabies is not limited to hairy areas of the body, but may be found in all areas. The more rapidly moving itch mite (up to an inch a minute) burrows beneath the skin evoking an allergic response characterized by itching. This itching is cyclic and often worse at night when the tissues are warmer and the lice are active. Because allergic reaction is necessary for symptoms to develop, symptoms are rare before 5 to 7 days after initial infection. Inspection of the vulvar skin will identify eggs and adult lice. Confirmation of the diagnosis can be made by microscopic inspection of material scraped from inflamed papules.

Itching of the perineum and perianal areas should also suggest pinworms (*Enterobius vermicularis*), skin changes due to Crohn's disease, anal fissures, or fistulae.

PRURITUS AND VULVODYNIA. Nonspecific pruritus and vulvodynia are perhaps the most frustrating vulvar complaints encountered in office practice. The profound itching of vulvar pruritus leads to uncontrollable scratching, which results in a repeating cycle of scratch, excoriation, healing, and itch that may lead to the development of what was called "lichen simplex chronicus," now called "hyperplastic vulvar dystrophy." Vulvodynia describes a conditions with chronic and extreme burning, discomfort, and stinging, resulting in dyspareunia and general disability. Both pruritus and vulvodynia are nonspecific symptoms that often lack definite findings. Causes for these symptoms include local infections, sexually transmitted diseases, vulvar dystrophies, lichen sclerosis, and epithelial neoplasia, including cancer. Even systemic disturbances such as diabetes, uremia, leukemia, and vitamin deficiencies may be at fault. Rarely, psychogenic processes may present in this manner.

Vulvar vestibulitis, also known as vestibular adenitis, presents with a history of progressively worsening vulvar tenderness and pain, leading to loss of function. These patients

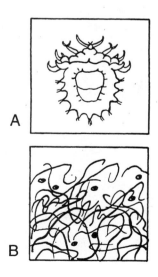

Figure 28.7. A. Phthirus pubis (the crab louse). **B.** Nits of the crab louse. (From Beckmann RB, Ling FW, Barzansky BM, et al. Obstetrics and gynecology. 2nd ed. Baltimore: Williams & Wilkins, 1995:294.)

give up tampon use and are unable to have intercourse because of the pain. Tenderness is localized to the posterior fourchette and vestibule. Careful inspection may reveal small punctate erythematous patches located in the area between the Bartholin's glands, hymeneal ring, and mid portion of the perineum. Gentle palpation with a cotton tip applicator will reproducibly map the area of involvement. The cause of this process is currently unknown.

Skin Changes and Dermatologic Disease

The skin of the vulva is susceptible to both dermatologic and systemic diseases. Psoriasis, seborrheic dermatitis and neurodermatitis, cutaneous candidiasis, and lichen planus may all affect the vulvar tissues. For many of these conditions, lesions elsewhere on the body may provide a clue to the diagnosis. The tissues of the vulva are also susceptible to acute cutaneous infections such as folliculitis, furunculitis, impetigo, and hidradenitis suppurativa.

In older patients, intense itching of the vulva may occur because of atrophic changes brought on by reduced estrogen levels. History will, of course, suggest estrogen deficiency, and inspection of the vulva will reveal a symmetrically reddened, smooth, and somewhat shiny look to the skin of the vulva and perineum. A maturation index, which is a relative percentage of basal, parabasal, and mature epithelium performed on a Pap smear specimen, may be helpful, but is rarely required. Biopsy will reflect the hypoplastic nature of this disease and help to differentiate this from lichen sclerosus (formerly known as "lichen planus atrophicus"), which has a similar gross appearance.

A thinned, atrophic-appearing skin, with linear scratch marks or fissures, is found in lichen sclerosus. The skin is often described as having a "cigarette-paper" or parchmentlike appearance. These changes frequently extend around the anus in a figure-eight configuration (Fig. 28.8). Atrophic changes result in thinning or even loss of the labia minora and

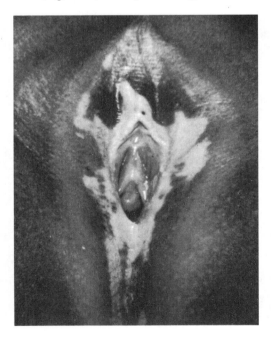

Figure 28.8. Clinical appearance of lichen sclerosus. (From Jones HW, Wentz AC, Burnett LS. Novak's textbook of gynecology. 11th ed. Baltimore: Williams & Wilkins, 1988:588.)

significant narrowing of the introitus. Fissures, scarring, and synechiae cause marked pain for some patients.

Hypertrophic vulvar dystrophy causes a thickening of the vulvar skin over the labia majora, outer aspects of the labia minora, and clitoral areas. The tissues may have a dusky red to thickened white appearance (Fig. 28.9). Fissuring and excoriations are common. Constant vigilance is required to watch for possible premalignant or malignant changes that often mimic these lesions and those of lichen sclerosis.

Disorders of the apocrine glands of the labia may also be a source of vulvar symptoms. In hidradenitis suppurativa, chronic blockage of these glands leads to itching and burning that progresses to abscess formation and ulceration (Fig. 28.10). These painful and tender lesions may coalesce, resulting in extensive scarring, chronic drainage, and sinus formation. When hidradenitis is suspected, a dermatologic consultation should be considered.

In patients with Fox-Fordyce disease, the apocrine glands become blocked with plugs of keratin. Intense itching and tiny flesh-colored papules (without erythema) are the hall-

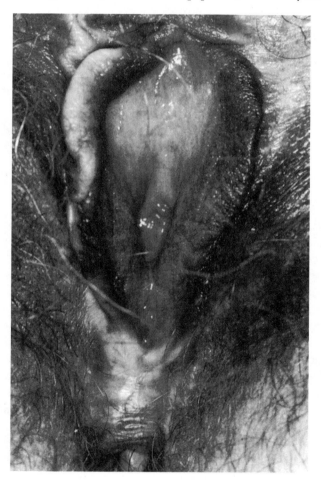

Figure 28.9. Hypertrophic vulvar dystrophy. (From Wilkinson EJ, Stone IK. Atlas of vulvar disease. Baltimore: Williams & Wilkins, 1995:36.)

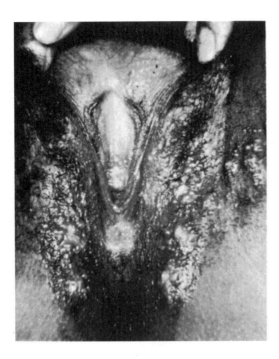

Figure 28.10. Hidradenitis suppurativa. (From Jones HW, Wentz AC, Burnett LS. Novak's textbook of gynecology. 11th ed. Baltimore: Williams & Wilkins, 1988:594.)

marks of this disorder. The itching that the patient reports is often inversely related to estrogen levels and, hence, is improved with pregnancy or estrogen-dominant oral contraceptives.

Vaginitis

Vaginal infections can be more than just the source of inconvenience and discomfort; they can represent a significant health risk. For example, patients with bacterial vaginosis are roughly nine times more likely to develop upper genital tract infections than those without the infection. Premature rupture of the membranes, premature delivery, chorioamnionitis, and postpartum endometritis are all more common in the presence of bacterial vaginosis. The incidence of bladder infections and postoperative cuff cellulitis is also increased. Awareness and treatment are, therefore, in the best interest of the patient.

Increased vaginal discharge is associated with an identifiable microbiologic cause in 80% to 90% of cases. Hormonal or chemical causes make up most of the remaining cases. Most vaginal infections result from three infectious causes: synergistic bacterial (bacterial vaginosis, nonspecific vaginitis), fungi (candidiasis), or protozoa, such as *Trichomonas* (trichomoniasis). Bacterial infections account for approximately 50% of infections, whereas fungi and *Trichomonas* infections account for roughly 25% each. Through history, gentle examination, and simple microscopic investigation, the cause of the patient's symptoms can be ascertained. The value of microscopic examination of vaginal smears cannot be overstated. For this reason, any patient who complains of vaginal discharge or irritation must be evaluated directly before therapy is suggested. Inaccurate diagnosis, or overtreatment of a physiologic condition, is doomed to fail and may even make the patient worse.

Table 28.2. Clinical Aspects of Common Vaginal Infections

Characteristic	Physiologic	Bacterial vaginosis	Candidiasis	Trichomoniasis
Symptoms				
Itching	−	−	++++	±
Burning	−	+	++	+
Dysuria	−	+	++	±
Discharge				
Amount	Slight	Moderate	Variable	Moderate
Color	Yellow-white	Gray-white	White	Yellow-**green**
Odor	−	+++	−	+
Character	Thin	Thin, homogeneous	**Thick, curdy**	**Frothy**
Adherence	Minimal	Moderate	**Strong**	Minimal
pH	**3.5–4.5**	**5–5.5**	**4–5**	**6–7**
Findings				
Gross	Normal	Minimal erythema	Erythema, excoriation	**Petechiae**
Microscopic	**Few white blood cells**	**"Clue cells"**	**Mycelia on KOH**	**Trichomonas**
"Whiff test"	−	++++	−	+

Boldfaced items are of particular help in making a differential diagnosis.

Examination of patients with complaints of increased vaginal discharge (leukorrhea), vaginal or vulvar irritation, or increased odor should include careful observation of the tissues as well as any discharge present. The location, color, consistency, odor, and pH of the discharge should be noted. The pH of the vaginal secretions is an often overlooked tool that may be very helpful in establishing the correct diagnosis (Table 28.2). Vaginal pH can be easily measured with commercially available pH tapes. Vaginal pH may be unreliable in the presence of blood or after recent douching or intercourse.

Wet preparations are made using one or two drops of normal saline and 10% KOH placed on separate slides. A small sample of the secretions obtained with a cotton-tipped applicator are then mixed with these solutions and a cover slip applied. Examination under low to medium power magnification will generally establish a diagnosis. A Gram stain may be performed on dried material, but is not as immediate and requires more supplies and experience. Culture of the cervix for possible sexually transmitted diseases or cervicitis should also be considered at the time of this examination.

Bacterial Vaginosis

Roughly one half of all vaginal infections are due to what is now termed bacterial vaginosis. Known by many names (Table 28.3), this change in vaginal ecology may affect up to 20% of women. This surprisingly high prevalence is supported by a number of studies and the observation that about one half of patients with bacterial vaginosis are asymptomatic or minimally symptomatic and thus the infection is not clinically apparent. This lack of symptoms is due to the lack of an inflammatory reaction; thus, the term "vaginosis" rather than "vaginitis." When symptomatic, bacterial vaginosis is characterized by a creamy, gray-white, adherent vaginal discharge, with an increase in vaginal odor. This odor is often "musty" or "fishy" in nature and is more noticeable after intercourse.

Table 28.3. Evolving Terminology of Bacterial Vaginosis

1894	Nonspecific vaginitis
1955	*Haemophilus* vaginitis
1963	*Corynebacterium* vaginitis
1980	*Gardnerella vaginalis* vaginitis
1982	Anaerobic vaginosis
1984	Bacterial vaginosis

Table 28.4. Changes Found in Bacterial Vaginosis

	Normal	Bacterial vaginosis
Bacteria (per mL)	10^9	10^{11}
pH	3.5–4.5	5–5.5 (up to 6.0)
Aerobic:anaerobic ratio	5:1	1000:1
H_2O_2 production	High	Low
Bacterial flora*		
Lactobacillus	95%	35%
Gardnerella	5%–60%	95%
Mobiluncus	0%–5%	50%–70%
Mycoplasma hominis	15%–30%	60%–70%

*Percent of women harboring each species.

Bacterial vaginosis is a polymicrobial process that involves the loss of normal lacto-bacilli, an increase in anaerobic bacteria (especially *Gardnerella vaginalis*, *Bacteroides* sp., *Peptococcus* sp., and *Mobiluncus* species), and a change in the chemical composition of the vaginal secretions. In addition to the changes shown in Table 28.4, high levels of mucinases, phospholipase A_2, lipases, proteases, arachidonic acid, and prostaglandins are all present. These are typical of the secretions found in draining abscesses elsewhere in the body. Amines (cadaverine and putrescine) are made through bacterial decarboxylation of arginine and lysine. These amines are more volatile at an alkaline pH, such as that created by the addition of 10% KOH or semen (roughly a pH of 7), giving rise to the odor found with the "whiff test" or reported by these patients following intercourse. It is thought that bacterial vaginosis develops 5 to 10 days after exposure to the involved bacteria. *Gardnerella* may be found in 90% of male partners of women with bacterial vaginosis. Hence, sexual transmission is postulated, although bacterial vaginosis can occur in virginal women.

Examination of women with bacterial vaginosis usually uncovers a creamy, adherent discharge covering normal-appearing genital tissues. Unlike physiologic discharge, which is regularly found in dependent portions of the vagina, the discharge seen in bacterial vaginosis uniformly coats the tissues. The discharge is gray-white and may be frothy in 10% of cases. Confirmation of the diagnosis is made by saline wet smear which shows more than 20% "clue cells." Clue cells are normal vaginal epithelial cells with small bacilli adherent to their surface, giving a ground glass appearance to the cytoplasm (Fig. 28.11). Gram stain, or stains used for urinary sediments, may help to identify these cells, but this is seldom necessary. The presence of a large number of inflammatory cells should suggest the possibility of cervical infection or *Trichomonas*. Diagnostic criteria for establishing the diagnosis of bacterial vaginosis are summarized in Table 28.5.

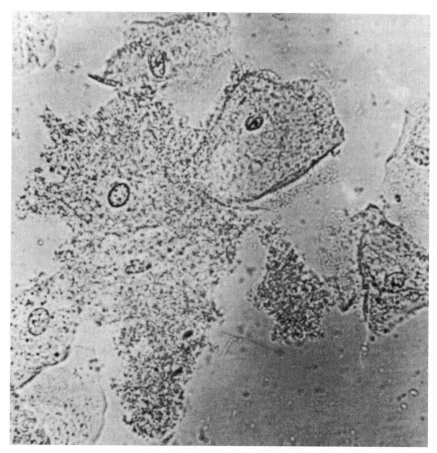

Figure 28.11. Microscopic appearance of bacterial vaginosis. (From Glass RH. Office gynecology. 4th ed. Baltimore: Williams & Wilkins, 1993:37.)

Table 28.5. Criteria for the Diagnosis of Bacterial Vaginosis

Three of the following
    Homogeneous, adherent discharge
    Vaginal pH of 5–5.5
    Positive "whiff" test (when mixed with 10% KOH)
    >20% clue cells under saline wet smear

Candida (Monilial) Vaginitis

Candida vaginitis accounts for between 25% and 40% of all vaginal infections. Some have estimated that 75% of women will experience at least one episode of candidal vulvovaginitis during their lifetime, and half of these will have one or more recurrences. The incidence of this infection has doubled over the past 20 years. Vulvovaginal candidiasis is caused by ubiquitous fungi found in the air or as common inhabitants of the vagina, rectum, and mouth. Most infections (80% to 95%) are caused by *Candida albicans,* with infections by *C. glabrata, C. tropicalis,* or others present in 5% to 20% of cases. Under normal circumstances, vaginal lactobacilli inhibit the growth of these fungi. When the normal ecosystem of the vagina is disturbed by stress, antibiotic use, pregnancy, diabetes, depressed immunity, contraceptive sponge use, and so forth, rapid fungal overgrowth may take place, reaching levels of 10^3 to 10^4 organisms per milliliter. Depressed cellular immunity, such as that caused by corticosteroids or AIDS, significantly increases the likelihood of infection. There appears to be a greater frequency of symptomatic infections around the time of menstruation. *Candida* infections are not considered sexually transmitted and are not associated with a greater risk of other infections. Vulvovaginal candidiasis is almost exclusively found between menarche and menopause.

Intense itching is the cardinal sign of fungal vulvovaginitis. External dysuria, dyspareunia, and vulvar burning are also common. Hypersensitivity to the organism may contribute to severity of symptoms found in even mild infections. Tissue erythema, edema, and excoriations are common. The discharge associated with these infections is ordinarily adherent, thick, and plaquelike, with a white to yellow color. It is generally odorless. The pH of the vagina is ordinarily normal. Microscopic examination of vaginal secretions will often show hyphae, but this may be facilitated with the use of 10% KOH which lyses white and red cells making the hyphae more apparent (Fig. 28.12). Fungal cultures with Nickerson or Sabouraud media can be made and should be positive in 24 to 72 hours.

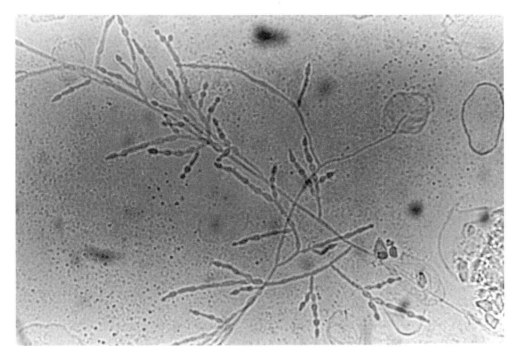

Figure 28.12. Microscopic appearance of vaginal monilia. Branching and budding of vaginal monilia distinguish it from lint or other foreign material. The use of 10% KOH lyses white blood cells and renders epithelial cells "ghostlike" making identification easier.

Trichomonas Vaginitis

Although decreasing in frequency owing to effective treatment and aggressive diagnosis, vaginal infections by *Trichomonas vaginalis* still account for up to 3 million cases of vaginitis each year in the United States. *Trichomonas vaginalis* is an anaerobic flagellate protozoan that lives only in the vagina, Skene's ducts, and urethra (male or female), and may be freely transmitted by sexual intercourse. Other species of *Trichomonas* are found in the rectum and oral pharynx, but do not cause vaginal infections. Studies have found that 30% to 80% of asymptomatic partners of women with *Trichomonas* infections will have a positive culture. The incubation period for *Trichomonas* infections is thought to be between 4 and 28 days. Because up to 15% of women may harbor the organism in an asymptomatic, carrier state, the exact time of exposure may be difficult to determine. Infection by *Trichomonas* organism is facilitated when vaginal pH becomes less acid. Therefore, the presence of blood, semen, or bacterial pathogens increase the risk of infection. Because of its predominately sexual transmission, the possibility of other sexually transmitted diseases should be considered and appropriate screening carried out.

Symptoms of *Trichomonas* infection vary, but may include vulvar itching or burning, copious discharge with a rancid odor, dysuria, and dyspareunia. The discharge associated with *Trichomonas* infections is generally thin, runny, and yellow-green to gray in color. In 25% of patients, the discharge will take on a "frothy" character. The vaginal pH is approximately 6 to 6.5 or above. Examination may reveal nonspecific edema or erythema of the vulva. Characteristic petechiae, or strawberry patches, on the upper vagina wall or cervix may be found in 10% to 15% of patients and are highly suggestive of the diagnosis.

The diagnosis is confirmed by microscopic examination of vaginal secretions suspended in normal saline (Fig. 28.13). *Trichomonas* is a fusiform protozoa slightly larger than a white blood cell. It has three to five flagella extending from the narrow end, which provide active movement that facilitates its identification. This motion is lost if the micro-

Figure 28.13. Microscopic appearance of *Trichomonas* infection. (From Jones HW, Wentz AC, Burnett LS. Novak's textbook of gynecology. 11th ed. Baltimore: Williams & Wilkins, 1988:572.)

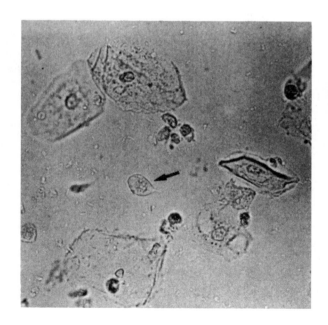

scope slide cools, there are large numbers of white blood cells present, or the pH of the saline used is acid. Culture for *Trichomonas* can be performed but is seldom necessary. Detection of *Trichomonas* by Pap smear results in an error rate of 50%. Monoclonal antibody kits are available but have not shown superiority over traditional diagnostic methods.

Chronic Vaginitis

The bane of health care providers and women alike are "chronic" vaginal infections. For these unfortunate patients, vaginal irritation, discharge, or other symptoms come to impinge on every aspect of their lives. Frustration on the part of the patient and provider, "doctor shopping," multiple visits, and multiple ineffective medications mark these patients. The causes of this problem are many, but incorrect diagnosis, reinfection, noncompliance, the presence of risk factors or behaviors, and inappropriate expectations may all play a role. These patients require frequent follow-up and careful evaluation at every visit. Each new episode of infection should be evaluated individually for its cause and predisposing factors. Alternate sources of excessive vaginal moisture, such as chronic cervical infections, must be evaluated. When only physiologic discharge and normal tissues are found, exploration for the presence of stresses, somatization, psychosocial changes, or abuse should be considered.

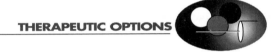

THERAPEUTIC OPTIONS

Vulvar Diseases

Asymptomatic small Bartholin's cysts require no therapy. Mild infections of the Bartholin's gland may respond to antibiotic or topical therapies. Broad-spectrum antibiotics are often successful in treating infections if abscess formation has not occurred. Warm to hot sitz baths will provide symptomatic relief and may promote pointing and drainage of small abscesses. Spontaneous drainage generally occurs in 1 to 4 days. When persistent, large, or particularly symptomatic abscesses occur, incision and drainage is indicated. Simple drainage of these abscesses is often associated with reoccurrence. Therefore, the placement of a Word catheter (a short, self-retaining stint) to form an epithelialized tract, packing with iodoform gauze, or surgical marsupialization of the gland, is often desirable, especially in patients who have already had recurrences. Recurrences still happen to 5% to 10% of patients following marsupialization. Excision of the gland, which is often difficult, is associated with significant risk of morbidity, including intraoperative hemorrhage, hematoma formation, secondary infection, scar formation, and dyspareunia. For these reasons, excision is not generally recommended.

Treatment of condyloma acuminata is frequently tedious, requiring multiple visits and close follow-up. Treatment is directed toward reducing further spread, reducing cancer risk, and cosmetic improvement. Complete eradication is unlikely and further spread remains a continuing possibility. Condyloma can be treated in the office by the application of 20% to 25% podophyllin resin in tincture of benzoin, podophyllotoxin (0.5% solution, Condylox), or bichloracetic and trichloroacetic acids (80% to 100% solution). Studies do not show definite superiority of one agent over another, although podophyllin is contraindicated for pregnant patients owing to systemic absorption. This systemic absorption limits the size of lesions that should be treated with podophyllin to less than 2 cm, and restricts its use to lesion on the vulva, not the vagina. Topical therapy cure rates are good (50% to > 75%), but recurrence generally exceeds 50% in 1 year. When a topical therapy is used, it should be applied carefully with the blunt or broken end of an applicator stick. The material should only be applied to the raised lesions. Some prefer to protect the adjacent skin by first applying a thin coating of petrolatum (Vaseline) around the base of the lesions. Podophyllin should be rinsed off the perineum in 30 minutes to 4 hours. With most topical therapy, slough of the treated lesions happens in 2 to 4 days. Scarring is rare. Reapplication of the topical agent is usually required, and should be carried out at a follow-up visit in 7 to 10 days. Patients may self-apply podophyllotoxin to external lesions by applying the medication for three consecutive days each week for up to 3 weeks. No matter what agent is used, if the lesions do not respond after several treatments, a re-evaluation of the diagnosis should be made. Injections with alpha-interferon or interferon gel have been advocated, but success is limited, side effects are many, and the treatment is expensive and time consuming, requiring multiple, frequent visits. Topical 5-fluorouracil (5-FU) may be applied two to three times a day by the patient, but significant chemical irritation often results. This is best reserved for severe cases and those followed by a consultant. Severe cases, those with multiple recurrences, and pregnant patients with condyloma often require surgical, laser, or other specialized therapy and warrant referral.

Molluscum contagiosum is treated by curettage of the base of the papule, followed by cautery with either ferric subsulfate (Monsel's solution) or 85% trichloroacetic acid. Cryosurgery or electrocautery may also be used but are more expensive and cumbersome.

Herpetic vulvitis causes a tremendous amount of morbidity for its sufferers. General therapy with analgesics and antipyretics is appropriate. Topical applications of 2% lidocaine for pain relief or an antimicrobial preparation to inhibit secondary infection may also be used as needed. Approximately 10% of patients will need hospitalization for pain control or management of urinary complications. Direct therapy consists of oral acyclovir (Zovirax, 200 mg five times a day for 7 to 10 days) begun as soon as the diagnosis is made. Topical acyclovir ointment (5%) applied three to six times a day for 7 days, applied using gloves or a finger cot to prevent autoinoculation of other sites, may also be used, but is less effective than systemic management. Treatment with acyclovir will shorten the period of viral shedding and may improve symptoms if begun early enough in the course of the infection. Suppressive therapy with 400 mg twice daily on a continuous basis for up to 12 months may be used in patients with frequent (> 6/year) recurrences. This prophylaxis significantly decreases both the frequency and severity of subsequent episodes by approximately 75%, but does not completely prevent them, nor prevents the patient from spreading the disease through viral shedding. Once prophylaxis is discontinued, the risk, frequency, and severity of recurrence may be unchanged.

Vulvar Irritation

Irritation of the vulva is common with most vulvar and vaginal pathologies. Simple treatment with cool sitz baths, moist soaks, or the application of soothing solutions such as

Burow's solution (Domeboro, aluminum acetate 5% aqueous solution, three to four times daily for 30 to 60 minutes) will be helpful. Patients should be advised to wear loose fitting clothing and keep the area dry and well ventilated. To dry the perineum after bathing, a hair dryer set on the lowest setting will provide drying without further irritation from a towel. Systemic therapy with antihistamines is useful for some conditions, especially at night when itching is often intense and sedation may be desirable. Topical use of fluorinated steroids to combat irritation should be limited, as a steroid-induced dermatitis may result from prolonged use. Crotamiton (Eurax) may be applied topically, twice daily, to suppress itching. Occasionally, the use of a topical anesthetic, such as 2% xylocaine jelly, may be required.

Contact dermatitis of the vulva is treated primarily by identification and removal of the offending substance. Wet compresses or soaks using Burow's solution (three to four times daily for 30 to 60 minutes), followed by air drying or drying with a hair dryer (on cool) will help relieve symptoms. Loose fitting clothing and a nonmedicated baby powder used sparingly may facilitate the drying process. Steroid creams, such as hydrocortisone (0.5% to 1%) or fluorinated corticosteroids (Valisone, 0.1%, Synalar, 0.01%) may be applied two to three times a day if needed. Antihistamines are of little benefit.

When atrophic change is the cause of irritation, estrogen replacement (either locally or systemically) is the treatment of choice. In patients with significant atrophic vulvar or vaginal changes, estrogen therapy may take up to 6 months to give satisfactory results. In the case of lichen sclerosus, local application of testosterone propionate (2%) in petrolatum (applied two to three times daily, diminishing to once or twice weekly when satisfactory results are obtained) is generally effective. Hypertrophic dystrophy is best treated with fluocinolone acetonide (0.025% or 0.01%), triamcinolone acetonide (0.01%), or similar corticosteroid applied two to three times daily. Fluorinated steroids should be used for short periods only, replacing them with hydrocortisone or nonsteroidal therapies when possible.

Pediculosis pubis and scabies require treatments aimed at both the adult parasites and also the eggs. Treatment with 1% permethrin (Nix cream) with a second application 10 days after the first is generally effective. Local treatment of two applications over 2 days of a 1% gamma-benzene hexachloride (lindane) lotion, shampoo, or cream (Kwell) is also effective. Lindane must be left in contact with the eggs for at least 1 hour to be effective. Lindane is contraindicated in pregnant and breastfeeding women. Even with effective treatment, itching from scabies may continue for several days after therapy, and may require antihistamine treatment. Bedding, clothes, towels, and the home environment require careful cleaning and disinfection to avoid reinoculation.

Patients with pruritus and vulvodynia present special management problems. As in most area of medical care, treatment is best based on establishing a correct diagnosis and instituting appropriate management. When symptomatic therapy must be used, improved local hygiene, tepid soaks, and astringent agents (such as Burow's solution) may all be effective in decreasing symptoms. Topical steroids, in small quantities and for a limited time only, may also be used.

Vulvar vestibulitis undergoes spontaneous improvement in between one third and one half of patients over the course of 6 months. Some have suggested withdrawal of oral contraceptives, but strong evidence for either causation or significant improvement is lacking. Topical steroids can be tried, but success is generally poor. Local anesthetics (2% lidocaine gel) can be used to improve symptoms or to allow intercourse, but the subsequent loss of pleasurable, as well as nociceptive sensation, is often unsatisfactory. Refractory cases may require surgical or laser excision, but risk scarring that may result is continuing disability.

Treatment of hidradenitis suppurativa consists of local therapy (sitz baths, incision and drainage, topical antibiotics) and systemic therapy with antibiotics or oral contraceptives. Local excision may be required in severe cases.

Vaginal Infections

Bacterial Vaginosis

Bacterial vaginosis and vaginitis can be treated with either oral or topical medications giving good results. Oral metronidazole (Flagyl, Protostat, 500 mg twice daily for 7 days) gives 90% to 100% cure rates. Oral ampicillin (500 mg every 6 hours for 7 days), tetracycline (250–500 mg twice daily for 7 days), or clindamycin (300–450 mg every 6 hours for 7 days) may also be used, but cure rates are poorer. Oral metronidazole is associated with the potential for systemic side effects including a metallic taste in the mouth and stomach upset. Because of a disulfiram-like reaction, patients must be warned to avoid alcohol intake during therapy.

Topical therapy for bacterial vaginosis can give excellent results with fewer risks of systemic side effects. Topical triple sulfa (cream or suppositories) has fallen out of favor, being replaced by topical clindamycin (2% cream) and metronidazole (0.75% gel). Both agents do have slight systemic absorption (1% to 5%), so systemic effects are possible, but remote. Topical clindamycin (5 g of cream, 100 mg of clindamycin) is applied nightly for 7 days, whereas topical metronidazole (5 g of cream, 37.5 mg of metronidazole) is applied twice daily for 5 days. Cure rates are comparable to oral therapy.

Currently, treatment of the patient's sexual partner is not advised, although it should be considered in cases of multiple infection, cervical or upper tract infections, concomitant or suspected sexually transmitted disease, or in women with recurrent bacterial vaginosis.

Candida Vulvovaginitis

The most common treatments for vaginal fungal infections are the synthetic imidazoles drugs (Table 28.6). These agent all provide good symptomatic relief and microbiologic cures. Triazole-based medications such as terconazole (Terazol) or fluconazole (Diflucan) can also be used. A small number (< 5%) of fungal infections will be resistant to imidazole therapy. These organisms are generally susceptible to triazoles. Side effects from either the imidazoles or triazoles are mild and relatively infrequent. Oral therapy with fluconazole (150 mg single dose) provides convenience, patient acceptance, and excellent cure rates. Some patients like the immediate soothing effects of topical agents, leaving much of the choice up to patient and physician preference.

Povidone-iodine, as a douche or gel, gentian violet (1%), and boric acid (600 mg capsules placed high in the vagina twice daily) are also reasonable therapies for vulvovaginal candidiasis.

Patients should be advised to keep the perineal area clean and dry, avoid tight or synthetic undergarments, and complete the prescribed course of therapy.

Despite good patient compliance, correct diagnosis, and effective medications, roughly

Table 28.6. Common Therapies for Vulvovaginal Candidiasis

Agent	Trade name	Dosage
Imidazoles		
Miconazole	Monistat	200 mg suppositories, qHS × 3 d
		2% cream, 5 g qHS × 7 d
Clotrimazole	Femcare	100 mg inserts, qHS × 7 d
	Gyne-Lotrimin	1% cream, 5 g qHS × 7 d
	Mycelex	
Butoconazole	Femstat	2% cream, 5 g qHS × 3 d
Tioconazole	Vagistat	6.5% ointment, 4.6 g HS
Triazoles		
Terconazole	Terazol	80 mg suppositories, qHS × 3 d
		0.8% cream, 5 g qHS × 3 d
		0.4% cream, 5 g qHS × 7 d
Fluconizole	Diflucan	150 mg single dose (oral)

30% of patients will experience a recurrence of symptoms within a month. The reason for this recurrence is unknown, but may be related to a continuing exposure, a change in host defenses (such as altered cellular immunity), or the ability of the fungus to burrow beneath the epithelium of the vagina, making cure more difficult. Topical suppressive therapy, oral nystatin, perianal creams, and medications for sexual partners have not been successful in reducing the recurrence rate. Oral suppressive therapy on a once a month basis does appear to lessen the frequency and severity for the small number of patients with chronic recurrences. Prophylactic use of antifungals during broad-spectrum antibiotic therapy or around the time of menstruation is debated, but may be appropriate based on the individual patient's history and needs. Frequent recurrences should suggest further evaluation of the patient for diabetes or immunosuppression.

Trichomonas Vaginitis

The standard treatment for *Trichomonas* vaginitis is metronidazole. Metronidazole may be used as a single-day oral treatment of 1 g in the morning and 1 g in the evening, or as a 250-mg dose every 8 hours for 7 days. Each gives comparable cure rates, but costs and side effects are lower with single-day therapy. Metronidazole is relatively contraindicated in the first trimester of pregnancy, when alternate therapies must be used. Alternate therapies include topical clotrimazole, povidone-iodine, or hypertonic (20%) saline douches. Because of its sexual transmission and association with other sexually transmitted diseases, it is recommended to treat asymptomatic sexual partners at the same time. Resistance to metronidazole is uncommon. Most treatment failures are actually due to reinfection or failure to comply with treatment.

Chronic Vaginitis

Great care must be exercised in the management of patients with "chronic vaginitis." Over-treatment, especially without a definite diagnosis is tempting, but risks making the problem worse. As noted above, the cornerstone of treatment is diagnosis. Once a possible cause is found, specific therapy is instituted with a great deal of emphasis on the need for compliance. The patient should be asked to return shortly after the course of treatment for re-evaluation, even if no symptoms are present. This allows objective tests of cure, underscores the need for compliance, and shows the degree of concern shared by the health care provider. Prolonged therapies, prophylaxis, or vaginal acidification may all be required. During this process it is important to remain vigilant for new infections, but also for signs of a "hidden agenda" such as abuse, fear of sexually transmitted disease, infidelity, or somatization, all of which can magnify symptoms of physiologic processes or provide an excuse for care. A frank explanation of the possibility of reinfection must be carried out in those with true recurrent infections. The possibility of additional sexual partners for the patient or her paramour should be explored in an appropriately nonjudgmental way.

HINTS AND COMMON QUESTIONS

When patients have painful vulvar ulcers due to herpes or other infections, the use of a "sore-throat" spray containing phenol will provide pain relief without having to touch the painful tissues. Use care in the amount of spray administered to avoid a contact vulvitis from the treatment itself.

Because 85% of Bartholin's gland infections occur during the reproductive years, other diagnoses including malignancy must be considered in women before menarche or after menopause.

Patients with significant vulvar irritation may have problems with painful urination. This may be lessened by having the patient void while sitting in warm water or while pouring warm water over the vulva.

Gentian violet (1%) is still a good local therapy for either candidiasis or herpes lesions because it is selectively fixed in areas where the epithelial barrier has been broken. Unfortunately, it also stains anything it touches, making it unpopular with patients, office staff, and spouses.

Some patients wish not to offend and will douche prior to coming to the office for treatment of a vaginal discharge. This renders most microscopic evaluations of little help. However, vaginal pH returns to its predouche state faster than the microscopic findings, making it potentially still worth obtaining.

Urethral prolapse in children and urethral caruncles in postmenopausal women, can mimic urethral or vulvar cancer. These lesions are soft, smooth, friable, and bright red. They often present with a history of discharge or bleeding. Although these usually respond to conservative therapy (estrogen in the older women; sitz baths and antibiotics in children), the possible need for biopsy to rule out cancer often means referral to a urologist or gynecologist.

Vulvar hematomas generally present with an obvious history of blunt trauma, such as a straddle injury or assault, but occasionally may result from sexual activities which are not volunteered in the initial history. Hematomas are generally self-limited to the affected labia and respond to pressure and ice packs. Rarely, large or expanding hematomas require consultation and possible surgical intervention.

Because estrogen therapy for atrophic vulvitis or vaginitis may take up to 6 months to give full relief, consideration should be given to adding vaginal moisturizers or lubricants. Newer products (such as Replens) act to hold moisture in the vaginal tissues so that use may be as infrequent as three to four times a week.

When performing microscopic examination of vaginal secretions, be careful not to get any of the 10% KOH solution on the microscope objective lens. Potassium hydroxide will quickly corrode the objective and ruin the microscope. Always use a cover slip when viewing wet preparations to minimize this possibility.

The best way to tell the difference between true clue cells and normal vaginal epithelium is by examining the edge of the cells. Normal epithelial cells have a ground glass appearance to the cytoplasm but do not have bacilli adherent to their surface. The adherent bacilli found on clue cells enhance the granular appearance of the cells, but more importantly blurs the cell margins. Therefore, true clue cells can be distinguished by their "fuzzy" borders as well as their granular appearance.

Topical metronidazole is currently available in two forms: one for dermatologic use and one for intravaginal use. The pH of these two preparations is very different, making it important to specify the form on the prescription to avoid significant chemical irritation.

It is sometimes difficult to differentiate between *Candida,* cotton lint (from a cotton tip applicator), and sweater fuzz when viewed under the microscope. Man-made fibers appear uniform and often look round or cylindrical. Cotton appears flat and ribbonlike. Neither will have the characteristic branches or small round spores that identify *Candida.*

With frequent recurrences of vulvovaginal candidiasis, consider checking for oral thrush or balanitis in an uncircumcised partner. Although uncommon, either could be the source of reinfection.

Is that motile object in the microscope *Trichomonas* or a sperm? Sperm are much small than white cells; *Trichomonas* organisms are larger.

One of the most recalcitrant sources of chronic vaginal discharges is often overlooked: the chronic use of tampons and pads. Frequently patients will get into a recurring cycle of discharge, with pad or tampon use that promotes infection or discharge, necessitating more pad or tampon use, and so forth. Convincing these patients that their own tampon use may be the problem can be very difficult. As difficult as it is, the cycle must be broken. Once it is, many patients with "chronic infections" will show marked improvement.

A useful adjunctive therapy for chronic vaginal infections is vaginal acidification. This favors the re-establishment of normal flora and inhibits colonization and growth of other species. Acidification can be accomplished through the use of commercial preparations (e.g., Amino-Cerv or Aci-Jel) or boric acid capsules or douches.

Yes, *Trichomonas* organisms can live for up to 6 hours on a wet surface and, therefore, could be a source of infection; however, because a moderately large inoculum is required, it is very unlikely that infections arise from towels, swimming pools, or toilet seats. We do know that *Trichomonas* organisms may be harbored asymptomatically for many years before being detected, making an accurate assessment of the source difficult. The net result is that finding a *Trichomonas* infection is not, in and of itself, evidence of infidelity.

Patients frequently ask about the advisability of douching. Most gynecologists favor not douching, but rather would rely on the vagina's natural cleansing action. Douching has been suggested to increase the risk of upper genital tract infection and endometriosis. Mechanical or chemical irritation may also result. If a patient **must** douche, it should be held to less than once a week and employ only mildly acidic water (1 tsp of vinegar in a quart of water) or plain, unscented, and unmedicated commercial products.

Occasionally a question will arise about the use of yogurt (consumption or douches) to treat or prevent vaginal "yeast" infections. The arguments for this are based on repopulating the vagina with "friendly" lactobacilli. Yogurt is tasty when eaten and douching with it will provide a soothing effect, but evidence of a true therapeutic benefit is lacking. For those patients who do wish to try this therapy, be sure to advise them to use "active culture" products, not those that have been pasteurized, which kills the bacteria. (Also, avoid those with fruit if douching.)

SUGGESTED READINGS

General Readings

American College of Obstetricians and Gynecologists. Vulvar Dystrophies. ACOG Technical Bulletin 139. Washington, DC: ACOG, 1990.

American College of Obstetricians and Gynecologists. Vulvovaginitis. ACOG Technical Bulletin 135. Washington, DC: ACOG, 1989.

Glass RH, Ed. Office Gynecology, 4th ed. Baltimore: Williams & Wilkins, 1992.

Goetsch MF. Vulvar vestibulitis: prevalence and histologic features in a general gynecologic practice population. Am J Obstet Gynecol 1991;164:1609.

Jones KD, Lehr ST. Vulvodynia: diagnostic techniques and treatment modalities. Nurse Pract 1994;19:34.

Kent HL, Wisniewski PM. Interferon for vulvar vestibulitis. J Reprod Med 1990;87:1138.

Mann MS, Kaufman RH, Brown D, Adam E. Vuvlar vestibulitis: significant clinical variables and treatment outcome. Obstet Gynecol 1991;79:122.

McKay M. Vulvodynia. J Reprod Med 1984;29:471.

Schover LR, Youngs DD, Cannata R. Psychosexual aspects of the evaluation and management of vulvar vestibulitis. Am J Obstet Gynecol 1992;167:630.

Solomons CC, Melmed MH, Heitler SM. Calcium citrate for vulvar vestibulitis: a case report. J Reprod Med 1991;36:879.

Stewart De, Reicher AE, Gerulath AH, Boydell KM. Vulvodynia and psychological distress. Obstet Gynecol 1994;84:587.

Bacterial Vaginosis

Eschenbach DA. Vaginal infection. Clin Obstet Gynecol 1983;26:186.

Eschenbach DA, Hillier S, Critchlow C, et al. Diagnosis and clinical manifestations of bacterial vaginosis. Am J Obstet Gynecol 1988;158:819.

Faro S. Bacterial vaginitis. Clin Obstet Gynecol 1991;34:582.

Fischbach F, Petersen EE, Weissenbacher ER, et al. Efficacy of clindamycin vaginal cream versus oral metronidazole in the treatment of bacterial vaginosis. Obstet Gynecol 1993;82:405.

Fleury FJ. Adult vaginitis. Clin Obstet Gynecol 1981;24:407.

Hillier SL, Lipinski C, Briselden AM, Eschenbach DA. Efficacy of intravaginal 0.75% metronidazole gel for the treatment of bacterial vaginosis. Obstet Gynecol 1993;81:963.

Ledger WJ. Historical review of the treatment of bacterial vaginosis. Am J Obstet Gynecol 1993;169:474.

Livengood CD III, McGregor JA, Soper DE, Newton E, Thomason JL. Bacterial vaginosis: efficacy and safety of intravaginal metronidazole treatment. Am J Obstet Gyencol 1994;170:759.

Reed BD, Eyler A. Vaginal infections: diagnosis and management. Am Fam Physician 1993;47:1805.

Summers P. Vaginitis in 1993. Clin Obstet Gynecol 1993;36:105.

Sweet RL, Gibbs RS: Infections of the Female Genital Tract, 3rd ed. Baltimore: Williams & Wilkins, 1995.

Specific References

Bartholin's Gland Infections
Aghajanian A, Bernstein L, Grimes DA. Bartholin's duct abscess and cyst: a case-control study. South Med J 1994;87:26.
Cheetham DR. Bartholin's cyst: marsupialization or aspiration? Am J Obstet Gynecol 1985;152:569.

Condyloma Acuminata
Bonnez W, Elswick RK Jr, Bailey-Farchione A, et al. Efficacy and safety of 0.5% podofilox solution in the treatment and suppression of anogenital warts. Am J Med 1994;96:420.
Friedman-Kien AE, Eron LJ, Conant M, et al. Natural interferon alpha treatment of condylomata acuminata. JAMA 1988;259:533.
Gabriel G, Thin RNT. Treatment of ano-genital warts. British Journal of Venerologic Diseases 1983;59:124.
Gall SA, Hughes CE, Trofatter K. Interferon for the therapy of condyloma acuminatum. Am J Obstet Gynecol 1985;153:157.
Gutman LT, St Claire KK, Everett VD, et al. Cervical-vaginal and intraanal human papillomavirus infection of young girls with external genital warts. J Infect Dis 1994;170:339.
Horowitz BJ. Interferon therapy for condylomatouss vulvitis. Obstet Gynecol 1989;73:446.
Kinghorn GR. Genital warts: incidence of associated genital infections. Br J Dermatol 1978;99:405.
Sillman FH, Sedlis A, Boyce JG. A review of lower genital intraepithelial neoplasia and the use of topical 5-fluorouracil. Obstet Gynecol Surv 1985;40:190.
Slater GE, Rumack BH, Peterson RG. Podophyllin poisoning. Systemic toxicity following cutaneous application. Obstet Gynecol 1978;52:94.
Vesterinen E, Meyer B, Cantell K, Purola E. Topical treatment of flat vaginal condyloma with human leukocyte interferon. Obstet Gynecol 1984;64:535.

Herpes Vulvitis
Baker DA. Herpes and pregnancy: new management. Clin Obstet Gynecol 1990;33:253.
Brennick J, Duncan L. Images in clinical medicine. Vulvar herpes simples infection. N Engl J Med 1993;90:38.
Bryson YJ, Dillon M, Bernsterin DI, Radolf J, et al. Risk of asquisition of genital herpes simplex virus type 2 in sex partners of persons with genital herpes: a prospective couple study. J Infect Dis 1993;167:942.
Bryson YJ, Dillon M, Lovett M, et al. Treatment of first episodes of genital herpes simplex virus infection with oral acyclovir: a randomized double-blind controlled trial in normal subjects. N Eng J Med 1983;308:916.
Cone RW, Swenson PD, Hobson AC, Remington M, Corey L. Herpes simplex virus detection from genital lesions: a comparative study using antigen detection (HerpChek) and culture. J Clin Microbiol 1993;31:1774.
deRuiter A, Thin RN. Genital herpes. A guide to pharmacological therapy. Drugs 1994;47:297.
Goldberg LH, Kaufman R, Kurtz TO, et al. Long-term suppression of recurrent genital herpes with acyclovir. A 5-year benchmark. Acyclovir Study Group. Arch Dermatol 1993;129:582.
Haddad J, Langer B, Astruc D, Messer J, Lokiec F. Oral acyclovir and recurrent genital herpes during late pregnancy. Obstet Gynecol 1993;82:102.
Johnson RE, Nahmias AJ, Magder LS, et al. A seroepidemiologic survey of the prevalence of herpes simples virus type 2 infection in the United States. N Eng J Med 1989;321:7.
Kaplowitz LG, Baker D, Gelb L. Prolonged continuous acyclovir treatment of normal adults with frequent recurrent genital herpes simplex virus infection. JAMA 1991;256:747.
Kawana T, Kawagol K, Takizawa K, Chen JT, Kawaguchi T, Sakamoto S. Clinical and virologic studies of female genital herpes. Obstet Gynecol 1982;60:456.
Mertz GJ, Critchlow CW, Benedetti J, et al. Double-blind placebo-controlled trial of oral acyclovir in first-episode genital herpes simplex virus infection. JAMA 1984;252:1147.
Mertz GJ, Jones CC, Mills J, et al. Long-term acyclovir suppression of frequently recurring genital herpes simplex virus infection: a multicenter double-blind trial. JAMA 1988;260:201.
Nilsen AE, Aasen T, Halsos AM, et al. Efficacy of oral acyclovir in the treatment of initial and recurrent genital herpes. Lancet 1982;2:571.
Randolph AG, Washington AE, Prober CG. Cesarean delivery for women presenting with genital herpes lesions. Efficacy, risks, and costs. JAMA 1993;270:77.
Straus SE, Seidlin M, Takiff HE. Effect of oral acyclovir treatment on symptomatic and asymptomatic virus shedding in recurrent genital herpes. Sex Transm Dis 1989;16:107.

Wald A, Benedetti J, Davis G, et al. A randomized, double-blind, comparative trial comparing high- and standard-dose oral acyclovir for first-episode genital herpes infections. Antimicrob Agents Chemother 1994;38:174.

Necrotizing Fasciitis

Cunningham DS, Cutler GB JR Spontaneous vulvar necrotizing fasciitis in Cushing's syndrome. South Med J 1994;87:837.

Farley DE, Katz VL, Dotters DJ. Toxic shock syndrome associated with vulvar necrotizing fasciitis. Obstet Gynecol 1993:82(suppl):660.

Nolan TE, King LA, Smith RP, Gallup DC: Necrotizing surgical infection and necrotizing fasciitis in obstetric and gynecologic patient. South Med J 1993;86:1363.

Vulvar Dystrophies

Bopusema MT, Romppanen U, Geiger JM, et al. Acitretin in the treatment of severe lichen sclerosus et atrophicus of the vulva: a double-blind, placebo-controlled study. Journal of the American Academy of Dermatology 1994;30:225.

Friedrich EG JR. Vulvar dystrophy. Clin Obstet Gynecol 1985;28:178.

Mann MS, Kaufman RH. Erosive lichen planus of the vulva. Clin Obstet Gynecol 1991;34:605.

Vulvodynia and Vestibulitis

Bornstein J, Pascal B, Abramovici H. Intramuscular β-interferon treatment for severe vulvar vestibulitis. J Reprod Med 1993;38:117.

Martius J. Eschenbach DA. The role of bacterial vaginosis as a cause of amniotic fluid infections, chorioamnionitis and prematureity: a review. Arch Gynecol Obstet 1990;247:1.

Read JS, Klebanoff MA. Sexual intercourse during pregnancy and preterm delivery: effects of vaginal microorganisma. The Vaginal Infections and Prematurity Study Group. Am J Obstet Gynecol 1993;168:514.

Sandler B. Lactobacillus for vulvovaginitis [letter]. Lancet 1979;2:791.

Soper DE, Bump RC, Hurt WG. Bacterial vaginosis and trichomoniasis vaginitis are risk factors for cuff cellulitis after abdominal hysterectomy. Am J Obstet Gynecol 1990;163:1016.

Spiegel CA. Bacterial vaginosis. Clin Microbiol Rev 1991;4:485.

Swedberg J, Steiner JF, Deiss F, Steiner S, Diggers DA. Comparison of single-dose vs. one-week course of Metronidazole for symptomatic bacterial vaginosis. JAMA 1985;254:1046.

Sweet RL. New approaches for the treatment of bacterial vaginosis. Am J Obstet Gynecol 1994;169:479.

Thomason JL, Gelbart SM, Scaglione NJ. Bacterial vaginoisis: current review with indications for asymptomatic therapy. Am J Obstet Gynecol 1991;165:1210.

Candida Vulvovaginitis

Forssman L, Milsom I. Treatment of recurrent vaginal candidiasis. Am J Obstet Gynecol 1985;152:959.

Horowitz BJ. Candidiasis: specification and therapy. Current Problems in Obstetrics Gynecology Fertility 1990;8:233.

Horowitz BJ, Edelstein SW, Lippman L. Sexual transmission of Candida. Obstet Gynecol 1987;69:883.

Javanovic R, Congema E, Nguyen H. Antifungal agents vs. boric acid for treating chronic mycotic vulvovaginitis. J Reprod Med 1991;36:593.

Milsom I, Forssman L. Repeated candidiasis: reinfection or recrudescence? A review. Am J Obstet Gynecol 1985;152:956.

Sobel JD. Epidemiology and pathogenesis of recurrent vulvovaginal candidiasis. Am J Obstet Gynecol 1985; 152:924.

Witkin SS. Immunologic factors influencing susceptibility to recurrent candidal vaginitis. Clin Obstet Gynecol 1991;34:662.

Trichomonas Vaginitis

Hager WD, Brown ST, Kraus SJ, et al. Metronidazole for vaginal trichomoniasis: Seven-day vs. single-dose regimens. JAMA 1980;244:1219.

Krieger JN, Tam MR, Steven CE, et al. Diagnosis of trichomoniasis. Comparison of conventional wet mount examination with cytologic studies, cultures, and monoclonal antibody staining of direct speciments. JAMA 1988;259:1223.

Lossick JG. Single-dose metronidazole treatment for vaginal trichomoniasis. Obstet Gynecol 1980;56:508.

McLellan R, Spence MR, Brockman M, Raffel L, Smith JL. The clinical diagnosis of trichomonasis. Obstet Gynecol 1982;60:30.

Thomason JL, Gelbart SM. Trichomonas vaginalis. Obstet Gynecol 1989;74:

Wolner-Hanssen P, Krieger JN, Stevens CE, et al. Clinical manifestations of vaginal trichomonas. JAMA 1989; 261:571.

Index